Hematology

Tony Jnosic

Hematology

edited by William S. Beck

fourth edition

The MIT Press
Cambridge, Massachusetts
London, England

This book was set in Times Roman by Achorn Graphic Services, Inc., and printed and bound by Halliday Lithograph in the United States of America

Library of Congress Cataloging in Publication Data

Main entry under title:

Hematology.

Includes bibliographies and index.

1. Blood—Diseases. 2. Hematology. I. Beck, William Samson, 1923– . [DNLM: 1. Hematologic Diseases. WH 100 H486]

RC633.H433 1985 616.1′5 84-21850

ISBN 0-262-02216-8 (hard)

0-262-52097-4 (paperback)

Contents

Preface to the Fourth Edition

Four years have passed since the last revision of this book. Once again the need for a new edition is clear and compelling. Lectures most extensively revised in this edition are the ones on vitamin B_{12} deficiency, the thalassemias, hemolytic anemias associated with membrane disorders, leukemia, the immunopathology of malignant lymphomas, platelets, and newer aspects of the protein interactions in blood coagulation. The last includes thrombomodulin, protein C, and other new clotting factors du jour.

The general outline remains as before. These are lectures—we resolutely call them that rather than chapters—that may be read by students in their own time, both as preparation for and reminder of discussions in lecture hall and laboratory. There is no intention here to preempt lectures and lecturers. Long experience in the hematology courses of Harvard Medical School and the Harvard–MIT Division of Health Sciences and Technology suggests that the lecture hour is now best used for illustration and expansion.

Again the lectures are in outline form. This seems to help with the organization of ideas, and it facilitates note taking. Nonetheless, we have tried to make the text in this edition even more readable than its predecessor. Decisions on what stays and what goes have not been easy—and in view of the moderate increase in pages it may be that the decisions made were insufficiently stringent.

Emphasis remains on physiology and pathophysiology. The systematic considerations of clinical abnormalities are meant to illustrate basic mechanisms. We mention therapy but its discussions are generally intended to make pathophysiologic points. Topics are treated in a traditional sequence—red cells, then white cells, then clotting—and we assume that lectures will be read in that sequence. However, cross-references are supplied for those who read the lectures in some other sequence.

I note again that authors of many of these lectures are indebted to those who lectured in former years and who contributed to earlier editions. Rather than adopt complex rules of authorship, we have chosen to acknowledge these fine predecessors in this preface. I acknowledge with thanks the stimulating past contributions of N. Abramson, A. Aisenberg, C. A. Alper, R. H. Aster, R. W. Colman, R. A. Cooper, D. Deykin, L. K. Diamond, B. G. Forget, B. Glader, H. A. Godwin, W. C. Moloney, P. R. Reich, G. K. Sherwood, J. T. Truman, and I. Umansky. I must also recognize the capable efforts of Alice Colby and Anne Ireland, who assisted in the preparation of the manuscript.

William S. Beck
February 1985

From the Introduction to the First Edition

In the present Harvard Medical School curriculum, hematology is one of a dozen blocks within the large one-year Pathophysiology course, which begins in the middle of the first year. For many years we have furnished our students in this course with syllabus materials and lecture notes. These notes have long been known as "the camel," which, as everyone knows, is an animal that looks as though it had been put together by a committee. When responsibility for the course came to me, the scanty lecture notes took the form of severe and often uninformative outlines. Students complained of the burdens of note taking, and some brought tape recorders. Accordingly lecturers were asked to flesh out their outlines, and our camel grew. It became apparent in time that the value of the syllabus would be enhanced by careful editing. The result is the present volume. The vast expansion of knowledge in the various branches of pathophysiology poses an increasingly difficult problem for those who would define the content of a core curriculum and establish standards and priorities for what is to be taught. It is my view that this difficult cause can be furthered only by the thoughtful preparation of texts such as this, for the very act of editing such a volume necessitates choices and permits correlations and overviews that are never quite possible when many and diverse individuals are responsible for a course of instruction.

The major goal of this endeavor is to improve the quality and usefulness of these notes as teaching instruments. It is our intention to revise this small volume frequently so it will retain the freshness and currency that characterized the informal syllabus materials of previous years.

Some believe it would now be appropriate to abandon formal lectures. I see much merit in that proposal. Surely medical students are capable of handling reading assignments. Surely they deserve exemption from having read to them lectures that they could as well read themselves. Still there is cause for regret about a step that would deny students an hour or two with colleagues who rate high as teachers, scientists, and personalities. How to make the best use of these hours will be the subject of experimentation and innovation in the years ahead.

In a sense, this volume is a successor to Ham's famous *Syllabus* and its revision by Page and Culver. Unlike the present book, however, the earlier syllabuses placed major emphasis on laboratory diagnosis. We hope that this volume will be useful to our students, both in the first- and second-year hematology courses and in later clinical years. We hope too that students and physicians beyond Harvard Medical School may find this a helpful review of hematology, one that may serve as a compendium and guide to the several large new textbooks of hematology.

William S. Beck
February 1973

Contributors

William S. Beck	Professor of Medicine, Harvard Medical School and Massachusetts General Hospital
H. Franklin Bunn	Professor of Medicine, Harvard Medical School and Brigham and Women's Hospital
William B. Castle	Francis Weld Peabody Faculty Professor of Medicine, Emeritus, Harvard Medical School
W. Hallowell Churchill, Jr.	Associate Professor of Medicine, Harvard Medical School and Brigham and Women's Hospital
Allen C. Crocker	Associate Professor of Pediatrics, Harvard Medical School and Children's Hospital Medical Center
Robert I. Handin	Associate Professor of Medicine, Harvard Medical School and Brigham and Women's Hospital
David C. Harmon	Instructor in Medicine, Harvard Medical School and Massachusetts General Hospital
Nancy L. Harris	Assistant Professor of Pathology, Harvard Medical School and Massachusetts General Hospital
James H. Jandl	George Richards Minot Professor of Medicine, Harvard Medical School
Samuel E. Lux	Professor of Pediatrics, Harvard Medical School and Children's Hospital Medical Center
David G. Nathan	Robert A. Stranahan Professor of Pediatrics, Harvard Medical School and Children's Hospital Medical Center and Dana Farber Cancer Institute
Stephen H. Robinson	Professor of Medicine, Harvard Medical School and Beth Israel Hospital
Robert D. Rosenberg	Professor of Medicine, Harvard Medical School, and Professor of Biology, Massachusetts Institute of Technology
David S. Rosenthal	Associate Professor of Medicine, Harvard Medical School and Brigham and Women's Hospital
Thomas P. Stossel	Professor of Medicine, Harvard Medical School and Massachusetts General Hospital

Hematology

LECTURE 1 Hematopoiesis and Introduction to the Anemias

William S. Beck

I. BIOLOGY OF HEMATOPOIESIS

Hematopoiesis is a series of consecutive events wherein the hematopoietic stem cell matures into functional blood cells. Its locus changes in the course of development.

A. Ontogeny

In the third week of human embryogenesis, mesenchymal cells in the yolk sac form clusters called *blood islands*. Peripheral cells of the islands join to form a primitive vascular system. Simultaneously central cells of the islands differentiate into elements that become detached and are carried off by the mounting stream of primitive plasma. These are the *yolk sac stem cells*. Some differentiate into *primitive erythroblasts*, the earliest hemoglobin-synthesizing cells. Unlike pronormoblasts of adult bone marrow, they do not mature into erythrocytes.

In the third month of embryonic life, yolk sac stem cells migrate to the liver, which then becomes the chief site of blood cell formation. Additional contributions are then made by the spleen, lymph nodes, and thymus. Hematopoiesis may continue in the liver until after birth. However, bone marrow hematopoiesis begins in the fourth lunar month and by the end of gestation is the major source of blood cells. The terms *medullary* and *extramedullary hematopoiesis* denote blood cell production by bone marrow and by tissues other than bone marrow, respectively.

At birth, medullary hematopoiesis occurs in almost every bone. Flat bones (sternum, ribs, skull, vertebrae, and innominates) retain most of their hematopoietic activity throughout life, but hematopoiesis progressively diminishes within the shafts of long bones. In the adult, it is limited to the ends of these bones. At times of increased demand for blood cells, active marrow reappears in these sites. With the exception of lymphocyte production, hematopoiesis in the adult occurs exclusively in bone marrow. As noted below, even lymphocytes derive from medullary precursors. Some extramedullary hematopoiesis persists at birth, but it rapidly diminishes, to resume only under abnormal circumstances. In such instances, liver and spleen are the major loci of extramedullary hematopoiesis. Curiously the thymus never resumes this embryonic function.

B. Phylogeny

Much has been learned of the physiology of blood from studies of the evolution of the hematopoietic system. Amphioxus and other primitive chordates lack blood cells. In some invertebrates, hemoglobin occurs in solution in plasma. The mature red cells of reptiles, birds, and fish contain nuclei, mitochondria, and ribosomes that are actively engaged in hemoglobin synthesis. The locus of adult blood-forming tissue varies in different species. For example, it is kidney in amphibia and teleosts; gonads in some fishes; liver in turtles; and tissues around the heart in sturgeon and paddlefish.

C. Mammalian bone marrow

The fine structure of bone marrow was not elucidated until recently. *Nutrient arteries* enter marrow cavities through bone foramina. Arteries branch into distributing arterioles that give rise to an endosteal bed of *sinusoids*. From the bed, sinuses travel in a radial direction toward the central longitudinal veins lying in the long axis of the bone. Hematopoietic tissue lies betwen the sinuses. *Erythropoiesis, granulopoiesis* (or *myelopoiesis*), and *thrombopoiesis* take place extravascularly in the marrow *stroma* outside the sinusoids. Rates of hematopoietic activity and blood supply are related. Sinusoidal walls have three layers: *endothelial cells, basement membrane,* and *adventitial cells*. Endothelial and adventitial cells are both mononuclear reticulum cells that are capable of phagocytosis (as will be discussed in lecture 2). Blood is present within the sinusoids, but intrasinusoidal materials (both diffusible and particulate) have free access to extrasinusoidal areas through gaps in the walls. Hematopoietic cells, having undergone maturation outside the sinusoids, enter the sinusoid at a critical moment in the maturation sequence. This critical event is termed the *release* of blood cells from marrow into blood. Its mechanism is poorly understood.

II. STEM CELLS

The marrow of adult mammals contains pluripotent *stem cells* that give rise to the several lines of differentiated blood cells—erythrocytes, granulocytes-monocytes, thrombocytes (platelets), and probably to lymphocytes of various kinds (T- and B-lymphocytes, plasma cells). Semantic confusion has arisen from the fact that the term *stem cell* has been used in three ways.

A. Definitions

1. Morphologic definition

One definition of the stem cell is as a *morphologic* entity. However, stem cells are few in number and they have still not been identified to everyone's satisfaction. Present evidence suggests, to the disappointment of some, that they are small mononuclear cells resembling lymphocytes. They are mobile cells, and many are normally present in the blood (about 1–5 per 10^5 nucleated cells). At certain times (e.g., after whole-body irradiation, during antigenic stimulation), the number in blood increases. As noted, waves of migration also occur during embryonic life.

2. Kinetic definition

The stem cell is also definable as a *kinetic* entity. The stem cell pool is characterized by its ability (1) to be self-renewing *and* (2) to give rise to further differentiated cells. Our knowledge of bone marrow function implies that such cells must exist. In kinetic terms, any cell with these properties is a stem cell, even if it is already partially differentiated.

To obviate confusion between kinetic and morphologic definitions, the noncommittal term α *cell* has been used in kinetic discussions in place of *stem cells*. An α cell is any cell that can replace itself *and* give rise to a more differentiated cell. The latter is termed an *n cell*. Discussions of bone marrow kinetics ordinarily deal with the behavior of *compartments* of cells. A compartment is defined as any distinct class of cells, whether the distinction is based on function, morphology, developmental stage, or other properties. The definition of the α cell just given is perhaps more accurately applied to the α cell compartment, for it is the compartment that renews itself and gives rise to further differentiated cells. This is the case because indeterminacy surrounds the behavior of the individual α cells, which may behave *asymmetrically* (α → α,n) or *symmetrically* (α → 2α or α → 2n). Thus, descriptions of the net behavior of a *population* of α cells must rest on statistical considerations since experimental difficulties obscure the behavior of any *single* stem cell.

3. Operational definition: CFU

This definition regards the stem as a *colony-forming unit* (*CFU*) in the various systems that made it possible for the first time to *assay* stem cells. In the first of these, devised by Till and McCulloch, suspensions of marrow cells are injected intravenously into heavily irradiated mice in which the spleen and marrow are reduced to stroma and are hematologically empty. In 8–10 days, discrete macroscopic colonies are observed in the animal's *spleen*, which has become a "home" for the wandering injected stem cells. Hence, the stem cell progenitors of these colonies were termed *CFU-S* (S for spleen).

a. CFU-S (CFU-GEMM)

Single stem cells (CFU-Ss) lodge in the spleen stroma and there, under the peculiarly specific influence of the *hematopoietic inductive microenvironment* (HIM), proliferate and differentiate into large colonies. At first, stem cells proliferate actively and produce minute clonal colonies of undifferentiated stem cells. After 5 days, specific differentiation takes place, and discrete colonies are seen macroscopically on the surface of the spleen and within its parenchyma.

Chromosome studies indicate that each colony is derived from a single stem cell. Colony enumeration permits a valid quantitative assay of the number of injected CFU-Ss. In this method stem cells are detected indirectly by observing the results of their proliferation and differentiation; hence CFU is a noncommittal or operational term applicable to colony-forming units from injected suspensions of marrow, spleen, or diverse materials.

The majority of spleen colonies (60–70%) contain only erythroid cells. Most of these are on the spleen surface. About 15% are megakaryocytic. These grow beneath the capsule. About 20% contain only granulocytic (myeloid) cells. These grow within the spleen. Presumably these differences in colony position reflect effects of the HIM. After 10 days, colonies may include more than one cell line—and more CFUs. This is evidence that the marrow stem cell is pluripotent, giving rise to each of the principal cell lines: granulocytic, erythrocytic, macrophages, and megakaryocytes. (As noted below, this has led to replacement of the term *CFU-S* with *CFU-GEMM*.) Some believe this cell also gives rise to other marrow elements, including lipocytes, fibrocytes, chrondrocytes, and osteocytes.

The HIM is currently under active study. It exists in bone marrow as well as spleen and is defined as an environment that (1) favors extensive expression of restricted cell functions, (2) permits exchange of information or molecules between stem cells and environment, and (3) permits necessary interactions among important cell types. Evidence for the existence of the HIM is summarized in table 1.1.

b. CFU-C (CFU-GM)

A second assay system for stem cells was eventually developed that employs culture methods. Such techniques were unreliable until it was found that media must be semisolid and contain a *stimulating factor* or *growth factor*. The first colonies obtained in culture consisted of myeloid cells and macrophages and depended on *colony-stimulating factor (CSF),* or *colony-stimulating activity (CSA),* which is readily provided by "feeder cells" or by addition of extracts of various cell types (macrophages, monocytes, activated lymphocytes, endothelial cells, certain fetal tissues, etc.). The presence of CSF disposes marrow stem cells to form clones of granulocytes and/or macrophages in 7–10 days. Two important cellulár sources of CSF are mononuclear leukocytes and stimulated T cells. When leukocytes are fractionated, the richest subcellular source of CSF is the cell membrane fraction. In the last few years many CSFs have been purified to apparent homogeneity. The properties of some of them and their confusing nomenclature is summarized in table 1.2.

A simple interpretation of the data is that hematopoietic cell development is regulated by a series of growth factors that are progressively restricted in their biological activities and target cells. For example, the recently cloned growth factor *interleukin-3* (IL-3) is indifferent to lineage, promoting growth and development of all myeloid progenitor cells. It also facilitates self-renewal of pluripotent (CFC-GEMM) stem cells, and can "immortalize" granulocyte precursors in vitro. One form of CSF, termed GM-CSF, is more restricted, stimulating proliferation and development of only granulocyte, macrophage and eosinophil colony-forming

Table 1.1
Evidence Indicating Existence of Hematopoietic Inductive Environment

(1) Transfused stem cells "home" to marrow and spleen of irradiated mice.
(2) Occasional failure of "take" after marrow transplantation between identical twins. This suggests defect in receptiveness of stroma.
(3) Delay of aplasia (termination of hematopoiesis) after heavy local irradiation and delay of resumption of hematopoiesis after ectopic implantation of hematopoietic tissue. This suggests that HIM must be destroyed or regenerated before permanent aplasia or resumption of hematopoiesis can occur—and that sustained stem cell proliferation requires intact stroma.
(4) Studies in two genetically anemic strains of mice, Sl/Sl^d and W/W^v, show dichotomy between stroma and stem cells. In Sl/Sl^d mice stroma is defective and incapable of supporting proliferation of normal stem cells. In W/W^v mice stem cells are defective and incapable of proliferating in normal stroma.
(5) Regional difference in ratio of erythroid and myeloid colonies in the spleens of irradiated mice infused with allogeneic stem cells. Presumably stroma has compartments, each supporting differentiation of stem cells in one or the other cell lines.
(6) Marrow-derived "fibroblasts" supposedly arising from stromal cells lack markers of hematopoietic stem cells. Fibroblasts and adipose cells or fat-filled macrophages may be instrumental in sustaining hematopoiesis in vitro.
(7) Ultrastructural evidence of close association between developing hematopoietic cells and stromal cells. The latter appear different for different cell lines.

cells and the proliferation, but not the subsequent development, of CFU-GEMM and the red cell progenitor to be discussed below, BFU-E. The growth factors G-CSF and M-CSF are even more restricted in their activities.

Firm evidence that two of these factors are distinct molecular species comes from data on the cloning and sequencing of the complementary DNA (cDNA) of GM-CSF. The amino acid sequence of GM-CSF was deduced from the cDNA sequence. GM-CSF is encoded by only one gene; hence reported differences in GM-CSF from different tissues probably reflect post-translational modifications. Interestingly, IL-3 can compete with GM-CSF for binding to its receptors. Thus, some multipotential stem cells, progenitor cells, and IL-3-dependent cell lines have both IL-3 and GM-CSF receptors. IL-3 can bind to both receptors, but GM-CSF can bind only to its own receptor. Since these two regulatory molecules appear to have distinct roles vis-à-vis self-renewal, proliferation, and development, it may be that the outcome of a response depends upon the relative concentrations of the two regulators and the number and accessibility of binding sites.

The discovery of the CFU-C, a second type of CFU, led to a new convention for naming CFUs. Now letters following the

Table 1.2
Biological Activities and Target Cells of Myeloid Growth Factors

Growth factor	Other names	Nature of response	Target cells: CFU-S	CFU-GM ↙ G	CFU-GM ↘ M	CFU-Eos	CFU-Meg	BFU-E
IL-3	BPA	Self-renewal	+	+	− ?	ND	ND	?
	HCGF							
	Multi-CSF	Proliferation	+	+	+	+	+	+
	MCGF							
	PCSF	Development	ND	+	+	+	+	+
GM-CSF	MG1-1GM	Self-renewal	ND	−	−	−	ND	−
	CSF	Proliferation	ND	+	+	+	−	+
		Development	ND	+	+	+	−	−
G-CSF	MG1-2	Self-renewal	ND	−	−	−	ND	−
	D-Factor	Proliferation	ND	+	+	+ ?	ND	−
	GM-DF	Development	ND	+	− ?	−	ND	−
M-CSF	CSF-1	Self-renewal	−	−	−	−	−	−
	L-cell CSF	Proliferation	−	− ?	+ +	−	−	−
	MG1-1M							
	CSA	Development	−	− ?	+	−	−	−

The table (adapted from *Nature* 309(1984): 746) is compiled from published data and is meant not to be a comprehensive survey of the field. + indicates a positive response, − a negative response, and ? an equivocal or controversial result. ND, not determined. The full names correponding to the growth factor abbreviations are as follows: IL-3, interleukin-3; BPA, burst-promoting activity; HCGF, hematopoietic growth factor; CSF, colony-stimulating factor; MCGF, mast cell growth factor; PCSF, P-cell-stimulating factor; GM-CSF, granulocyte/macrophage colony-stimulating factor; MG1-1GM, macrophage/granulocyte inducer–granulocyte macrophage; G-CSF, granulocyte colony-stimulating factor specific; MG1-1M, macrophage/granulocyte inducer–macrophage specific; CSA, colony-stimulating activity; CSF-1, colony-stimulating factor-1. The target cells are: CFU-S, colony-forming unit–spleen, multipotential stem cells; BFU-E, burst-forming unit–erythroid, a primitive erythroid progenitor cell assayed in vitro; CFU-GM, granulocyte/macrophage colony-forming unit which has ability to form G (granulocytes), M (macrophages), or mixed colonies in vitro; CFU-Eos, eosinophil colony-forming unit; CFU-Meg, megakaryocyte colony-forming unit. BFU-E, CFU-GM, CFU-Eos and CFU-Meg form part of the so-called "committed" progenitor-cell compartments.

hyphen symbolize which cell lines arise from the CFU. CFU-S, now termed CFU-GEMM (see above), is more pluripotent than CFU-C, now termed CFU-GM, for granulocyte and macrophage. We now say that CFU-GM is *committed* to the production of granulocytes and macrophages. The terms *commitment* and *determination* signify unipotentiality—that is, capable of maturation only within a single line. A committed precursor cell has acquired responsiveness to a specific "poietin" (for example, CSF, erythropoietin, and so on). Figure 1.1 depicts a current model of differentiation in the granulocyte-macrophage (monocyte) pathway. Note the hierarchy of CFUs with varying degrees of commitment. More will be said of this model in lecture 17.

c. CFU-E and BFU-E

Culture methodology employing plasma clots (or methylcellulose plates) soon led to the discovery *CFU-E,* a colony-forming unit

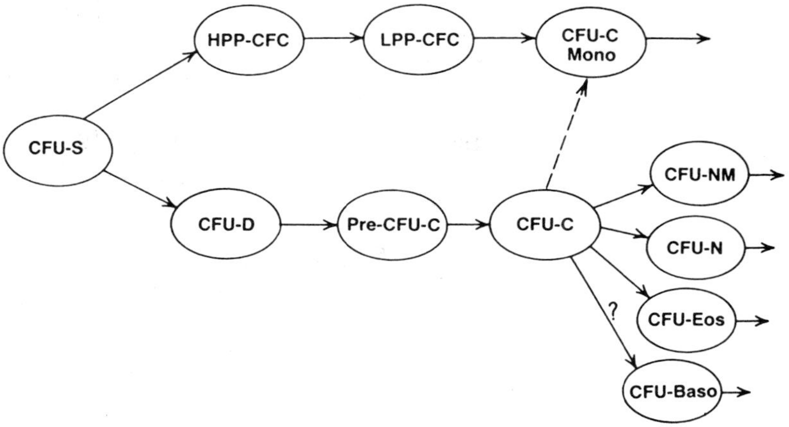

Fig. 1.1
This model depicts a concept of differentiation in the granulocyte/monocyte pathway, presenting a hierarchy of cells with varying degrees of commitment and proliferative potential. Abbreviations: CFU-S: pluripotent stem cell; CFU-D: colony-forming unit diffusion chamber; Pre-CFU-C: pre-colony-forming unit culture; HPP-CFC: high proliferative potential CFC; LPP-CFC: low proliferative potential CFC; CFU-C: colony-forming unit culture; CFU-C Mono: monocytic colony-forming unit culture; CFU NM: neutrophil/macrophage colony-forming unit; CFU-N: neutrophil colony-forming unit; CFU-Eos: eosinophil colony-forming unit; CFU-Baso: basophil colony-forming unit; CFC: colony-forming cell. (By permission of Dr. Peter Quesenberry)

committed to erythropoiesis that forms tiny erythroid colonies of 8–64 cells, and the more primitive *BFU-E,* a burst-forming unit, also committed to erythropoiesis and apparently a precursor of the *CFU-E,* that forms irregular macroscopic erythroid colonies (''bursts'') containing thousands of cells. Both forms are dependent on the presence of *erythropoietin.* BFU-E responds to erythropoietin by differentiating into CFU-E. Some data indicated that the ability of BFU-E to proliferate and differentiate in culture also depends on a helper effect of added *T lymphocytes,* but subsequent work implicated *monocytes,* which are stimulated by T lymphocytes.

Major progenitors of hematopoietic cells and their lineages are summarized in table 1.3 and figure 1.1. The relation of CFU-GEMM to lymphocytes remains uncertain. Since (1) spleen colonies lack lymphocytes and (2) a stem cell chromosome marker can be found in spleen colony cells *and* lymphoid cells repopulating lymphoid organs, it appears that CFU-GEMM and lymphoid cells derive from a common precursor, a more primitive totipotential stem cell termed *CFU-LM* (*LM* for lymphoid-myeloid). Although this concept is not yet firmly established, it is included in the model in figure 1.2. (Also see figure 23.2).

Table 1.3
Some Hematopoietic Progenitor Cells

Term	Required stimulus	Detected by	Postulated role
CFU-GEMM (CFU-S)	HIM of certain mouse tissues; IL-3	Spleen colony assay	Pluripotent stem cell
CFU-GM (CFU-C)	Several CSFs from "feeder cells," tissue extracts, leukocyte extracts, urine, etc.	Colony formation in conditioned agar medium	Committed progenitor of granulopoiesis
BFU-E	Erythropoietin, helper T lymphocytes	Colony formation in plasma clot culture	Committed progenitor of erythropoiesis (early)
CFU-E	Erythropoietin	Colony formation in plasma clot culture	Committed progenitor of erythropoiesis (late)
CFU-Meg	Thrombopoietin	Colony formation in plasma clot culture	Committed progenitor of thrombopoiesis

d. CFU-Meg

The progenitor of megakaryoctyes, the *CFU-Meg,* also derives from the CFU-GEMM. Their differentiation is also influenced by the HIM. A regulatory hormone termed *thrombopoietin* is believed to control platelet production. As described in lecture 27, megakaryocytopoiesis and platelet production are stimulated by *thrombocytopenia* (low platelet count in blood) and suppressed by *thrombocytosis* (high platelet count).

B. Summary of current model

Although each type of CFU is a distinct progenitor cell, only the CFU-LM (if validated) is a truly totipotent stem cell. CFU-GEMM is still pluripotent and thus uncommitted. CFU-GM, CFU-Meg, CFU-Eos, BFU-E, and CFU-E are unipotent near-descendants committed to differentiation along a specific line. These unipotent CFUs require only a stimulus to launch their maturation by blastic transformation and further differentiation. The stimulus is a humoral poietin. *Erythropoietin* is the specific stimulus for unipotent stem cells committed to erythropoiesis. Mounting evidence indicates the importance of specific growth factors in the differentiation of stem cells committed to granulopoiesis and thrombopoiesis, respectively.

Various other factors influence different phases of hematopoiesis. *Thymus* or *T lymphocytes* may promote hematopoiesis by increasing the CFU-GEMM proliferation rate and inducing differentiation. *Chalones* are low-molecular-weight, tissue-specific, species-nonspecific substances that can be isolated from mature granulocytes and that in some laboratories purportedly inhibit the proliferation of more differentiated granulocyte precursors. Their role is unknown. A *colony-inhibiting activity* (CIA) has been described that blocks production or release of CSA by mononuclear phagocytes. It appears to be *lactoferrin,* an iron-binding glycoprotein found in the granules of mature granulocytes. It is further dis-

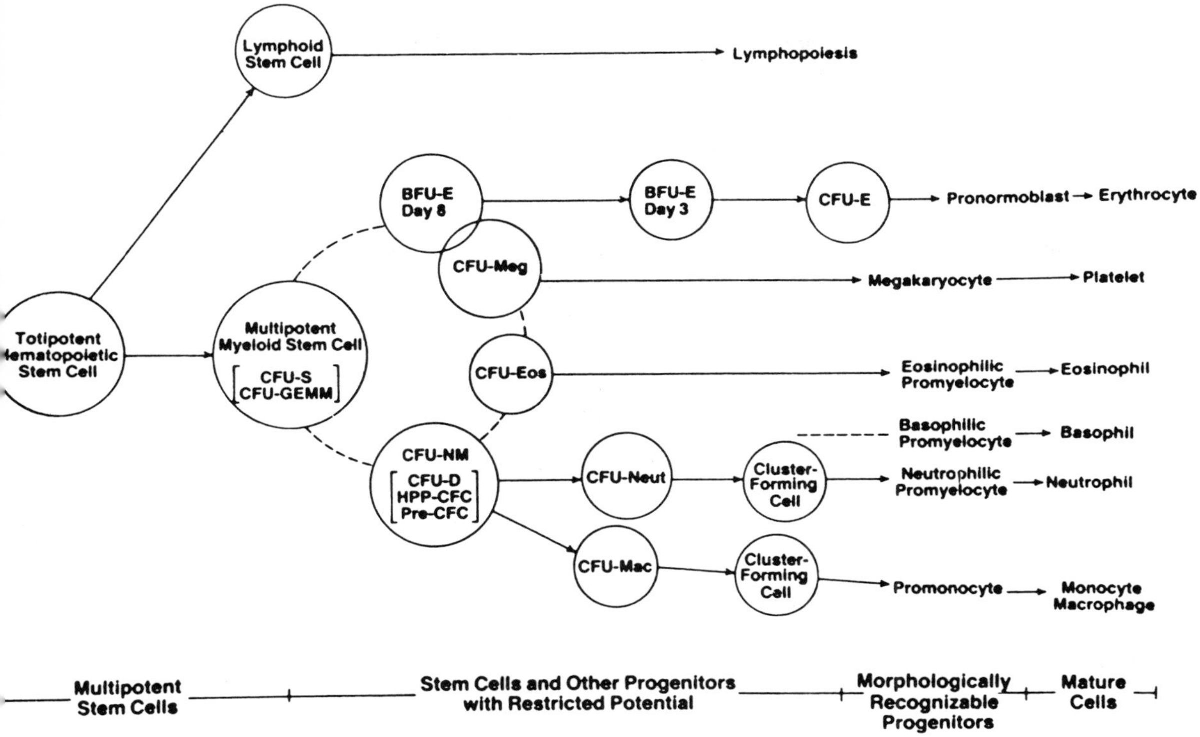

Fig. 1.2
A model of the cellular anatomy of hematopoiesis. Hematopoiesis is viewed as a series of steps that begins with a hematopoietic stem cell. This cell gives rise to lymphoid as well as myeloid elements and eventually all the differentiated cells of circulation. Stem cells with restricted potential are referred to as committed stem cells and include erythroid burst-forming units (BFU-E), megakaryocytic colony-forming units (CFU-Meg), eosinophilic colony-forming units (CFU-Eos), and neutrophil/macrophage colony-forming units (CFU-NM). Progenitors closely related to CFU-NM include those capable of giving rise to colonies in diffusion chambers (CFU-D), colony-forming cells with great proliferative potential but that give rise only to macrophages and monocytes (HPP-CFC), and the so-called pre-CFC. More differentiated progenitors include the mature or day 3 erythroid burst-forming unit, as well as colony-forming units capable of giving rise only to neutrophils (CFU-Neut) or macrophages (CFU-Mac). These latter two types of colony-forming cells are to be distinguished from their even more mature relatives that give rise to clusters of cells. It is these cells that occur just before the morphologically recognizable myeloblasts and neutrophilic promyelocytes and promonocytes. Eosinophilic colony-forming cells also give rise to eosinophilic promyelocytes. The megakaryocyte, the earliest morphologically recognizable cell of the platelet differentiation pathway, has a nuclear proliferative potential similar to that of the erythroid colony-forming unit (CFU-E), which lies immediately before the first recognizable erythroid cell, the pronormoblast.

The dotted line in this figure reflects the fact that the molecular and cellular events that lead from a multipotent to a committed stem cell are unknown. (By permission of Dr. John W. Adamson) cussed in lecture 17. *Prostaglandins* of the E series (PGE_1 and PGE_2) are potent inhibitors of CFU-GM proliferation; those of the F series are often stimulatory. The effects of PGE can be overcome with CSF. In addition *regulatory cell-cell interactions,* involving immunocompetent cells, modulate the proliferation and differentiation of stem cells.

C. Functional states

Stem cells have been profitably studied by *"suicide" techniques* in which actively dividing cells take up enough tritiated thymidine to cause radiation-induced "suicide." In such experiments most pluripotent CFU-GEMMs are spared. Thus pluripotent stem cells are in two functional states: a large majority that are in a quiescent state and a small minority that are actively proliferating. The former cells, which can exchange reversibly with the latter, comprise a dormant bone marrow reserve, which is said to be in the G_0 phase (see below). A potent factor causing resting CFU-GEMM to become active is depopulation of the marrow.

Under the influence of the HIM, pluripotent stem cells are irreversibly transformed to unipotent committed or determined progenitors of erythropoiesis or granulopoiesis (or other cell lines) (figure 1.3). Like pluripotent stem cells, unipotent committed cells are partitioned between resting and proliferating compartments; however, far more of them are actively proliferating. A "poietin" acts by inducing them to differentiate further.

These arrangements for hematopoiesis and stem cell differentiation with their diverse controls have obvious survival value. Pluripotent stem cells essential for continuing hematopoietic function are elegantly protected from external influences that might lead to their depletion. They respond mainly to local factors that influence their numbers. Committed progenitor cells, on the other hand, must be able to respond to external influences bearing information from other organ systems.

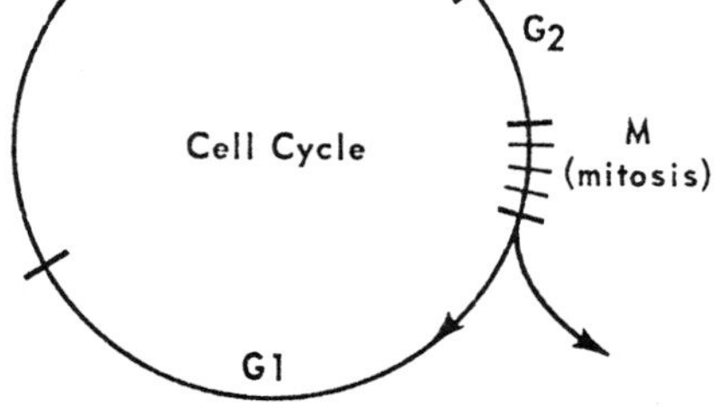

Fig. 1.3
Phases in life cycle of a typical proliferating bone marrow cell.

III. CYTOKINETICS

Cytokinetics is the study of the kinetics of proliferating cell populations. It is concerned with the behavior of cell compartments, each of which can be characterized in terms of its kinetic parameters: size (the numbers or mass of cells), transit time, and flux.

A. Modes of proliferative behavior

1. Constantly proliferating

Some cells (e.g., germinative cells of epidermis, cryptepithelial cells of intestinal mucosa, and stem cells of bone marrow) are constantly proliferating. Metabolic activities in these cells are devoted primarily to replication. Derangements of these cells or their regulators can lead to serious illnesses.

Constantly proliferating cells serve to replace the mature cells of a *maturation series* that are continuously being lost to attrition.

2. Nonproliferating

Nonproliferating cells, that is, cells that cannot divide, are typified by neurons and muscle cells. In humans most tissues consist largely of differentiated cells in this category. Metabolic activities in such cells are devoted primarily to specialized functions.

3. Proliferating on demand

Some cells proliferate only when called upon to do so—as in wound healing, the regeneration occurring after partial extirpation of an organ or repletion of nutritional deficiency. Many cells (e.g., parenchymal cells of liver, kidney, exocrine glands, and other organs) have a proliferative potential that may seem surprising in view of their specialized functions.

B. Patterns of proliferation

The cytokinetics of bone marrow cells may be divided into *erythrokinetics, granulokinetics,* and *thrombokinetics*. Bone marrow cells, like other proliferating cells, may have two patterns of behavior.

1. Steady-state pattern

In the steady state, proliferation is at a constant rate. Bone marrow cells in the steady state proliferate at a rate equaling the rate at which cells in the peripheral blood are removed. The proliferating population thereby keeps the population of mature blood cells constant. The existence of such steady-state kinetics implies the existence of a feedback control loop. Elements of the loop will be described later.

2. Non-steady-state pattern

Under physiologic or pathologic conditions to be described, proliferative behavior may be altered so that cell production rates rise or fall. It is not possible to predict the consequences of a change in the number of cells in a proliferating cell compartment unless the new proliferation rate is specified. Thus, a compartment of proliferating bone marrow cells containing twice the normal number will provide new cells at the normal rate if the enlarged cell population proliferates at half the normal rate.

C. Biologic mechanisms

1. Definitions

The term *proliferation* is often used loosely in discussions of bone marrow function. It should refer to cell division alone; however, it sometimes implies cell division plus differentiation and maturation. It signifies a change in numbers and thus is not a property of the steady state. *Differentiation* is the process whereby a dividing cell gives rise to progeny that differ from it qualitatively. A differentiating cell has a higher *potentiality* level than the differentiated cell. Some genes of pluripotent parent cells are repressed in the course of differentiation. Thus differentiation, which occurs only in dividing cells, represents a change in gene expression that is attributable to reprogramming of the genome. *Maturation* refers to the specialization that is associated with *accumulation of gene products* (e.g., hemoglobin in erythroid cells, immunoglobulins in plasma cells) and *refinement of structure* (e.g., loss of erythrocyte nucleus, segmentation of granulocyte nucleus). In a sense, it is a quantitative change. It is initiated by differentiation but does not require cell division; in fact, it is accompanied by loss of the ability to divide.

2. Cell division cycle

Studies of synchronized cells in culture have shown that the life cycle of a cell has four phases, as shown in figure 1.3: phase M, the period of mitosis (about 0.5–1 hr); phase G_1, the postmitotic or presynthetic gap (about 10 hr); phase S, the period of DNA synthesis and chromosome replication (about 9 hr); and phase G_2, the postsynthetic or premitotic gap (about 4 hr). The total *generation time,* or *time of cycle* (T_c), of a typical proliferating bone marrow cell is about 24 hr (though T_c varies with stage of maturation). As noted, a resting or nonproliferating cell is in phase G_0. Knowledge of the cell cycle provides useful insights into the interpretation of cytokinetic techniques and the planning of chemotherapy for leukemia and other proliferative disorders (see lecture 21).

D. Techniques for studying marrow

As in other areas of hematology, available techniques may be roughly divided into simple methods that can be employed in a clinical setting and elaborate methods that require the research laboratory or some other special facility. Almost every patient with a hematologic disease raises problems of cytokinetics. Is bone marrow function active, hypoactive, or hyperactive? Is marrow activity effective in the sense that it leads to delivery of cells into the blood? The following are methods for judging the level of bone marrow activity. Techniques for assessing specific aspects of marrow function (erythrokinetics, granulokinetics, thrombokinetics, etc.) will be discussed later. Table 1.4 summarizes the kinds of information obtainable from examination of the bone marrow.

Table 1.4
Kinds of Information Obtainable from Examination of Bone Marrow

Procedure	Property	Examples of abnormal states
Bone marrow aspiration	Degree of cellularity	Decreased in hypoplastic or aplastic anemia Increased in reactive states (leukocytosis, erythrocytosis) and proliferative disorders (leukemia, myeloma, etc.)
	Relative preponderance of erythroid and myeloid precursors (E/M ratio)	Increased when erythropoiesis increased (polycythemia) or when myelopoiesis decreased (hypoplastic neutropenia) Decreased when erythropoiesis decreased (hypoplastic anemia, pure red cell aplasia) or when myelopoiesis increased (leukemia, leukocytosis)
	Presence of megakaryocytes	Present in normal marrow and in immune-mediated thrombocyopenia (ITP) Absent in leukemia and other myelophthistic states
	Morphology of erythrocyte precursors	Abnormal in megaloblastic and hypochromic anemias
	Morphology of granulocyte precursors	Abnormal in leukemia, myeloid metaplasia
	Presence of foreign cells:	
	Nests of cancer cells	Metastatic cancer
	Granulomas	Tuberculosis sarcoid, etc.
	Lymphocytes and lymphoblasts	Lymphoma and lymphocytic leukemia.
	Plasma cells	Multiple myeloma and severe infection
	Storage cells	Gaucher's disease and other lipidoses
	Evaluation of iron stores	Decreased in iron deficiency Increased in iron-loading disorders and defective iron reutilization
	Other procedures:	
	Bacteriological culture	Positive in tuberculosis, brucellosis, other infections
	Chromosome studies	Abnormal in chronic myelocytic leukemia, etc.
	Special stains	Useful in usual proliferative and metabolic disorders
Bone marrow biopsy	Detects all of the above, although morphology of individual cells not as clearly delineated as in aspirate. However, *architecture is preserved.*	
	Therefore, biopsy more accurately detects:	
	Marrow/fat ratio	Increased in marrow hyperplasia Decreased in aplastic anemia
	Fibrosis	Present in myelofibrosis
	Vasculitis	Present in lupus erythematosus, acute vasculitis, etc.
	Plasma cells	See above
	Granulomas and cancer cells	See above

1. Examination of bone marrow

a. By aspiration

Bone marrow is most commonly removed by aspiration from the posterior iliac spine, sternum, or vertebral spine (figure 1.4). Aspiration disturbs marrow architecture. Hence, this technique is employed primarily to determine types of cells present and their relative numbers. Smears are ordinarily stained with Wright's stain or Wright plus Giemsa's stain. Excess aspirated marrow in the clotted specimen may then be sectioned, stained with H&E (hematoxylin and eosin), and examined for tumor cells or otherwise studied. Stained smears of bone marrow aspirates are subjected to the following studies: (1) determination of the E/M ratio, that is, the ratio of the erythroid cell total to myeloid cell total (normal ratio is 1:3); (2) differential count; (3) search for abnormal cells; (4) evaluation of iron stores in reticulum cells (see lecture 6); and (5) kinetic studies to be described below.

b. By biopsy

Alternatively, marrow may be sampled in a coherent piece with a biopsy needle. When decalcified, sectioned, and stained with H&E, this specimen reveals the undisturbed marrow architecture. Since marrow cells stained with H&E are often difficult to identify, it is customary to smear a biopsy specimen on a cover slip before placing it in formalin. The Wright's stained "touch prep" or "imprint" is useful in facilitating cell identification.

2. Activity of marrow

a. Cellularity

A marrow aspirate that is richly cellular implies normal or increased marrow activity. However, the degree of cellularity does not indicate whether marrow activity is effective.

b. Average maturity

Marrow is studied for a shift in average maturity of a cell line using morphologic criteria. By inference, a "shift to left" signifies a rising ratio of dividing to nondividing cells.

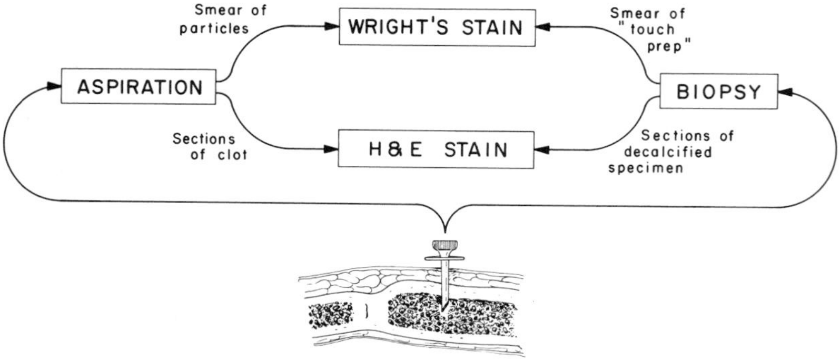

Fig. 1.4
Diagrammatic summary of usual methods for clinical examination of bone marrow.

c. Mitotic index

The *mitotic index* (*MI*) is the percentage of cells in mitosis relative to the total number of cells in a closed compartment. It is affected by duration of mitosis and duration of resting stage (G_0). An elevated MI usually implies increased proliferation, though when mitosis is prolonged, as in megaloblastic anemia, its significance needs careful interpretation. When bone marrow is examined in a clinical setting, the MI is usually only approximated. Normally, it is 1–2%.

When "mitotic figures" (cells in metaphase) are counted in tissue culture preparations after addition of colchicine (which blocks mitosis in metaphase), one can calculate a *stathmokinetic index*.

d. Rate of DNA synthesis

This determination requires techniques for assaying the incorporation of ^{3}H-dThd into cellular DNA. This method is based on assumptions that the ^{3}H of ^{3}H-dThd is nonexchangeable after DNA is labeled, DNA turnover is due solely to cell division and cell death, and ^{3}H-dThd is not diluted unpredictably by varying pools of endogenous unlabeled dThd. Application of the technique is difficult in vivo. However, if a cell culture is exposed to a brief pulse of ^{3}H-dThd and the percentage of labeled mitotic figures followed, it is found that none is labeled initially since only cells in the S phase incorporate ^{3}H-dThd. As these cells move into mitosis, the percentage increases sharply. A second wave of mitosis in 20–24 hr permits assessment of T_c. The duration of S (T_s) divided by generation time (time of cycle, T_c) equals the *labeling index,* which is the percentage of cells labeled if all the cells are proliferating. The extent to which the labeling index falls short of expectation (T_s/T_c) is a measure of nonproliferating cells in G_0.

IV. PHYSIOLOGY OF ERYTHROPOIESIS

A. The erythron

1. Definition

The term *erythron* refers to the combined population of erythrocytes and their precursors, whether immature or mature, in blood or in bone marrow, or at intravascular sites. The term emphasizes that erythrocytes and their precursors—whether circulating or fixed—have a functional unity, however much they are dispersed.

2. Quantitative aspects

Data on the numbers of cells in fixed and circulating components of the erythron are summarized in table 1.5. The circulating adult erythrocyte compartment is by far the largest. The pool of reticulocytes in bone marrow is about the same size as the pool of reticulocytes in blood.

Table 1.5
Components of the Erythron in a Normal 70-kg Human

Cell type	Cell number/kg ($\times 10^9$)	Relative number	Estimated volume of each cell (μm^3)	Total volume of cell compartment (ml)		Approximate transit time (days)
Marrow						
Nucleated cells	5.3	1.7	250	88	6% in marrow	5.0
Reticulocytes	8.2	2.7	120	44		2.8
Blood						
Reticulocytes	3.1	1.0	100	23	94% in blood	1.0
Erythrocytes	307	100	90	2,000		120

Adapted from C. A. Finch, *Blood* 50(1977): 699.

B. Erythrocyte maturation

The stem cell pool of the marrow continually generates a supply of cells committed to erythropoiesis, which yield, in turn, a series of nucleated erythroid precursors. These undergo 4 divisions in about 4 days, during which nuclear and cytoplasmic maturation take place (figure 1.5). Thus they are called *maturational divisions*. Each division yields a smaller cell. Size reduction—from about 25 μm to about 9 μm—is due largely to reduction in absolute nuclear size.

1. Cytoplasmic maturation

The *pronormoblast* is rich in polyribosomes and actively engaged in the synthesis of protein (mainly hemoglobin). A Golgi apparatus and mitochondria are present. Wright's stain reveals marked basophilia. With maturation, the hemoglobin content of the cytoplasm increases and the content of ribosomes (and RNA) de-

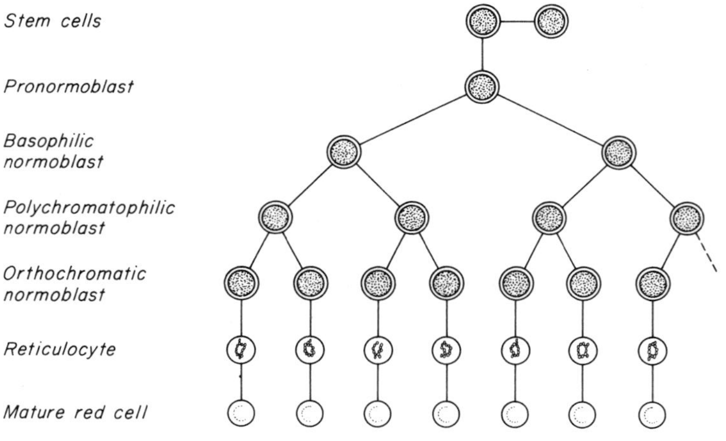

Fig. 1.5
Scheme of erythropoiesis. Number of divisions may be larger or smaller. Dotted line indicates intramedullary cell death (i.e., ineffective erythropoiesis).

creases in linear fashion. The staining reaction changes from the blue of the *basophilic normoblast* to the lavender of the *polychromatophilic normoblast* to the orange-pink of the *orthochromatic normoblast*. Electron micrographs of these cells reveal bundles of *microtubules*, clumps and individually dispersed *ferritin* molecules (see lecture 6), and occasional membrane-bound aggregates of ferritin called *siderosomes*.

2. Nuclear maturation

In the early stages, nuclear chromatin is loosely arranged in fine aggregates and a nucleolus is present. As maturation progresses, nuclear chromatin becomes clumped, condensed, and more basophilic by a process called *pyknosis*, and the nucleolus disappears. Following the fourth maturational division, pyknosis accelerates and nuclear chromatin becomes maximally compressed. The nucleus is then ejected from the cell.

3. The reticulocyte

The *reticulocyte* is the cell that remains after ejection of the nucleus from the orthochromatic normoblast. Although anucleate, it contains polyribosomes and later monoribosomes (hence, it actively synthesizes globin) and mitochondria (hence, it synthesizes heme and utilizes oxygen). In a Wright's stained smear, the reticulocyte is slightly larger than a mature erythrocyte and is identifiable by a slight diffuse basophilia that is termed *polychromatophilia*. The reticulocyte is so named because exposure to a supravital stain (brilliant cresyl blue or new methylene blue) causes cytoplasmic organelles to clump into an easily recognized blue-staining reticulum. Although reticulocytes can be recognized by their polychromatophilia (especially when their numbers are increased) in a routine blood smear, supravital staining is necessary if reticulocytes are to be accurately counted.

Maturation of a reticulocyte to an adult erythrocyte takes 24–48 hr. In the course of maturation, mitochondria and ribosomes disappear—and the cell thereby loses the capacity for hemoglobin synthesis and oxidative metabolism. Ribosomal RNA is degraded ultimately to extracellular ribonucleosides.

Most maturing erythrocytes enter the blood as reticulocytes. Release of reticulocytes from the marrow involves a poorly understood process of physical extrusion through gaps in the walls of marrow sinusoids. The reticulocyte level of blood is the most commonly used clinical index of erythropoietic activity (see below). About 1% of the circulating erythrocyte mass is generated by normal marrow each day. Hence, the normal reticulocyte "count" is 1%. Note the difference between the reticulocyte count, expressed as a percentage of the erythrocyte count (the usual mode), the absolute reticulocyte count per cubic millimeter, and the "reticulocyte index," which corrects the reticulocyte percentage for abnormalities in the hematocrit (assuming that the normal hematocrit is 45%).

4. Ineffective erythropoiesis

As indicated in figure 1.5, cell death may occur within the marrow during the maturation sequence. Normally about 10% of the maturing cells die in this way, though some say the number is smaller. To the extent that erythropoiesis fails to deliver cells to the blood, it is termed *ineffective*. In certain diseases (e.g., megaloblastic anemia), the extent of ineffective erythropoiesis is abnormally great, and relatively few red cells reach the blood despite intense erythropoietic activity.

C. Regulation

The rate of erythropoiesis is governed by the rate of oxygen transport to the tissues, which is the product of oxyhemoglobin concentration and cardiac output. (This relation and the effects on it of blood viscosity and blood volume are discussed further in lecture 20.) When oxygen transport decreases, erythropoiesis increases.

The existence of a feedback loop between erythropoietic marrow and tissues was postulated by Paul Bert in 1878, who found that survival of Andean natives at high altitudes was dependent on increased erythropoiesis. Later work revealed that low tissue pO_2 stimulated erythropoiesis. Since anemia leads to a decrease in tissue pO_2, this discovery explained both the compensatory increase in erythropoiesis in most anemias and the homeostatic balance between red cell production and destruction.

1. Erythropoietin

Early in the twentieth century, Carnot and DeFlandre postulated that a humoral agent adjusts erythropoiesis in response to tissue pO_2. The suggestion received experimental support in 1950 when Reissmann showed that inducing hypoxia in one of a pair of parabiotic rats increases red cell production in both rats. The agent, named *erythropoiesis-stimulating factor* (*ESF*) or *erythropoietin,* was finally demonstrated in 1953 by Erslev in the serum of anemic rats.

a. Properties

Sheep and human erythropoietins were finally purified after much difficulty. The molecule has a carbohydrate content of 50–60% and a sialic acid content of 10–15%. The mol. wt. of human material is 39,000. Precise information on chemical structure is lacking. Desialation results in total loss of biological activity when assayed in vivo but not when assayed in vitro. The discrepancy is due to the fact that asialoerythropoietin (like other asialoglycoproteins) is rapidly cleared from blood by hepatic cells. The carbohydrate portion of the molecule may convey specificity in the recognition of target cell receptors.

b. Source

Erythropoietin is found in both plasma and urine. Early studies on nephrectomized rats suggested that it is produced in the kidneys, but later work showed that small amounts are produced by extrarenal tissue. Extrarenal production in anephric animals and patients rises in response to tissue hypoxia. Thus the renal oxygen sensor and the renal erythropoietin-producing cell both have extrarenal alternatives. To date, attempts to identify which renal cells or structures synthesize erythropoietin have been unsuccessful.

c. Locus of action

Erythropoietin selectively stimulates erythropoiesis in bone marrow by stimulating early committed cells (BFU-E and CFU-E) to differentiate into pronormoblasts. The mechanism of action is not understood in detail. There is some evidence that erythropoietin binds to membrane surface receptors and thereby stimulates synthesis of messenger RNA and perhaps cyclic AMP and cyclic GMP in erythropoietin-responsive cells.

d. Physiologic role

Early workers were uncertain whether erythropoietin is a "panic mechanism" that is called into play only when anemia is present or whether there is a slow, constant baseline erythropoietin effect in normal subjects. The following evidence suggests that the latter view is correct: (1) elevation of the red cell mass to supranormal levels by hypertransfusion decreases erythropoiesis; (2) antierythropoietin antibodies lead to aplasia of marrow erythroid elements; (3) some erythropoietin is found in normal urine; and (4) erythropoietin levels rise in serum and urine in most anemias—but not in most patients with the anemia of renal disease (see lecture 3). A convenient reliable erythropoietin assay suitable for routine clinical use is not yet available.

e. Assay

The benchmark assay for erythropoietin is still a tedious procedure that quantifies incorporation of ^{59}Fe into hemoglobin in hypertransfused mice in which endogenous erythropoietin production is suppressed. Development of a radioimmunoassay was delayed for years pending purification of the hormone. Such assays are at last available; their use in clinical settings is beginning.

2. Erythropoietic response to anoxia

a. Early events

When anoxia is brought about by sudden anemia (as happens after hemorrhage), there occurs first a premature release of marrow reticulocytes (see table 1.3). These so-called *shift reticulocytes* are recognizable in the blood as large polychromatophilic cells. They take longer to mature than the ordinary circulating reticulocytes of normal blood. The accelerated release of reticulocytes from marrow under hypoxic conditions may be mediated by erythropoietin, but a separate *reticulocyte release factor* has been postulated.

b. Later events

Erythropoietin secretion leads to increased activity of erythroid marrow, which may lead to compensation of the anemia (i.e., to a normal hemoglobin level despite continued blood loss). If it does, there is a new steady state at a higher level of marrow activity. The marrow can increase its activity in this way to about 10 times the normal level. There is a corresponding rise in the blood reticulocyte count. A few normoblasts may enter the blood when the marrow is stressed further. If marrow cannot keep up with rate of blood loss, the hemoglobin level decreases. Sustained anoxia leads to centrifugal expansion of erythroid marrow throughout the skeleton and sometimes to extramedullary erythropoiesis. The signals leading to the expansion of erythroid marrow at the expense of fatty marrow are not known.

D. Erythrokinetics

Diagnosis of the underlying cause of anemia requires an appraisal of the patient's "erythrokinetics." The following methods are employed in the clinical evaluation of erythrokinetics.

1. Red cell production

Effective red cell production may be judged by (1) the *reticulocyte count,* perhaps the single most useful piece of information in analysis of anemia; (2) the *erythroid/granulocytic (E/G)* or *erythroid/myeloid (E/M) ratio* in marrow smears, a useful substitute for the unavailable data on the total number of erythroid cells in marrow, which is meaningful only when granulocyte production is normal; and (3) the study of *ferrokinetics,* quantitative data on the traffic of iron, which are rarely available in the clinic. This methodology will be discussed in lecture 6.

2. Red cell destruction

Red cell destruction may be judged from (1) measurements of *red cell life span* and (2) studies of the *rate of hemoglobin catabolism.* These techniques will be discussed in lectures 7 and 11.

V. THE ANEMIAS

A. Definition

Anemia must be defined circumspectly. Ordinarily it refers to a decrease in the total number of circulating erythrocytes, a decrease in the concentration of hemoglobin in blood, or a decrease in the hematocrit compared to a normal group. But the normal population must be relevant. A hemoglobin level that is normal at sea level is relatively low at high altitudes. Also the hematocrit may be a deceptive parameter. In hypovolemia (decreased blood volume), red cell mass may be decreased, but plasma volume is also decreased. Thus, the hematocrit may remain normal. In physiologic hypervolemia (as occurs in pregnancy), blood volume is increased and hematocrit decreased, but red cell mass is actually increased. Hence, a definition of anemia must encompass the functional competence of blood to deliver oxygen to tissues.

B. Clinical features

1. Significance of adaptation

Signs and symptoms depend significantly on the rate of onset of anemia. In anemia due to acute hemorrhage, a 30% decrease in red cell mass may lead rapidly to circulatory collapse and death. In slowly developing anemia of equal severity, symptoms may be few. This means that the body adapts to anemia and that the process of adaptation take time. Adaptation consists of a combination of mechanisms that increase the oxygen-delivering capacity of a decreased amount of hemoglobin. It includes (1) acceleration of the heart rate and respiratory rate; (2) increased cardiac output; and (3) a "shift to the right" in the oxygen saturation curve that is now known to be mediated by an increase in red cell 2,3-diphosphoglycerate (see lecture 8). As a result of these adaptations, a patient can tolerate without symptoms a slowly developing 50% decrease in red cell mass.

2. Signs and symptoms

Signs and symptoms in a patient with anemia are those of the underlying disorder (if one is present) *and* those due to anemia per se. The latter may be classified into three groups: (1) those due to decreased oxygen transport (fatigue, syncope, dyspnea, angina pectoris, widespread impairment of organ function in GI, GU, and other body systems, etc.); (2) those due to decreased blood volume (pallor, postural hypotension, etc.); and (3) those due to increased cardiac output (palpitation, with pulse pressure, "hemic" heart murmurs, onset of congestive heart failure, etc.).

C. Classification

Anemias have been classified in many ways. The two most useful ways are based on (1) the morphology of the average red cell and (2) the pathophysiologic mechanism responsible for the red cell deficit. Neither scheme is wholly satisfactory. In the following lists, references are given to lectures in which disorders are discussed.

1. By red cell morphology

This classification is useful because it leads from the initial laboratory data on a patient's mean red cell size and chromicity (i.e., mean hemoglobin concentration in red cells) to a consideration of disease categories most likely responsible. Classification is based on two of the three *red cell indexes*.

MCV denotes the mean corpuscular volume of red cells (normal = 85–100 μm^3). It is calculated by the formula

$$\text{MCV} = \frac{\text{vol. packed RBC (1/1)} \times 1{,}000}{\text{RBC count/mm}^3\ (\times 10^{12})}$$

MCHC denotes mean corpuscular hemoglobin concentration (normal = 31–35 g/100 ml):

$$\text{MCHC} = \frac{\text{hemoglobin (g/100 ml)}}{\text{vol. packed RBC (1/1)}}.$$

A third red cell index, *MCH*, or mean cell hemoglobin (normal = 27–34 pg/red cell), is noted here although it is less useful in the classification of anemias than the MCHC:

$$\text{MCH} = \frac{\text{hemoglobin (g/100 ml)}}{\text{RBC count/mm}^3\ (\times 10^{12})}.$$

Note that MCV is a measure of volume; MCHC, of concentration; and MCH, of mass.

a. Normocytic-normochromic anemias: MCV = 85–100; MCHC = 31–35

1. Acute bleeding.
2. Hemolytic anemias (lectures 11–14).
   a. Extracorpuscular defects, immune and nonimmune.
   b. Intracorpuscular defects, membrane, metabolic, and hemoglobinopathic.
   c. Combined defects.
3. Marrow failure associated with hypoproliferation of hematopoietic cells (lecture 3).
   a. Aplastic anemia.
   b. Pure red cell aplasia.
   c. Anemia of chronic renal failure.
   d. Anemia of endocrine disease.
   e. Toxic depression of bone marrow.
   f. Myelophthisic anemia.

b. Microcytic-hypochromic anemias: MCV = <85; MCHC = <30

1. Iron deficiency (lecture 6).
2. Sideroblastic anemias.
   a. Refractory.
   b. Reversible.
   c. Pyridoxine-responsive.

c. Macrocytic-normochromic anemias: MCV = >100; MCHC = 31–35

1. Megaloblastic anemias (lectures 4–5).
   a. Vitamin B_{12} deficiency.
   b. Folic acid deficiency.
   c. Others.
2. Nonmegaloblastic macrocytic anemias (lecture 5).

2. By pathophysiologic mechanism

This classification fosters understanding of the disease process in kinetic terms. Its major shortcoming is the fact that some anemias are due to more than one pathophysiologic mechanism. Often one mechanism predominates early in the course but another supervenes. In practice these complications should be borne in mind.

a. Increased red cell loss.

1. Bleeding, acute and chronic.
2. Hemolytic anemias (lectures 11–14).

b. Decreased red cell production

1. Marrow failure associated with hypoproliferation of hematopoietic cells (lecture 3).
2. Marrow failure associated with ineffective erythropoiesis.
   a. Impaired hemoglobin synthesis: the hypochromic anemias (lecture 6).

b. Impaired DNA synthesis: the megaloblastic anemias (lectures 4–5).

D. Approach to patient

The diagnosis of anemia, like the diagnosis of any other disease, rests on the information derived from a careful history, physical examination, and laboratory evaluation. A history of drug ingestion or exposure to other toxic substances must be recorded in detail. A family history of anemia makes a genetic disorder likely, and a history of previous anemia in the patient suggests either an inherited disorder or persisting cause (e.g., menorrhagia in the female). Racial and geographic derivations are pertinent in certain hemoglobinopathies (hemoglobin S or C) and red cell metabolic disorders (G-6-PD deficiency). Signs or symptoms of inflammation, evidence of a bleeding tendency, splenic enlargement and lymphadenopathy provide important diagnostic clues. Chronic leg ulcers are sometimes seen in hemolytic disease. Epithelial changes including flattening of the nails and glossitis occur in iron deficiency. A depapillated tongue and neurologic signs of posterior and lateral column disease are found with vitamin B_{12} deficiency. As indicated above, the basic approach to the differential diagnosis of anemia depends on the laboratory. After anemia has been detected by a hematocrit or hemoglobin determination, a blood film should be carefully examined and red cell indexes (MCV and MCHC) obtained. A reticulocyte count should be obtained early, along with the plasma iron concentration and iron-binding capacity. These determinations usually permit the physician to characterize the functional abnormality of the erythron and indicate what other information is needed for a more specific diagnosis.

SELECTED REFERENCES

Cline, M. J., and Golde, D. W. Cellular interactions in haematopoiesis. *Nature* 277(1979): 177.

Erslev, A. J. Humoral regulation of red cell production. *Blood* 8(1953): 348.

Graber, S. E., and Krantz, S. B. Erythropoietin and the control of red cell production. *Ann. Rev. Med.* 29(1978): 51.

Miller, M. E., et al. Plasma levels of immunoreactive erythropoietin after acute blood loss in man. *J. Clin. Invest.* 67(1981): 702.

Nathan, D. G., et al. Human erythroid burst-forming unit: T-cell requirement for proliferation *in vitro*. *J. Exp. Med.* 147(1978): 324.

Quesenberry, P., and Levitt, L. Hematopoietic stem cells. *New Eng. J. Med.* 301(1979): 755, 819, 868.

Sherwood, J. B., and Goldwater, E. Radioimmunoassay of erythropoietin. *Brit. J. Haematol.* 48(1981): 359.

Zuckerman, K. S. Human erythroid burst-forming units: Growth *in vitro* is dependent on monocytes, but not living lymphocytes. *J. Clin. Invest.* 67(1981): 702.

LECTURE 2 Reticuloendothelial (Mononuclear Phagocyte) System, Lymphatic System, and Spleen

William S. Beck

I. INTRODUCTION

The *reticuloendothelial system* (*RES*), the *lymphatic system,* and the *spleen* have certain features in common: they are of major hematologic importance in health and disease; they are complex and many faceted, with shared or overlapping functions; and they all pose unsolved basic problems. The following discussion gives emphasis to hematologic aspects and is intended only as an introductory guide. The text will call attention to later lectures that deal with immunologic and other aspects of these systems.

II. RETICULO-ENDOTHELIAL SYSTEM

A. Definition

The term *reticuloendothelial system,* or *RES,* was introduced in 1924 by Aschoff to designate those scattered body cells that avidly take up vital dyes. The definition later came to include cells taking up injected particulate matter (i.e., India ink, iron, etc.). Anatomically the system consists of the (1) *fixed macrophages,* or *reticulum cells,* of spleen, lymph nodes, bone marrow, and liver (Kupffer cells); (2) *free macrophages,* or *histiocytes,* in spleen, lymph nodes, lung, serous cavities, and other tissues; (3) *endothelial cells* lining *sinusoids* (or *sinuses*) in liver, bone marrow, spleen, and lymph nodes (plus similar cells in the adrenal and pituitary glands); and (4) circulating *monocytes* of blood.

Because later work showed that each of these cell types arises from the blood *monocyte,* which in turn derives from precursors in the bone marrow, the system was renamed *mononuclear phagocyte system,* or *MPS*. The terms *RES* and *MPS* are now used interchangeably, although some authorities restrict the RES to fixed cells and exclude free macrophages and monocytes. This text will employ the older term, RES, and will define its component cells as above. Functionally RES cells are distinguishable by their ability to ingest particulate matter by the process of *phagocytosis*. In addition they play significant roles in *humoral defense* and *metabolism*.

B. Distribution and size

Its component cells are so widely distributed that investigators have facetiously suggested that the body is simply an inert matrix designated to support the RES. Its size is not precisely known. In the rat, each of the three major organs of the RES (spleen, liver, and bone marrow) has been estimated to contain 10^9 RES cells. A normal human spleen contains about 1.4×10^{11} cells. If it is assumed that half the cells in the human spleen are RES cells (as in the rat) and that liver and bone marrow contain an equal number of RES cells, the RES of a normal person must then consist of 2×10^{11} cells. Thus it is of substantial size.

C. Characteristics of major cell types

As noted above, the three major cell types are reticulum cells, free macrophages or histiocytes, endothelial cells, and monocytes. In tissues these cells are usually associated with *lymphocytes* and *plasma cells* (or *plasmacytes*). Properties of RES cells are investigated by three methods: (1) study of morphology by techniques of histology, cytochemistry, phase microscopy, and electron microscopy; (2) study of structural transitions in health and disease; and (3) study of functional properties in health and disease. The following is a brief description of the major cell types.

1. Fixed macrophages (reticulum cells)

A typical inactive fixed macrophage (reticulum cell) is a large cell, with a diameter of more than 20 μm. In stained imprints, the abundant cytoplasm is pale blue and homogeneous in appearance. The relatively small nucleus is usually round. Blue nucleoli are usually present. They are capable of phagocytosis and may be sites of abnormal accumulations of proteins, lipids, and other materials (see lectures 6 and 25).

Fixed macrophages apparently are in dynamic equilibrium with free mobile macrophages. They occur in so-called *lymphoreticular tissues* (spleen and lymph nodes) and bone marrow. Such tissues are interlaced with a reticular fibrillary network that ramifies throughout the tissue. They also include: the macrophages of the liver (Kupffer cells), which have a characteristic stellate appearance; pulmonary alveolar macrophages; and perhaps osteoclasts. Some secretory macrophages may not be phagocytic and, strictly speaking, may not be part of the RES.

A comment is in order on the relation between reticulum cells and pluripotent stem cells (lecture 1) in the light of past claims that reticulum cells (or other RES cells) can undergo transition into lymphocyte precursors and other cell types. That matter is still unsettled. But it is clear that neither the reticulum cell nor the sinusoidal endothelial cell is identical with the pluripotent stem cell—labeling data having shown that these cells lack the kinetic and migratory properties required of a competent hematopoietic stem cell. Rather, as shown in figure 1.2, fixed and free macrophages arise from the following maturation sequence: pluripotent stem cell (CFU-GEMM) → CFU-GM → CFU-Mac → promonocyte → monocyte → macrophage.

2. Free macrophages

Free macrophages are large lysosome-filled wandering cells (diameter up to 50 μm) with functions resembling those of primary fixed macrophages, or reticulum cells. Direct evidence of their bone marrow origin is suggested by chromosome studies of pulmonary macrophages in patients transplanted with marrow from donors of the opposite sex.

3. Endothelial cells

The endothelial cell component of the RES was originally thought to include only the sinusoid-lining cells of lymph nodes and spleen and the endothelial cells of the capillaries of liver, bone marrow, adrenals, and pituitary. Later models included the endothelial cells of all blood vessels.

Endothelial cells are connected with one another (and with surrounding reticulum cells) by a fiber lattice. Thus they resemble specialized reticulum cells. The loose arrangement of the cells in spleen, bone marrow, and lymph nodes differs from that of the endothelium in ordinary blood vessels in that they rest upon a basement membrane distinctive for its defective strandlike character.

Electron microscopic study of cells lining sinusoids reveals *clefts* between and among extensions of these cells. These surround *pores* that begin at the sinusoid surface and become continuous with similar clefts between adjacent reticulum cells. The presence of these intercellular clefts (and the absence of obturating basement membranes) is characteristic of sinuses and helps to explain their high permeability.

4. Monocytes

As noted above, the blood monocyte is the precursor of fixed and free macrophages in tissues. The mature monocyte is a large motile cell (diameter 12–20 μm) with a characteristic indented nucleus, lacy chromatin, grayish-blue cytoplasm in Wright's stained smears, and very fine pinkish granules. Living monocytes adhere avidly to glass surfaces and display cytoplasmic spreading. Electron microscopy reveals a well-developed Golgi complex and numerous mitochondria, lysosomes, and microtubules. Monocytes are discussed further in lecture 17.

D. Functions of RES

The major functions of the RES are phagocytic, immunologic, and secretory. In spleen and lymph nodes, RES cells are in close proximity to immunologically reactive cells. In liver and bone marrow, however, RES cells are adjacent to hepatocytes and hematopoietic cells, respectively. This may mean that the functions of RES cells differ in different locations.

1. Clearing function

The capacity of the RES for engulfing particulate material, denatured plasma proteins, and effete or damaged cells is called its *clearing function*. Such ingestion can lead to rapid killing and destruction of bacteria or red cells or to indefinite storage of particles such as silica, carbon, and thorium dioxide. This RES function is a fundamental body defense mechanism. Its impairment by disease can have disastrous consequences.

2. Immunologic functions

Tissue macrophages play a key role in the antigen-induced blastic transformation of lymphocytes. This involves (1) a preliminary processing of foreign or pathogenic antigens by macrophages; (2) enhancement of lymphocyte proliferation by secretion of mitogenic protein, B and T cell differentiation factors, T cell activating factor, and other products; (3) secretion of multiple substances involved in tissue organization and repair; and (4) subsequent regulation by the activated lymphocyte of microbicidal and cytocidal functions of the macrophage.

3. Secretory functions

In addition to the products just mentioned, macrophages secrete enzymes that hydrolyze tissue components (lysosomal proteases, collagenase, nucleases, etc.), products involved in body defense (muramidase, complement components, interferon, etc.), products that modulate other cells (angiogenesis factors, low-molecular weight chemotactic factor, CSF, etc.), and various other products (pyrogen, transferrin, transcobalamin II, thromboplastin, etc.).

E. Techniques for studying the RES

1. Measurement of clearing capacity

The *clearing capacity* of the RES can be quantified in animals by injecting increasing doses of particulate materials such as carbon, saccharated iron oxide, colloidal gold, or thorium dioxide. Such experiments show that (1) with increasing doses, the rate of particle clearance approaches a maximal clearance rate asymptotically; (2) maximal clearance rates of different colloids are not the same; and (3) the maximal clearance rates (expressed as milligrams cleared per 100 g body weight) differ from species to species. This variation is a function of spleen and liver weight.

2. Blockage of the RES

The clearing function of the RES can be blocked to a variable extent by injection of suspensions of particulate matter such as carbon. There is some blockage specificity in that clearance of one substance by the RES (e.g., carbon) may not be blocked by prior injections of another substance (e.g., thorotrast). The mechanism of blockade specificity is unknown. It may reflect saturation of phagocytes (or a specific population of them) or depletion of serum factors needed to facilitate phagocytosis (*opsonins*). The actual site of particle clearance in the RES is influenced by many factors—rate of blood flow, possible presence of local tissue damage, nature of the particles, and so forth. As we shall see, the spleen has a special capacity to clear mildly damaged red cells from the circulation. More severely damaged red cells are removed mainly by the liver. More will be said of these RES functions in later discussions of red cell destruction (lectures 11 and 12) and phagocytosis (lecture 18).

3. Visualization of the RES

Since cells of the RES are identifiable by their ability to ingest particulate matter, many early workers studied tissue distributions of radioactive colloidal particles. Such particles when injected intravenously are rapidly cleared from the blood and trapped by the RES in the liver, spleen, and bone marrow. These observations led to the development of external scanning techniques that employ radioactive colloids to delineate the structure and functional integrity of organs rich in RES cells. The use of short-lived radionuclides greatly reduces the radiation dose. Use of radionuclides that decay rapidly increases the yield of emitted photons and improves the spatial resolution of scanning procedures without increasing the radiation dose. Finally, advances in radiation detection methods have permitted both visualization of a specific organ system and its functional evaluation.

a. Scanning liver and spleen

Nuclear medicine services currently scan the liver and spleen by injecting technetium-99m sulfur colloid. The usual dose of 2 mCi gives a whole-body radiation dose of only 0.008–0.03 rad and a critical organ dose of 0.3–0.6 rad to the liver. An image of liver and spleen is thus readily obtained (figure 2.1). Focal defects due to neoplasm, cysts, abscesses, and so forth appear as circumscribed areas of decreased uptake. Diffuse diseases cause mottling. With increasing severity of hepatocellular disease, more colloid is shunted to other parts of the RES.

b. Special methods for scanning spleen

A second method used in scanning the spleen exploits a physiologic process peculiar to that organ—the sequestering of damaged red cells (i.e., heat-damaged red cells, labeled with a suitable gamma-emitting nuclide such as rubidium-81). The type of red cell damage is not the critical factor in producing sequestration; the degree of damage is. If damage is too great, cells are sequestered in the liver or are destroyed by intravascular hemolysis; if too slight, the cells accumulate in the spleen too slowly.

Splenomegaly is the most frequently encountered abnormality in spleen scanning. Space-occupying lesions are also demonstrable. These include abscess, lymphomatous involvement, and granulomatous lesions of sarcoid. Evidence of splenic infarction may also be seen.

The term *functional asplenia* refers to failure of the spleen to develop on image. This is usually due to failure of the radionuclide to reach the spleen's macrophages because of reduced perfusion to the spleen (as may result from elevated blood viscosity during a sickle cell crisis). After resolution of such crisis with resulting improvement in arterial perfusion, radionuclide is again delivered in sufficient quantity.

c. Scanning bone marrow

Attempts to scan and thereby quantify bone marrow have been less successful. Current efforts to scan that organ employ two

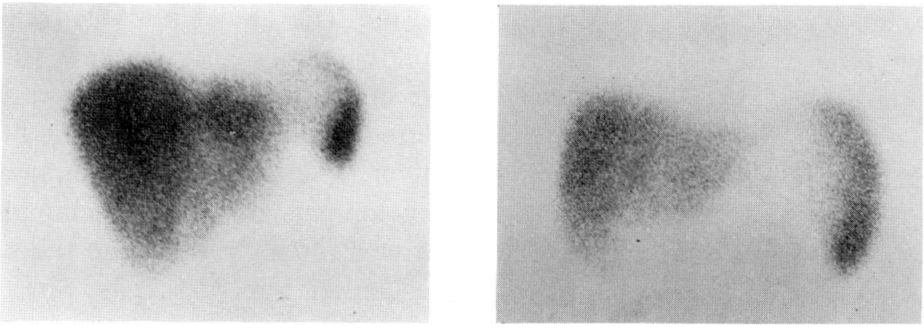

A B

Fig. 2.1
Image of liver and spleen scan. Patients were previously injected with 6 mCi of technetium-99m sulfer colloid: *A,* normal subject; *B,* patient with splenomegaly associated with hepatic cirrhosis. (Courtesy of Dr. D. A. McKusick)

physiologic processes peculiar to bone marrow: the accumulation (1) of colloids labeled with ^{99m}Tc, ^{113m}In, or ^{198}Au by marrow RES cells and (2) of transferrin-bound ^{59}Fe by marrow erythroid cells—a process that will be discussed in lecture 6.

III. LYMPHATIC SYSTEM

A. Description

The *lymphatic system* consists principally of *lymphatic capillaries, ducts,* and *lymph nodes*. The small lymphatic capillaries in body tissues are separated from the capillaries carrying blood. They make up a complex network of fragile distensible vessels, resembling veins, that collect *lymph,* the watery extravascular fluid of tissues, and conveys it to the blood. Their function is drainage, not perfusion or circulation; thus they end blindly in tissues. Lymphatic capillaries unite to form progressively larger vessels that converge finally in two main channels, the *thoracic,* or *left lymphatic duct,* and the *right lymphatic duct* (figure 2.2). Lymphatic vessels, like blood vessels, are present in nearly every tissue. An exception is the bone marrow, which contains no lymphatic vessels.

Lymph nodes are bean-shaped bodies occurring at intervals along the larger lymphatic vessels and ranging from 1 to about 15 mm in diameter. Despite an occasional solitary node, most nodes occur in groups or chains that are known by regional names, for example, *inguinal, axillary, supratrochlear,* and *cervical* groups, which are superficial; and *mesenteric* and *retroperitoneal* groups, which are deep. Each group receives the lymph draining from a particular body area.

B. Lymph node structure

The gross internal structure of a typical lymph nodes is shown in figure 2.3. The *hilus* is a slight depression through which pass

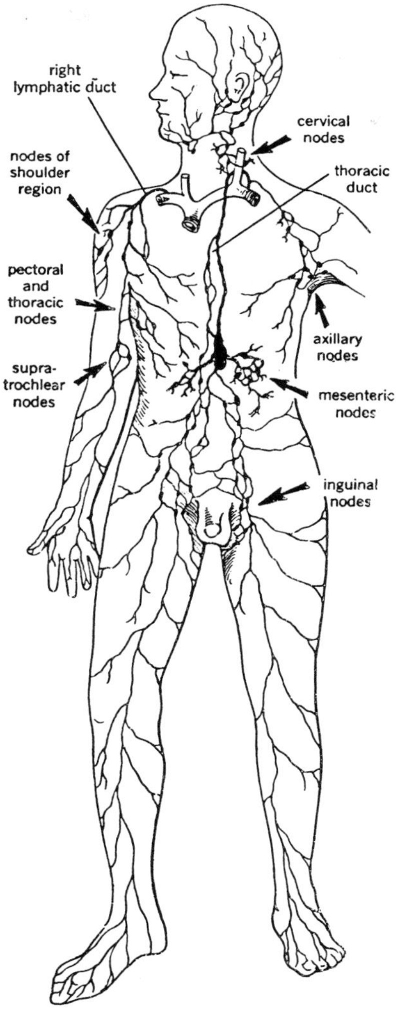

Fig. 2.2
Human lymphatic system. (From W. S. Beck, *Human Design: Molecular, Cellular, and Systematic Physiology,* New York: Harcourt Brace Jovanovich, 1971).

blood and lymphatic vessels. The outer covering is a *capsule* of connective tissue from which fibrous *trabeculae* proceed into the substance of the node, dividing it into irregular, freely communicating spaces. Suspended with this framework is the *reticular framework.* Its most loosely meshed areas are the *sinusoids,* through which the lymph percolates. RES cells line the sinusoids. The cut section of a node shows an outer *cortex* and an inner *medulla.* Both consist of *lymphoid tissue.* However, the cortex contains lymphatic *nodules,* or *secondary follicles,* temporary structures whose appearance varies with their state of activity. (Similar nodules occur in the spleen and throughout the body in

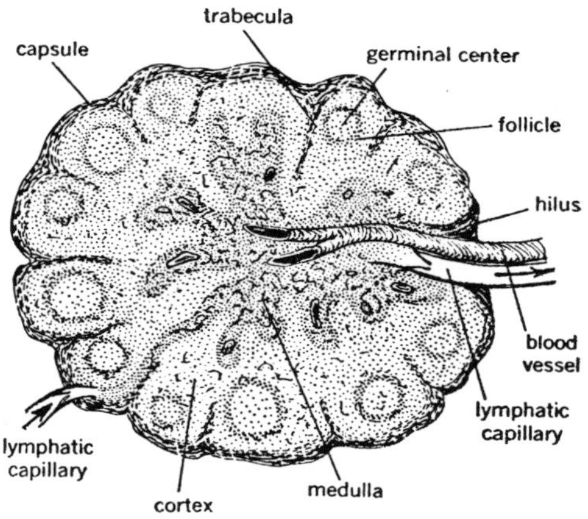

Fig. 2.3
Gross structure of a lymph node. (Compare with figure 23.1.) (From W. S. Beck, *Human Design: Molecular, Cellular, and Systematic Physiology,* New York: Harcourt Brace Jovanovich, 1971)

regions of *diffuse* lymphoid tissue, as in the walls of the intestine and respiratory passages.) Nodules are made up of masses of lymphocytes of various ages arranged in a characteristic pattern. When appropriately stimulated, the central portions of the nodules can produce new *lymphocytes*. Hence, they are *germinal centers*. Lymph entering a node via an afferent lymphatic vessel at the hilus circulates through the sinusoids and leaves by efferent vessels. In passing through the node, it picks up the lymphocytes arising in germinal centers.

C. Lymphoid cells

1. Lymphocytes

The familiar lymphocyte in stained blood smears is a small round cell with a characteristic dark nucleus and a thin, pale or blue rim of cytoplasm lacking distinct granules. Similar cells are found in the lymph nodes, spleen, bone marrow, and other tissues—indeed more than a kilogram of lymphocytes are found outside blood, lymph nodes, and bone marrow. All of these cells are called lymphocytes because they have similar morphology, but we now recognize this group to be functionally heterogeneous.

As shown in figure 1.1, lymphocyte precursors are believed to arise from the pluripotent hematopoietic stem cell (CFU-LM). The earliest recognizable lymphocyte precursor is the *lymphoblast,* a larger mononuclear cell with basophilic cytoplasm. This cell matures into a smaller *prolymphocyte,* which has coarse, clumped chromatin with distinct open spaces. The prolymphocyte then evolves into a *mature lymphocyte,* which may be large, intermediate, or small in size. These are the most numerous cells in lymphoid tissues, which contain all three sizes. Normally blood lymphocytes are intermediate or small.

As we shall discuss in detail later (lectures 17, 22, and especially 23), the seemingly homogeneous population of small lymphocytes consists of at least two types, so-called *T lymphocytes* or *T cells* (thymus derived) and *B lymphocytes* or *B cells* (bursa or bursa-equivalent derived). These cells play key roles in the immune system and hence are said to be immunocompetent.

a. T lymphocytes

The undifferentiated precursors of T cells migrate from the bone marrow during fetal life (and perhaps throughout life) to the cortex of the thymus, where a high rate of cellular proliferation and turnover prevails. During their stay there lymphocytes become immunocompetent—that is, each cell acquires the ability to respond to a single antigenic determinant. Immunocompetent T lymphocytes leave the thymus and settle in distinct anatomical loci in peripheral lymphoid tissues, spleen, and lymph nodes (figure 2.4). Some T lymphocytes travel constantly from lymph nodes and spleen back into efferent lymphatics and from there into the venous and arterial circulation. T cells leave the circulation in the postcapillary venules, percolate through the tissues, and eventually reenter the lymphatics. If in the course of its journey the T cell encounters the specific antigen with which it can interact, it may then undergo *blastic transformation,* proliferate, and develop into a clone of cells, some of which become the effector cells that mediate specific cellular immunity. Other clone members may persist as "memory cells" for subsequent encounters with the same antigen.

b. B lymphocytes

The lymphoid cell line that eventually gives rise to plasma cells develops differently. In birds the precursors of plasma cells migrate from the bone marrow to the *bursa of Fabricius,* a lymphoepithelial organ, where they become immunocompetent. The anatomical equivalent of the bursa in mammals is not yet definitely identified. Many believe it is the bone marrow. Immunocompetent B cells migrate to spleen and lymph nodes where they occupy distinct sites in the cortex of lymphoid follicles. As shown in figure 2.4, B cells are found in the superficial cortex of the node, the follicles (germinal centers), and the medullary cords.

2. Plasma cells

Plasma cells (*plasmacytes*) originate in two ways (see figure 23.2): (1) by a *maturation* pathway (B-immunoblast → plasmacytoid lymphocyte → plasmacyte) that derives from the stem cell (figure 1.1) and (2) through *blastic transformation of B lymphocytes* by antigenic stimulation. The product of both pathways is an enlarged cell with cytoplasmic basophilia (due to RNA in the endoplasmic reticulum so prominent in electron micrographs), eccentric positioning of the nucleus in the cell, and characteristic

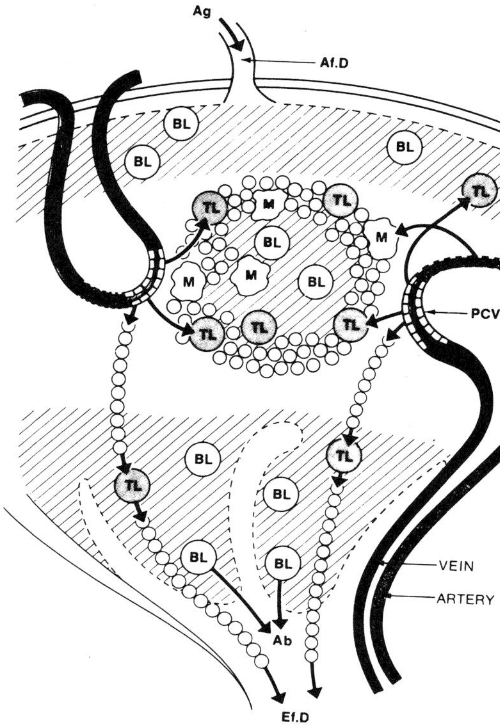

Fig. 2.4
Diagram of lymph node showing characteristic loci of various cells. Abbreviations used: TL, T lymphocyte; BL, B lymphocyte; M, macrophage; Ag, antigen; Ab, antibody; Af. D, afferent lymphatic duct; Ef. D, efferent lymphatic duct; PCV, postcapillary venule. The crosshatched zones represent areas populated by B lymphocytes. Areas containing open circles represent T lymphocyte regions. T lymphocytes circulate in close proximity to macrophages, allowing interaction between these cells and specific antigen. (From C. G. Craddock et al., *New Eng. J. Med.* 285(1971): 380, reprinted by permission)

coarsening of chromatin masses that is actively engaged in immunoglobulin synthesis (see lectures 23 and 24).

D. Functions

1. Filtration of lymph

Lymph nodes remove foreign particles from lymph before it enters the blood. All lymph passes through at least one node. In its tortuous course through a node, it is cleansed of bacteria, dead cells, and other foreign particles by simple mechanical filtration and by phagocytic RES cells. This function is especially important when lymph is infected. Unless infection is severe, it is eliminated by the first node or group of nodes in the pathway of the lymph.

2. Production of lymphocytes

As noted, lymph nodes are centers for the proliferation of lymphocytes and other immunocompetent cells, sometimes termed *immunocytes*. Antigens arriving at a node stimulate such cell production.

IV. SPLEEN

A. Structure

The *spleen* is a discrete organ with both lymphoid and RES elements. Indeed it comprises the largest collection of lymphocytes and RES cells in the body. It is beneath the diaphragm, behind and to the left of the stomach. It is covered by peritoneum and held in position by peritoneal folds. Like a lymph node, it has a connective tissue capsule from which trabeculae extend inward. Both capsule and trabeculae contain a few smooth muscle fibers. They are less prominent in humans than in dogs and other animals, in which the capsule is contractile.

The spaces between trabeculae contain three types of splenic pulp: *white pulp, red pulp,* and *marginal zone* (figure 2.5). All are distinguishable to the naked eye on cut section.

White pulp consists of scattered *follicles* with germinal centers and the *periarterial lymphatic sheaths,* sleeves of loose reticular connective tissue that is packed with lymphocytes and free macrophages. The sheaths surround arteries as they enter the splenic parenchyma.

Sheaths are surrounded by a poorly defined region between white and red pulp called the marginal zone. It is made up of a reticular meshwork with narrow interstices, blood vessels, and free cells. Many arteries terminate within it.

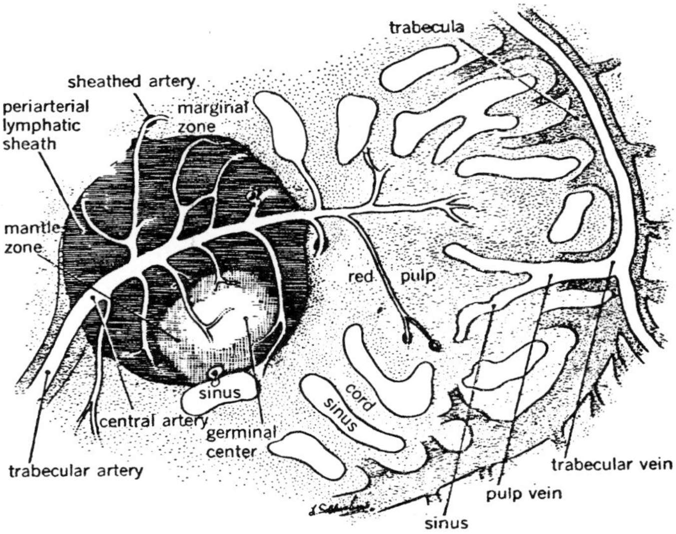

Fig. 2.5
Diagram of organization of blood vessels in spleen. (From L. Weiss, in R. Greep, ed., *Histology,* New York: McGraw-Hill, 1965, used by permission)

Red pulp consists primarily of *vascular sinusoids* (or *sinuses*) that are separated by *cords*. Both are vascular spaces lined by RES cells arrayed upon a lattice-like reticular framework. Sinuses are thin-walled, cucumber-shaped, venous vessels that anastomose freely and form the first stage of the efferent circulation. Cords are bands or septums of reticular fibers that separate sinuses. Many arterial vessels terminate in them.

B. Pathway of circulation

Arterial blood entering the spleen follows a complex pathway before emerging as venous blood. The main *splenic artery* has many branches, called *trabecular arteries*. These enter the white pulp as the *central arteries,* which also have many branches. Some terminate in the white pulp; later branches terminate in the marginal zone; still later branches terminate in the red pulp. Those that acquire lymphatic sheaths before terminating in the white pulp are termed *sheathed arteries*. A few arteries communicate directly with sinuses. Two routes are taken by blood passing through the spleen. A small portion of it passes directly into the sinusoids—or into the cords at a point that affords free and immediate transfer into the sinuses. Blood taking this pathway has a virtually unobstructed route to the venous collecting system and out of the spleen via the *splenic veins*. This is the *rapid transit pathway* or closed portion of the splenic blood flow. Essentially it bypasses the cords. A larger portion of the blood empties into the cords of the red pulp. (The substantial amount that empties into the white pulp and marginal zone finds its way into the cords.) Blood in the cords must navigate the circuitous and macrophage-lined cordal compartments before penetrating the narrow holes through which it gains access to the sinuses. This is the *slow transit pathway* or open portion of the splenic blood flow. In traversing this pathway through the spleen, blood is brought into intimate contact with the phagocytic RES cells of white pulp, marginal zone, and red pulp.

C. Functions

The spleen is not essential for life, and serious disturbances do not usually follow splenectomy. However, some of the events occurring after splenectomy have yielded clues to the spleen's functions.

1. Hematopoietic functions

The spleen's hematopoietic functions in the embryo were mentioned in lecture 1. As a result of its embryonic capability the spleen retains the ability to initiate hematopoietic functions into adult life. The phenomenon of extramedullary hematopoiesis in the spleen occurs in varied and unusual situations. The major example of splenic hematopoiesis in the adult is the poorly understood idiopathic or agnogenic myeloid metaplasia (see lecture 19).

2. Culling function

The culling function (also termed *hemoclastic function*) refers to the spleen's ability to destroy by phagocytosis aged or imperfect red blood cells. In this role, the spleen acts as an inspector, scrutinizing circulating red cells and removing the few that, so to speak, fail to meet specifications. Such selective destructions are facilitated by the unique splenic circulation. As blood passes through the white pulp, plasma tends to be skimmed off, and the cells are concentrated. This phenomenon, coupled with the slow transit open circulation pathway, leads to stasis of flow, so that opportunities for phagocytosis of old or damaged red cells by RES cells increase. Even after passage through the cords, red cells may remain for some time in the sinusoids. There the glucose supply is rapidly diminished and the oldest cells fail to survive. The red cells are thereby subjected to additional culling. In sum, the materials removed by the spleen in normal subjects include senescent red cells, acanthocytes, and those particles or bodies removed by "pitting" (see below). Materials removed in disease include spherocytes, sickled red cells, hemoglobin C red cells, antibody-coated red cells, white cells, platelets, and microorganisms.

3. "Pitting" function and reticulocyte conditioning

The "pitting" function of the spleen refers to its ability to remove particles from intact red cells without destroying them. Such particles include the siderotic granules of siderocytes (see lecture 6), Howell-Jolly bodies, Pappenheimer bodies, Heinz bodies (see lecture 13), and so forth. This function results from the pinching off of particle-containing portions of red cells that are having difficulty squeezing through the pores between cords and sinusoids. The pinched-off red cell reseals itself but, because its membrane surface area is reduced, it becomes a *spherocyte* (see lectures 11 and 13). Some of these cells appear thereafter to have had a bite taken from them.

The intricate splenic filter, which receives 5% of the blood volume each minute, makes the spleen a "training camp" for reticulocytes. Reticulocytes that have excess membrane or weak surface charges are preferentially retained by the spleen. During their sojourn, they are molded, pitted, or if beyond repair culled out.

4. Immunologic functions

As noted above, lymphocytes leave the thymus in early life and colonize the spleen and lymph nodes. Lymphocytes found in the adult spleen are partly sequestered blood-borne lymphocytes. The spleen is rich in lymphocytes and RES cells and plays an active part in antibody synthesis and other defense mechanisms. When blood enters the spleen, *soluble antigens* are skimmed off with the plasma and enter the right-angled arterioles supplying the germinal centers of the white pulp. *Particulate antigens* lodge first in the red pulp and are transported across the marginal zone into the germinal center, where IgM antibody response begins. When the splenic microcirculation is impaired, as in sickle cell anemia, or when the spleen has been removed, the antibody response to intravenous antigen is blunted. *Tuftsin* and *properdin,* two plasma proteins that serve as opsonins (see lecture 18) and that fall in concentration after splenectomy, are synthesized in the spleen.

5. Clearance function

Because of its unique circulation, the spleen is the major site of clearance of poorly opsonized microorganisms. (The liver clears the bulk of well-opsonized bacteria from the blood.) Ninety percent of the blood entering the spleen is dumped into the "open circulation" of the red pulp, and the blood is then forced into the sinuses. This means the blood cells and other particles contained in the blood are required to percolate along the fine meshwork of the splenic cords until they can squeeze through tiny 0.5 μm to 2.5 μm pores between endothelial cells lining the walls of the venous sinuses to enter the venous circulation and leave the spleen. This meandering microcirculation allows time for splenic phagocytes to remove even poorly opsonized bacteria.

6. Reservoir function

The spleen serves as a store or reservoir of platelets. In dogs, cats, and guinea pigs, it also serves as a reservoir of red blood cells, which tend to accumulate in the sinuses during sleep. The cells are ejected back into the blood under stress or under the influence of epinephrine. Recent studies have cast doubt on the importance of this function in normal humans. A healthy adult human spleen contains only 20–30 ml of blood. Although pooling of red cells does not normally occur in the spleen, 20–30% of the platelet mass is sequestered in the normal spleen. With massive splenomegaly, up to 30% of the red cell mass and 80—90% of the platelet mass may be pooled in the spleen.

7. Endocrine function

The spleen exerts poorly understood controls over the number of red cells, white cells, and platelets in the blood. Some have suggested that the spleen secretes one or more hormones that affect the rates of blood cell production in the bone marrow.

D. Pathophysiology

1. Consequences of splenectomy (the hyposplenic state)

Asplenia (i.e., absence of the spleen) is due to surgical removal performed in an otherwise normal individual who has suffered traumatic rupture or in the therapy of various hematologic disorders. In sickle cell anemia repeated spontaneous splenic infarction of the spleen may lead to "autosplenectomy" in childhood (see lecture 9). Functional asplenia may also occur in newborn infants and in various conditions leading to RES blockage (e.g., chronic hemolysis in which erythrophagocytosis blocks the splenic RES cells). Clinically the diagnosis is confirmed by spleen scan.

Splenectomy, or "hyposplenism," usually leads to typical changes in the blood: (1) a rise in platelet and granulocyte counts, sometimes reaching alarming peaks in 10 days and then subsiding to nearly normal values; (2) absolute lymphocytosis and monocytosis; (3) appearance of Howell-Jolly bodies and other red cell inclusions; (4) appearance of many target cells and spiculated red cells ("burr" cells); (5) slight increase in reticulocyte count; and (6) appearance of giant platelets. In about 10% of normal individuals, small *accessory spleens* occur in the mesentery in the region of the splenic hilum or elsewhere. They may enlarge after splenectomy and rarely may cause relapse of the hematologic condition for which the spleen was originally removed.

Hyposplenic (or splenectomized) children are vulnerable to overwhelming, often fatal, pneumococcal infection. Older patients are more likely to have acquired immunity to the different types of pneumococcus.

A wide variety of conditions and spleen sizes are associated with hyposplenism. Atrophic spleens are noted in ulcerative colitis, celiac disease, dermatitis herpetiformis, thyrotoxicosis (Graves' disease), and hemorrhagic thrombocythemia and as a result of therapeutic irradiation and after radiocontrast studies with thorium dioxide (Thorotrast®). The spleen may be normal sized or large in sickle cell anemia, sarcoidosis, and amyloidosis and with the use of high-dose corticosteroids.

E. Splenomegaly

A small number (3–5%) of normal subjects have palpable spleens. The major systemic causes of splenic enlargement are summarized in table 2.1. In addition, splenomegaly is rarely due to an intrinsic

Table 2.1
Major Causes of Splenomegaly

Disorders of lymphatic system	**Macrophage disorders**
Reactions to viral infections (e.g., infectious mononucleosis, infectious hepatitis)	"Work hypertrophy" secondary to immune response in bacterial infections (e.g., subacute bacterial endocarditis, miliary tuberculosis)
Reactions to connective tissue disorders (e.g., systemic lupus erythematosus, Felty's syndrome)	"Work hypertrophy" secondary to chronic hemolysis (e.g., hereditary spherocytosis, lecture 13)
Lymphoproliferative disorders (e.g., lymphocytic leukemia, lymphoma)	Lipidoses (e.g., Gaucher's disease, lecture 25)
Infiltrative disorders	Histiocytoses (e.g., Letterer-Siwe disease, lecture 25)
Myeloproliferative disorders, (e.g., myeloid metaplasia, polycythemia vera)	**Venous congestion**
Amyloidosis	Splenic or portal vein thrombosis
Sarcoidosis	Hepatic cirrhosis
Gaucher's disease	
Metastatic cancer	

Table 2.2
Major Indications for Splenectomy

To control (or stage) basic disease
Hereditary spherocytosis
Immunothrombocytopenia
Immunohemolysis
Hodgkin's disease
To correct chronic or severe hypersplenic symptoms
Hairy cell leukemia
Felty's syndrome
Myeloid metaplasia
Thalassemia major
Gaucher's disease
Hemodialysis splenomegaly
Splenic vein thrombosis

abnormality such as splenic cyst. The pattern obtained on scanning an enlarged spleen is shown in figure 2.1B. Table 2.2 summarizes the major medical indications for splenectomy.

F. Hypersplenism

The term *hypersplenism* is noted for its imprecision. Classically the clinical state given this name is characterized by (1) reduction in the blood of red cells, platelets, granulocytes, or any combination thereof; (2) splenomegaly of any cause; (3) adequately cellular bone marrow (i.e., marrow is compensating adequately in response to cytopenia); and (4) correction of this picture by splenectomy. Since this picture is not always complete, a better definition might be a situation in which the spleen is better out than in. Much evidence suggests that the major cause of blood cytopenias is splenic hypersequestration of blood cells.

SELECTED REFERENCES

Aster, R. H. Pooling of platelets in the spleen: Role in the pathogenesis of "hypersplenic" thrombocytopenia. *J. Clin. Invest.* 45(1966): 645.

Chen, L-T. Microcirculation of the spleen: An open or closed circulation? *Science.* 201(1978): 157.

Coleman, C. N. Functional hyposplenia after splenic irradiation for Hodgkin's disease. *Ann. Int. Med.* 96(1982): 44.

Eichner, E. R. Splenic function: Normal, too much, and too little. *Am. J. Med.* 66(1979): 311.

Erickson, W. D., et al. The hazard of infection following splenectomy in children. *Am. J. Dis. Child.* 116(1976): 1.

Hosea, S. W., et al. Opsonic requirements for intravascular clearance after splenectomy. *New Eng. J. Med.* 304(1981): 245.

Jandl, J. H., et al. Proliferative response of the spleen and liver to hemolysis. *J. Exp. Med.* 122(1965): 299.

Pearson, H. J. The born-again spleen, return of splenic function after splenectomy for trauma. *New Eng. J. Med.* 298(1978): 1389.

Weiss, L. A scanning electron microscopic study of the spleen. *Blood.* 43(1974): 665.

Weiss, L., and Tavassoli, M. Anatomical hazards to the passage of erythrocytes through the spleen. *Semin. Hematol.* 7(1970): 372.

LECTURE 3 Normocytic Anemias

William S. Beck

I. INTRODUCTION

The differential diagnosis of anemia in a patient whose MCV and MCHC are within normal limits and whose reticulocyte count is not elevated requires consideration of the several normocytic-normochromic anemias. Most are associated with hypoproliferative bone marrow failure. The term *bone marrow failure* refers to failure of the marrow to deliver blood cells into the blood, that is, failure of effective hematopoiesis. A patient with marrow failure may have an empty (hypocellular) marrow or a full (normocellular to hypercellular) marrow. In the latter case, erythropoiesis is taking place, but it is ineffective. An experienced hematologist can usually predict whether the marrow of a patient with marrow failure is hypocellular or hypercellular. But he is sometimes surprised, and a bone marrow aspiration or biopsy is essential if a precise diagnosis is to be made.

This lecture summarizes the major anemias of bone marrow failure. Although diverse, they share certain features: (1) they are common; (2) they are among the least well understood of all hematologic disorders; and (3) often, but not always, they have a poor prognosis. Even though they are not always curable, therapy is often beneficial. The recent successful transplantation of bone marrow in certain cases has been an advance of importance and promise.

II. APLASTIC ANEMIA

Aplastic anemia is a disorder (or group of disorders) characterized by the diagnostic triad (1) cellular depletion and fatty replacement of bone marrow, (2) pancytopenia, and (3) delayed plasma iron clearance. The second and third elements of the triad are sequelae of the first. It is due to toxic or unknown factors that injure stem cells and impair their capacity to renew themselves. Some evidence suggests that in some cases the microenvironment necessary for stem cell proliferation may have become unsatisfactory.

A. Terminology

By the 1930s clinicians had found that liver extract and iron benefited many anemias, and they began to classify anemias as either *responsive* or *refractory* (or, alternatively, *regenerative* or *aregenerative*). The classification went no further because until the late 1930s, bone marrow was almost never examined ante mortem. It was customary in those days to apply the term *aplastic anemia* to all instances of refractory anemia with pancytopenia. Thus the term was applied to a functional rather than a morphologic state of the bone marrow.

In 1941, Bomford and Rhoads attempted to classify the refractory anemias on the basis of bone marrow architecture and cellularity observed post mortem. Interestingly some cases of refractory anemia were found to be associated with a full bone marrow that was normocellular or hypercellular; others were associated with an empty or hypocellular (or aplastic) marrow. Despite the diversity of associated marrow pictures, the imprecise terms *refractory anemia* and *aplastic anemia* have continued in vogue, as synonyms of each other and of pancytopenia. This usage has complicated the scientific literature. In the present discussion, the term *aplastic anemia* will be reserved for pancytopenia due to morphologic and functional *hypoplasia* of the marrow. It could be argued that *hypoplastic anemia* is a more appropriate term than *aplastic anemia* since the marrow is never totally aplastic (total aplasia would probably be incompatible with life) and since the pathologic process is often patchy, with island-like foci of normocellular or even hypercellular marrow present.

B. Etiologic classification

1. Drugs and chemicals

Many chemical agents are known to cause aplastic anemia. Many more are suspected to do so from circumstantial evidence, but proof is lacking. Agents capable of depressing bone marrow can be divided roughly into two groups (see table 3.1): (1) those that regularly produce marrow hypoplasia if the dose is sufficiently large and (2) those that occasionally (frequently or infrequently) produce hypoplasia.

a. Benzene

Benzene exposure is a well-known cause of marrow suppression, aplasia, and occasionally leukemia. It was the first clear-cut specific causal agent, having been identified in the rubber tire industry. Previously many industrial workers had been fatally exposed. Benzene has since been incriminated in many hematologic abnormalities, sometimes uncritically, and it remains a serious problem for industrial medicine. It has been claimed that pancytopenia may occur years after actual exposure to benzene. Many benzene-related chemicals (e.g., toluene, trinitrotoluene, DDT) are also suspected of causing aplastic anemia.

b. Chloramphenicol

Today the agents causing aplastic anemia are more commonly pharmacologic then industrial. Chloramphenicol is a widely used antibiotic that is the best studied of the agents causing aplastic anemia. The drug is a nitrobenzene derivative that commonly causes a brief, reversible suppression of the bone marrow in many (perhaps all) exposed patients. Patients with this dose-related disorder exhibit anemia and sometimes thrombocytopenia, decrease in reticulocytes, increase in serum iron, and vacuolization of bone

Table 3.1
Agents Associated with Aplastic Anemia

Those regularly producing marrow hypoplasia if dose is sufficient		
Ionizing radiation		
Benzene and derivatives (toluene, etc.)		
Cytostatic agents (6-mercaptopurine, busulfan, melphalan, vincristine, etc.)		
Other poisons (inorganic arsenic)		
Those occasionally associated with marrow hypoplasia		
Class	Relatively frequent	Infrequent
Antimicrobial	Chloramphenicol Organic arsenicals Penicillin, tetracyclines	Streptomycin Amphotericin B Sulfonamides Sulfisoxazole (Gantrisin®)
Anticonvulsant	Methylphenylethylhydantoin (Mesantoin®) Trimethadione (Tridione®)	Methylphenylhydantoin Diphenylhydantoin (Dilantin®) Primidone
Analgesic	Phenylbutazone	Aspirin
Antithyroid		Carbimazole Tapazole $KClO_4$
Hypoglycemic		Tolbutamide (Orinase®) Chlorpropamide (Diabinese®)
Antianxiety		Chlorpromazine (Thorazine®) Chlordiazepoxide (Librium®)
Insecticide		DDT Parathion
Miscellaneous		Colchicine Acetazolamide (Diamox®) Hair dyes CCl_4, Bi, SCN

marrow cells. Rarely (in 1 of every 15,000 treated subjects) chloramphenicol causes prolonged, self-sustaining, often fatal marrow aplasia. This disorder seems dose independent. Many of its victims have had previous exposure to the drug. There is now evidence that reversible marrow suppression is due to the ability of chloramphenicol to inhibit mitochondrial protein synthesis. This irreversible suppression, like certain other forms of aplastic anemia, is a defect of the stem cells that renders them incapable of dividing and differentiating (see below). Study of this serious medical problem has been limited by the lack of an animal model.

c. Other agents

Many agents (see table 3.1) are suspected of causing aplastic anemia because patients with the disease have been previously exposed to them. Some of these are common household chemicals. In most cases, it is possible to do no more than guess at their importance, especially in cases of commonly used drugs such as aspirin. Despite the pitfalls inherent in any effort to incriminate a specific agent, a serious search should always be attempted. The history should cover the patient's work, hobbies, cosmetics, and daily activities, as well as medications.

2. Radiation

High radiant energies (x-rays, γ-rays, and neutrons), from laboratory or reactor accidents or from deliberate therapeutic exposure affect all tissues in which cell turnover is rapid. These include the germinal epithelium of the gonads, the bone marrow hematopoietic cells, and the intestinal epithelium. Intensive radiation kills cells in each of these tissues, and death of the patient may follow acute marrow aplasia or intestinal ulceration. If the patient survives a critical 3–6 week period, surviving stem cells slowly produce marrow regeneration. If stem cells are damaged, regeneration may be incomplete, and permanent marrow hypoplasia with pancytopenia results. Injury to the microvasculature of marrow may be the fundamental defect in this situation. This injury is believed to alter the stromal microenvironment and thereby interfere with marrow regeneration.

3. Infection and immunologic rejection

Aplastic anemia is a complication of several infections, especially viral hepatitis and miliary tuberculosis. This suggests that an immunologic mechanism may be responsible for marrow aplasia in these cases. This is supported by occasional cases of aplastic anemia following transfusion of whole blood or bone marrow into immunologically deficient children with graft-versus-host rejection of stem cells. In such cases treatment with immunosuppressive drugs might be justified. Alternatively viruses may directly attach or suppress stem cells. Such a mechanism was observed in marrow culture systems in recent cases in which a parvovirus was implicated as the causal agent of aplastic anemia.

4. Constitutional factors

The term *constitutional aplastic anemia* is applied to a poorly understood group of congenital disorders or syndromes. *Fanconi's anemia* is a familial marrow hypoplasia that appears in the first decade of life and is accompanied by multiple congenital abnormalities in other tissues—bone, kidney, spleen, and skin. There is a high incidence of later leukemia and other neoplasms.

5. Idiopathic

In about half of the patients with aplastic anemia, an etiologic agent cannot be implicated. These are termed *idiopathic,* though it is likely that many are due to exposure to occult pollutants that have not yet been identified.

6. Paroxysmal nocturnal hemoglobinuria (PNH)

PNH is a rare disease in which red cell membranes and perhaps membranes of other formed elements are abnormal, with resulting hemolytic anemia and other phenomena. It frequently develops as a complication of marrow aplasia and, like other aplastic disorders, may terminate in acute leukemia. Conversely aplastic anemia can develop in the course of PNH. PNH will be discussed in lectures 13 and 21.

C. Pathophysiologic mechanisms

1. Defects of stem cells, suppressor T cells, and HIM

Although the pathogenesis of bone marrow failure in aplastic anemia is not known, there seems little doubt that it is a result of defective function in a compartment of pluripotent stem cells. Provocative supporting data have come from the marrow culture techniques described in lecture 1. These studies show (1) low CFU-GM counts in some aplastic marrows; (2) suppression of CFU-GM of normal marrow when co-cultured with the aplastic marrow; (3) lack of such suppression by other aplastic marrows; and (4) normal CFU-GM counts in a few cases. In a recent culture study of 21 patients with aplastic anemia, 12 displayed no obvious cause for the low CFU-GM numbers (these may have had defective HIMs); 3 had suppressor T cells that inhibited CFU-GMs; 3 had inhibiting serum antibodies against marrow CFU-GMs; and 3 had defects of CSF (2 had CSF inhibitors and 1 had low CSF levels). Thus there is a diversity of pathogenetic mechanisms. Presumably therapy with antithymocyte globulin is more likely to be successful when suppressor T cells are operating. Bone marrow transplant should be more effective when CFU-GMs are present with a defective HIM. These results clearly imply that aplastic anemia is several diseases with common clinical features.

2. Defects of DNA or DNA repair

Abnormal DNA (multiple strand breaks) has been observed in lymphocytes of patients with aplastic anemia. This pattern, which may be due to defective DNA repair enzymes, may be responsible for observed maturation defects (e.g., some macrocytic red cells, increased levels of fetal hemoglobin).

3. Increased erythropoietin levels

The high erythropoietin levels that result from aplastic anemia may accelerate the maturation and release of marrow elements. This may account for occasional macrocytosis in aplastic anemia.

D. Clinical features

The onset is often insidious but it may be acute. Clinical manifestations include the sequelae of pancytopenia: (1) signs of anemia (see lecture 1); (2) thrombocytopenic bleeding (especially when infection is present), though purpura is often not severe; and (3) susceptibility to infection as a result of neutropenia. (More will be said of neutropenia in lecture 19.) The reticulocyte count is low, and reticulocytes may appear immature. Hemolysis is not prominent, but as in many other normocytic-normochromic anemias, red cells are somewhat short-lived. Often there is moderate anisocytosis and poikilocytosis. In some patients, especially children, red cells may contain increased levels of fetal hemoglobin. The marrow is hypocellular. A biopsy is needed in addition to an aspiration. The marrow consists of strands of reticulum with small clusters of lymphocytes, reticulum cells, and plasma cells in large areas of acellular stroma and fat.

Serum iron is always elevated, often to the point of 100% saturation of transferrin. (The characteristic "ferrokinetics" of aplastic anemia will be described in lecture 6.) In aplastic anemia iron disappears from the plasma slowly, does not reappear in the red cells, and does not localize in the marrow but is taken up instead by the parenchymal cells of the liver. Splenomegaly is usually not present. When it is present, one should seek a specific cause such as leukemia, lymphoma, miliary tuberculosis, lupus erythematosis, or metastatic carcinoma.

E. Therapy

The therapeutic mainstays of aplastic anemia are (1) avoidance of suspected offending chemical agents; (2) careful hygiene (e.g., use of soft toothbrush, avoidance of needles, etc., to minimize minor bleeding); and (3) transfusion with red cells.

1. Transfusion

The purpose of transfusion is to buy time until a remission occurs. Unfortunately this happens rarely in adults. Transfusions should be kept to a minimum in order to avoid hepatitis, hemosiderosis, and isoimmunization. Chronic anemia is well tolerated, and it is rarely necessary to raise hemoglobin above 8–9 g/100 ml. In severel aplastic anemia, this goal can be met with about 2 units of blood every 2 weeks. Careful cross-matching is necessary to avoid immunization with minor blood groups. Washed or frozen red cells are used to avoid immunization to transfused white cells and platelets. Total body iron is about 3,500 mg, and the body has no way of eliminating excess iron. Since 1 unit of blood contains about 250 mg of iron, 15 transfusions more than double body iron.

Transfused platelets are used when necessary, but they inevitably lead to isoimmunization. They are best reserved for life-threatening thrombocytopenic bleeding (see lectures 16 and 27). Leukocyte transfusions have not yet proved reliable. All transfusions should be avoided when bone marrow transplantation is contemplated.

2. Corticosteroids

Corticosteroids are used primarily for their "capillary-tightening" effect in minimizing capillary bleeding. They do not stimulate hematopoiesis. The rise in white count is more likely due to the effect of steroids in blocking egress of white cells from blood to tissues (see lecture 19).

3. Marrow stimulants

Since the work of Shahidi and Diamond in 1959, androgens in high doses have been widely used in aplastic anemia. Somehow androgens stimulate erythropoiesis and sometimes leukopoiesis and thrombopoiesis. The erythropoietic effect of androgen is mediated in other disorders at least in part by an increase in erythropoietin activity. This cannot be the mechanism in aplastic anemia because erythropoietin levels are already high. When favorable results are obtained with testosterone, they may appear only after several months. Prolongation of therapy (up to 20 months) improves results. Good remissions are obtained in a number of cases. Some responses have been short-lived. Another androgen, oxymetholone, is more effective when given in large doses. Striking remissions are obtained in occasional testosterone-resistant cases. $CoCl_2$ and phytohemagglutinin have been tried as marrow stimulants with unimpressive results.

4. Antithymocyte globulin (ATG)

In an increasing number of cases, ATG (derived from horses immunized against thymocytes) has produced excellent and prolonged remission. As noted above, ATG therapy fails in many cases. It inevitably causes serum sickness.

5. Bone marrow transplantation

Marrow transplantation would be ideal therapy if it could be done successfully. In fact, *syngeneic transplantation* (i.e., donor and recipient are identical twins) has been attempted in a number of cases. Some of these transplants led to prompt engraftment; others took many months or required chronic immunosuppression and marrow reinfusion. The successes, incidentally, support the view that aplastic anemia is a disorder of bone marrow stem cells. It also appears that the insult producing that failure is transient.

Allogeneic transplantation of marrow (i.e., donor and recipient genetically dissimilar but matched in major histocompatibility antigens, or HLAs) has presented great difficulties and has led to rejection in 30–40% of cases. Before the recognition in the mid-1960s of the importance of the HLAs and the mixed lymphocyte culture (MLC) technique for compatibility assay, allogeneic transplant invariably failed. Supportive therapies available at that time for maintaining life while engraftment was taking place were grossly inadequate. It was regularly found that when bone marrow cells from a nonidentical donor were infused into a recipient, problems arose not only from graft rejection but also from the reaction of immunocompetent cells in the marrow grafts against recipient's tissues (i.e., "graft-versus-host disease," or GVHD), manifested by skin rash, diarrhea, increased susceptibility to infection, and, ultimately, destruction of engrafted marrow. Even when HLAs matched, half the patients developed GVHD of varying severity. This indicates the probable existence of other histocompatibility loci of importance in tissue tolerance. A higher rate of success has recently been achieved by employing vigorous methods of abolishing the patient's immune response in order to prevent graft rejection, and continuing immunosuppression after the transplant to modify or prevent GVHD. Methods used included total body irradiation, high doses of immunosuppressive drugs such as cyclophosphamide, and and antilymphocyte serum. In addition, massive supportive therapy (including a sterile environment) are employed. By such methods, as well as by careful matching of the donor recipient, recent results have been much more encouraging, although the proportion of patients responding varies from series to series. So far, all reported series have been retrospective. Nonetheless, substantial problems remain, and clinics undertaking such therapy for aplastic anemia are likely to have many failures until research sharpens skills and deepens knowledge.

6. Splenectomy

Splenectomy is indicated if active hemolysis is present (i.e., if the transfusion requirement is increasing and red cell sequestration in the spleen can be shown by scanning methods). Some have held that splenectomy has an ill-defined beneficial effect in aplastic anemia even in the absence of hemolysis. The claim is controversial. Splenectomy does lead to better responses to platelet transfusions, especially after the appearance of platelet isoantibodies.

F. Prognosis

Useful statistics are difficult to obtain. Many large series have been reported but with frequent changes in supportive therapy, some involving methods of red cell or platelet transfusion, it is difficult to apply published survival data to cases at hand. About a quarter of the patients with idiopathic aplastic anemia survive 5 years. These may be the less severely affected patients. Severe anemia is a bad prognostic sign. Most patients die of infection and hemorrhage. A few develop acute leukemia.

III. PURE RED CELL APLASIA

A. Terminology

Pure red cell aplasia (PRCA) is an uncommon disorder characterized by isolated loss of erythroid precursors in the bone marrow. Synonyms include ''erythroblastic hypoplasia,'' ''erythroblastopenia,'' ''erythroid hypoplasia,'' and ''Diamond-Blackfan syndrome.'' PRCA was recognized as an entity distinguishable from aplastic anemia in 1922. It has received increasing attention because of the interesting implications of specific erythropoietic failure and of its possible relation to autoimmunity and thymic tumors. However, it is observed in both association with and the absence of other diseases. The disorder may be acute or chronic. Both groups include hereditary and acquired cases.

B. Acute type

A self-limited form of erythroid aplasia occurs in both hematologically normal and abnormal individuals. Typically pallor develops rapidly in a patient with preexisting hemolytic anemia (e.g., hereditary spherocytosis, drug-induced hemolytic anemia). The episode is usually introduced by a mild febrile illness.

Laboratory examination reveals a sometimes severe anemia,

low reticulocyte count, normal or low serum bilirubin, and normal white count and platelet count. The bone marrow early shows depletion of all erythroid elements. During the early stage of spontaneous recovery, bone marrow displays many early erythroid cells. A brisk reticulocytosis ensues. The recovery phase may be associated with bone pain resulting from bone marrow expansion. In patients who were previously splenectomized for hemolytic anemia, the recovery phase may be associated with an outpouring of nucleated red cells. This ''erythroblastic crisis'' may reflect the lack of an essential extramedullary site for final maturation of immature erythroid cells.

The cause of such acute crises of red cell production is unknown. They have been related to virus infections such as infectious mononucleosis, primary atypical pneumonia, and influenza. They have also been related to certain drugs, especially diphenylhydantoin (Dilantin®) and chloramphenicol (Chloromycetin®). Pathophysiologic mechanisms are not known.

C. Chronic type

1. Constitutional

In this rare disorder, chronic isolated erythroid hypoplasia occurs early in childhood. Presumably, it is congenital or hereditary. Etiology and pathogenesis are not known. Anemia is first observed at age 2 weeks to 2 years. Later signs, including congestive heart failure, hepatomegaly, and splenomegaly, are reversed by transfusion. Subsequently liver damage may be induced by transfusion hemosiderosis, serum hepatitis, and cardiac cirrhosis. Irreversible hepatomegaly and splenomegaly may come to dominate the clinical picture. Normochromic-normocytic anemia with absolute reticulocytopenia is the rule. White count and platelet count are normal or slightly decreased. Secondary hypersplenism may cause pancytopenia, but examination of the bone marrow distinguishes that condition from the pancytopenia of marrow aplasia. The marrow is cellular. There is erythroid hypoplasia and a low E/M ratio. Remaining erythroid cells are immature. Myeloid cells and megakaryocytes appear normal.

Transfusions and corticosteroid therapy have been useful in the management of many patients. Some develop prolonged remissions, but many later need further therapy. Many deaths are due to complications of therapy.

2. Acquired

PRCA arising for the first time in an adult is assumed to be acquired, though this conclusion may be questionable. It is an uncommon and fascinating disease of adults over 50, characterized by isolated erythroid hypoplasia and an association in half the cases with thymic tumors. Females predominate over males (2:1) in the group with pure red cell aplasia and thymoma; males dominate in the group without thymoma. Association with thymoma (usually a noninvasive spindle cell thymoma) suggests that an immunologic mechanism is involved in the etiology or pathogenesis. Thymic hyperplasia or thymoma is found in association with seemingly unrelated "immunologic" diseases such as myasthenia gravis, hypogammaglobulinemia, and rheumatoid arthritis. The possibility that red cell aplasia is caused by immunologic rejection of erythroid tissue is supported by striking erythropoietic responses to therapy with corticosteroids and immunosuppressive agents and by direct demonstration of autoantibodies against mature red cells (i.e., immunohemolytic anemia), immature erythropoietic cells, and unrelated tissue components. Krantz and coworkers have demonstrated an IgG antibody in the serum of patients with PRCA and with and without a thymoma against bone marrow erythrocyte precursors. A patient of the author's has an IgG antibody that prevents BFU-E formation by circulating stem cells. Her own rate of BFU-E formation is restored to normal in vitro when her serum is replaced by normal serum.

When a thymic tumor is present, thymectomy is useful in preventing possible malignant extension and promoting reactivation of the bone marrow, though it is sometimes difficult to judge its benefits. Remissions occur in 25%, both with and without thymomas, but half of these are sustained without further therapy. It is sometimes difficult to decide how intensively one should look for an occult thymoma in a patient with PRCA. Exploratory thoracotomy is usually not undertaken unless x-ray or CT-scan evidence is found of a thymic tumor.

The role of a thymoma in PRCA is unclear. Some evidence suggests that the tumor secretes the antierythroblast antibody, disappearance of the antibody having been demonstrated after thymectomy in one case. However, thymoma may be only one manifestation of a generalized immune deficiency syndrome.

IV. ANEMIA OF CHRONIC RENAL FAILURE

A. Introduction

Chronic renal failure, whatever its cause, is invariably associated with anemia, the extent of which is roughly proportional to the severity of the uremia, but exceptions are observed. The anemia of renal failure is attributable to several diverse mechanisms that affect red cell production and destruction.

B. Pathophysiologic mechanisms

1. Hydremia

The hematocrit or hemoglobin concentration reflects both red cell mass and plasma volume. The latter varies widely in renal failure.

Therefore, the extent of dehydration or hydremia should be known before hematocrit and hemoglobin can be interpreted.

2. Hemolysis

Red cell life span in patients with chronic renal failure is shortened. The defect is extracorpuscular since patients' red cells survive normally when injected into healthy recipients and normal red cells have a shortened life span in uremic recipients (see lecture 11). The relation between blood urea nitrogen and red cell life span appears linear. Normalization of red cell life span often follow intensive dialysis. Changes in red cell membrane ATPase and glutathione stability have been described in red cells suspended in uremic plasma, and the burring of red cells in uremia has been shown to be caused by a nondialyzable, heat-labile plasma factor. These may contribute to metabolic impairment and hemolysis. Another factor is mechanical disruption of metabolically fragile red cells by an abnormal microvasculature.

3. Ineffective erythropoiesis

Iron turnover is normal, but iron utilization is often subnormal. The interpretation of decreased iron utilization is difficult, since it can reflect both erythroid hypoplasia and ineffective red cell production. Since bone marrow examination does not reveal erythroid hypoplasia, the decrease in iron utilization in chronic renal failure is attributed to ineffective erythropoiesis. Intensive dialysis improved iron utilization. Thus, uremia decreases the viability both of mature red cells and their progenitors.

4. Deficiency states

Iron may be limiting because of blood loss from the gastrointestinal or female generative tract or in the hemodialysis coil. Renal inflammatory lesions may lead to low serum iron because of defective reutilization of iron (see lecture 6). In a rare patient with nephrosis, the urinary loss of transferrin may lower iron-binding capacity and impair the metabolic cycling of iron. Folic acid deficiency should be suspected and prevented in patients undergoing intensive dialysis since folic acid is dialyzable.

5. Bleeding

Purpura and gastrointestinal and gynecologic bleeding occur in a third or half of all uremic patients. Such loss of blood contributes to the development of anemia. The mechanism of the bleeding tendency is poorly understood. Thrombocytopenia, when present, is rarely of a magnitude to explain spontaneous blood loss. However, platelet function, as evaluated from bleeding time, platelet adhesiveness, and other platelet function tests, is commonly abnormal (see lecture 27). Since these patients are often closely monitored, iatrogenic blood loss may also be significant.

6. Responsiveness to erythropoietin

Nephrectomized uremic animals ordinarily can respond to the administration of erythropoietin with increased erythroid activity. However, in a few uremic human subjects (and animals) treated with erythropoietin, the response is subnormal and inversely proportional to the degree of uremia.

7. Failure of erythropoietin production

The role of the kidney in the synthesis or release of erythropoietin was discussed in lecture 1. The site of its production in the kidney remains unclear. Several authors studying decreased granularity of the juxtaglomerular apparatus in hypoxia conclude that it reflects erythropoietin release. In chronic renal disease, the degree of impairment in erythropoietin release and the extent of bone marrow compensation vary widely. In some cases the rate of red cell production is well maintained, possibly because of inappropriate secretion of erythropoietin in the injured kidney or extrarenal erythropoietin secretion. In severe cases, erythropoietin production ceases almost completely. Intensive dialysis does not restore production.

C. Clinical features

Manifestations of renal failure depend on the underlying disorder. However, pallor and anemia are universally present. The anemia is normocytic-normochromic, and usually slightly reticulocytopenic. A few red cells are deformed, some with multiple tiny spicules and others with gross shape changes and loss of volume. These cells have been called, respectively, *schistocytes* (or *burr cells*) and *helmet cells* (or *triangular cells*). The total and differential leukocyte count and platelet count are usually normal, but the underlying disorder may modify the picture. The bone marrow may appear somewhat hypoplastic, but characteristically it is nearly normal in appearance. The normality is spurious because, in the context of a reduced hemoglobin concentration, a normal bone marrow should display a compensatory increase in erythroid activity.

D. Therapy

Anemia is often mild to moderate, and no therapy is necessary. Ideal therapy would be dialysis and erythropoietin administration. The former is now in use; the latter is still experimental. Androgens have been useful in some cases. Transfusion is employed judiciously and with restraint.

V. ANEMIA OF ENDOCRINE DISEASE

Many hormones (in addition to erythropoietin) participate in the regulation of erythropoiesis, and patients lacking such hormones often develop hypoplastic anemia. Since erythropoietin production is controlled by tissue oxygen tension, it is indirectly influenced by hormones that affect oxygen equilibrium. Hormones that affect enzymes and protein synthesis also affect synthesis of hemoglobin and production of red cells. The hormones most often involved in the development of hypoplastic anemia are those of the pituitary, thyroid, adrenal cortex, and gonads.

A. Anemia of pituitary deficiency

Hypophysectomy in an experimental animal leads to the development of a moderate hypoplastic anemia owing to loss of adenohypophyseal hormones. Of these, the thyroid-stimulating hormone seems most important since the anemia of hypophysectomy resembles the anemia of thyroidectomy. Growth hormone is said to be capable of stimulating red cell production in animals, but the physiologic role of this effect is not clear. In human subjects, pituitary dysfunction or pituitary ablation leads to normochromic-normocytic anemia. Red cell life span is normal, but bone marrow examination and ferrokinetic studies disclose relative bone marrow failure and moderate hypoplastic anemia. Relacement therapy with combination of thyroid, adrenal, and gonadal hormones usually reverse the anemia.

B. Anemia of thyroid disease

1. Hypothyroidism

The mechanism of anemia observed in patients with myxedema or other hypothyroid disorders is not always clear-cut since the conditions may be complicated by nutritional deficiencies. However, many hypothyroid patients have hypoplastic anemia that is unresponsive to therapy with iron, vitamin B_{12}, or folic acid and that is similar to the normochromic-normocytic, reticulocytopenic anemia of thyroidectomized animals. In this disorder, red cell life span is normal, and ferrokinetics indicates hypoactive but effective marrow function. The anemia in hypothyroid subjects is mild to moderate with a hemoglobin concentration rarely less than 8–9g/100 ml. The decrease in erythroid bone marrow activity is often too small to be morphologically demonstrable. The hematocrit may not accurately reflect the reduction of bone marrow activity and red cell mass since plasma volume is decreased in hypothyroidism. This may result in temporary aggravation of "anemia" after thyroid replacement therapy since plasma volume is restored to normal before red cell mass. Although the characteristic anemia of hypothyroidism is normochromic-normocytic, the anemia observed may be microcytic-hypochromic due to iron deficiency resulting from (1) menorrhagia, a frequent complication; (2) achlorhydria, present in half the anemic patients; or (3) intestinal malabsorption of iron.

The anemia may also be macrocytic. Occasionally hypothyroidism coexists with true pernicious anemia (see lecture 4). More often, the coexisting megaloblastic anemia is due to poor dietary intake of folic acid or intestinal malabsorption.

2. Hyperthyroidism

Despite the erythropoietic effect of thyroid hormones in experimental animals, patients with hyperthyroidism or thyrotoxicosis rarely have elevated hemoglobin concentration. However, since the erythroid activity of the marrow and the turnover of plasma and red cell iron are above normal, an increase in plasma volume may keep the hematocrit within normal limits. Red cell life span is moderately shortened in patients with thyrotoxicosis. In a few severe cases, iron utilization is subnormal.

C. Anemia of adrenal disease

Adrenalectomy in animals causes a mild anemia responsive to therapy with corticosteroids or erythropoietin. A similar normochromic-normocytic anemia occurs in Addison's disease, but because of the concomitant reduction in plasma volume, the hemoglobin and hematocrit do not reflect the true red cell mass. The basis of this anemia and the erythropoietic effect of ACTH and cortical hormones (in physiologic amounts) is not known.

D. Anemia of gonadal disease

The erythropoietic effect of androgen is well known and extensively utilized in the treatment of patients with various types of refractory anemia. Castration of the male animal causes a decrease in the rate of red cell production until hemoglobin concentration and red cell mass become stabilized at levels approximating those of the normal female. In pharmacologic doses, androgens are potent stimulators of red cell production. They act by enhancing either the production of erythropoietin or its effect on the bone marrow.

VI. MYELOPHTHISIS

A. Definition

The term *myelophthisis* denotes a situation in which bone marrow has been replaced by nonmarrow elements. Common invaders of the bone marrow cavity are leukemic cells, tumor cells, infectious granulomas, fibrous tissue, and lipid storage cells. It is commonly said that the resulting anemia is due to simple mechanical replacement of bone marrow. However, the pathophysiology is probably more complex. For example, the anemia may be due in part to local competition betrween invading cells and hematopoietic cells for essential nutrients. There is also evidence that metastatic tumor lesions or granulomas may secrete substances that are inhibitory to surrounding marrow cells. It is of interest in this regard to note that some of the same peripheral blood alterations found in patients with metastases to the bone marrow are also observed in patients who have metastatic cancer without marrow involvement.

B. Clinical features

Typical clinical features of myelophthisis include (1) normocytic-normochromic anemia with reticulocytopenia; (2) *leukoerythroblastic reaction*, in which the white blood cell count is elevated and many immature white cells and nucleated red cells are in the blood (to be discussed in lecture 19); (3) marked anisocytosis and poikilocytosis of the red cells with teardrop forms; and (4) a low, normal, or high platelet count, often in association with bizarre or giant platelets. The diagnosis rests on histologic demonstration of the invading cells in a bone marrow biopsy.

SELECTED REFERENCES

Abdou, N. I., et al. Heterogeneity of pathogenetic mechanisms in aplastic anemia: Efficacy of therapy based on in vitro results. *Ann. Int. Med.* 95(1983): 43.

Ajlouni, K., and Doeblin, T. D. The syndrome of hepatitis and aplastic anemia. *Brit. J. Haematol.* 27(1974): 345.

Buckner, C. D., et al. Human marrow transplantation—current status. *Prog. Hematol.* 8(1973): 299.

Cronkite, E. P. Radiation-induced aplastic anemia. *Semin. Hematol.* 4(1967): 273.

Erslev, A. J. Hematopoietic stem cell disorders—aplastic (Section 3). In Williams, W. J., et al., eds., *Hematology*, 3d ed., New York: McGraw-Hill, 1983, pp. 151–170.

Hirst, E., and Robertson, T. I. The syndrome of thymoma and erythroblastopenic anemia: A review of 56 cases including 3 case reports. *Medicine* 4(1967): 225.

Kagen, W. A., et al. Studies on the pathogenesis of aplastic anemia. *Am. J. Med.* 66(1979): 444.

Scott, J. J., et al. Acquired aplastic anemia. *Medicine* 37(1959): 119.

Sieff, C. Pure red cell aplasia. *Brit. J. Haematol.* 54(1983): 331.

Storb, R., et al. One-hundred-ten patients with aplastic anemia treated by marrow transplantation in Seattle. *Transplant Proc.* 10(1978): 135.

Thomas, E. D., et al. Bone marrow transplantation. *New Eng. J. Med.* 292(1975): 832, 895.

Yunis, A. A., and Bloomberg, G. R. Chloramphenicol toxicity: Clinical features and pathogenesis. *Prog. Hematol.* 4(1964): 138.

LECTURE 4 Megaloblastic Anemias I. Vitamin B_{12} Deficiency

William S. Beck

I. INTRODUCTION

Lecture 1 pointed out that the major categories of anemia due to bone marrow failure include (1) microcytic-hypochromic anemias (discussed in lecture 6); (2) normocytic-normochromic anemias (lecture 3), and (3) megaloblastic anemias. This lecture considers the megaloblastic anemias.

Macrocytic anemias (anemias in which the MCV exceeds 100) can be nonmegaloblastic or megaloblastic. The former group includes disorders (e.g., alcoholism, certain hemolytic anemias) in which red cell size is increased but marrow and blood do not display megaloblastic changes. Such changes are found in marrow and blood in the latter group. Megaloblastic anemias are divisible into (1) those due to vitamin B_{12} (cobalamin) deficiency; (2) those due to folate deficiency; and (3) those unresponsive to vitamin B_{12} or folic acid. Vitamin B_{12} and folate deficiency, in turn, have many specific causes. Pernicious anemia, for example, is but one cause of vitamin B_{12} deficiency. Care should be taken not to employ "megaloblastic anemia," "vitamin B_{12} deficiency," and "pernicious anemia" as interchangeable synonyms as many writers do.

In this lecture, we shall first discuss the features of megaloblastic anemias in terms applicable to all cases of such anemias. We shall then discuss vitamin B_{12} deficiency, first in general terms and then in terms of its specific causes. The same sequence will be followed for folate deficiency and its specific causes. This sequence has been followed because it parallels the physician's approach to the ordinary patient with anemia. The approach should consist in completing the following steps: (1) recognize the presence of anemia; (2) determine whether it is caused by bone marrow failure; (3) determine whether it is megaloblastic anemia; (4) elucidate the broad etiological category (i.e., vitamin B_{12} deficiency, folate deficiency, etc.), as outlined in table 4.1; (5) elucidate the specific etiological mechanism; and (6) treat the patient and observe the response to treatment.

II. MEGALOBLASTIC ANEMIA PER SE

A. Terminology

Megaloblastic anemia is a widely used though imprecise term for a group of disorders having in common a characteristic pattern of morphologic and functional abnormalities in blood and bone marrow. The pattern is due to impairment of DNA synthesis by any of several causes. The term is imprecise because (1) the condition

Table 4.1
Etiologic Classification of the Megaloblastic Anemias

Category	Etiologic mechanisms
Vitamin B_{12} deficiency	
A. Decreased intake	Poor diet, lack of animal products, strict vegetarianism
	Impaired absorption
	Pernicious anemia
	Gastrectomy (total and partial)
	Destruction of gastric mucosa by caustics
	Anti-IF antibody in gastric juice
	Abnormal intrinsic factor molecule
	Intrinsic intestinal disease
	Familial selective malabsorption (Imerslund's syndrome)
	Illeal resection, ileitis
	Sprue, celiac disease
	Infiltrative intestinal disease (lymphoma, scleroderma, etc.)
	Drug-induced malabsorption
	Competitive parasites
	Fish tapeworm infestations (*Diphyllobothrium latum*)
	Bacteria in diverticula of bowel, blind loops
	Chronic pancreatic disease
B. Increased requirement	Pregnancy
	Neoplastic disease
	Hyperthyroidism
C. Impaired utilization	Enzyme deficiencies
	Abnormal serum vitamin B_{12} binding protein
	Lack of TC II
	Nitrous oxide administration
Folate deficiency	
A. Decreased intake	Poor diet, lack of vegetables
	Alcoholism
	Infancy
	Hemodialysis
	Impaired absorption
	Intestinal short circuits
	Steatorrhea
	Sprue, celiac disease
	Intrinsic intestinal disease
	Anticonvulsants, oral contraceptives, other drugs
B. Increased requirement	Pregnancy; infancy
	Hyperthyroidism
	Hyperactive hematopoiesis
	Neoplastic disease; exfoliative skin disease
C. Impaired utilization	Folic acid antagonists: MTX, Triamterene, Trimethoprim
	Enzyme deficiencies
Unresponsive to vitamin B_{12} or folate therapy	Metabolic inhibitors
	Purine synthesis: 6-mercaptopurine, 6-thioguanine, azathioprine
	Pyrimidine synthesis: 6-azauridine
	Thymidylate synthesis: 5-fluorouracil

Table 4.1

Category	Etiologic mechanisms
	Deoxyribonucleotide synthesis: hydroxyurea, cytosine arabinoside, severe iron deficiency
	Inborn errors
	Lesch-Nyhan syndrome
	Hereditary orotic aciduria
	Deficiency of formininotransferase, methyltransferase, etc.
	Unexplained disorders
	Pyridoxine-responsive megaloblastic anemia
	Thiamine-responsive megaloblastic anemia
	Erythremic myelosis (Di Guglielmo's syndrome)

may be unassociated with anemia and (2) through usage the adjective *megaloblastic* and the noun *megaloblast* have acquired different connotations. ''Megaloblastic'' denotes an abnormal morphologic pattern in *any* of the cell lines in bone marrow. Its normal antithesis is ''normoblastic.'' Thus, one speaks of megaloblastic erythropoiesis, granulopoiesis, or thrombopoiesis. In contrast, ''megaloblast'' through usage refes only to cells of the erythroid series. In 1880 Ehrlich gave the name *megaloblast* to the abnormal erythroid precursors found in pernicious anemia. He thought these cells belonged to a cell series separate and distinct from that of normal erythroid precursors, which were termed *normoblasts*. Now we regard megaloblasts as functionally and morphologically abnormal normoblasts. The abnormality of an individual cell is usually irreversible, but the overall megaloblastic character of the blood and bone marrow is rapidly reversible in most cases.

In this lecture, ''megaloblasts'' denotes any maturation stage of the megaloblastic erythroid series (the series is promegaloblast → basophilic megaloblast → polychromatophilic megaloblast → orthochromatic megaloblast → adult macrocyte). Specific maturation stages are referred to by their full names. The term *megaloblastic* refers to morphologic and functional patterns in erythrocyte, granulocyte, and platelet precursors. Indeed, the term *megaloblastic* may be usefully applied to similarly affected cells of the buccal and vaginal mucosa and other tissues. The process wherein normoblastic cells become megaloblastic is termed *megaloblastic transformation*.

B. Megaloblastic transformation

1. Morphology

The following descriptions deal with the morphology of individual megaloblastic cells in Wright's stained smears of bone arrow aspirates (figure 4.1A)

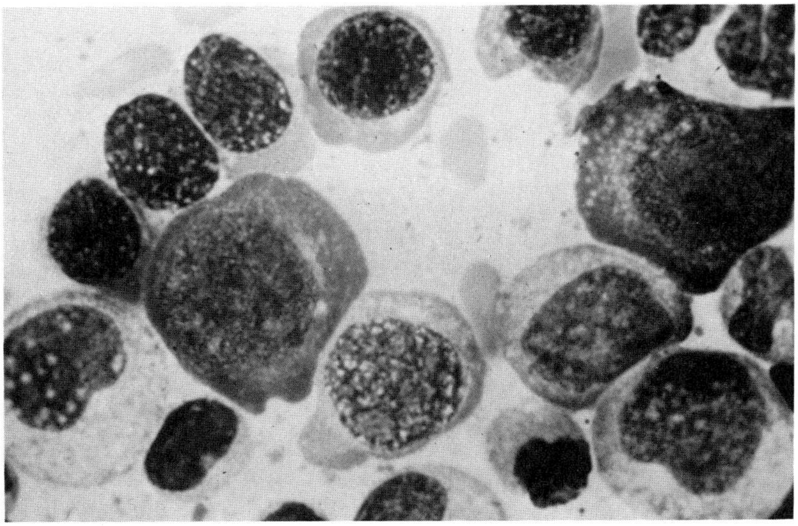

A

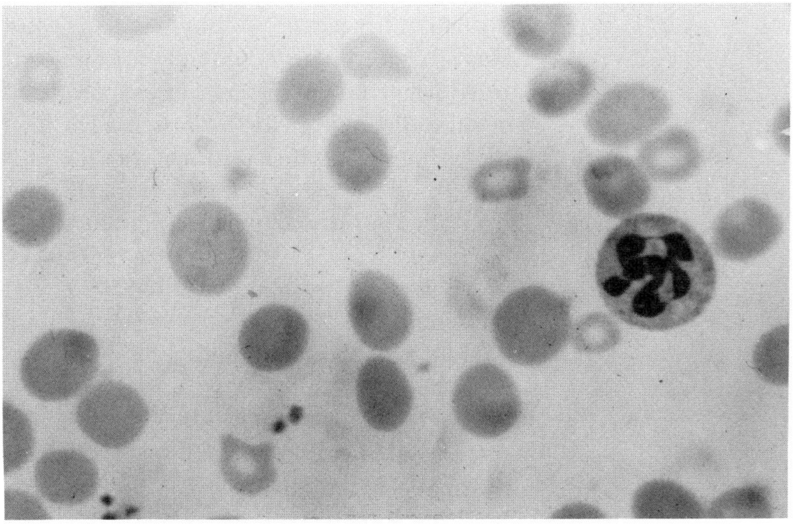

B

Fig. 4.1
Appearance of megaloblastic bone marrow (*A*) and blood (*B*).

a. Megaloblastic red cell precursors

Megaloblastic erythroid cells at all stages of development are larger than corresponding cells of the normoblastic series and often have a higher than normal ratio of cytoplasmic area to nuclear area. Promegaloblasts, the most immature of the series and the most easily recognized, display a brilliantly colored, deeply basophilic, granule-free cytoplasm and a lavender-tinted chromatin with a characteristic open and fine-grained, or particulate, texture that contrasts with the ground-glass texture of the fibrous or strandlike pronormoblast chromatin. Large blue nucleoli and a prominent perinuclear halo may be present.

As the cell matures, the chromatin retains its granular texture and is slow to form coarse, deeply basophilic clumps. Development of a dense pyknotic nucleus like that of an orthochromatic normoblast either fails to occur or is delayed. With the appearance of hemoglobin, the apparent maturity of the cytoplasm contrasts with the apparent immaturity of the nucleus—a feature termed *nuclear-cytoplasmic asynchronism* or *dissociation*. In mild or incipient megaloblastic anemias, or in megaloblastic anemias associated with iron deficiency and other conditions, the bone marrow may contain partially developed or intermediate megaloblasts.

b. Megaloblastic white cell precursors

Such cells also display nuclear-cytoplasmic asynchronism and apparent enlargement, the most striking enlargement occurring at the metamyelocyte stage. A *giant metamyelocyte* has a relatively large nucleus, sometimes bizarre in shape, with a characteristic ragged or uneven chromatin pattern. The nucleus takes stain poorly and may be pinched off in several places, in apparent anticipation of the hypersegmentation of the mature neutrophil. The cytoplasm appears more immature (i.e., more basophilic and freer of granules) than that of a normal metamyelocyte. Comparable changes may be found in myelocytes and in band forms. The characteristic hypersegmented neutrophil of the peripheral blood will be described below.

c. Megaloblastic megakaryocytes

These cells may also be abnormally large. Granulation of the cytoplasm may be deficient. The nucleus is sometimes bizarre, showing numerous distinct and unattached lobes that give the cell an exploded appearance. It should be noted that megakaryocytes are often not distinctly abnormal in appearance.

2. Mechanism

It has been established that (1) megaloblasts contain a substantially increased amount of RNA and a normal or slightly increased amount of DNA per cell, the former presumably accounting for the cytoplasmic basophilia; and (2) tritiated thymidine (^{3}H-dThd) is readily incorporated into the DNA of megaloblasts and, thus, DNA synthesis can occur. These results suggest that the megaloblasts is a cell in a state of "unbalanced growth" owing to impaired synthesis of one or more deoxyribonucleotides, the precursors of DNA. As in the unbalanced growth pattern observing other species, DNA replication and cell division are blocked while synthesis of cytoplasm (RNA and protein) proceeds normally; hence the RNA/DNA ratio rises.

a. Pathway of DNA synthesis

It had been anticipated that cells in which DNA synthesis is impaired by vitamin B_{12} deficiency (e.g., bone marrow cells) would be found to contain a cobalamin-dependent ribonucleotide reductase resembling that of lactobacilli inasmuch as the metabolic and growth behavior of vitamin B_{12}-deficient lactobacilli closely resembles that of vitamin B_{12} deficient marrow cells (elevated RNA/DNA ratios, unbalanced growth, etc.). However, the scheme of RNA and DNA synthesis in animal cells (figure 4.2), like that in *E. coli,* includes a cobalamin-independent reductase in which nonheme iron performs the hydrogen-transferring function performed by cobalamin in the lactobacillus system. As discussed below, the actual role of cobalamin in DNA synthesis is described by the "methylfolate trap theory" according to which vitamin B_{12} deficiency results in sequestration of tetrahydrofolate in the form of N^5-methyltetrahydrofolate, which cannot be utilized in the critical thymidylate synthetase reaction (see figure 4.7).

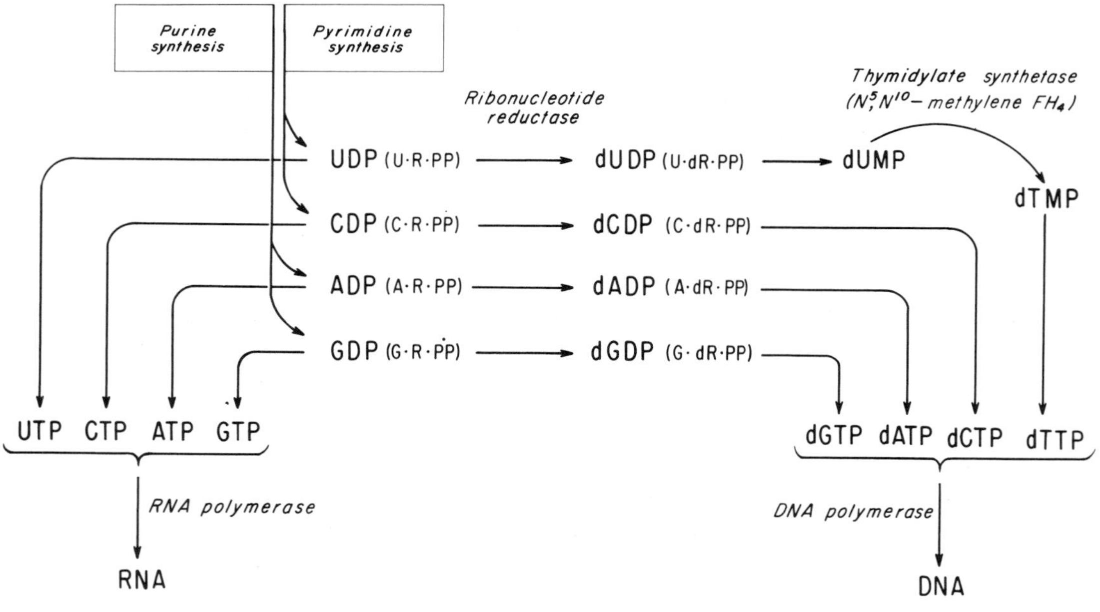

Fig. 4.2
Pathways of nucleotide and nucleic acid synthesis in *Escherichia coli* and animal cells. (From W. S. Beck, *Vitamins and Hormones* 26(1968): 395)

b. Deficiency of dTTP: "thyminelessness"

Until recently it was believed that the only major consequence of vitamin B_{12} deficiency, folate deficiency, and other disorders causing megaloblastosis is impairment of dTTP biosynthesis, with resulting impairment of DNA synthesis. This, it was held, was the critical defect that led to the unbalanced growth state, whether in bacteria or animal cells, and to loss in the capacity for cell division, with eventual cell death. This phenomenon is still an important mechanism in the megaloblastic state, but it is not the whole story.

c. Uracil misincorporation into DNA

In view of data showing extensive DNA fragmentation in megaloblastic cells, a phenomenon that would be difficult to explain entirely on the basis of thyminelessness, a new view of megaloblastic transformation held that there is an increase in dUMP (and dUTP) levels in cells unable to convert dUMP to dTMP (figure 4.3). As a result there is a sharp increase in the dUTP/dTTP ratio. Since DNA polymerase does not distinguish between dUTP and dTTP, uracil is incorporated into DNA in place of thymine. An editorial enzyme, uracil-DNA-glycosylase, detects misincorporated uracils and excises them. Since there is insufficient dTTP for satisfactory repair, DNA is fragmented, with resulting impairment in cell division and cell death. This theory, which is now amply supported, has interesting biological implications.

First, it suggests that a cell's level of dUTPase, the enzyme normally responsible for preventing accumulation of dUTP, may in part explain the fact that the degree of impairment of DNA synthesis varies from cell line to cell line in megaloblastic anemia. (Usually it is more severe along the erythrocyte precursors than along granulocyte precursors).

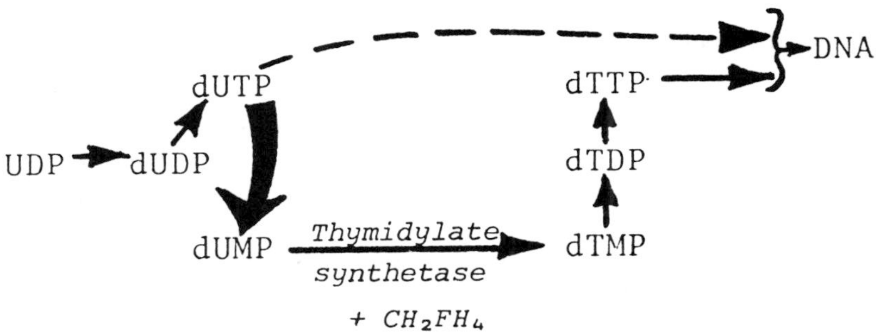

Fig. 4.3
Enzymatic machinery for exclusion of uracil from DNA. The pyrophosphatase, *dUTPase*, destroys dUTP (by converting it to dUMP) before it can serve as substrate for DNA polymerase. *Uracil-DNA-glycosylase* removes uracil *from* DNA that was misincorporated in place of thymine, or that arose from cytosine by deamination.

Second, it is clear that the role of uracil-DNA-glycosylase in normal cells is to excise the uracils arising from an occasional deamination of cytosine in DNA. Such an event would be mutagenic since it would alter the genetic code. If DNA were synthesized with a substantial amount of misincorporated uracil in place of thymine (which does not alter the genetic code), the glycosylase would be overwhelmed and play a harmful role since repair would be inadequate.

C. Clinical features

1. General symptoms

The following description includes manifestations that are common to all of the megaloblastic anemias. (Features associated with specific syndromes will be given later.) The anemia is often severe but because it develops slowly may produce few symptoms until the hematocrit reaches a low level. When symptoms appear, they are the usual symptoms of anemia: weakness, palpitation, ease of fatigue, light-headedness, and shortness of breath. Congestive heart failure may supervene. Patients characteristically demonstrate pallor and slight jaundice.

2. Blood

a. Red cells

Red cells display striking variations in size and shape and are normochromic (unless iron deficiency coexists) and macrocytic with MCVs ranging from 100 μm^3 to more than 140 μm^3. *Macroovalocytes,* oval-shaped red cells up to 14 μm in diameter, are characteristically present (figure 4.1B). The reticulocyte count is lower than normal, in both absolute terms and terms of percentage. Red cell changes become more severe as the anemia worsens. When the hematocrit is low (i.e., $<20\%$), nucleated red cells may appear in the blood. Such cells show typical megaloblastic features—indeed, frank promegaloblasts are occasionally found.

b. Neutrophils

Many have more than 4 segments (figure 4.1B). Some have up to 16 segments. These *macropolycytes* may be very large. Typically, more than 5% of the neutrophils have 5 or more segments. On the basis of early concepts such as Arneth's that equated cell age with lobe count, such cells have been considered older than normal. In fact, hypersegmentation of neutrophils is more likely due to an abnormality of nuclear division or of the chromatin itself.

3. Bone marrow

Aspirated bone marrow is cellular. The megaloblastic changes described above may be seen in erythrocyte, granulocyte, and platelet precursors, though frequently major changes are only in the erythroid series. The E/M ratio typically rises from 1:3 to 1:1. Megaloblastic granulopoiesis is more evident in situations such as infection, in which increased granulocyte production is called forth. In typical severe megaloblastic anemia, most of the erythroid cells are promegaloblasts. Many mitotic figures (i.e., cells in metaphase) are found among them. Unless iron deficiency is present, iron in reticulum cells is commonly increased.

4. Chemical changes in body fluids

Changes secondary to megaloblastic anemia per se include the following: (1) slight to moderate increases in serum bilirubin and iron; (2) marked elevation in serum lactic dehydrogenase (isozymes 1 and 2) and muramidase; (3) occasional decrease in serum potassium that may worsen dangerously in the early stages of repletion therapy; and (4) decreased serum uric acid.

D. Cytokinetics

1. Erythrokinetics

Whatever its cause, megaloblastic anemia is associated with two pathophysiologic abnormalities: *ineffective erythropoiesis* and moderate *hemolysis* of circulating erythrocytes.

a. Ineffective erythropoiesis

The presence of ineffective erythropoiesis is indicated by (1) a marked increase in the number of erythroid precursors in bone marrow and in the ratio of erythroid precursors to released erythrocytes; (2) an increase in plasma iron turnover to 3–5 times the normal level, with normal iron uptake by individual erythroid precursors (see Figure 6.4); (3) a decreased rate of reappearance of labeled plasma iron in peripheral blood erythrocytes; (4) indirect evidence of intramedullary destruction of megaloblasts, which includes: (i) the high serum levels of lactic dehydrogenase (isozymes typical of erythroid precursors) and muramidase (from leukocyte precursors); (ii) increase in production of "early-labeled peak" bilirubin (see lecture 7) and endogenous carbon monoxide; (iii) the ease with which megaloblasts undergo autohemolysis in vitro compared to normoblasts; and (iv) the fact, noted above, that marrow reticulum cells phagocytize megaloblastic erythroid precursors.

b. Hemolysis

Ineffective erythropoiesis is associated with intramedullary hemolysis. A substantial degree of extramedullary hemolysis also occurs. This is indicated by studies showing that erythrocyte lifespan is moderately decreased (to one-half to one-third normal) when patient erythrocytes are tested in a normal subject. Thus, an intracorpuscular defect is present. Decreased survival or normal erythrocytes in untreated patients suggests the presence of an extracorpuscular defect as well.

2. Ferrokinetics

Ferrokinetic abnormalities are (1) elevated plasma iron; (2) elevated plasma iron turnover; (3) decreased incorporation of plasma iron into circulating hemoglobin; (4) accumulation of iron in marrow reticulum cells; and (5) increased iron stores in the liver (hepatic siderosis) and other tissues. Unlike the situation in uncomplicated iron overload, radioiron moves rapidly in megaloblastic anemia from the plasma to the marrow. After a period of retention there, it is slowly released, most of it moving to the liver.

3. Leukokinetics

Inadequate bone marrow production or delivery of myeloid cells probably accounts for their decreased numbers in the blood. The elevated serum muramidase in megaloblastic anemia is due to an increased rate of myeloid cell destruction in the marrow; thus, the mechanism of leukopenia is "ineffective granulopoiesis," due presumably to defective DNA synthesis in granulocyte precursors.

4. Thrombokinetics

"Ineffective thrombopoiesis" also occurs in megaloblastic anemia. This state is characterized by an increased megakaryocyte mass in the bone marrow with a decreased rate of platelet production. Thus, the pathophysiology of ineffective thrombopoiesis parallels that of ineffective erythropoiesis and leukopoiesis.

According to Harker and Finch, the term *ineffective thrombopoiesis* should be restricted to situations in which daily platelet production per nuclear megakaryocyte unit is less than half of that expected. Their data showed that in subjects with megaloblastic anemia, mean daily platelet production averaged 6 (platelets per nuclear unit) compared with a normal rate of 49. Megakaryocyte mass was 4 times normal, but platelet production was 40% of normal. Hence, platelet production was only 10% of that expected from the megakaryocyte mass.

E. Etiology

Table 4.1 summarizes the major categories of megaloblastic anemia according to etiologic mechanism. Vitamin B_{12} deficiency and folic acid deficiency are the most common causes, each deficiency having many possible causes. Both deficiencies result in a tissue coenzyme deficiency that is correctable by repletion of the lacking vitamin. Repletion is followed by reversion of megaloblastic hematopoiesis to normal. The table also lists megaloblastic anemias that are unresponsive to therapy with vitamin B_{12} and folic acid. This group and the megaloblastic anemias of folic acid deficiency will be discussed in lecture 5.

III. VITAMIN B_{12} VITAMINOLOGY

A. Historical notes

Classic studies of pernicious anemia (PA) have led to much of our present knowledge of both vitamin B_{12} and folic acid. Until the demonstration by Minot and Murphy (1926) of the successful treatment of PA by liver feeding, the disease was frequently fatal. The efficacy of liver treatment implied that the disease is a deficiency state, but its appearance in individuals taking normal diets was unexplained until Castle discovered in 1929 that intestinal absorption of the anti-PA principle of liver—a dietary and therefore "extrinsic factor"—requires prior binding to an "intrinsic factor" secreted in the stomach. An individual with PA synthesizes little or no intrinsic factor; therefore, the resulting vitamin deficiency is a conditioned one caused by impairment of an absorptive mechanism whose biologic novelty sets vitamin B_{12} apart from other vitamins. Potent liver extracts soon replaced liver feeding in the treatment of PA, but difficulties plagued investigators attempting to purify the anti-PA principle of liver. For example, lack of a naturally occurring animal disease resembling PA meant that purification studies could be guided only by tedious assays performed on PA patients in relapse.

After the unsuccessful attempts of two decades to purify liver principle by E. J. Cohn and coworkers, discoveries of the following factors by workers in the fields of bacterial and animal nutrition led to the discovery of vitamin B_{12}; (1) *LLD factor,* a factor in yeast and liver extracts that is essential in the nutrition of *Lactobacillus lactis* Dorner and other microorganisms; (2) *animal protein factor,* a factor obtained from tissue extracts and animal feces that promotes growth of pigs and poultry receiving only vegetable rations; and (3) a *ruminant factor,* lack of which causes a wasting disease of ruminants grazing in cobalt-poor pastures and replacement of which can be effected by oral feeding of cobalt salts (or by dusting cobalt on pastures), parenteral cobalt being ineffective. The discovery and crystallization of vitamin B_{12} by E. L. Rickes and associates (1948) of Merck Laboratories followed the astute observation by Shorb of proportionality between the nutrient activity of liver extracts in cultures of *L. lactis* Dorner and their therapeutic activity in PA. The resulting simple microbiological assay facilitated purification and identification of the vitamin. Animal protein factor and cobalt-dependent ruminant factor were then identified with vitamin B_{12}.

B. Nutritional aspects

1. Sources

Vitamin B_{12} is synthesized only by certain microorganisms. Wherever it is found in nature, it can be traced to microorganisms growing in soil, sewage, water, intestine, or rumen. Animals depend ultimately upon microbial synthesis for their vitamin B_{12} supply. Foods in the human diet that contain vitamin B_{12} are essentially those of animal origin—meat, liver, fish, eggs, and milk. Although nitrogen-fixing bacteria associated with leguminous plants are vitamin B_{12} dependent, vitamin B_{12} has not been found in plant tissues.

The most intensive natural synthesis of vitamin B_{12} occurs in rumen bacteria. Of the microorganisms that synthesize the vitamin, many do so in quantities just sufficient for their needs. However, organisms such as the rumen organism *Propionibacterium shermannii* and the antibiotic-producing molds *Streptomyces griseus* and *Streptomyces aureofaciens* synthesize amounts sufficient to make them feasible commercial sources. Some microorganisms that cannot synthesize vitamin B_{12} (e.g., *L. lactis, L. leichmannii*) require an exogenous supply and hence are useful in the microbiologic assay of vitamin B_{12}. Other microorganisms cannot synthesize vitamin B_{12} and appear not to require it (e.g., *Escherichia coli*).

2. Daily requirements

The average daily diet in Western countries contains 5–30 μg of vitamin B_{12}. Of this, 1–5 μg is absorbed. Total body content is 1–5 mg in an adult man. Of this, approximately 1 mg is in the liver. Kidneys are also rich in the vitamin. Vitamin B_{12} has a daily rate of obligatory loss approximating 0.1% of the total body pool size.

The daily dietary requirement is 2–5 μg; hence, a deficiency state will not develop for several years after cessation of vitamin B_{12} ingestion. Because of the buffering effects of body stores, it has been difficult to obtain precise data on the normal daily requirement.

C. Chemical aspects

1. Structure

The chemical structure of vitamin B_{12} was elucidated in 1955 by Hodgkin following skillful x-ray crystallographic analysis. The structure displays several unique features (figure 4.4, formula I). The cyanocobalamin molecule (mol. wt. 1,355) has two major portions: (1) a planar group, which bears a close but imperfect resemblance to the porphyrin macroring (shown in figure 7.1); and (2) a nucleotide, which lies nearly perpendicular to the planar group (formula II). The porphyrin-like moiety contains four reduced pyrrole rings (designated A–D) that link to a central cobalt atom whose two remaining coordination positions are occupied by a cyano group (above) and a 5,6-dimethylbenzimidazolyl moiety (below the planar group). With one exception, the pyrrole rings are connected to one another by methine carbon bridges similar to those found in porphyrins. The exception is the direct linkage between the α-carbons of rings A and D. The macroring of vitamin B_{12} and related compounds is termed *corrin;* the major corrin derivatives are known generically as *corrinoid* compounds. Both corrin and porphin macrorings are synthesized from δ-aminolevulinic acid.

2. Nomenclature

Many corrinoid compounds are known. Some occur naturally; others have been prepared synthetically. Compounds were early given trivial names (e.g., vitamin B_{12}). Even the semisystematic term *cobalamin* was introduced before chemical structure was known. After much confusion, approval was given in 1973 to a

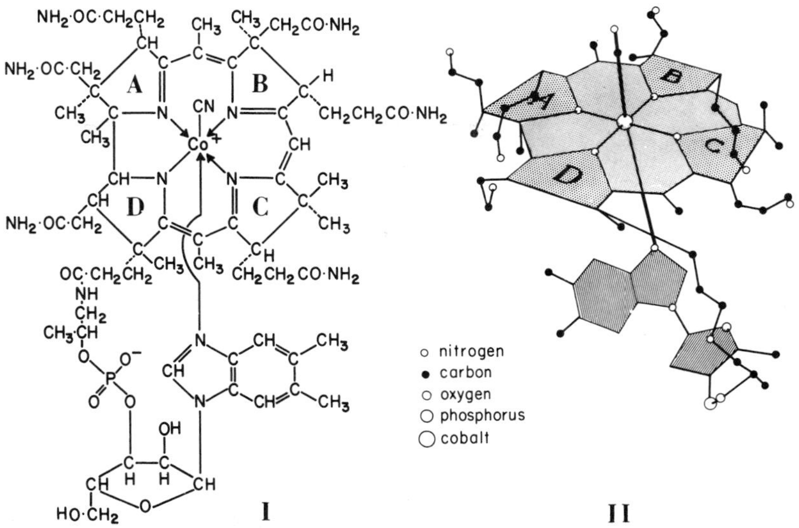

Fig. 4.4
Chemical structure of vitamin B_{12}; *formula I,* molecular structure of cyanocobalamin; *formula II,* semidiagrammatic representation of three-dimensional structure showing relations of planar and nucleotide moieties. Hydrogen atoms and a number of oxygen atoms are omitted. (From W. S. Beck, *New Eng. J. Med.* 266(1962): 708)

system of names and abbreviations. Table 4.2 lists these terms for the four compounds found in the human body. In this system vitamin B_{12} becomes cyanocobalamin. In other compounds, the cyano ligand is replaced by another moiety.

The four compounds of importance in animal cell metabolism are the vitamin *cyanocobalamin* (CN-Cbl) and its analogue *hydroxocobalamin* (OH-Cbl) and the two coenzyme forms *adenosylcobalamin* (AdoCbl) and *methylcobalamin* (MeCbl). In AdoCbl, a 5′-deoxyadenosyl moiety is the ligand of cobalt above the plane (figure 4.5). This coenzyme, discovered by H. A. Barker in studies of the isomerization of glutamate by bacterial extracts, was

Table 4.2
Names of Cobalamins Found in Human Body

Semisystematic name	Abbreviation	Systematic name
Cyanocobalamin[a]	CN-Cbl	α-(5,6-dimethylbenzimidazolyl)-cyanocobamide
Hydroxocobalamin	OH-Cbl	α-(5,6-dimethylbenzimidazolyl)-hydroxocobamide
Adenosylcobalamin	AdoCbl	α-(5,6-dimethylbenzimidazolyl)-adenosylcobamide
Methylcobalamin	MeCbl	α-(5,6-dimethylbenzimidazolyl)-methylcobamide

a. Also called vitamin B_{12}.

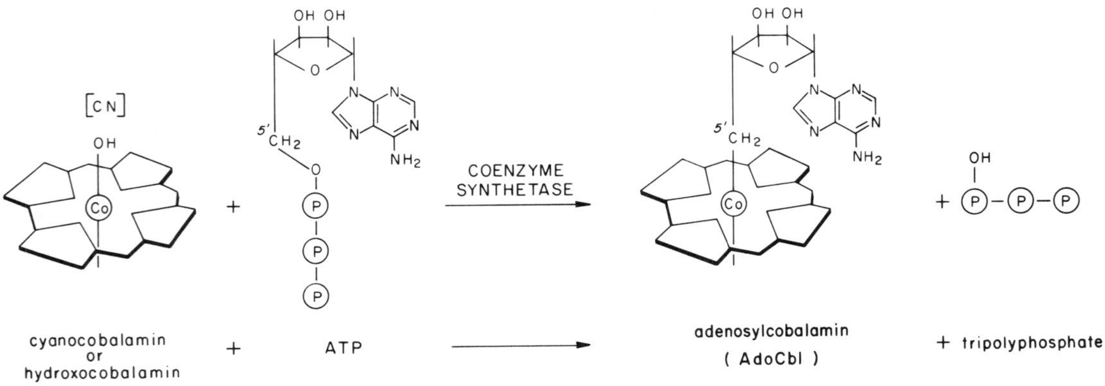

Fig. 4.5
The coenzyme synthetase system in which ATP adenosylates cobalamin to form adenosylcobalamin. The reaction requires a thiol and a reduced flavin or ferredoxin. Reducing agents are required in a preliminary step that converts tervalent cobalt of cobalamin (termed cob(III)alamin) through the bivalent state (cob(II)alamin) to the univalent state (cob(I)alamin), which has nucleophilic properties. (From W. S. Beck, in W. J. Williams, et al., *Hematology*, 3d ed., New York: McGraw-Hill, 1983)

soon identified as the main storage form of vitamin B_{12} in mammalian liver. In adenosylcobalamin, the 5′-methylene carbon atom of the 5′-deoxyadenosyl moiety is linked directly to the cobalt atom. In MeCbl, the ligand of cobalt is a methyl group. In both coenzyme forms the carbon-cobalt bond is labile to light, cyanide, and acid. It is likely that cyanocobalamin occurs only from the attack by cyanide on coenzyme forms and other cobalamins. Methylcobalamin occurs in small amounts in liver but is the major cobalamin in blood plasma.

D. Metabolic functions

1. AdoCbl-dependent reactions

AdoCbl functions as an acceptor-donor of hydrogen in two types of reactions. In AdoCbl-dependent isomerizations, hydrogen transfer is *intra*molecular—that is, the transferred hydrogen originates in one portion of the substrate molecule and ends in another. On the coenzyme, hydrogen is carried by C-5′ of the adenosyl group. For example, the *methylmalonyl CoA mutase* reaction occurs as follows:

$$\underset{\text{methylmalonyl CoA}}{CH_3\text{—}\overset{\overset{\text{COCoA}}{|}}{CH}\text{—}COOH} \overset{\text{AdoCbl}}{\rightleftharpoons} \underset{\text{succinyl CoA}}{\overset{\overset{\text{COCoA}}{|}}{CH_2}\text{—}CH_2\text{—}COOH}$$

The cobamide-dependent mutation (or isomerization) of methylmalonyl CoA, one of two AdoCbl-dependent reactions demon-

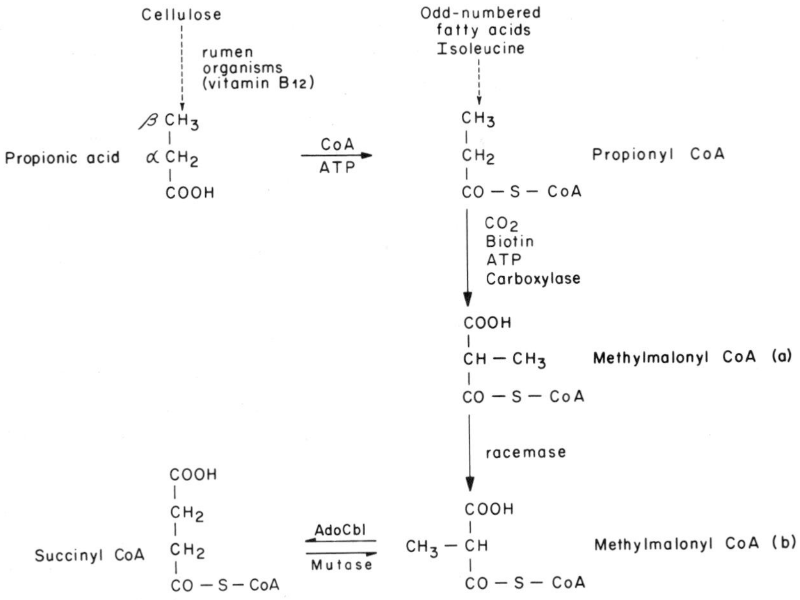

Fig. 4.6
Pathway of propionic acid metabolism.

strated thus far in animal tissues, is a step in the pathway of propionic acid catabolism (figure 4.6). Propionic acid is metabolized in animal tissues by a biotin-dependent carboxylation of propionyl CoA to methylmalonyl CoA, an α-carboxy derivative of propionyl CoA. After a racemization step, methylmalonyl CoA mutase catalyzes the reversible conversion of methylmalonyl CoA to its β-carboxy isomer, succinyl CoA, which after deacylation enters the tricarboxylic acid cycle.

The other AdoCbl-dependent enzyme in animal cells, leucine 2,3-aminomutase, is of uncertain significance. It catalyzes the conversion of β-leucine to leucine.

A second type of cobamide-dependent reaction (though one that does not occur in human or other animal cells) is the *reduction* of ribonucleotides in which hydrogen transfer is *inter*molecular—that is, AdoCbl transfers hydrogen (on C-5′) from the -SH group of an outside reductant (thioredoxin) to the C-2′ of the substrate. In the ribonucleotide reductase reaction, ribonucleotides are converted to deoxyribonucleotides, the precursors of DNA. Interestingly, this type of ribonucleotide reductase occurs only in vitamin B_{12}-requiring lactobacilli, *Euglena gracilis,* and a few other vitamin B_{12}-dependent microorganisms. The ribonucleotide reductase of animal cells (and *E. coli*) is cobalamin-independent. This enzyme relies on an atom of nonheme iron instead of a vitamin B_{12} coenzyme.

2. MeCbl-dependent reactions

Methylcobalamin participates in the cobalamin-dependent synthesis of methionine in bacteria and animal cells according to the scheme in figure 4.7. This pathway, one of several pathways of methionine synthesis, serves primarily as a means for converting N^5-methyltetrahydrofolate to tetrahydrofolate (see lecture 5). It has recently been shown that nitrous oxide (N_2O) impairs this enzyme by promoting the oxidation of cob(I)alamin to cob(III)alamin, thereby depleting the level of MeCbl and producing a state resembling vitamin B_{12} deficiency. N_2O treatment thus offers a useful new research tool.

3. Role of vitamin B_{12} in animal cell metabolism

As noted above, an explanation for the role of vitamin B_{12} in animal cell DNA synthesis finally won acceptance after long controversy. According to the so-called "methylfolate trap" theory, vitamin B_{12} deficiency slows the cobalamin-dependent pathway of methionine synthesis (figure 4.7). As a result, folate is sequestered as N^5-methyltetrahydrofolate, a form that is unavailable to the critical thymidylate synthetase reaction (figure 4.2). Other evidence favoring this theory includes the following abnormalities said to occur in vitamin B_{12} deficiency: (1) altered partitioning of tissue folate compounds; (2) elevated serum N^5-methyltetrahydrofolate levels; and (3) increased excretion of formiminoglutamic acid after histidine loading in some subjects. One more item of supporting evidence is discussed in lecture 5.

In summary, the two metabolic systems impaired in human vitamin B_{12} deficiency are (1) methylmalonyl CoA isomerization, and thus propionate catabolism; and (2) methionine methyl syn-

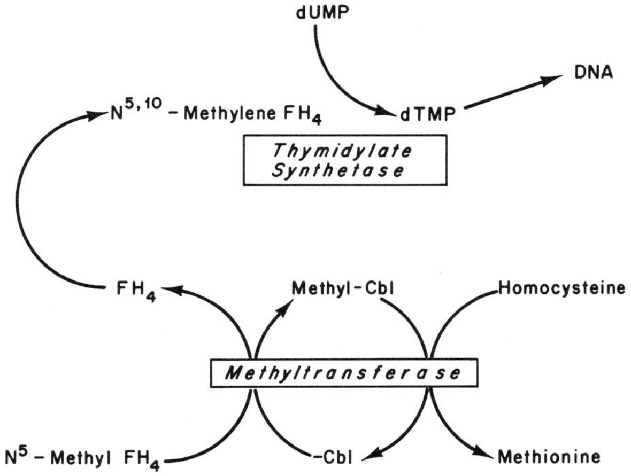

Fig. 4.7
Diagram of relation between N^5-methyltetrahydrofolate: homocysteine methyltransferase and thymidylate synthetase. In vitamin B_{12} deficiency, folate is sequestered as N^5-methyltetrahydrofolate. This ultimately deprives thymidylate synthetase of its folate coenzyme (N^5, N^{10}-methylene FH_4) and thereby impairs DNA synthesis.

thesis, and thus tetrahydrofolate regeneration. Impairment of DNA synthesis undoubtedly accounts for megaloblastic erythropoiesis and related phenomena. Trapping of folate as N^5-methyltetrahydrofolate impairs thymidylate synthesis, which depresses DNA synthesis, and causes accumulation of dUTP, which causes uracil misincorporation into DNA. This mechanism may also underlie the neurological damage of human vitamin B_{12} deficiency. However, impairment of methylmalonyl CoA metabolism may also be involved. Nondividing nerve cells are not engaged in DNA synthesis, though the cells that make myelin do divide. Neurologic symptoms are prominent in vitamin B_{12}-deficient sheep, for which propionate metabolism is of greater importance than it is in humans. Vitamin B_{12}-deficient humans excrete abnormal quantities of methylmalonate and, according to a recent report, propionate and acetate.

E. Physiologic aspects

1. Intestinal absorption: the intrinsic factor mechanism

Intrinsic factor (IF), a protein normally present in human gastric juice, is necessary for the absorption of the ileum of ingested cobalamins. Following discovery of IF by Castle in 1929, efforts to purify it were complicated by the need before the advent of radioactive vitamin B_{12} to use a patient in relapse as an assay system. Substantial purifications were finally achieved in 1973 by the use of affinity chromatographic methods. This elegant work opened a new era in the study of IF and other vitamin B_{12}-binding proteins.

a. Structure of IF

Human IF is an alkali-stable glycoprotein that binds a molecule of cobalamin (cyano-, hydroxo-, or adenosyl- derivative) with high affinity. The mol. wt. is about 44,000 (human IF) and 50,000–59,000 (hog IF). IF contains about 15% carbohydrate. When bound to vitamin B_{12}, IF forms dimers. Bound vitamin alters the conformation of IF, producing a more compact form that is more resistant to proteolytic digestion (although free IF is more resistant to proteolysis than once believed). To date human IF has been sequenced to a total of 84 amino acid residues out of 340.

b. Vitamin B_{12}-binding proteins of gastric juice

Gastric juice contains several vitamin B_{12}-binding proteins (table 4.3). Only one possesses IF activity (such activity being defined as the capacity to promote intestinal absorption of vitamin B_{12}).

Electrophoresis reveals two immunologically nonidentical binders or classes of binders, one with slow and one with rapid mobility, that have been designated, respectively, *S-protein* and *R-protein*(s). IF activity resides in the S-protein.

IF is secreted by the parietal cells of the fundic mucosa in the human, guinea pig, cat, rabbit, and monkey, by the chief cells in the rat and by glandular cells of the pylorus and duodenum in the

Table 4.3
Major Vitamin B_{12}-Binding Proteins

Source	Protein(s)	Function	Class[a]
Gastric juice	Intrinsic factor (IF)	Promotes absorption of vitamin B_{12} in ileum	S
Gastric juice	"Haptocorrin" "Cobalophilin(s)"[b]	May be involved in formation of IF-B_{12}; binds cobalamin analogues	R
Plasma	Transcobalamin I (TC I)[b]	May participate in plasma transport of vitamin B_{12}	R
Plasma	Transcobalamin II (TC II)	Promotes entry of vitamin B_{12} into cells	S
Plasma (and granulocytes)	Transcobalamin III (TC III)[b]	Unknown	R

a. Based on electrophoretic mobility: R, rapid; S, slow.
b. As noted in text these names have been proposed for R proteins, and some have recommended that the term *transcobalamin* be restricted to what is now termed transcobalamin II.

hog. Its secretion is enhanced by histamine, metacholine, and gastrin. IF secretion usually parallels HCl secretion.

c. R-proteins

R-proteins are now recognized to be a class of immunologically identical proteins that are found in serum, leukocytes, saliva, gastric juice, milk, and virtually all body cells. R-proteins have been given different names—transcobalamin I (TC I) and III (TC III); and granulocyte binder. Genetic evidence suggests that these are all one protein with one structural gene since two brothers lacked the protein in all body fluids and granulocytes. Various groups have proposed that R-protein(s) be named *haptocorrin* and *cobalophilin,* but these terms are not yet universally accepted. R-proteins are currently receiving intensive study. We shall return to them in discussions of plasma vitamin B_{12} transport proteins and serum vitamin B_{12} assays.

2. Locus and mechanism of vitamin B_{12} absorption

Vitamin B_{12} derivatives in food are liberated by peptic digestion in the stomach and bound there by IF. The stable IF-B_{12} complex encounters specific mucosal receptors in the microvilli of the ileum. A specific site on the IF molecule (other than the vitamin B_{12} binding site) attaches to a receptor. Attachment requires neutral pH, Ca^{++}, or other divalent cations, but no energy. Mucosal receptors accept IF-B_{12} in preference to free IF and are readily saturated. The IF receptor has been isolated and purified. It contains 2 subunits, and the similarity of its amino acid sequence to that of IF suggests that it arose by gene duplication.

The model in figure 4.8 has been proposed for the attachment of IF-B_{12} complex to IF receptor. As the IF-B_{12} complex has a tendency to form oligomers, the binding of complex to receptor may be analogous to the formation of an IF oligomer. Vitamin B_{12} (without IF) is ultimately transferred to portal vein blood.

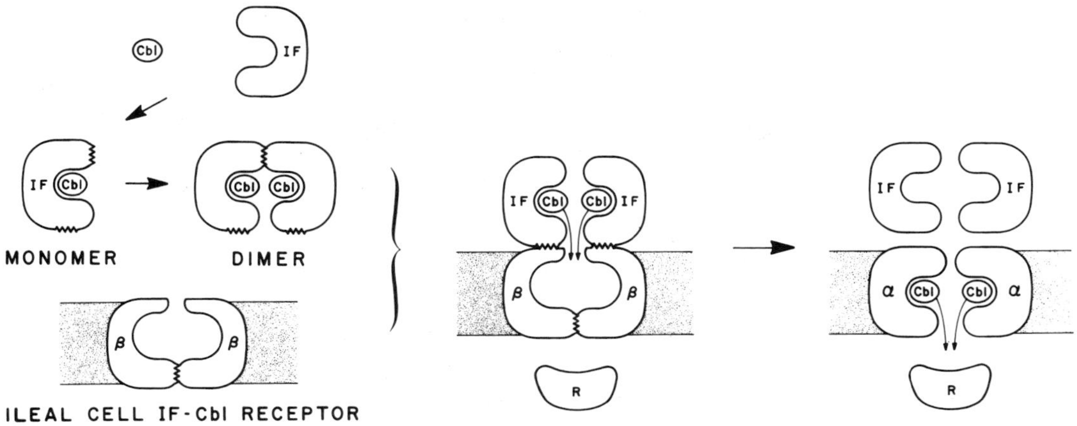

Fig. 4.8
A hypothetical model for the binding of IF-B_{12} complex to IF receptor. The complex forms a pseudooligomer with its "relative," the IF receptor. It probably attaches to the β subunit of the receptor, which then undergoes conformational change to α. Intracellular R-proteins then accept Cbl from α. (Adapted from R. Gräsbeck, in B. Zagalak and W. Friedrich, eds., *Vitamin B_{12}: Proceedings of the Third European Symposium on Vitamin B_{12} and Intrinsic Factor,* New York: Walter de Gruyter, 1979, p. 743)

3. Antibodies to IF

Two types of anti-IF antibodies occur. *Blocking antibodies* prevent binding of vitamin B_{12} by IF and show little species specificity. Antibodies of this type occur in some individuals receiving hog IF by mouth. *Binding antibodies* combine with IF-B_{12} complex but also with free IF without impairing its ability to bind vitamin B_{12}. Both types of antibodies occur in sera of some patients with PA.

4. Clinical assay of vitamin B_{12} absorption and IF

Following the observation that increasing the dose of parenteral vitamin B_{12} leads to excretion of increasing percentages of the dose in the urine. Schilling showed that a large parenteral dose (1 mg) of nonradioactive vitamin B_{12} given 2 hr after oral administration of radioactive vitamin B_{12} increases excretion of radioactive vitamin B_{12}, presumably by blocking vitamin B_{12} binding sites in plasma and liver. Thus, vitamin B_{12} absorption can be assayed by studies of urinary excretion following oral administration—an advance over methods requiring stool analysis.

In the *Schilling test* (part I), a fasting patient is given 0.5 μCi (0.5–1.0 μg) ^{57}Co-cyanocobalamin by mouth at time zero. A 24 hr urine collection is begun. At 2 hr, 1 mg of nonradioactive cyanocobalamin is administered intramuscularly. This is the "flushing" dose. An adequate sample of pooled urine is assayed for radioactivity. If excretion of radioactivity is low (<7%), the Schilling test (part II) is performed (in no less than 5 days) by the same procedure except that 60 mg of hog IF is given orally with the radioactive vitamin B_{12}. If poor excretion in part I was due to IF deficiency, the result in part II should be normal. If excretion is still abnormal, other explanations must be found for malabsorption of vitamin B_{12}. The kidneys excrete cyanocobalamin and inulin in a similar manner, and radioactive vitamin B_{12} has been used in measurements of the glomerular filtration rate. Renal disease with impaired glomerular filtration may delay excretion of radioactivity in the Schilling test.

5. Transport of vitamin B_{12} in plasma

Normal plasma contains 150–650 pg/ml of vitamin B_{12} (normal range varying with method and laboratory), all of which is protein bound. The three major vitamin B_{12}-binding proteins of plasma are usually designated *transcobalamin I* (TC I), *transcobalamin II* (TC II), and *transcobalamin III* (TC III). Their properties are summarized in table 4.4. Interest in these proteins has expanded dramatically in recent years. Known functions of the transcobalamins are two: (1) prevention of loss of cobalamins in urine, sweat, and other body secretions; and (2) transport of cobalamins through cell membranes. However, as noted below, they undoubtedly have other functions.

a. TC I and TC III

TC I and TC III are essentially identical R-proteins. The recommended names *haptocorrin* and *cobalophilin* do not imply a specific transport function. Probably TC III is an isoprotein of TC I that is unsaturated with vitamin B_{12} and therefore less charged. Both appear to arise from granulocytes, but R-proteins also arise

Table 4.4
Properties of Vitamin B_{12}-Binding Proteins of Plasma

Property	TC I	TC II	TC III
Electrophoretic mobility (pH 8.6)	α_1	$\alpha_2\beta$	α_2
Molecular weight	120,000[a]	38,000[b]	120,000
Cobalamin binding capacity (μg/mg)	12.2	28.6	12.2
Protein type (R or S)	R	S	R
Salic acid, residues/mole	18	0	11
Portion of plasma vitamin B_{12} bound (approx.)	75%	25%	0%
Portion of binder unsaturated (approx.)	50%	98%	—
Half-life of TC-B_{12} complex	9–12 days	12 hr	60–90 min
Reacts with			
Anti-TC II	No	Yes	No
Anti-TC I	Yes	No	Yes
Anti-saliva R-protein	Yes	No	Yes

a. Isolated R-proteins have a "true" mol. wt. of 63,000–72,000, but in gel filtration and gel electrophoresis values of approximately 120,000 are obtained due to high carbohydrate content (~40%)
b. Some evidence has suggested that TC II consists of two peptides of mol. wt. 38,000 and 27,000.

from salivary and gastric glands. All R-proteins possess the same amino acid sequence, differences among them being attributable to variations in carbohydrate moieties. Much of the plasma TC III appears to arise from granulocytes in vitro after blood has been collected—that is, during clotting. Thus, the content of R-proteins differs in plasma and serum. TC III levels may rise in granulocyte disorders (leukemias, myeloproliferative disorders, etc.). TC I levels rise in malignant diseases (hepatoma, metastatic breast cancer, etc.). The fact that TC III contains less sialic acid than TC I may explain its low plasma level. Like other asialoglycoproteins, it may be cleared rapidly by hepatic cells. This may also account for excretion of some cobalamin in bile. Of the amount so excreted, about 75% is reabsorbed by IF-mediated mechanisms.

Within cells, R-proteins promote uptake of vitamin B_{12} by mitochondria and other organelles.

R-proteins differ from TC II and IF in the specificity of their binding sites. This property, which is discussed below, may give them a role in the binding and disposition of biologically inert and potentially harmful cobalamin analogues and corrins.

b. TC II

When a small amount of vitamin B_{12} enters the blood (portal and systemic), it is taken up first by TC II. Indeed, more than 90% of *recently* absorbed vitamin B_{12} is carried by TC II. TC II-B_{12} complex is then cleared from plasma rapidly (in hours); vitamin and protein moiety disappear at comparable rates.

TC I, in contrast, carries most of the vitamin B_{12} in plasma and is cleared from plasma slowly (half-life of 9–12 days). Nevertheless, a quarter of the circulating vitamin B_{12} continues to be carried by TC II long after its intestinal absorption.

The nonessentiality of TC I as a transport protein is puzzling. Congenital absence of TC I is harmless, but severe megaloblastic anemia occurs in infants lacking TC II. Only TC II can promote cellular uptake of vitamin B_{12}. Vitamin B_{12} is taken up by many cells, which possess specific surface receptors for TC II-bound vitamin B_{12} that are analogous to the IF-B_{12} receptors of ileal cells. Uptake involves pinocytosis followed by lysosomal degradation of TC II. Hepatic cells have an especially high affinity for TC II-bound vitamin B_{12}. The source of human TC II is not yet known. Inconclusive data suggest synthesis in the liver and in the monocyte-macrophage system. There is evidence that TC II (and sometimes TC I) may occasionally form complexes in the serum with immunoglobulins.

TC II levels decrease in chronic myeloproliferative disorders and occasionally in pernicious anemia. The sum of the levels of unsaturated TC I and TC II—sometimes called serum *unsaturated B_{12} binding capacity* (UBBC) and largely contributed by TC II—may be decreased in cirrhosis and hepatitis.

6. Assay of serum vitamin B_{12}

The microbiologic assay of serum vitamin B_{12} (using such cobalamin-dependent organisms as *Lactobacillus leichmannii* and *Euglena gracilis*) was largely supplanted in the 1960s by a radioisotope dilution assay (RIDA) employing a vitamin B_{12}-binding protein. The fact that this assay gave higher results than the microbiological assay was recently explained by the discovery in serum (and then in tissue) of a class of vitamin B_{12} *analogues* that are not recognized as vitamin B_{12} by microorganisms but are assayed as vitamin B_{12} by RIDA procedures when the binder is R-protein but not when it is IF. In other words, the relatively low binding specificity of R-proteins produces a falsely high value in serum vitamin B_{12} assays. This discovery led to RIDA methods using IF as binder that yield results in agreement with those of microbiological assays. In addition it raised several interesting questions that still lack answers: (1) What is the source and fate of these analogues? (2) Do they have pathophysiological significance? (3) Is it the role of R-proteins in gastric juice to bind these compounds, which may be of dietary origin, in order to minimize their absorption in the intestine? (4) Is it the role of granulocyte R-protein (TC III) to prevent the dissemination of these analogues, which may escape exclusion in the intestine, by binding them and delivering them to hepatocytes, which retain and eventually excrete them? These matters are now under active study.

IV. VITAMIN B_{12} DEFICIENCY

A. Clinical features

The clinical picture of human vitamin B_{12} deficiency includes the nonspecific manifestations of megaloblastic anemia and its sequelae—glossitis, elevated serum LDH, weight loss, and so forth—that occur as well in folic acid deficiency and the following specific features that make possible the diagnosis of vitamin B_{12} deficiency, irrespective of the underlying cause: (1) neurologic abnormalities; (2) decreased serum vitamin B_{12} level; (3) methylmalonicaciduria; and (4) characteristic response to vitamin B_{12} therapy and lack of response to therapy with physiologic doses of folic acid.

1. Neurologic syndrome

The neurologic syndrome of vitamin B_{12} deficiency is classically said to consist of symmetrical paresthesias in feet and fingers with associated disturbances of vibratory sense and proprioception, progressing to spastic ataxia with "subacute combined system" disease of spinal cord, that is, degenerative changes of the dorsal and lateral columns. In fact, the picture is more often chronic than subacute and more varied and complex. Typically, it develops late in untreated PA, and if not treated it becomes irreversible. Significantly and surprisingly it can occur in the absence of megaloblastosis.

Early pathologic changes in the cord consist of focal swelling of individual myelinated nerve fibers. Lesions later coalesce into larger foci involving many fiber systems. Clinical signs include cerebral abnormalities, irritability, somnolence, "megaloblastic madness," and perversion of taste, smell, and vision with central scotomata and occasional optic atrophy. Tobacco amblyopia, a curious visual disorder in vitamin B_{12}-deficient smokers, has been attributed to the tendency of cyanide in tobacco smoke to convert a meager supply of vitamin B_{12} coenzyme to metabolically inert cyanocobalamin. As noted earlier, the mechanism of neurological involvement is unknown. Proposed theories include (1) chronic cyanide intoxication; (2) synthesis and incorporation into myelin of "funny fatty acids" owing to competition between acetyl CoA and accumulated methylmalonyl CoA in the biosynthetic pathway of fatty acids; and (3) depression of the methionine synthetase system in nervous tissue with consequent impairment of myelin synthesis.

2. Decreased serum vitamin B_{12} level

Decreased serum vitamin B_{12} level is a decisive diagnostic datum. As noted above, the normal range is 150–650 pg/ml. Clinical signs generally begin to appear when the serum level is below 100. Serum folate is elevated when serum vitamin B_{12} is depressed unless there is coexisting folate deficiency.

3. Methylmalonic-aciduria

Methylmalonicaciduria is a sensitive index of vitamin B_{12} deficiency except in the rare cases in which it is due to inborn error. Normal subjects excrete only trace amounts of methylmalonate, that is, 0–3.5 mg/24 hr. Levels are variably elevated in vitamin B_{12} deficiency, sometimes to 300 mg or more per 24 hr. Vitamin B_{12} therapy restores excretion patterns to normal. In practice, the assay of urinary methylmalonate is rarely necessary.

4. Response to therapy

Vitamin B_{12} therapy of vitamin B_{12} deficiency produces an abrupt reticulocyte crisis that begins several days after the start of therapy (figure 4.9). Reversal of clinical abnormalities then ensues. A partial response follows large (i.e., pharmacologic) doses of folic acid (i.e., 5 mg/day), though the hematocrit is not fully restored to normal and patients previously without neurological symptoms may suffer an acute onset of such symptoms. However, small (i.e., physiologic) doses of folic acid (i.e., 200–400 μg/day) produce no response in vitamin B_{12} deficiency, whereas they produce good responses in folic acid deficiency.

B. Specific syndromes

1. Introduction

Deficiency of vitamin B_{12}, as of all other vitamins, may result from inadequate dietary intake, defective intestinal absorption, abnormally increased requirements, or impaired utilization in the tissues (see table 4.1).

Deficiency of vitamin B_{12} results from *poor diet* only rarely. Re-

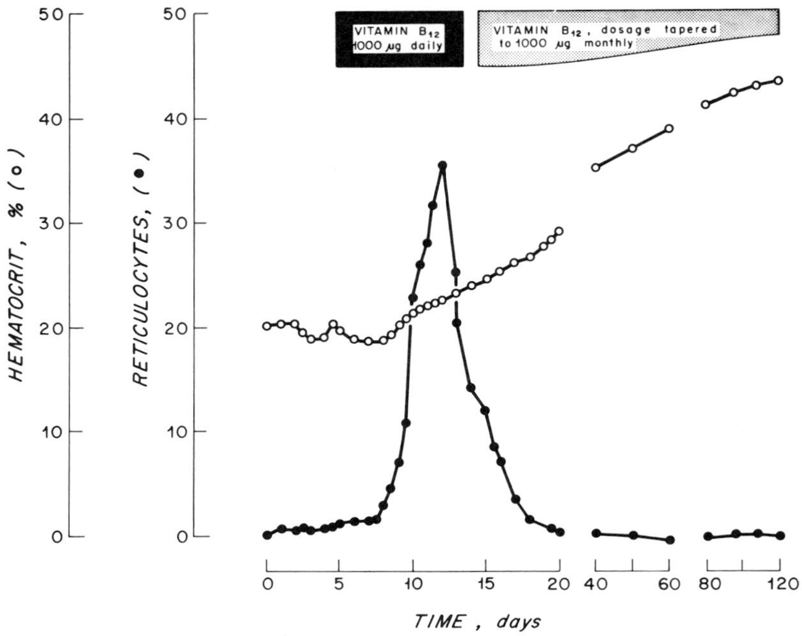

Fig. 4.9
Time course of reticulocyte count and hematocrit level during treatment of pernicious anemia with vitamin B_{12}. (From W. S. Beck and M. Goulian, in J. R. DiPalma, ed., *Drill's Pharmacology in Medical Practice,* 4th ed., New York: McGraw-Hill, 1971, chapter 51)

ported instances have occurred mainly in vegetarians who also avoid all dairy products and eggs. Occasionally it is associated with severe general malnutrition.

Vitamin B_{12} deficiency is most often the result of *diminished intestinal absorption* of various etiologies. The most common cause is pernicious anemia, to be discussed below, in which a gastric mucosal defect decreases IF synthesis. Other and less common causes include: (1) total (occasionally subtotal) gastrectomy; (2) pancreatic disease, in which lack of proteases in the duodenum appears to interfere with formation of the IF-B_{12} complex; (3) overgrowth of intestinal bacteria that occurs in the "blind loop" syndrome, strictures, anastomoses, diverticula, and other conditions producing intestinal stasis; (4) parasitic infestation with the vitamin B_{12}-utilizing fish tapeworm *Diphyllobothrium latum,* a common condition in Scandinavian countries; and (5) organic disease of the ileum that interferes with vitamin B_{12} absorption despite the presence of adequate IF. The large vitamin B_{12} reserve must be depleted before the deficiency syndrome develops. Hence, several years may pass before the appearance of deficiency symptoms after total gastrectomy or cessation of treatment in pernicious anemia. Vitamin B_{12} deficiency due to *increased requirements* occurs mainly in pregnancy, presumably arising from the superimposition of fetal demands upon a background of poor nutrition. No examples are known in which a tissue deficiency of vitamin B_{12} arises from failure of activation or antimetabolites.

2. Pernicious anemia

a. Terminology

The old name "pernicious anemia" (PA) is now reserved for the once fatal condition resulting from defective secretion of IF by cells in the fundus and upper part of the body or the stomach. Vitamin B_{12} therapy makes it quite unpernicious. The term *pernicious anemia* is often wrongly used as a synonym for vitamin B_{12} deficiency, of which PA is but one cause, or of megaloblastic anemia, of which vitamin B_{12} deficiency is one cause. In recognition of the fact that PA was first described in 1855 at Guy's Hospital by Thomas Addison, the term *Addisonian pernicious anemia* is sometimes used to distinguish true PA from "non-Addisonian-pernicious anemia" (i.e., vitamin B_{12} deficiency arising from other causes).

b. Etiology

A genetic basis for PA is suggested by the high incidence of the disease in Scandinavians, a relatively inbred population. Also, minor abnormalities (e.g., achlorhydria) are reported in relatives of patients. The disorder is basically a chronic atrophic gastritis that eventually compromises IF (and HCl) secretion. The discovery that 55–70% of the patients have binding or blocking anti-IF antibodies in serum and gastric juice suggests an underlying autoimmune process. But although such antibodies can block IF function (if they enter the intestine), there is no evidence that they are responsible for cessation of IF synthesis. Also, anti-IF antibodies occur in the serum of patients with diabetes mellitus, thyroid disease, and other diseases in the absence of PA. It is of interest that serum from PA patients often contains antibodies against gastric parietal cell cytoplasm and thyroid acinar cell cytoplasm. Both antibodies also occur in Hashimoto's thyroiditis and rarely in normals. In sum, evidence is still lacking that these phenomena are related to the initiation or perpetuation of the basic gastropathy of PA. Nor is it clear how the process is instigated by genetic determinants.

c. Clinical features

PA occurs typically in 40–70-year-old north Europeans of fair complexion, with one notable exception: there is an unusually early onset of PA in black American (and South African) women, 21% of whom are under 40. There is a slow onset of (1) megaloblastic anemia and related phenomena; (2) neurologic changes (in some but not all patients); (3) other specific signs of vitamin B_{12} deficiency (low serum vitamin B_{12}, methylmalonicaciduria); (4) a striking response of reticulocytes and hematocrit to therapy with vitamin B_{12}; and (5) partial response to high doses of folic acid (5 mg) but not to physiologic doses (200–400 μg). Diagnostic features are (6) achlorhyria after histamine stimulation; (7) decreased vitamin B_{12} absorption in the first part of the Schilling test that is corrected in the second part by oral IF; and (8) increased incidence of associated gastric carcinoma, myxedema, and rheumatoid arthritis.

d. Therapy

Patients with PA require the life-long administration of vitamin B_{12}. Ordinarily, it is given parenterally at monthly intervals after reserves have been repleted.

3. "Juvenile pernicious anemia"

So-called juvenile pernicious anemia includes four entities: (1) true PA with failure of IF secretion, which is extremely rare in children; (2) congenital IF lack, with no other associated abnormality of gastric secretion; (3) production of a biologically inert IF; and (4) familial selective malabsorption of vitamin B_{12} (i.e., absorption of other nutrients is normal) with normal secretion of IF and HCl in the stomach. Presumably, there is a defect of specific mucosal receptors for the IF-B_{12} complex. The disorder is familial (recessive) and is associated with proteinuria. The Schilling test indicates decreased absorption of vitamin B_{12} uncorrected by IF.

SELECTED REFERENCES

Babior, B. M., ed. *Cobalamin: Biochemistry and Pathophysiology,* New York: Wiley, 1975.

Beck, W. S. Deoxyribonucleotide synthesis and the role of vitamin B_{12} in erythropoiesis. *Vitamins and Hormones* 26(1968): 413.

Beck, W. S. Metabolic features of cobalamin deficiency in man (Chapter 9). In Babior, B. M. ed. *Cobalamin: Biochemistry and Pathophysiology,* New York: Wiley, 1975, pp. 403–450.

Beck, W. S. Metabolic aspects of vitamin B_{12} and folic acid (Chapter 34); The megaloblastic anemias (Chapter 47). In Williams, W. J., et al., eds., *Hematology,* 3d ed., New York: McGraw-Hill, 1983, pp. 311–331, 434–465.

Castle, W. B. The conquest of pernicious anemia (Chapter 10). In Wintrobe, M. M., ed., *Blood, Pure and Eloquent: A Story of Discovery, of People, and of Ideas,* New York: McGraw-Hill, 1979, pp. 283–318.

Chanarin, I. *The Megaloblastic Anemias,* 2d ed., Oxford: Blackwell, 1979.

Dolphin, D., ed. *B_{12}*. Vol. 1: *Chemistry*. Vol. 2. *Biochemistry and Medicine,* New York: John Wiley, 1982.

Gräsbeck, R. Soluble and membrane-bound vitamin B_{12} transport proteins. In Zagalak, B., and Friedrich, W., eds., *Vitamin B_{12}: Proceedings of the Third European Symposium on Vitamin B_{12} and Intrinsic Factor. University of Zurich, March 5–8, 1979. Zurich, Switzerland,* New York: Walter de Gruyter, 1979, pp. 743–764.

Kolhouse, J. F., et al. Cobalamin analogues are present in human plasma and can mask cobalamin deficiency because current radioisotope dilution assays are not specific for true cobalamin. *New Eng. J. Med.* 299(1978): 785.

Zagalak, B., and Friedrich, W., eds. *Vitamin B_{12}: Proceedings of the Third European Symposium on Vitamin B_{12} and Intrinsic Factor. University of Zürich, March 5–8, 1979. Zürich, Switzerland,* New York: Walter de Gruyter, 1979.

LECTURE 5 Megaloblastic Anemias II. Folic Acid Deficiency

William S. Beck

I. FOLIC ACID VITAMINOLOGY

A. Historical notes

In 1891 Sir Frederick Gowland Hopkins's classic studies of the pigments of butterfly wings led to the isolation of xanthopterin and leucopterin, yellow and white pigments that were not characterized until 1940 when Wieland showed them to be members of a novel group of heterobicyclic compounds, the *pterins* or *pteridines*. Many pteridines are found in nature as free compounds; the metabolic role of some of them was recognized only recently. Their most important role was appreciated only after the discovery of folic acid.

Converging lines of nutritional research led to the recognition of folic acid and its related derivatives in the mid-1940s. The first began in 1931 with the description of the "Wills factor," an antianemia principle of yeast. Subsequently reported unidentified factors included "vitamin M," an antianemia principle of liver, yeast, and brain; "vitamin B_c," a liver factor that prevents macrocytic anemia in chicks; "Norit eluate factor," a factor that supports the growth of *Lactobacillus casei*; and finally "folic acid," the name given to a substance from spinach leaves that promotes growth of *Lactobacillus casei* and *Streptococcus lactis R*, later renamed *Streptococcus fecalis R*. Each factor was subsequently identified as pteroylmonoglutamic acid or one of its derivatives. In 1948 crystalline folic acid was obtained from liver and its structure confirmed by organic synthesis.

Although experimental folic acid deficiency was known to produce megaloblastic anemia, it was early recognized that folic acid is not the antipernicious anemia principle of liver. Confusion arose early when folic acid therapy was found to provide notable reticulocyte responses in PA. Hemoglobin regeneration was incomplete, however, and relapses and neurologic complications occurred during treatment. Liver extracts active in PA were then found by direct assay to contain little or no folic acid. Thus, it was recognized that vitamin B_{12} deficiency is the basis of the megaloblastic anemia of PA and that folic acid deficiency is a distinctive cause of megaloblastic anemia.

B. Chemical aspects

1. Structure and nomenclature

Folic acid is the trivial name for *pteroylmonoglutamic acid* (figure 5.1), parent compound of the large family of compounds known collectively as "folate" or "folates." The molecule contains three moieties: (1) a pteridine derivative; (2) a *p*-aminobenzoic acid residue; and (3) an L-glutamic acid residue. The combination of the

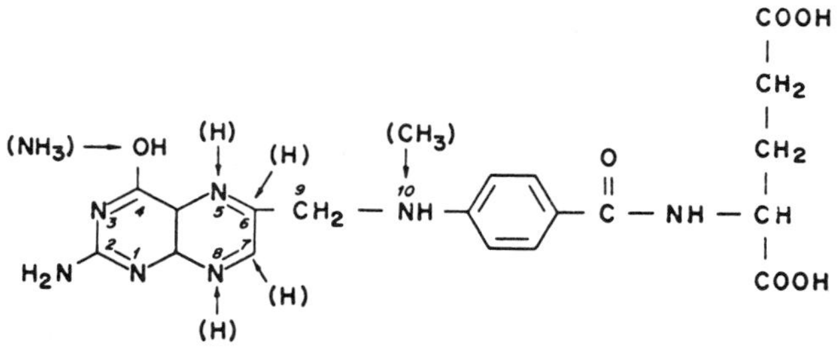

Fig. 5.1
Chemical structure of folic acid (pteroylmonoglutamic acid). Substituents in parentheses are attached to molecules in the several chemical derivatives described in the text.

first two comprises pteroic acid, the systematic name of which is N-(2-amino-4-hydroxypteridin-6-ylmethyl)-*p*-aminobenzoic acid. The corresponding acyl radical is termed pteroyl; hence, folates are pteroylglutamates.

2. Classification of derivatives

a. By number of glutamate residues

Folic acid occurs in nature largely in the form of *polyglutamates,* in which multiple glutamic acid residues are attached by peptide linkage to the γ-carboxyl group of the preceding glutamic acid residue. Pteroylmonoglutamate is often simply termed *pteroylglutamate.* Higher forms are termed *pteroyldiglutamate, pteroyltriglutamate*, and so forth. The synthetic folic acid used therapeutically is pteroylmonoglutamate. Pteroylmonoglutamate is designated by the symbols *PteGlu* or *F* (folic acid). For simplicity, we shall use the latter except in referring to polyglutamates, which are abbreviated $PteGlu_2$, $PteGlu_3$, and so forth.

b. By oxidation level

Folic acid occurs at three levels of oxidation: (1) folic acid (F); (2) 7,8-dihydrofolic acid (FH_2); and (3) 5, 6, 7, 8-tetrahydrofolic acid (FH_4). The reduction of F to FH_4 is a necessary prerequisite to participation of folic acid in enzyme reactions. In this reduction, F is reduced first to FH_2, which is then reduced to FH_4. In animal cells, both reactions are catalyzed by a single NADPH-linked enzyme, *dihydrofolate reductase.* A notable property of dihydrofolate reductase is its extreme sensitivity to folate analogues containing a 4-amino group (figure 5.1) such as aminopterin and amethopterin, later renamed methotrexate (MTX), which are avidly bound and inhibitory at concentrations as low as 10^{-9}M. Indeed, MTX binds 10,000–50,000 times more tightly to the reductase than does its natural substrate. This is a major reason for their cytotoxic action as antileukemic agents.

c. By identity of one-carbon group

The folate family consists largely of FH_4 derivatives bearing a "one-carbon" substituent. Such as compound may be symbolized as "C-FH_4." The varieties of "C-FH" differ in the identity of the one-carbon substituents of FH_4 (figure 5.2). Known one-carbon substituents of FH_4 are the following:

formyl	—CHO	methylene	—CH_2—
hydroxymethyl	—CH_2OH	methenyl	—CH=
methyl	—CH_3	formimino	—CHNH

Note that three oxidation levels of carbon are represented among the one-carbon units (formyl, hydroxymethyl, and methyl) and that only one type (formimino) contains nitrogen.

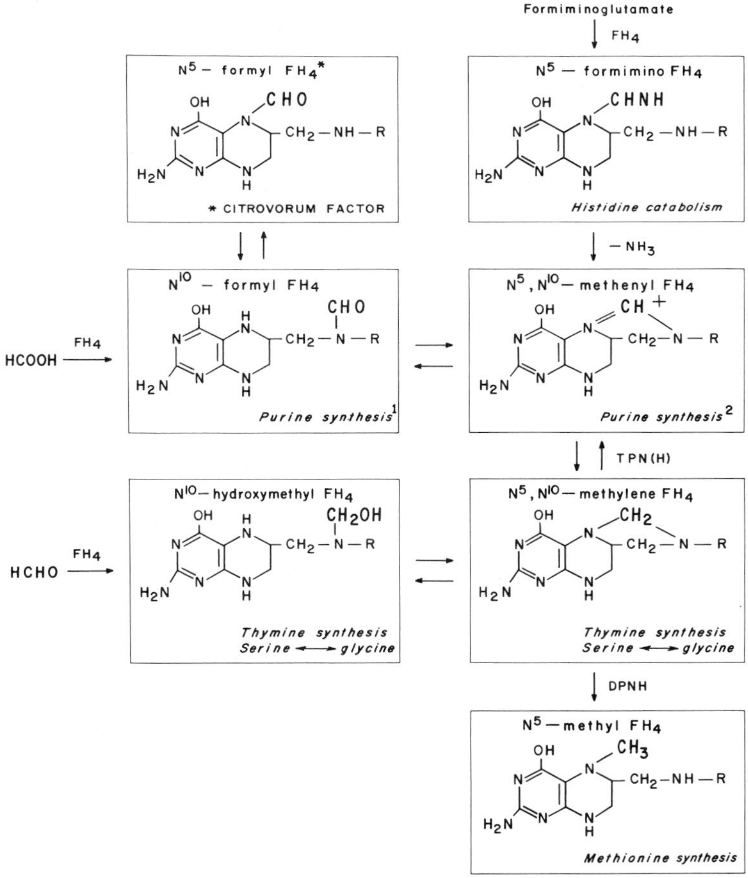

Fig. 5.2
Derivatives of tetrahydrofolic acid (FH_4), their interconversions, and the metabolic pathways in which they participate. One-carbon substituents are shown in boldface. *Purine synthesis*[1] refers to the step in purine synthesis in which 5-amino-4-imidazolecarboxamide ribotide is converted to 5-formamino-4-imidazole carboxamide ribotide; *purine synthesis*[2] refers to the conversion of glycinamide ribotide to formylglycinamide ribotide. (From W. S. Beck, *New Eng. J. Med.* 266(1962): 765)

d. By locus of one-carbon group

It is seen in figure 5.2 that one-carbon units attach to N^5 or N^{10} or both and that specific enzymes interconvert many of these compounds.

e. By degree of stability

Most reduced derivatives of folic acid are sensitive to oxidation in air and hence are unstable, especially under autoclave conditions. A notable exception is N^5-formyl FH_4, a compound isolated from liver and yeast soon after the discovery of folic acid. It was first recognized as a growth factor for *Leuconostoc citrovorum* (later renamed *Pediococcus cerevisiae*) and thus was named "citrovorum factor." (Other of its trivial names are "leucovorin" and "folinic acid.") Prior to the identification of its structure, a relation to folic acid was established by the observation that citrovorum factor levels, low in the urine of folate-deficient rats, are increased by folic acid.

f. By microbiologic activity

Folate derivatives differ in their ability to serve as nutrients for microorganisms. Table 5.1 summarizes these specificities for three important assay organisms. It is noteworthy that the major form of folate in human serum is N^5-methyl FH_4, which is assayed with *Lactobacillus casei*.

C. Nutritional aspects

1. Sources

The many folate compounds are widely distributed in nature. Green leaves are rich sources and presumably the sites of active synthesis. The richest vegetable sources are asparagus, broccoli, spinach, and lettuce, each of which contains >1 mg of folate per 100 g dry weight. Folates are also found in liver, kidney, yeast, and mushrooms. The vitamin is synthesized by many bacteria. Sulfonamide drugs attack bacteria by interfering competitively with the incorporation of *p*-aminobenzoic into pteroic acid, an intermediate that reacts with glutamate in the presence of ATP to form pteroylglutamate. The major product of the natural synthetic pathway is 7,8-dihydrofolate.

Determination of food folate requires extraction procedures that avoid destruction of labile reduced forms. Since precautions have

Table 5.1
Activity of Various Folate Derivatives as Bacterial Nutrients

Folic acid derivative	*Pediococcus cerevisiae*[a]	*Streptococcus fecalis*	*Lactobacillus casei*
FH_4 and most derivatives except N^5-methyl FH_4 (form of folate in serum)	+	+	+
F and pteroyl*di*glutamates	−	+	+
N^5-methyl FH_4 (form of folate in serum), N^5-methyl FH_2 and pteroyl*tri*glutamates	−	−	+

a. Formerly named *Leuconostoc citrovorum*. Citrovorum factor is the trivial name given to N^5-formyl FH_4, a stable compound essential for the growth of *L. citrovorum*. Note that of the three organisms, only *L. casei* is supported by N^5-methyl FH_4, the folate derivative found in serum.

not always been observed, published values of folate content in foods are often unreliable. Also, results of folate determinations are influenced by the assay method used. As noted in table 5.1, for example, *S. fecalis* is indifferent to N^5-methyl FH_4 or short polyglutamates. Unless pretreated with *conjugase*, higher polyglutamates are unavailable to all assay organisms.

An average daily American diet prepared without special precautions and treated with conjugase contains approximately 200 μg of folate by *S. fecalis* assay and an additional 400–500 μg of folate active only with *L. casei*. Values are approximately one-fourth as high without conjugase treatment. The folate in some vegetables (broccoli, lettuce, asparagus) is almost entirely in polyglutamate form. Monoglutamate *L. casei*-active folate activity in cow's milk averages 55 μg/l. Excessive cooking, particularly with large amounts of water, can remove or destroy a high percentage of the folate in foods.

2. Daily requirements

The minimum daily adult requirement for folic acid, or its derivatives, is approximately 50 μg. As noted above, the average diet contains several times this amount in the form of various folate compounds, some of which may be unavailable. Body reserves of folic acid are relatively much smaller than those of vitamin B_{12}. When a subject receiving a normal intake is switched to a daily intake of 5 μg/day, megaloblastic anemia develops in about 4 months. Folic acid requirements are increased during growth, in pregnancy, and, as will be noted later, in a number of disease states.

D. Metabolic functions

In metabolism, FH_4 is a catalytic self-regenerating acceptor-donor of one-carbon units in reactions involving one-carbon transfers from a carbon-containing donor, X-C, to an acceptor, Y:

$$\begin{array}{lllll} \text{X-C} & + \text{FH}_4 & \rightarrow \text{FH}_4\text{-C} & + \text{X} \\ \text{FH}_4\text{-C} & + \text{Y} & \rightarrow \text{Y-C} & + \text{FH}_4 \\ \hline \text{Sum: X-C} & + \text{Y} & \rightarrow \text{Y-C} & + \text{X} \end{array}$$

The metabolic systems of animal tissues known to require folic acid coenzymes are summarized in table 5.2. It should be noted that folic acid coenzymes are in the form of polyglutamates (see below).

1. Thymidylate synthesis

The reaction, impairment of which in human folate deficiency produces major clinical manifestations, is thymidylate synthesis. Methylation of deoxyuridylate to thymidylate, catalyzed by the enzyme thymidylate synthetase, is an essential preliminary step in the synthesis of DNA (see figure 4.6). The coenzyme of this reaction, N^5, N^{10}-methylene-tetrahydrofolate, is unique among folate

Table 5.2
Metabolic Systems Requiring Folic Acid Coenzymes in Animal Cells

System	Related transformations of folic acid coenzymes
Serine $\rightleftarrows$ glycine	Serine + FH_4 $\rightleftarrows$ N^5,N^{10}-methylene FH_4 + glycine
Thymidylate synthesis	Deoxyuridylate (dUMP) + N^5,N^{10}-methylene FH_4 $\rightarrow$ FH_2 + thymidylate (dTMP)
Histidine catabolism	Formiminoglutamate + FH_4 $\rightarrow$ N^5-formimino FH_4 + glutamate
Methionine synthesis[a]	Homocysteine + N^5-methyl FH_4 $\rightarrow$ FH_4 + methionine
Purine synthesis[1]	Glycinamide ribotide + N^5,N^{10}-methenyl FH_4 $\rightarrow$ FH_4 + formylglycinamide ribotide
Purine synthesis[2]	5-amino-4-imidazole carboxamide ribotide + N^{10}-formyl FH_4 $\rightarrow$ FH_4 + 5-formamido-4-imidazole carboxamide ribotide

a. Pathway also requires a vitamin B_{12} derivative (methylcobalamin).

coenzymes because it transfers a one-carbon group *and* serves as hydrogen donor in reducing the transferred group to a methyl group. The reaction generates FH_2 (table 5.2), which must be reduced again to FH, by dihydrofolate reductase before it can again be utilized as a coenzyme. Thus, the following "thymidylate synthesis cycle" exists, in which the hydroxmethyl carbon of serine is transformed into the methyl carbon of thymine as FH_4 is regenerated from FH_2 at the expense of NADPH:

$$\text{Serine} + FH_4 \rightarrow N^{10}\text{-hydroxymethyl } FH_4 + \text{glycine}$$
$$N^{10}\text{-hydroxymethyl } FH_4 \rightarrow N^5,N^{10}\text{-methylene } FH_4 + H_2O$$
$$\text{dUMP} + N^5,N^{10}\text{-methylene } FH_4 \rightarrow FH_2 + \text{dTMP}$$
$$FH_2 + \text{NADPH} + H^+ \rightarrow FH_4 + \text{NADP}^+$$

Limitation of thymidylate synthesis in folic acid deficiency impairs DNA synthesis with resulting megaloblastic transformation.

2. Histidine catabolism

Interference with the breakdown of histidine (figure 5.3) and its catabolic product, formiminoglutamic acid (abbreviated FIGlu), in folic acid deficiency has no morbid effects, but it provides the basis for a test that has been used in the diagnosis of folic acid deficiency. When insufficient FH_4 is present to accept the formimino group, FIGlu accumulates, appears in the urine, and is easily detected. Urocanic acid, a prior intermediate in the same pathway, is also excreted in the urine in folic acid deficiency. Sensitivity is increased with a large oral loading dose (20 g) of histidine. Normal persons excrete little or no FIGlu. The highest levels of FIGlu excretion occur in subjects receiving folic acid antagonists.

3. Purine synthesis

Deficiency of folate also diminishes the folate-dependent conversion of 5-amino-4-imidazole carboxamide ribotide (AICAR) to 5-formamido-4-imidazole carboxamide ribotide. AICAR accumulates and is excreted in the urine in excessive amounts in the partially

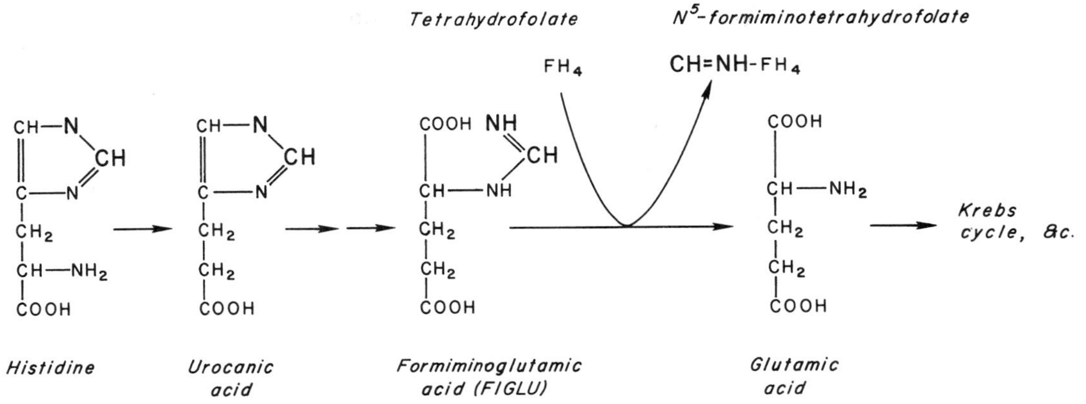

Fig. 5.3
Pathway of histidine catabolism, showing synthesis and FH_4-dependent degradation of FIGlu. (From W. S. Beck, in W. J. Williams et al., *Hematology,* New York: McGraw-Hill, 1972)

degraded form 5-amino-4-imidazole carboxamide. No clinical manifestations have thus far been related to the block in purine synthesis. FIGlu and AICAR are occasionally excreted in pure vitamin B_{12} deficiency, possibly because lack of vitamin B_{12} may depress the vitamin B_{12}-dependent pathway of methionine synthesis in which N^5-methyl FH_4 is converted to FH_4 (figure 4.7). For this reason, some workers have decried the specificity of the FIGlu test. When FIGlu excretion is elevated in vitamin B_{12} deficiency, however, further study often reveals coexisting folate deficiency. In the author's experience, FIGlu excretion is not abnormal in most vitamin B_{12}-deficient subjects.

4 Role of free pteridine

In the light of the metabolic functions of folic acid, it is of interest that the free pteridine, *tetrahydrobiopterin*, has been identified as the coenzyme of the enzymatic hydroxylation of phenylalanine to tyrosine, of the oxidation of long-chain alkyl ethers of glycerol to fatty acids, and perhaps of other reactions, for example, the 17-α-hydroxylation of progesterone. FH_4 is weakly active in these systems in vitro but appears to have no such functions in vivo.

E. Physiologic aspects

1. Significance of folylpolyglutamates

Recent studies of these naturally occurring peptides have shown that (1) all or most cells contain folate in polyglutamate form and contain a *synthetase* for converting folylmonoglutamates to polyglutamates; (2) despite this fact, plasma folate consists exclusively and conspicuously of the monoglutamate N^5-methyl FH_4; (3) the substrate of synthetase is FH_4, not N^5-methyl FH_4; (4) folylpolyglutamates greatly predominate over folylmonoglutamates within cells; (5) folylpolyglutamates exist in reduced and substituted forms even as folylmonoglutamates do; (6) multiple polyglutamate chain lengths exist in all cell types; and (7) although most cells contain folylpolyglutamate synthetase and conjugase, the lysosomal locus of the latter serves to separate these enzymes in the cell.

Folylpolyglutamates (and their reduced and substituted forms) are the active coenzymes of folate-dependent enzyme reactions (e.g., thymidylate synthetase and N^5-methyl FH_4–methionine methyltransferase). In vitamin B_{12}-deficient humans, the ratio of polyglutamates to monoglutamates is decreased. This pattern evidently signifies a failure of folylpolyglutamate synthesis in vitamin B_{12} deficiency. This is probably due to the accumulation or "trapping" of folate as N^5-methyl FH_4, which is a poorer substrate for folylpolyglutamate synthetase. This supports the "methylfolate trap" theory of how vitamin B_{12} deficiency impairs DNA synthesis (lecture 4).

2. Intestinal absorption

The mechanism of intestinal absorption of folate is imperfectly understood. The proximal jejunum is the principal site of folate absorption. Within minutes of an oral 1-mg dose of folylmonoglutamate, material active with *S. fecalis* and *L. casei* can be detected in plasma. Peak values are reached in 1–2 hr.

Orally administered ^{3}H-folylmonoglutamate and ^{3}H-folylheptaglutamate both increase plasma folate comparably. Since plasma contains only folylmonoglutamate, folylpolyglutamate must be hydrolyzed during intestinal absorption. Although such data may not accurately reflect the disposition of food folate, which is largely in polyglutamate form, it does not appear that much of this folate is nutritionally available. Nonetheless, studies with ingested labeled polyglutamates indicate that fecal losses are greater as the length of the poly-γ-glutamyl side chain increases.

The existence of "*conjugases*" that convert polyglutamates (once called folate "conjugates") to monoglutamate has long been recognized. Yet the precise role of these peptidases in connection with intestinal absorption is still unclear. According to one theory, folylpolyglutamate is hydrolyzed within the lumen of the intestine, and the monoglutamate product is absorbd subsequently. Another holds that hydrolysis occurs on or at the brush border of the intestinal cell, with subsequent transport, reduction, and methylation of the monoglutamate. A third theory is that polyglutamate enters the epithelial cell intact, hydrolysis occurring as an intracellular process followed by transport of the hydrolytic product.

3. Metabolism

When a small dose of tritiated folic acid (^{3}H-F) is administered intravenously, 60% is cleared from the plasma in one circulation time and 90–95% is removed in 3 min. The rapidity of clearance suggests either that uptake is active or that it is passive and cells contain binding substances of high affinity—or, perhaps more likely, that folate is both absorbed actively and bound intracellularly. An active transport system for folate is suggested by the slow rate of cellular penetration of 4-amino folate analogues. The nature of intracellular folate binders is discussed below.

Folates are found in all body tissues. The principal form of the vitamin in serum, red cells, and liver is N^5-methyl FH_4; about a third of the serum folate is N^5-methyl FH_2. As noted above, a large portion of the folate in red cells and liver is in the form of polyglutamates. Total body folate has not been measured. That it is at least several milligrams may be surmised from nutritional data.

A portion of folate turned over each day is degraded to *p*-amino-benzoylglutamate and other cleavage products, which along with some intact folate, N^5-methyl FH_4, and citrovorum factor are excreted by the kidney.

4. Folate-binding proteins

Until recently, it was not clear whether a portion of the folate in serum is protein bound. Since serum folate is largely dialyzable (and excretable by kidney), it seemed that any binder must be a weak one that leaves most serum folate unbound. Experiments with high-specific activity ^3H-F and ^3H-methyl FH_4 finally produced evidence of some folate binding by a serum protein. Normal serum binds less than 10% of the serum folate (average, 45 pg/ml) and folate-deficient serum binds greater amounts (average, 333 pg/ml). This elevation appears early in the course of folate deficiency and falls promptly after treatment with folic acid. Such changes reportedly are not observed in vitamin B_{12} deficiency. Folate-binding protein from folate-deficient serum appears to consist of two proteins (or classes of proteins) one with a mol. wt. in excess of 200,000, the other with a mol. wt. of 50,000. Similar material is also found in human milk and lymphocyte membranes. A membrane-derived intracellular folate-binding protein may regulate uptake of folate into cell and serve as a storage site for folylpolyglutamates. The binding protein has many properties in common with β-lactoglobulin, the folate-binding protein of cow's milk.

II. FOLIC ACID DEFICIENCY

A. Clinical features

The clinical picture of human folic acid deficiency includes nonspecific manifestations of megaloblastic anemia similar to those observed in vitamin B_{12} deficiency (see lecture 4)—megaloblastic hematopoiesis, glossitis, cytologic abnormalities in various types of epithelium, elevated serum LDH, and so forth—and the following specific features that make possible the diagnosis of folic acid deficiency, irrespective of the underlying cause: (1) decreased serum folate level: (2) decreased red cell folate level; (3) elevated excretion of FIGlu after a loading dose of histidine; (4) full clinical response to therapy with physiologic doses of folic acid; (5) abnormally rapid disappearance from the serum of an intravenously injected standard dose of folic acid; and (6) decreased urinary excretion of radioactivity following a standard oral dose of ^{3}H-F. Features suggestive, but not diagnostic, of folic acid deficiency in a patient with megaloblastic anemia are (7) lack of neurologic changes of the type seen in vitamin B_{12} deficiency; (8) normal serum vitamin B_{12} and urine methylmalonic acid levels; and (9) a history of circumstances almost certain to lead to folic acid deficiency, for example, poor diet, frank malabsorption, or alcoholism.

1. Decreased serum folate level

The serum folate assay, a microbiologic procedure employing *L. casei* (ATCC 7469), is the most reliable method for the definitive diagnosis of folic acid deficiency, although satisfactory radioisotope dilution assays are now available. A typical range of normal is 6–20 ng/ml. Serum folate levels are low (<3) in folic acid-deficient subjects.

2. Decreased red cell folate

Although assay of red cell folate is said to provide a better assessment of the level of folate coenzymes in tissue than serum folate, the test is not widely used clinically. The normal range is 165–600 ng/ml of packed cells. Folic acid-deficient subjects in one study had levels of 24–135 (mean, 74).

3. Elevated FIGlu excretion

The elevated FIGlu excretion after a histidine-loading dose provides a useful and simple test for folic acid deficiency. However, as noted above, it is less specific diagnostically than the serum folate determination. It becomes abnormal later than serum folate and thus gives a better measure of tissue coenzyme levels. Its greatest usefulness is in subjects taking antifolate drugs, in whom serum folate levels may be normal and tissue coenzyme levels drastically reduced.

4. Response to therapy

The occurrence of a full therapeutic response following administration of a "physiologic" dose of folic acid (i.e., 200–400 μg daily) distinguishes folic acid deficiency from vitamin B_{12} deficiency, in which a response to folic acid occurs only after "pharmacologic" doses (i.e., 5 mg daily). Unlike the patient with PA, who cannot assimilate the needed vitamin from food, the folic acid-deficient patient is likely to have a spontaneous response to dietary folic acid unless the hospital diet is restricted in vegetables and liver. Thus, a long control period, which includes the administration of vitamin B_{12} in small doses, is necessary for definitive diagnosis by this method.

B. Specific syndromes

Major causes of folic acid deficiency, summarized in table 4.1, are considered here under the headings (1) decreased intake; (2) increased requirements; and (3) blocked activation.

1. Decreased intake

a. Poor diet

Because the amount of folic acid in the diet is not greatly in excess of the nutritional requirement and because body folate reserves are relatively small, folic acid deficiency develops rapidly in individuals taking an inadequate diet. As mentioned, loss of food folate through excessive cooking may also cause folic acid deficiency, especially among disadvantaged peoples who live on finely divided foods such as rice. Megaloblastic anemia occurring in chronic liver disease is usually due to folic acid deficiency resulting from poor diet and impaired hepatic storage of folic acid. Nutritional folic acid deficiency is often associated with multiple vitamin deficiencies. In such patients, a significant history of gross dietary inadequacy is usually easy to obtain.

b. Malabsorption

The importance of intestinal malabsorption as a cause of folic acid deficiency was established by investigators using test procedures that assess by microbiologic or isotopic techniques the concentration of folate in the serum, urine, or stool following an oral test dose of the vitamin. These include (1) comparison of the microbiologically assayed time course of urinary folic acid activity after parenteral and oral administration of 5 mg of folic acid; (2) microbiologic determination of serum folate activity after a standard oral dose of folic acid; (3) determination of urinary radioactivity after an oral dose of ^{3}H-F (40 μg/body weight) accompanied by a parenteral flushing dose of 15 mg of unlabeled folic acid; and (4) assay of fecal radioactivity after an oral dose of ^{3}H-F. Each of the procedures has advantages and disadvantages.

Various forms of malabsorption are common causes of folic acid deficiency. *Nontropical sprue* (adult celiac disease) is now recognized to be a generalized disorder of absorption in children or adults that is related to the ingestion of wheat protein (i.e., gluten) or its glutamine-rich polypeptide components. Patients display many signs of malabsorption, including weight loss, iron deficiency, osteomalacia, decreased prothrombin levels, and so forth. The diagnosis rests on (1) clinical evidence of folic acid deficiency; (2) a response to therapy with a gluten-free diet; (3) a jejunal biopsy showing villous atrophy and other changes that are characteristic if not pathognomonic; (4) steatorrhea; and (5) demonstrable malabsorption of folic acid. Folic acid treatment corrects the deficiency without affecting the absorptive defect.

Tropical sprue, in many ways similar to nontropical sprue, is a malabsorptive disorder of unknown etiology with a wide spectrum of clinical manifestations. It occurs frequently and endemically in the tropics—notably the West Indies, the Indian subcontinent, and southeast Asia—and can be acquired by residents of temperate climates who go to the tropics; sometimes it persists long after return from the topics. It may be due in part to deficiency of dietary folate, the malabsorption resulting from secondary gastrointestinal changes. Treatment with folic acid alone usually reverses all abnormalities, including defective folate absorption.

Other causes of malabsorption are noted in table 4.1. Low serum folate levels in patients receiving diphenylhydantoin (Dilantin®) have been attributed to a reversible drug-induced malabsorption of pteroylpolyglutamate. Oral contraceptives have recently been shown to block deconjugation of pteroylpolyglutamate in certain women.

2. Increased requirements

a. Pregnancy

Anemia is diagnosed by unique criteria in pregnancy because the physiologic hydremia accompanying gestation decreases hemoglobin concentration by a few grams per 100 ml despite a concurrent increase in total hemoglobin mass. Large surveys of pregnant women show that anemia of pregnancy is common and is due (in order of decreasing frequency) to combined deficiency of iron and folic acid; combined deficiency of iron, folic acid, and vitamin B_{12}: iron deficiency alone; iron and vitamin B_{12} deficiency; and folic acid deficiency alone. Thus, although anemia is commonly due to multiple nutritional deficiencies, two-thirds of anemic women are folic acid deficient during pregnancy, and folic acid deficiency is the major cause of megaloblastic anemia during pregnancy. Its frequency is attributable to low reserves of folic acid and the fact that pregnancy increases daily requirements for folic acid 5–10-fold, especially in the last trimester. The presence of multiple fetuses, poor diet (a frequent result of anorexia or nausea), infection, and lactation may further increase requirements. An unexplained phenomenon is the capacity of the fetus to take up folic acid (and other nutrients) at the expense of the mother, even when the available supply is markedly reduced. Despite controversy, most workers agree that routine folic acid supplementation is desirable during pregnancy because not only folic acid requirements are increased but clinical evidence suggests an association between severe folic acid deficiency and complications of pregnancy other than anemia, for example, abruptio placenta, embryopathology, spontaneous abortion, and bleeding.

b. Hyperactive hematopoiesis

The requirement for folic acid rises sharply in hemolytic anemias associated with acute or chronic overactivity of the bone marrow (lectures 10–14). Indeed, megaloblastic changes may appear in the bone marrow almost simultaneously with the onset of a severe acute hemolytic process.

c. Neoplastic disease

Moderate to severe folic acid deficiency is frequently observed in patients with neoplastic disease, especially metastatic cancer and the leukemias. The deficiency presumably reflects competitive utilization of the vitamin by tumor cells, a phenomenon that resembles the preemption of maternal nutrients by a fetus. However, other explanations for deficiency in a given patient may be valid, among them poor diet, cachexia, malabsorption, and hepatic insufficiency.

3. Blocked activation

a. Folic acid antagonists

The 4-aminopteroylglutamates Aminopterin® and methotrexate are powerful inhibitors of dihydrofolate reductase that can cause deficiency of folate coenzymes in tissues within hours. Other enzymes of folic acid metabolism are inhibited only weakly. Major toxic effects of these drugs are: (1) necrotic mouth lesions; (2) ulcerations of the esophagus, small intestine, and colon with abdominal pain, vomiting, and diarrhea; (3) megaloblastic anemia and subsequent bone marrow hypoplasia and pancytopenia; and (4) a miscellany of effect including alopecia and increased sensitivity to infection. Citrovorum factor effectively counteracts the actions of methotrexate and is useful in the treatment of toxicity.

b. Vitamin C deficiency

Because the metabolic relations of folic acid and vitamin C are unresolved, vitamin C deficiency merits comment in a discussion of folate-responsive megaloblastic anemias resulting from impaired reduction of folic acid. The anemia accompanying scurvy has no characteristic pattern. Usually, it is normoblastic, due to hemolysis or tissue bleeding, with resulting iron deficiency. Occasionally it is megaloblastic. The megaloblastic anemia appears in some patients to respond to therapy with ascorbic acid alone and in others to folic acid alone. Despite reports of response to ascorbic acid therapy, it is usual for ascorbic acid therapy to be ineffective until folic acid is given. The following data have suggested that ascorbic acid participates in the reduction of folic acid to FH_4: (1) dietary deficiency of vitamin C may cause an otherwise barely adequate intake of folic acid to become insufficient; (2) in scurvy, oral vitamin C augments the erythropoietic effect of 125 μg of folic acid given daily; and (3) in experimental megaloblastic anemias induced in monkeys by folic acid and vitamin C deficiencies, citrovorum factor is more active erythropoietically than folic acid. Such a double deficiency is the presumed basis for megaloblastic anemia in infants fed exclusively on unsupplemented formulas containing dried milk deprived of vitamin C in the manufacturing process. Despite these findings, a biochemical role for ascorbic acid in the reduction of folic acid remains to be established. It is more likely that ascorbic acid increases the stability of FH_4 and its derivatives.

III. MEGALOBLASTIC ANEMIA UNRESPONSIVE TO VITAMIN B_{12} OR FOLIC ACID

Megaloblastic anemia is occasionally unaccompanied by vitamin B_{12} or folic acid deficiency and fails to respond to therapy with either vitamin. In some cases, folic acid or vitamin B_{12} deficiency coexists with megaloblastic anemia but is not responsible for it. These relatively uncommon occurrences arise in three situations (see table 4.1): (1) therapy with an antimetabolite drug that interferes with DNA synthesis; (2) inborn error of metabolism; and (3) refractory megaloblastic anemia of undetermined etiology.

Except for the dysplastic features to be described, megaloblasts in these marrows generally resemble those in vitamin-deficiency megaloblastic anemia. It can be assumed, therefore, that the defect in all is an impaired capacity to duplicate DNA at a normal rate.

A. Antimetabolite drugs

The many antimetabolites employed in the chemotherapy of leukemia, lymphoma, and solid tumors include agents that block the synthesis of DNA, either as a solitary effect or in concert with similar effects on RNA or protein synthesis. Agents that block DNA synthesis inhibit either single or multiple steps in the biosynthetic pathway. We shall consider here only major examples of each class of agents. Notes on their chemotherapeutic applications will be found in lectures 21 and 22. Consideration is also omitted of agents (like methotrexate) that block DNA synthesis by mechanisms that are neutralized by simultaneously administered folic acid or citrovorum factor. These were discussed above.

1. Inhibitors of purine synthesis

The most commonly employed purine analogues are the thiopurines, *6-mercaptopurine* (6-MP), *thioguanine* (6-TG), and *azathiopurine* (Imuran®). Although much is known about the multiple sites of action of the thiopurines and their nucleotide derivatives, the mechanism of their chemotherapeutic effects is not precisely known. For example, (1) 6-MP competes with hypoxanthine for a binding site in inosinic acid pyrophosphorylase and is itself converted to thioinosinic acid (TIMP), which inhibits the conversions of inosinic acid (IMP) to xanthylic acid (XMP) and adenylic acid (AMP); (2) 6-MP is incorporated into RNA and DNA; and (3) TIMP mimics AMP and GMP as a feedback inhibitor of the first step of purine synthesis, in which phosphoribosylamine is formed from glutamine and phosphoribosylpyrophosphate. These considerations suggest that the thiopurines can inhibit RNA and DNA synthesis; they can be incorporated into both nucleic acids, thereby causing malfunctions of the several forms of nucleic acid; and they can inhibit coenzyme formation and function, thereby interfering with cell metabolism. The main toxic effects of the thiopurines are bone marrow depression with resulting leukopenia, anemia, and thrombocytopenia. Before hypoplasia occurs, the marrow is megaloblastic. Serum folate and vitamin B_{12} levels are normal, and vitamin therapy is unavailing. The megaloblastosis, usually mild, disappears when drugs are withdrawn. If thiopurines interfere equally with the synthesis of RNA and DNA, the appearance of megaloblastosis suggests that effects on DNA synthesis are physiologically more critical than those on RNA synthesis.

2. Inhibitors of pyrimidine synthesis

Two groups of chemotherapeutic agents block the synthesis of pyrimidine nucleotides: (1) those that block methylation of deoxyuridylate (dUMP) to deoxythymidylate (dTMP) and (2) those that block de novo synthesis of the pyrimidine ring. The former includes *5-fluoro-2'-deoxyuridine* (FUdR), the deoxyribonucleoside of 5-fluorouracil (FU). The thymine deficiency produced by the inhibitory FUdR (or its in vivo product, FdUTP) on thymidylate synthetase is in part the basis of its chemotherapeutic action. Interestingly FdUTP is incorporated into DNA (like dUTP) in place of dTTP. It is also attacked by dUTPase (like dUTP), as discussed in lecture 4. Consequently when dUTPase levels are exceeded, both FU and U (uracil) are misincorporated into DNA, and both are excised by uracil-DNA-glycosylase with resulting DNA fragmentation. Administration of FUdR produces a mild megaloblastic anemia along with other toxic effects in rapidly proliferating tissues—glossitis, diarrhea, and so forth. Bone marrow eventually becomes hypoplastic.

The second category of inhibitors of pyrimidine synthesis is exemplified by *6-azauridine* (6-AzUR). It blocks the conversion of orotidylic acid to uridylic acid (figure 5.4) and may occasionally produce megaloblastosis associated with the accumulation of renal excretion of orotic acid and orotidine.

3. Inhibitors of deoxyribonucleotide synthesis

Two antitumor agents that appear to act by inhibiting ribonucleotide reductase, the enzyme that catalyzes the reductive conversion of ribonucleotides to deoxyribonucleotides (see figure 4.5),

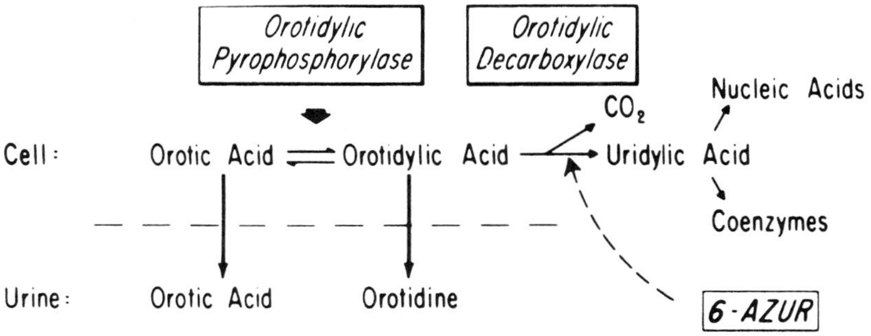

Fig. 5.4
Terminal portion of de novo pathway of pyrimidine synthesis, showing locus of action of 6-azauridine (6-AzUR). Dashed lines indicate inhibition.

are 1-β-D-*arabinofuranosylcytosine* (ara-C, cytosine arabinoside) and *hydroxyurea*. Ara-C is a nucleoside in which the sugar component is arabinosyl, an analogue of both ribosyl and deoxyribosyl. It is believed to block the conversion of CDP to dCDP and inhibit DNA polymerase. It produces severe megaloblastosis that is indifferent to vitamin therapy. Hydroxyurea also produces marked megaloblastosis. It inhibits the reductive conversion of CDP to dCDP by complexing with the nonheme iron prosthetic group of ribonucleotide reductase.

B. Inborn errors

1. Hereditary orotic aciduria

Hereditary orotic aciduria is a rare disorder of pyrimidine metabolism manifested by severe megaloblastic anemia refractory to vitamin therapy, growth impairment, and the renal excretion of orotic acid in large quantities. The disease has been described in several children in whom orally administered preparations of uridylic and cytidylic acids produced clinical improvement with reduction of orotic aciduria. The defect is attributable to a genetically determined block in either the orotidylic pyrosphosphorylase and orotidylic decarboxylase reactions or both (figure 5.4).

2. Errors of folate metabolism

Inborn errors have been reported in folate absorption, folate interconversion (e.g., FH_2 reductase deficiency, N^5, N^{10}-methylene FH_4 reductase deficiency), and folate utilization (e.g., N^5-methyl FH_4-homocysteine methyltransferase deficiency, glutamate formiminotransferase deficiency). Although rare, inborn errors should be considered in patients who are not vitamin B_{12} deficient and who display (1) very low serum folate levels and poor response to oral folate; (2) mental retardation; (3) extreme elevation of serum folate level; (4) excessive urinary excretion of homocysteine or FIGlu; or (5) megaloblastic anemia in infancy. In most cases, the diagnosis is established by enzyme assays in fibroblast cultures of skin biopsy material.

C. Unexplained disorders

There remains a group of disorders associated with megaloblastic transformation, sometimes of severe degree, that does not respond to therapy with vitamin B_{12} or folic acid and that has not yet been associated with an enzyme deletion or defect (but which may nevertheless result from such a defect).

1. Pyridoxine-responsive anemia

The rare disorder of hemoglobin synthesis known as pyridoxine-responsive anemia is discussed in lecture 6. It is mentioned here because about 20% of such cases are associated with megaloblastosis. The mechanism of megaloblastic transformation in these cases is unknown. Since pyridoxine and folic acid both participate in the serine-glycine interconversion (see table 5.2), it is conceivable that a defect of this enzyme induces a requirement for pharmacologic doses of pyridoxine in the absence of which folic acid metabolism is impaired. In attempting to classify these complex disorders, Vilter pointed out that each type is characterized by variable combinations of ring sideroblasts, excess body iron, and refractory megaloblastic erythropoiesis. All are presumably due to metabolic errors—some hereditary and sex-linked, others apparently acquired. Megaloblastic changes are usually confined to the erythroid series. Thus, unless there is associated folic acid or vitamin B_{12} deficiency, hypersegmented neutrophils are not observed in the blood. Megaloblastosis is often atypical with dysplastic features (binucleate cells, clover-leaf nuclei, etc.). Serum lactic dehydrogenase is only moderately elevated. When megaloblastic transformation is severe and extensive, the disorder is indistinguishable from erythremic myelosis.

2. Erythremic myelosis (Di Guglielmo's syndrome)

Erythremic myelosis is considered elsewhere (lecture 19). It is mentioned here because it is associated with severe refractory megaloblastic anemia. Its major features are: (1) abnormal proliferation of erythroid and myeloid precursors in marrow; (2) dysplastic and megaloblastic PAS-positive erythroid precursors in blood, marrow, and tissues (e.g., large multinucleate cells, cloverleaf nuclei) and bizarre red cell morphology; (3) anemia due to ineffective erythropoiesis and variable hemolysis; (4) sideroblastic features; (5) elevated serum vitamin B_{12} levels in many but not all patients; (6) a tendency to appear as a complication or evolutionary stage of refractory anemia, polycythemia vera, or myelocytic leukemia; (7) a tendency to evolve into acute myelocytic leukemia; and (8) a notably poor response to therapy with antimetabolites, vitamin B_{12}, or folic acid. The nature and pathogenesis of erythremic myelosis are as unclear as those of the other refractory megaloblastic anemias. The writer suspects that in these disorders the bone marrow has acquired a hardy clone of somatically mutated cells in which the defect is loss of one or another of the enzymes in the pathway of DNA synthesis, for example, ribonucleotide reductase, thymidylate synthetase, DNA polymerase, or deoxyribonucleotide kinase.

SELECTED REFERENCES

Beck, W. S. — Megaloblastic anemias (Chapter 47). In Williams, W. J., et al., eds. *Hematology,* 3d ed., New York: McGraw-Hill, 1983, pp. 434–465.

Coleman, N., and Herbert, V. — Folate binding proteins. *Ann. Rev. Med.* 31(1980): 433.

Cox, E. V. — The anemia of scurvy. *Vitamins and Hormones* 26(1968): 635.

Erbe, R. W. — Inborn errors of folate metabolism. *New Eng. J. Med.* 293(1975): 753.

Herbert, V. — Experimental nutritional folate deficiency in man. *Trans. Am. Assoc. Phys.* 75(1962): 307.

Hild, D. H. — Folate losses from the skin in exfoliative dermatitis. *Arch. Int. Med.* 123(1969): 51.

Kisliuk, R. L., and Brown, G. M., eds. — *Chemistry and Biology of Pteridines. Proceedings of the Sixth International Symposium on the Chemistry and Biology of Pteridines, La Jolla, California, September 25–28, 1978,* New York: Elsevier North-Holland, 1978.

Lindenbaum, J. — Aspects of vitamin B_{12} and folate metabolism in malabsorption syndromes. *Am. J. Med.* 67(1979): 1037.

Reynolds, E. H., et al. — Anticonvulsant therapy megaloblastic haemopoiesis and folic acid metabolism. *Quart. J. Med.* 35(1966): 521.

Smith, L. H., Jr. — Hereditary orotic aciduria—pyrimidine auxotrophism in man. *Am. J. Med.* 38(1965): 1.

LECTURE 6 Hypochromic Anemias I. Iron Deficiency and Excess

William S. Beck

I. INTRODUCTION

A. Major mechanisms of anemia

As noted in lecture 1, anemia may be due either to increased loss of red cells (as in hemorrhage or hemolysis) or decreased production of red cells. Increased loss or destruction is associated (at least in early stages) with effective erythropoiesis and marrow hyperproliferation, as manifested by elevation of the reticulocyte count. Anemias due to decreased red cell production are associated with low reticulocyte counts. This category includes anemias associated with ineffective erythropoiesis (as in hypochromic and megaloblastic anemia) or hypoproliferative defects of the erythroid marrow (as in aplastic anemia or myelophthisis).

This lecture concerns the *hypochromic anemias,* a group of disorders in which the primary defect is a quantitative decrease in hemoglobin synthesis. DNA synthesis and the capacity for cell division are not primarily at fault.

B. MCHC and microcytosis

Whatever the reason for impairment of hemoglobin synthesis, the main result is a decreased mean cell hemoglobin concentration (MCHC). A useful hypothesis holds that in the course of erythroid maturation, cell divisions continue to occur until the MCHC of the developing cell reaches a certain critical value. In hypochromic anemia, one or more extra divisions may occur because the MCHC is depressed. Since each cell division reduces cell size, abnormal extra divisions yield red cells of abnormally small mean corpuscular volume (MCV). This state is termed *microcytosis*. The converse situation, in which fewer divisions occur, results in *macrocytosis*.

C. Major causes of hypochromic anemia

1. Impaired heme synthesis

1. Unavailability of iron for synthetic process.
   a. Iron deficiency.
   b. "Pyridoxine-responsive" anemia and the several related "sideroblastic" anemias.
   c. Lead poisoning.
2. Defective iron reutilization.

2. Impaired globin synthesis

1. α thalassemia.
2. β thalassemia.

II. IRON METABOLISM

A. Total body iron

Body iron is repeatedly reutilized; hence, daily intake and loss are small. Quantitative considerations are therefore uniquely important for an understanding of iron metabolism and its pathophysiology.

1. Amount

The average adult body contains a total of about 4 g of iron; the range is 2–5 g. For convenience, we shall consider that a 70-kg man contains 50 mg/kg or 3.5 g.

2. Compartments in 70-kg man

	Total (g)	% of total
1. Hemoglobin iron	2.3	66
2. Tissue iron	1.1	33
a. Available, or storage, iron (ferritin, 0.5; hemosiderin, 0.5)	1.0	29
b. Nonavailable, or essential, iron (myoglobin, 0.14; cytochromes, catalase, 0.01)	0.15	4
3. Plasma, or transport, iron	0.004	0.1

B. Nutritional requirements

The minuteness of daily iron losses, revealed in classic studies of McCance and Widdowson in 1936 and confirmed by balance studies using ^{59}Fe, implies that daily iron intake is equally minute. Otherwise the body would accumulate iron.

1. Content in diet

The average diet contains considerably more iron than is needed, though exact amounts are in dispute. Moreover, much of the nonheme iron in the diet is relatively unavailable unless enhancers such as ascorbic acid are present. Typical Western diets contain about 6 mg elemental iron per 1,000 calories. Hence, an adult consuming a 2,500-calorie diet ingests about 15 mg/day. Appreciable amounts of iron can come from iron cooking pots. Despite the seeming excess of dietary iron over need, iron deficiency is common in the world's populations, and many countries have chosen to fortify flour, infant formulas, and other foods with medicinal iron. In Sweden today, 42% of all ingested iron comes from fortification. This and other factors (popularity of self-administered ascorbic acid, use of iron prophylaxis in pregnancy, etc.) have decreased the incidence of iron deficiency but have alarmed those who fear the effects of increased iron intake in individuals with undiagnosed hemochromatosis and other iron-loading disorders (see below).

2. Amount absorbed

A normal individual absorbs 4–10% of the total iron ingested; an average normal figure is 6%. Hence, about 1 mg of iron is absorbed daily. Much work has been done on percentages of iron absorbed from different foodstuffs. Percentages vary notably, being low for eggs, liver, and leafy vegetables and high for muscle, fish, and soybeans.

3. Factors affecting daily requirement

a. Menstruation

Mean blood loss is 44 ml/menstrual period. Since 1 ml of blood contains about 0.5 mg of iron, normal menstrual losses average 22 mg/month or 0.7 mg/day, but in many women losses are as high as 2 mg/day. Menstrual losses tend to rise with increasing age and parity.

b. Pregnancy

In the second and third trimesters of pregnancy, the daily requirement is 4–6 mg. In an average normal pregnancy iron loss is spared by cessation of menstruation (saving = 280 days × 0.7 = 196 mg). But expansion of the mother's hemoglobin mass requires 480 mg of additional iron, and formation of the placenta, cord, and fetus requires another 390 mg. Actual loss of blood at delivery—about 660 ml of whole blood (560 ml in the placenta and 100 ml in the lochia)—wastes 330 mg. Thus the total iron cost of pregnancy (over and above normal basal requirement of 1.0 mg/day) = 480 + 390 + 330 − 196 = about 1,004 mg, or 3.6 mg/day. Since storage iron equals about 1,000 mg, a single pregnancy without supplemental iron inevitably exhausts stores. Lactation also increases iron losses.

c. Growth

Requirements are proportionately greater in infancy (3–24 months) than at any other age. They are also high in childhood and adolescence, especially in girls at the time of menarche.

C. Intestinal absorption

1. Locus

Iron is mainly absorbed in the duodenum and upper jejunum, though some absorption occurs in the stomach, ileum, and colon.

2. Regulation

Since the diet contains 10–20 times the amount of iron absorbed, body iron levels can be kept constant only through mechanisms that regulate the amount of iron absorbed in the small intestine. These mechanisms are not fully understood.

Absorption of iron by intestinal mucosal cells occurs in two phases: *uptake* of iron from lumen into cells and *transfer* of iron across cells into circulation. Ferrous iron (Fe^{++}) in the intestinal lumen enters readily into the mucosal cells of the duodenum and upper jejunum. There it is oxidized to ferric iron (Fe^{+++}), some of which complexes with the protein *apoferritin* to yield *ferritin*. The remainder complexes with *apotransferrin* to form *transferrin*, or a transferrin-like protein (see below)—some of it in minutes, the rest in the course of 12 to 24 hours. Transferrin appears to be the carrier in this transfer process. When the cells are sloughed away at the end of their 1- or 2-day life span, their residual iron is lost with them.

The rate of transfer of mucosal cell iron into the bloodstream is somehow governed by the body's iron requirements. Granick proposed a model, now known as the *mucosal block theory,* according to which the ferritin-apoferritin system in mucosal cells controls the amount of iron absorbed. In iron deficiency absorption increases. When iron deficiency is corrected, absorption returns to normal. The agency that transmits to the cells information on body iron stores is still unknown. Some evidence suggests it is a pool of tissue iron. Many reports suggest that such a system, if it exists, is fairly inefficient. For example, as iron ingestion increases, iron absorption increases, although the percentage absorbed decreases. Also, though the traffic of iron from mucosal cells into the body does increase in iron deficiency, exceptions cloud the picture. For example, little iron is absorbed in idiopathic steatorrhea (despite severe iron deficiency), and iron absorption rises despite lack of need in the disease called primary hemochromatosis.

3. Factors claimed to affect absorption

a. Amount of iron in diet

As noted, the proportion of iron absorbed decreases as the level of dietary iron increases; however, the absolute amount of iron absorbed increases.

b. Form of iron in diet: "bioavailability"

Heme iron, derived chiefly from the myoglobin and hemoglobin in meat, is apparently absorbed by a mechanism different from that for inorganic and nonheme iron. Heme is absorbed as such; the iron is freed of the porphyrin ring after it has been taken up by the mucosal cell. Phytates, oxalates, and phosphates in the intestinal lumen precipitate inorganic iron and decrease its absorption but have no effect on heme iron. Substances in various cereals (bran, wheat, and maize) also bind nonheme iron, as do tannins in tea and polyphenols in spinach and other vegetables. Nonheme iron absorption is enhanced by sugars and ascorbic acid (see below).

c. Pancreatic secretions

Some evidence suggests that exocrine pancreatic secretions depress iron absorption and their lack increases iron absorption. For example, iron absorption and tissue iron may be increased in pancreatic disease. The role of the pancreas remains unclear.

d. "Gastroferrin"

An iron-binding substance in gastric juice has been claimed to facilitate iron absorption in the intestine. Another substance, the protein gastroferrin, is said to bind a portion of dietary iron, thereby making it unavailable for absorption and preventing excess iron intake. In view of these conflicting reports, the role of gastric factors is unclear.

e. Hydrochloric acid

Fe^{+++} is less well absorbed than Fe^{++}, and a great or lessor portion of luminal inorganic iron is reduced in the gut before being absorbed. Clinical evidence suggests that HCl in the gut enhances absorption of Fe^{+++} but not of Fe^{++} or Hb (food) iron. Since inorganic Fe^{+++} is insoluble at pH > 5 (forming $Fe(OH)_3$), it has been postulated that HCl solubilizes Fe^{+++}, making it available for absorption.

f. Chelation

An alternative theory of HCl action is based on its role in *chelation*. Like other metallic ions, iron in solution represents a concentration of + charges that facilitate close contact and ready interaction between molecules. Covalent bonds from iron go to 6 corners of an octahedron. Iron is normally coated with a shell of H_2O molecules that are replaceable by other molecules and ions called *ligands*. Ligands also complex with the several stable and unstable oxidation states of iron. Such complexes vary in stability depending on the ligands. Small changes in the ligand may lead to large changes in the character of the iron complex.

Chelation is a process that results in the formation of stable heterocyclic rings as a consequence of ligand attachment. Simple *monodentate* ligands (e.g., acetate, chloride, NH_3) satisfy only one coordination site of a metal cation and form-charged soluble complex ions. *Bidentate* ligands (e.g., $H_2N—NH_2$) satisfy two coordination sites but not with one cation because of strain. Therefore, there is bridging (e.g., $Fe—H_2N—NH_2—Fe$) and, in turn, the formation of lattices. Other lattice-building ligands are OH^- and $PO_4^=$. When *polydentate* ligands combine to form strain-free heterocyclic rings, the resulting structure is a stable structure called a chelate. For example,

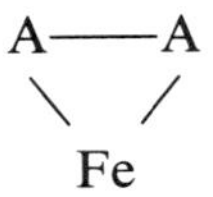

Many such examples are found among the derivatives of hydroxamic acid:

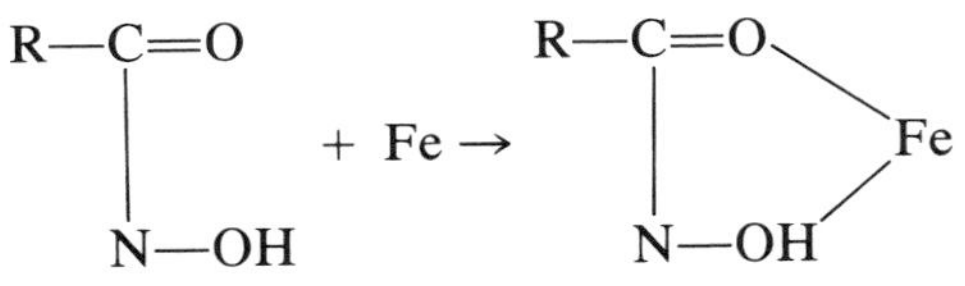

The bacterial *ferrioxamines* (figure 6.1) are, in effect, three linked hydroxamic acid derivatives. The drug *desferrioxamine* (Des-

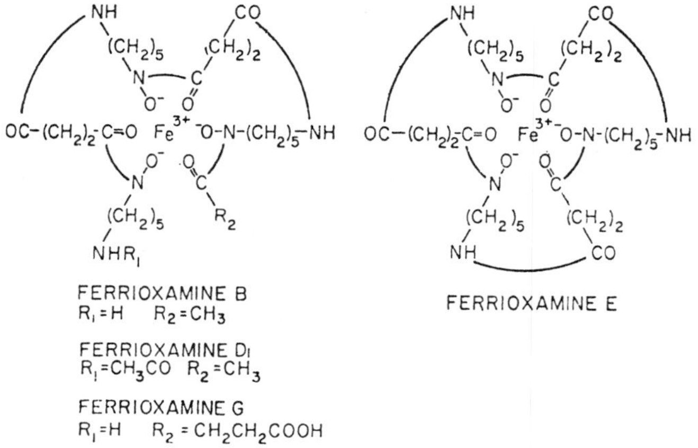

Fig. 6.1
Structure of ferrioxamines B, D_1, G, and E. (From V. Prelog, in F. Gross, ed., *Iron Metabolism: An International Symposium,* Berlin: Springer-Verlag, 1964, p. 73)

feral®), a potent and specific iron-chelating agent, is essentially an iron-free ferrioxamine. The iron-binding constant is 10^{30}.

Nonheme Fe^{+++} chelates readily with sugars, amino acids, and polyols (e.g., ascorbic acid). Some have proposed that iron is transported across the intestinal mucosal cell membranes as a soluble iron chelate. This may account for the capacity of agents such as sugars, amino acids, and other organic acids (including ascorbic acid) to promote iron absorption. These are chelating agents; some are also reducing agents. The chelating and reducing functions of these ligands are both important promoters of iron absorption. HCl also promotes chelation of iron. Once chelates have formed at a low pH, they remain soluble at an acid or alkaline pH.

D. Transport

1. Transferrin

All body iron is combined (chelated) with one or another protein. Plasma iron is carried in association with the specific iron-binding β_1-globulin *transferrin.*

a. Properties

Transferrin is a single polypeptide chain of mol. wt. 80,000 on which are arranged 2 identical branched carbohydrate chains, each anchored to an asparaginyl residue and terminating in sialic acid. The protein is 6.2% carbohydrate by weight. Half-life of transferrin in vivo is 8 days. Asialotransferrin is cleared more rapidly, though early work suggested that asialotransferrin may be an unusual asialoglycoprotein in this respect. Species differences may have been responsible.

Each molecule binds 2 Fe^{+++} ions with high affinity ($K = > 10^{30}$). For each Fe^{+++} bound, a suitable anion must be bound.

When available, HCO_3^- is the favored anion. Although there are chemical differences between the two binding sites, iron binding is essentially a random process, and release of iron to erythroid cells is an all-or-none phenomenon. After much controversy, it appears that the 2 Fe^{+++} are equivalent, the two sites being equivalent as iron donors. However, diferric transferrin is a better iron donor than monoferric transferrin.

The carbohydrate chains may be involved in the binding of transferrin to specific *transferrin receptors* on the erythroid cell surface. When colorless apotransferrin binds iron, the complex undergoes conformational change and becomes salmon-pink. One g of apotransferrin binds 1.25 mg of iron. Normal plasma concentration of apotransferrin and transferrin (combined) is 1–2.5 mg/ml. At least 18 genetic variants of transferrin are known.

Transferrin is required for the growth of many cell lines in culture. It is also a growth factor for fetal cells.

b. Transferrin receptor

Transferrin receptors are found in large numbers on the surfaces of erythroid cells and placenta, both of which have high iron requirements. Receptors have also been found recently on cultured non-hemoglobin-producing cells, both malignant and nonmalignant. Although their iron requirements are low, the density of surface receptors is high. The receptor protein is a glycoprotein of mol. wt. 180,000, with two equal subunits.

c. Physiologic role

Iron that has crossed the intestinal mucosal cell enters the blood and is there bound to plama transferrin (figure 6.2). Normal *serum iron* concentration is 100–150 μg/100 ml. Normal total *iron-binding capacity* (IBC) of serum (i.e, the total amount of iron that can be bound to the sum of apotransferrin and transferrin present) is 300–400 μg/100 ml. Thus circulating transferrin is normally about one-third saturated. Intravenously injected inorganic iron is rapidly bound to transferrin. Since unsaturated capacity for the total blood volume is about 10 mg (3–4 mg is already bound), injection of more than 10 mg iron can have serious toxic effects.

2. Plasma-to-cell cycle

In the *plasma-to-cell cycle*, a transferrin molecule attaches with high affinity to 1 of more than 250,000 transferrin receptors present on the surface of an erythroid precursor cell (but absent from mature erythrocytes). It has long been held that Fe^{+++} leaves transferrin and enters the cell, leaving the transferrin on the surface. It is now known that iron enters cells in two ways (figure 6.3): (1) by an interaction of specific surface receptors with transferrin involving bicarbonate ion that leaves transferrin externalized and (2) by a pinocytosis-like process wherein the transferrin-iron complex is taken into the cell, iron is released, and some transferrin is internalized. The former mechanism is quantitatively more important.

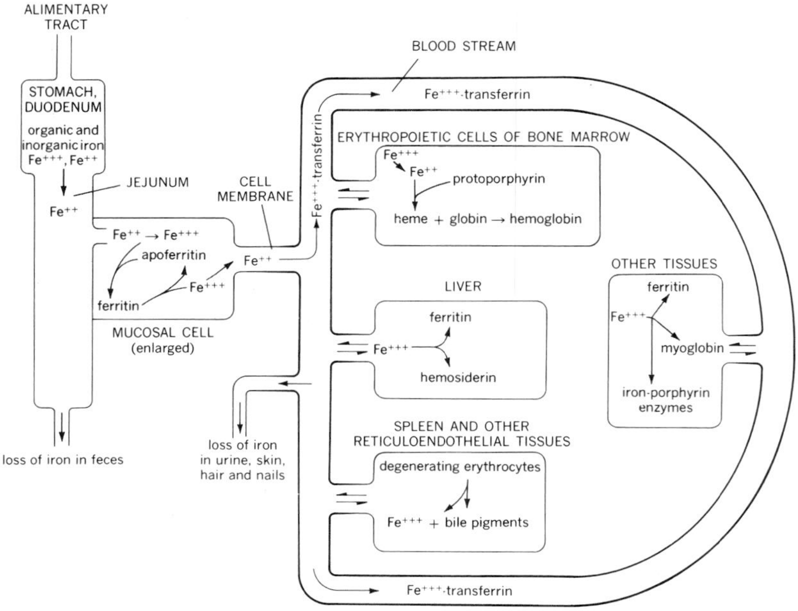

Fig. 6.2
Scheme of iron metabolism. (From W. S. Beck, *Human Design: Molecular, Cellular, and Systematic Physiology,* New York: Harcourt Brace Jovanovich, 1971)

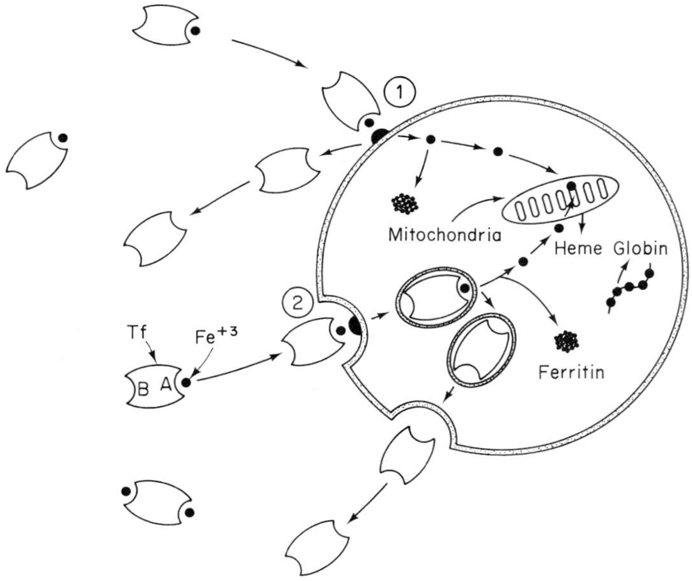

Fig. 6.3
Diagram of the incorporation of iron and the synthesis of heme and globin to the immature red cell. The nucleus is omitted. Two mechanisms of iron delivery are shown. In one, a molecule of iron-laden transferrin approaches a receptor on the cell surface. Binding to the receptor requires an anion (bicarbonate). In the other, there is pinocytosis of the transferrin iron complex. (From A. J. Erslev and T. G. Gabuzda, *Pathophysiology of Blood,* 2d ed., Philadelphia: W. B. Saunders, 1979)

When free apotransferrin is returned to the plasma, it can serve again in iron transport. Developing red cells thus have a specific capacity to extract iron from plasma. Although the erythroid marrow receives only 5% of the cardiac output, it extracts 85% of the circulating iron. The remainder goes to parenchymal organs, notably the liver and, if present, the placenta. Interestingly, transferrin and transferrin receptors are found on the surfaces of breast carcinoma cells but not on the cells of normal breast or benign lesions.

The *percentage saturation* of plasma transferrin is an important determinant of the fate of circulating iron. At low saturation, only marrow (and placenta) can extract iron from plasma. At high saturation, the liver takes up more iron. Plasma transferrin levels rise in chronic iron deficiency and drop in hypochromia associated with defective reutilization of iron (see below). Recent work shows that induction of hepatic transferrin synthesis in iron deficiency is regulated directly by an increase in transferrin messenger RNA.

E. Utilization and storage

Injected ^{59}Fe goes to the erythron and to sites of iron storage. However, labeled iron does not mix uniformly with storage iron, and therefore it cannot be used in short-term experiments to measure pool size of storage iron.

1. Storage iron

As noted above, about 30% of body iron is in storage form. The bulk of it is distributed equally between *ferritin* and *hemosiderin,* which are present in RES cells and parenchymal cells of many organs. About one-third is in the marrow; the rest is in spleen, muscle, and so forth.

a. Ferritin

Ferritin is formed from the combination of iron and apoferritin (figure 6.4). It is a complex molecule consisting of an iron core surrounded by 24 apparently identical spherical peptide subunits of mol. wt. about 18,500. Apoferritin has a mol. wt. of about 440,000. The iron content of ferritin is variable; it averages 3,000 atoms per molecule but can reach 4,500 atoms. Thus, the iron can add 35% to the weight of the protein shell. Ferritin has a readily identifiable appearance in electron micrographs.

Organ-specific and species-specific (iso)ferritins differing in electrophoretic mobility are now recognized. Ferritin iron is readily mobilized by the body when needed, but the mechanism of its mobilization is not clear. Until recently, ferritin was considered an exclusively intracellular protein. It is now known to occur in serum. As noted below, the serum ferritin assay is a new valuable tool for evaluating iron stores.

b. Hemosiderin

Hemosiderin was first recognized as an amorphous iron-containing granular substance in tissues. The granules are much larger than

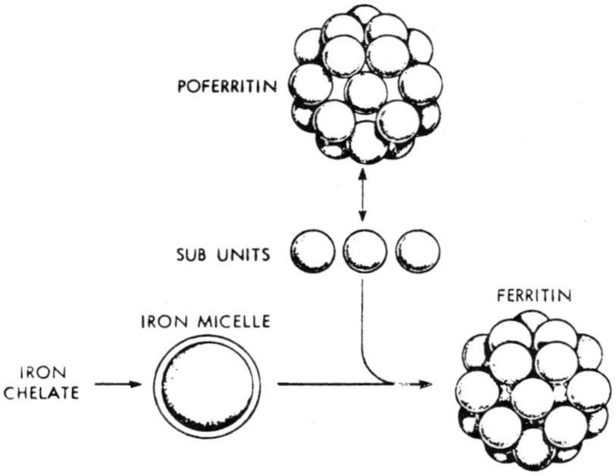

Fig. 6.4
Model showing structure and reconstitution of ferritin. The equilibrium for the dissociation of apoferritin monomers into subunits is assumed to favor the monomer, but removal of subunits by introduction of micellular iron can shift the equilibrium in the direction of ferritin formation. (From R. R. Crichton, *New Eng. J. Med.* 284(1971): 1413)

ferritin molecules and are easily seen by light microscopy, especially when stained with Prussian blue. Hemosiderin is a variable and complex substance formed by aggregation and polymerization of nonferritin micellar iron with natured and denatured protein. Evaluation of the hemosiderin content of liver and RES cells with Prussian blue stain is the best method of assessing body iron stores.

2. Intracellular events

Iron in erythroid cells stimulates apoferritin synthesis. Some of it forms ferritin (figure 6.3). Some goes to mitochondria, the loci of heme synthesis. Insertion of iron into protoporphyrin to form heme is catalyzed in mitochondria by *ferrochelatase* (*heme synthetase*), an enzyme system that requires globin and glutathione (-SH). The scheme in figure 6.3 accounts for the appearance of Prussian blue-stained preparations of marrow. In such preparations, approximately 40% of the normoblasts contain small scattered ferritin granules, which appear to be iron storage depots on which the cell can draw as heme synthesis proceeds. At completion of maturation, the iron has gone, leaving apoferritin. Cells containing such deposits are called *sideroblasts* (or, if not nucleated, *siderocytes*). Absence of sideroblasts from marrow is a sign of iron deficiency. Production of heme and globin within the immature cell is precisely balanced, and a decrease in synthesis of either is associated with a parallel decrease in production of the other. However, iron uptake by cells is not regulated, and iron accumulates abnormally if there is a block in porphyrin synthesis (as occurs in "sideroblastic" anemias). Cells in which such iron accumulation has occurred contain large iron clusters of various sizes that are visible with or without special iron stains. These sideroblasts usually contain much more iron than the normal variety. In the sideroblastic anemias, heme synthesis is blocked. Mitochondria become engorged with iron and burst, producing a distinctive *ring sideroblast* (figure 6.5).

3. Cell-to-plasma cycle

The *cell-to-plasma cycle* follows the breakdown of red cells at the end of their life span. Since 1% of the total number of circulating red cells breaks down each day, the amount of iron liberated from hemoglobin catabolism is 20–25 mg—the same amount required normally for hemoglobin synthesis each day. (Recall that only 1 mg of iron is ingested and lost each day.) Iron liberated from hemoglobin catabolism remains temporarily in the RES cells. As already noted, assessment of their iron content (by an iron stain) is the best clinical assay of body iron content. As this iron slowly leaves the RES cell, it is again bound by circulating transferrin and returned to the erythroid marrow. Thus, the cycle is as shown in diagram 6.1.

F. Ferrokinetics

Kinetic studies, employing ^{59}Fe, are utilized clinically less frequently than the pioneers of the 1950s expected. They are now used mainly for research purposes, though occasionally they are of practical value in locating sites of extramedullary erythropoiesis.

1. Plasma iron clearance

The clearance from plasma of intravenously injected ^{59}Fe (mixed with serum before injection) is a complex function of time, and several different ways of expressing this complexity have been developed. Over short intervals (1–2 hr), the ^{59}Fe clearance curve is approximately a single exponential function, whose negative slope increases when either serum iron is decreased or when erythroid

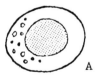

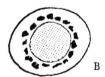

Fig. 6.5
Types of sideroblasts. *A,* deposits of ferritin; *B,* mitochondrial loading with ring configuration.

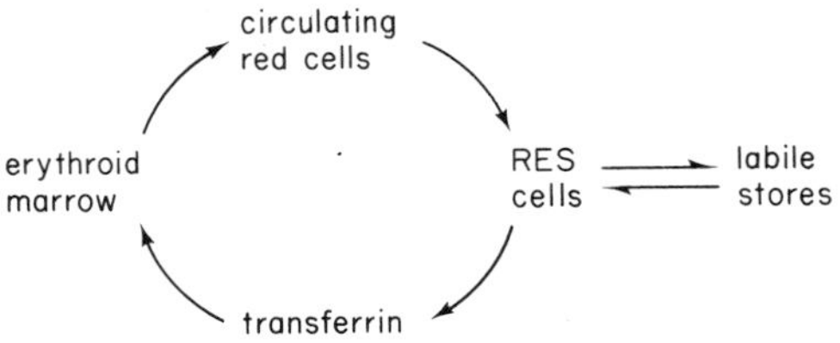

Diagram 6.1

activity is increased. Conversely, it is reduced when the serum iron is increased or erythroid activity is decreased. The normal half-clearance time is approximately 90 min.

2. Plasma iron turnover (PIT)

The PIT is a measure of the total amount of iron leaving the plasma per unit time. It depends on the size of the circulating iron pool (plasma iron concentration in μg/ml × total plasma volume). It can be expressed in several ways (per hemoglobin mass, blood volume, body weight, etc.) but is most usefully expressed per 100 ml of whole blood per day:

$$\text{PIT (mg iron/100 ml blood/24 hr)} = \frac{\text{plasma iron } (\mu\text{g/100 ml}) \times (100 - \text{Hct})}{T_{1/2}\ (\text{min}) \times 100}$$

Normal PIT is 0.6–0.8 mg/100 ml/day. PIT is a measure of iron taken up by erythroid cells and nonerythroid elements. Appropriate calculations permit correction for nonerythron iron turnover. Thus, total *red cell iron turnover* (RCIT) can be accurately assessed. PIT rises in proportion when erythroid marrow activity increases. PIT correlates well with actual red cell production as long as the serum iron remains between 70 and 200 μg/100 ml.

3. Red cell iron utilization rate

That portion of marrow activity leading to actual production of variable red cells may be estimated from the percentage of injected ^{59}Fe in the circulating red cell mass 10–14 days after the injection. This is the *red cell iron utilization rate*. Thus, the PIT may be used as an index of *total erythropoiesis*, and the red cell iron utilization (a percentage) times the red cell iron turnover (derived from the PIT) is an index of *effective erythropoiesis*. For convenience, the values of these parameters are usually expressed in relation to the basal level.

4. Organ localization

In addition to the reappearance pattern and time course of incorporation of ^{59}Fe into hemoglobin, the scanning of isotope distribution over various organs (in the intact subject) permits further characterization of abnormal erythropoiesis by demonstrating specific patterns of ineffective or extramedullary erythropoiesis, marrow aplasia, or hemolysis. The graphs in figure 6.6, which depict the 20-day time courses of marrow, liver, spleen, and blood radioactivity after injection of ^{59}Fe, illustrate these principles in a normal subject and in certain disease states.

5. Serum ferritin

Even though ferritin accounts for only a small fraction of the iron in serum, its concentration is stable and its level proportional to the much larger amount of storage iron in solid tissues. The development of a convenient radioimmunoassay for serum ferritin thus provided a reliable and noninvasive method for evaluating body

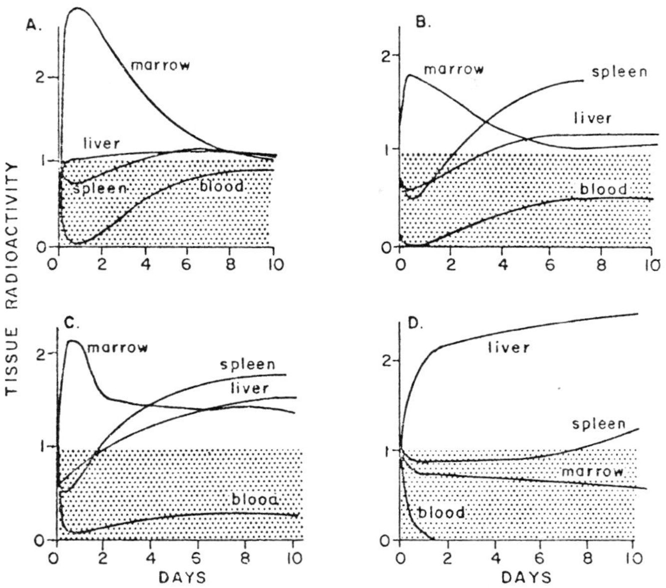

Fig. 6.6
Typical ferrokinetic studies in health and disease. The ordinate value of 1 represents the level of radioactivity immediately after an intravenous ^{59}Fe injection. The blood curve reflects the reappearance of incorporated ^{59}Fe in circulating red cells. If red cell iron utilization were 100%, the curve would reach the 1 level again. *A, normal pattern:* rapid marrow uptake and redelivery of ^{59}Fe as hemoglobin; *B, pattern in hemolytic anemia* (hereditary spherocytosis): rapid marrow uptake and redelivery of ^{59}Fe but less than 60% of injected iron appears in red cells because of splenic destruction of newly formed cells; *C, pattern in ineffective erythropoiesis* (megaloblastic anemia): rapid marrow uptake, but poor redelivery with less than 40% iron utilization because of intramedullary erythroid cell destruction (the other curves suggest splenic uptake of newly produced cells and liver uptake of ^{59}Fe because of high serum iron); *D, pattern in aplastic anemia:* no marrow uptake with 0% iron utilization in hemoglobin synthesis (^{59}Fe is deposited in parenchymal liver cells). (From C. A. Finch, et al., *Medicine* 49(1970): 17)

iron stores. This test along with assays for serum iron and IBC permits a greater degree of diagnostic discrimination. The ferritin in serum arises from the breakdown of iron-containing macrophages of the RES in the liver, spleen, and bone marrow, which derive their iron content largely from senescent red cells.

Serum ferritin levels, in contrast to other measures of iron status such as hemoglobin and serum iron, are usually good indexes of iron stores. The concentration of serum ferritin is about 100 ng/ml in the newborn, rising for about a month to 350 ng/ml, and then declining to 30 at age 6 months, where it remains through puberty. In adults, the concentration reflects the relatively larger iron reserves of males. In one series of men and women from which anemic individuals were excluded, mean levels were 140 and 39 ng/ml, respectively. A normal serum ferritin in most, but not all, instances denotes normal iron stores.

In iron deficiency the concentration is below 12 ng/ml. Concentrations above 200 ng/ml are sometimes (but not always) found in conditions with increased iron stores, such as thalassemia major and hemochromatosis. High serum ferritin levels inappropriate for the level of body iron stores are often seen in malignancy and conditions associated with tissue damage, for example, acute and chronic hepatitis, gastric carcinoma, and other malignant conditions, Hodgkin's disease, and acute myelocytic leukemia.

III. IRON DEFICIENCY

Iron deficiency is a common clinical state in which total body iron is diminished.

A. Stages

Deficiency occurs in sequential stages (figure 6.7). In *latent iron deficiency,* a stage omitted from some classifications, serum ferritin reveals that body stores are moderately decreased although there is no anemia, no decrease in serum iron, no increase in iron-binding capacity, and no decrease in transferring saturation. Free erythrocyte protoporphyrin is normal.

In *iron depletion,* stores are exhausted or nearly so, but anemia is still not present. Serum iron may be normal or only slightly decreased and IBC is normal or slightly increased, so that transferrin saturation is normal or nearly so. However, low serum ferritin levels signify sharply decreased iron stores.

Iron-deficient erythropoiesis (also called *iron deficiency without anemia*) is a more advanced stage characterized by decreased or

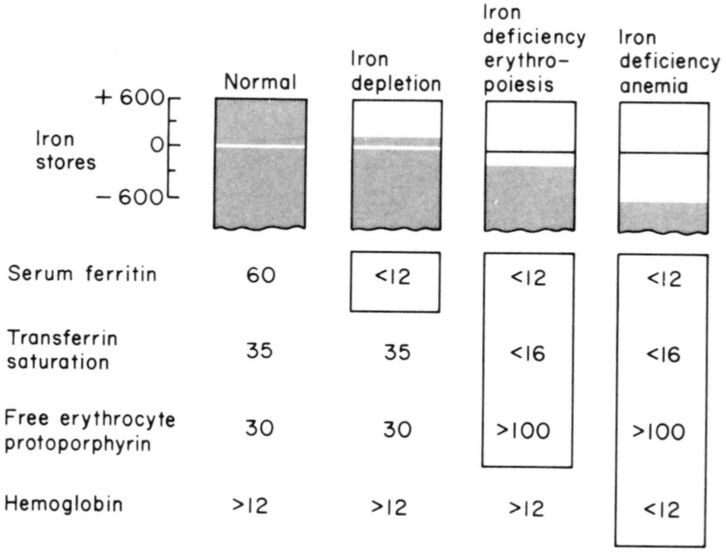

Normal
Iron depletion
Iron deficiency erythropoiesis
Iron deficiency anemia
+600
Iron stores
0
−600
Serum ferritin
60
<12
<12
<12
Transferrin saturation
35
35
<16
<16
Free erythrocyte protoporphyrin
30
30
>100
>100
Hemoglobin
>12
>12
>12
<12

Fig. 6.7
The stages of iron deficiency.

absent storage iron, low serum iron, elevated IBC, and low transferring saturation (<16%), but normal (or nearly normal) hemoglobin or hematocrit levels. If anemia is present, it is mild and normocytic-normochromic. Free erythrocyte protoporphyrin is elevated and serum ferritin minimal.

Iron-deficiency anemia is an advanced stage characterized by decreased or absent iron stores, low serum iron, elevated IBC and low transferrin saturation, elevated free erythrocyte protoporphyrin, low serum ferritin, and low hemoglobin or hematocrit level, with microcytosis-hypochromia.

B. Incidence

Iron deficiency is one of the commonest of medical disorders, though the precise incidence is hard to judge because differing diagnostic criteria are used in population surveys. Many studies judge iron nutrition by hemoglobin levels, but as noted above, this practice overlooks deficient individuals without anemia. Probably 10–30% of the world population is deficient in iron. In underdeveloped countries, it is a major public health problem, severely limiting work tolerance and productivity. In Western countries, it is the most common nutritional deficiency, affecting mainly women, children, and the poor.

C. Historical notes

Clinical signs of iron deficiency were recognized by the ancients; a good description appeared in an Egyptian papyrus of 1500 B.C. of what was probably a case of ancylostomiasis. *Chlorosis,* or "green sickness," was well known to European physicians after the midsixteenth century. Iron salts were used in France in the midseventeenth century along with other remedies, including phlebotomy.

D. Causes

1. Inadequate intake

a. Newborn period

It is most often the result of inadequate iron content of unsupplemented milk diets. Prolonged breast or bottle feeding leads to iron deficiency unless supplemental iron is given. During the first year of life, a full-term infant requires 160 mg of iron for erythropoiesis (a premature infant requires 240 mg). About 50 mg of need is met by red cell destruction that occurs physiologically during the first weeks of life. The remainder comes from the diet.

b. Childhood

During periods of rapid *growth,* diet may provide insufficient iron. Other factors, such as intestinal *parasites,* may also be present.

c. Adults

In order to maintain iron balance, the adult male needs to absorb only about 1 mg of iron daily from the diet; hence, iron deficiency in men is only rarely due to dietary deficiency alone. The major cause in men is bleeding (see below). Intestinal malabsorption of iron is an uncommon cause of iron deficiency except in specific malabsorption syndromes (sprue, etc.) or after gastrointestinal surgery. Half of all patients with subtotal gastrectomy develop iron deficiency in later years.

2. Excessive loss

Bleeding is the most common cause of iron deficiency in adult men and postmenopausal women. When bleeding is occult, it is usually from the GI tract (from lesions such as hiatus hernia, neoplasms, esophageal varices). In adult women, iron deficiency is most commonly due to iron losses in *menstruation* and losses in current or previous *pregnancies* that were never repleted. Internal iron loss in kidneys or lungs occurs rarely. In *hemoglobinuria,* iron is retained temporarily in proximal tubular cells but is lost when cells slough off into urine. It is diagnosed by Prussian blue stain of the urinary sediment.

E. Clinical manifestations

1. General symptoms

Clinical manifestations of iron deficiency are in two categories: those related to anemia and impaired O_2 delivery and those unrelated to hemoglobin concentration, which largely reflect decreases in tissue levels of iron-dependent enzymes. Symptoms also include those due to primary disorder (e.g., an anatomic lesion leading to bleeding). A curious and poorly understood manifestation of iron deficiency is the so-called *pica syndrome*, a perversion of the appetite that leads to bizarre practices such as ice-eating (pagophagia), dirt-eating (geophagia), and so forth. Abnormal gnawing behavior occurs in iron-deficient rodents.

2. Epithelial changes

These have been ascribed to deficiency of intracellular iron enzymes. It was once believed that these proteins were never diminished while stores still contain iron. However, recent work shows that even mild iron deficiency depresses cytochrome *c* levels in intestinal mucosa and muscle. The following types of epithelial changes occur.

a. Angular stomatitis and glossitis

Atrophic changes in epithelium of tongue and corner of mouth are common in iron deficiency. They are more severe in old subjects and in those on a poor diet.

b. Postcricoid esophageal web

Esophageal webbing is due to atrophic degeneration and keratinization of esophageal epithelium with infiltration by inflammatory cells. Such lesions may become malignant. They occur in certain iron-deficient females. The condition gives rise to dysphagia (Plummer-Vinson syndrome) or may be asymptomatic. Not all patients with webs have iron deficiency, but many did in the past. Webs are not common in iron deficiency. Only 7% in a large British series had dysphagia. They are more uncommon in the United

States and are extremely rare in Africa despite its high incidence of iron deficiency. Such data raise questions whether iron deficiency or other genetic and environmental factors cause webbing.

c. Achlorhydria and atrophic gastritis

Histamine-fast achlorhydria is found in many patients with iron deficiency anemia. Many of these have gastric parietal cell antibodies in serum. Proposed explanations are (1) iron deficiency is the initial event that produces atrophic gastritis with achlorhydria; and (2) mucosal atrophy is the initial event and iron deficiency is secondary, being the result of impaired absorption (and intermittent mucosal bleeding).

d. Koilonychia

Flattening or concavity of the nails is seen in severe iron deficiency anemia. Nails return to normal on treatment with iron. Incidence varies in different studies.

3. Bone marrow

Marrow shows erythroid hyperplasia with characteristic underhemoglobinized "ragged" normoblasts. Iron is decreased in RES cells. In severe iron deficiency, megaloblastic features are commonly present that respond to iron therapy alone. This is attributable to the fact that ribonucleotide reductase (see figure 4.2) contains an essential nonheme iron atom.

4. Blood cells

Red cells are eventually hypochromic and then microcytic. A few are target cells. Poikilocytosis is prominent in severe cases. The reticulocyte count is low. Platelets may be increased or decreased.

Iron-deficient children have decreased percentages of T lymphocytes and impaired incorporation of ^{3}H-thymidine by stimulated lymphocytes in culture. These lymphocyte abnormalities may account for the lower incidence of positive skin tests to various antigens.

Neutrophil function is depressed with decreased capacity to kill *E. coli* or *Staph, aureus* in vitro.

5. Other metabolic changes

Serum iron, IBC, transferrin saturation, and serum ferritin are affected as shown in figure 6.7. Other reported changes in iron deficiency are increased catecholamine levels; abnormality in thyroid hormone metabolism (decreased conversion of T4 to T3 in tissues); impaired ability to maintain body temperature; depressed muscle function, probably due to formation of excess lactate, probably as a result of depletion of the iron-containing mitochondrial enzyme α-glycerophosphate oxidase.

6. Therapeutic response

Significant increase in hemoglobin and reversal of other metabolic abnormalities should follow adequate iron therapy (see below).

F. Therapy

Principles of treatment are (1) correct the underlying disorder; (2) administer the amount of iron needed; and (3) observe the response to treatment. Many preparations of oral iron are available.

The usual daily dose is 100–200 mg elemental iron, which is conveniently given as ferrous sulfate, 300 mg, 3 times daily. Parenteral iron is given when the patient is intolerant of all forms of oral iron, rapid response is required, bleeding continues, or when the patient has a gastrointestinal disorder that may be aggravated by iron. In parenteral treatment, calculation should be made of iron deficit and dosage planned accordingly since an overdose cannot be corrected.

Further insight is gained by observing the response to iron therapy. The usual therapeutic dose increases erythrocyte production to about twice normal regardless of the severity of the anemia since production is limited by the 20–40 mg of iron absorbed plus the iron derived from the turnover of circulating cells. Parenteral iron may increase production to about 4 times normal initially, but within a week the response rate is similar to that of oral iron. In following the response to therapy, the increase in hematocrit is a more useful index than the reticulocyte count.

IV. OTHER CAUSES OF HYPOCHROMIA

A. Thalassemias

These are a group of genetically determined disorders in which the synthesis of the α or β chain of globin is impaired. Usually, they are associated with hypochromia and elevated or normal serum iron (see lecture 10).

B. Defective iron reutilization

Strangely this common disorder—perhaps the most common type of anemia—lacks a suitable name. It is also known as "anemia of chronic disease" even though many associated disorders are not chronic, and "anemia of inflammation." In infection or nonbacterial inflammation (as in rheumatoid arthritis or neoplasm), mild normocytic-normochromic anemia (hematocrit in the 30s) is common, though MCV and MCHC are depressed in some patients. The serum iron level often falls precipitously from normal in these conditions, and transferrin synthesis in the liver may be depressed. Therefore the serum IBC falls slowly over a period of weeks. Serum iron is low, averaging 30 but ranging from 10 to 70 μg/100 ml; IBC is moderately depressed, averaging 200 μg/100 ml. Thus saturation is 10–25%. Ferrokinetic studies show a PIT of 1–2 times normal. This pattern is diagnostically helpful as it contrasts with the raised transferrin level of uncomplicated iron deficiency, but often there is difficulty in its interpretation. Serum ferritin levels are often helpful in distinguishing this situation from iron deficiency. A normal or elevated ferritin concentration excludes inadequate iron stores and may obviate the need for a bone marrow examination. A depressed ferritin concentration signifies depressed iron stores and justifies iron therapy. However, as noted, serum ferritin may be raised in acute or chronic liver disease and in infectious and malignant conditions. Where doubt remains, the most reliable test of iron deficiency is still a Prussian blue stain of bone marrow aspirate.

This is a complex disorder in which at least three mechanisms play a variable role. The major mechanism is a decrease in the iron supply for hemoglobin synthesis due to an unexplained block in the release and reutilization of iron from the RES cell. There results an increase in stainable RES iron, depressed plasma iron and transferrin saturation, a decrease in sideroblasts, an increase in red cell protoporphyrin, and mild hypochromia of circulating red cells. A second mechanism is moderately increased destruction of circulating red cells, sometimes complicated by such events as intravascular fragmentation associated with vasculitis and/or intravascular clotting. The reduction in the rate of cell survival increases the iron requirements of the erythroid marrow and thereby accentuates the consequences of the block in iron release. A third mechanism, less well documented, is an inappropriately low level of erythropoietin production, which is unexplained. One theory has been the low levels of thyroid hormones in starvation, inflammation, and infection.

V. IRON OVERLOAD

Iron overload (iron-loading disorders) is a state in which total body iron is increased.

A. Causes

1. Inappropriate increase in intestinal absorption of iron.
   a. Idiopathic hemochromatosis.
   b. Various iron-loading anemias (sideroblastic anemias, thalassemia).
2. Grossly excessive oral administration of iron over a prolonged period.
   a. Excessive medicinal iron.
   b. South African Bantus (who ingest 100–200 mg of iron daily in beer and food cooked in iron pots).
3. Excessive blood transfusion (in patients with chronic bone marrow failure).

B. Specific disorders

1. Hemochromatosis

Idiopathic hemachromatosis is an inherited iron-loading disease associated with increased intestinal absorption of iron.

a. Description

Clinical features, although not pathognomonic, include lethargy, weight loss, loss of libido, abdominal pain, joint pain, and symptoms related to the onset of diabetes. Prominent physical signs include a darkened skin color, hepatomegaly, testicular atrophy, loss of body hair, arthropathy, and heart failure. An early manifestation in young adults may be cardiac failure. A family history of liver disease, hepatocellular carcinoma, or idiopathic hemochromatosis strongly suggests the diagnosis of idiopathic hemochromatosis in a given patient.

b. Diagnosis

Diagnostic criteria include demonstration of increased total body iron stores in parenchymal locations and evidence of tissue damage. IBC and serum ferritin levels are increased. Parenchymal distribution of iron, as distinguished from RES overload (as occurs in various anemias), is suggested by the presence of >4 mg of iron in a 24-hr urine collection after the intramuscular injection of 0.5 gm of desferrioxamine (in subjects with normal renal function). Liver biopsy definitively confirms the increase in parenchymal iron and permits assessment of tissue damage. The major diagnostic problem is in distinguishing idiopathic hemochromatosis and alcoholic liver disease with excess hepatic iron. It was once thought that a minor degree of stainable hepatic iron indicates excess body iron stores. Now it is recognized that stainable iron is common in normal and cirrhotic livers. Those with alcoholic cirrhosis and increased stainable iron include patients with (1) relatively normal iron stores whose liver iron concentration does not exceed twice the upper limit of normal and (2) markedly increased total body iron stores. The majority of such patients probably have idiopathic hemochromatosis as well as alcoholism. Only in these subjects is phlebotomy of benefit. When diagnosis is in doubt, iron stores should be assessed by phlebotomy and family members should be studied.

c. Therapy

Removal of iron by repeated phlebotomy has modified the prognosis and clinical course of idiopathic hemochromatosis. Aside from cardiac death in the early phase of treatment, mortality is now due chiefly to late hepatoma.

2. Sideroblastic anemias

This heterogeneous group of confusingly named chronic disorders is marked by diverse clinical and biochemical manifestations that reflect multiple underlying pathogenetic mechanisms. All are characterized by iron loading and hypochromic anemia.

a. Description

The majority of patients with sideroblastic anemia display the following features: (1) anemia, either hypochromic or dimorphic; (2) erythroid hyperplasia of the marrow, often with varying degrees of megaloblastic change, and clear evidence of sideroblastic features (i.e., significant number of ring sideroblasts); (3) increased iron stores in the RES cells (nearly always present); (4) hyperferremia with an increase in percentage saturation of transferrin; (5) increased PIT with subnormal red cell iron utilization; (6) decreased levels of various enzymes in mitochondria of erythroid precursors; and (7) hematologic response to pyridoxine therapy in a few cases.

b. Classification

1. Refractory sideroblastic anemias (primary, idiopathic).
   a. Hereditary (sex-linked hypochromic anemia).
   b. Acquired.
2. Reversible sideroblastic anemias (secondary).
   a. Toxins, drugs, ethanol, lead, and so forth.
   b. Other diseases (lymphoma, myeloma, myeloproliferative disease, etc.).
3. Pyridoxine-responsive anemia.

VI. ACUTE IRON POISONING

Iron poisoning is one of the commonest causes of fatal poisoning in young children who find and ingest an excessive quantity of therapeutic iron. The major clinical features are as follows: (1) a sequence of stages with abdominal disturbance followed by apparent improvement followed by shock, coma, and death; (2) metabolic acidosis and hypovolemia; and (3) extreme elevation of serum iron. Desferrioxamine therapy may be life saving. Desferrioxamine is also useful in diminishing tissue ferritin and hemosiderin in the various iron-loading disorders, if given in adequate doses and by continuous pump infusion.

SELECTED REFERENCES

Aisen, P., and Brown, E. B. — Structure and function of transferrin. *Prog. Hematol.* 9(1975): 25.

Aoki, Y. — Multiple enzymatic defects in mitochondria in hematological cells of patients with primary sideroblastic anemia. *J. Clin. Invest.* 66(1980): 43.

Bothwell, T. H., et al. — *Iron Metabolism in Man,* Oxford: Blackwell, 1979.

Charlton, R. W., and Bothwell, T. H. — Iron absorption. *Ann. Rev. Med.* 34(1983): 55.

Cook, J. D., and Finch, C. A. — Assessing iron status of a population. *Amer. J. Clin. Nutr.* 32(1979): 2115.

Crosby, W. H. — Pica: A compulsion caused by iron deficiency. *Brit. J. Haematol.* 34(1976): 341.

Hallberg, L., et al. — An analysis of factors leading to a reduction in iron deficiency in Swedish women. *Bull. World Health Org.* 57(1979): 947.

Halliday, J. W., and Powell, J. W. — Serum ferritin and isoferritins in clinical medicine. *Prog. Hematol.* 11(1979): 229.

Harris, J. W., and Kellermeyer, R. W. — Iron metabolism and iron-lack anemia (Chapter 2). In *The Red Cell—Production, Metabolism, Destruction: Normal and Abnormal,* rev. ed., Cambridge, MA: Harvard University Press, 1970, pp. 64–148.

Jacobs, A., and Worwood, M. *Iron in Biochemistry and Medicine,* New York: Academic Press, 1974.

Lee, G. R. The anaemia of chronic disease. *Semin. Hematol.* 20(1983): 61.

Modell, B. Advances in the use of iron-chelating agents for the treatment of iron overload. *Prog. Hematol.* 11(1979): 267.

Muller-Eberhard, U., ed. Iron excess: Aberrations of iron and porphyrin metabolism. *Semin. Hematol.* 14(1977): 1–262.

Seligman, P. A. Structure and function of the transferrin receptor. *Prog. Hematol.* 13(1983): 131.

LECTURE 7 Hypochromic Anemias II. Heme Metabolism and the Porphyrias

Stephen H. Robinson

I. HEME BIOSYNTHESIS

A. Normal pathways

Porphyrinogens, porphyrins, and *heme* are comprised of a ring of four pyrrole nuclei. Degradation of heme, with cleavage of the α-methene bridge, leads to the linear tetrapyrrole structure of the bile pigments (figure 7.1).

1. Site of synthesis

Most heme is synthesized as the prosthetic group of hemoglobin in erythroid precursors in bone marrow. However, some heme formation occurs in virtually all tissues (cytochromes, catalase and other heme enzymes, myoglobin, etc.). Liver is the second most important site of porphyrin and heme synthesis.

2. Sequence of biosynthetic steps

Formation of δ-*aminolevulinic acid* (ALA) from glycine and succinyl CoA is the major rate-limiting step in heme biosynthesis. This is mediated by the mitochondrial enzyme *ALA synthetase*. It is regulated by end-product repression and possibly also direct end-product inhibition by heme. It requires pyridoxal phosphate as a cofactor and is linked to aerobic metabolism via the Krebs cycle intermediate succinyl CoA.

The pyrrole *porphobilinogen* (PBG) is fomed by a condensation

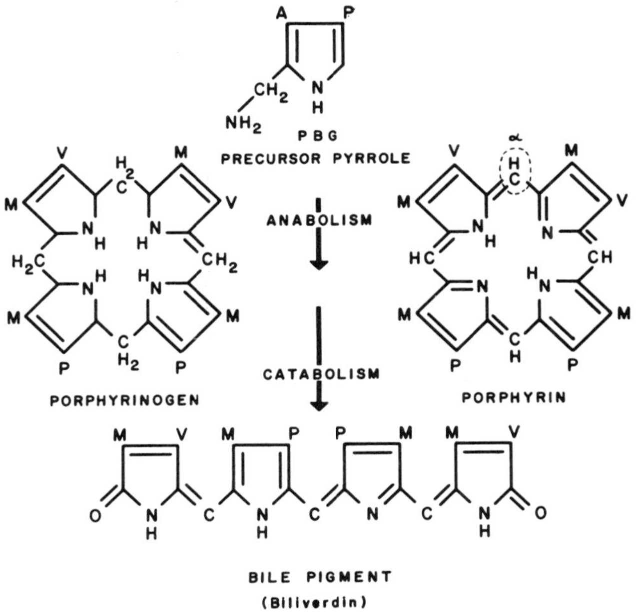

Fig. 7.1
Structure of porphobilinogen, protoporphyrinogen, protoporphyrin, and biliverdin. Bile pigment is formed by cleavage of the α-methene bridge in Fe-protophorphyrin (heme).

of 2 ALAs that is catalyzed by ALA dehydrase. PBG yields a red color when tested with Ehrlich's aldehyde reagent (*p*-dimethylaminobenzaldehyde). The color is not extractable into either chloroform or butanol. These procedures comprise the modified *Watson-Schwartz test*. A positive test in urine is characteristic of acute intermittent porphyria. *Uroporphyrinogen* (UROgen) is formed by condensation of 4 PBGs. In the presence of only *UROgen synthetase,* the isomer UROgen I is formed. As shown in figure 7.2, this is a blind alley since heme is derived only from the UROgen III isomer. Normally, when UROgen synthetase and *UROgen cosynthetase* are both present, virtually all UROgen is of the type III isomer. This intermediate is then converted to heme.

Coproporphyrinogen (COPROgen) is formed from UROgen by decarboxylation of the acetic acid side chains to methyl groups on each pyrrole nucleus. *Protoporphyrinogen* (PROTOgen) is formed from COPROgen III by oxidation of the propionic acid side chains on the two topmost pyrroles to vinyl groups. Because PROTOgen has 3 types of side chain (methyl, propionic acid, and vinyl), there are 15 possible isomers of PROTOgen, as compared to only 4 for UROgen and COPROgen. PROTOgen 9 is formed from COPROgen III. Porphyrinogens, not porphyrins, are the physiologic intermediates in heme biosynthesis. Porphyrinogens are reduced, unstable, colorless tetrapyrroles that are readily and irreversibly oxidized to porphyrins. Porphyrins are resonating molecules (see figure 7.1), with alternating single and double bonds. Largely because of this property, they are colored (red), fluoresce (red) in UV light, and are highly stable. Normally, little porphyrin is formed. However, porphyrins are formed when excess porphyrinogen production occurs, as in many of the *porphyrias*.

Once formed, porphyrins cannot be rereduced to porphyrinogens. They are lost from the heme biosynthetic pathway and are excreted in bile or urine. The single exception is *protoporphyrin* (PROTO) 9, which is formed physiologically from PROTOgen 9 in the presence of the enzyme *PROTOgen oxidase*. PROTO 9 is then chelated with iron under the influence of the enzyme *ferrochelatase* (*heme synthetase*) to yield heme. When formed in excess, PROTO is excreted via the bile into the feces. *Coproporphyrin* (COPRO) is found mainly in the feces, but some occurs in urine when produced in excess. *Uroporphyrin* (URO) is found primarily in urine.

Like ALA synthetase, ferrochelatase, PROTOgen oxidase, and COPROgen oxidase are mitochondrial enzymes. The physical proximity of these enzymes perhaps facilitates direct end-product inhibition of ALA synthetase by heme. The intermediate biosynthetic reactions occur in the soluble fraction of the cell. In erythroid but not hepatic cells, ferrochelatase, in addition to ALA synthetase, has a major regulatory role in heme biosynthe-

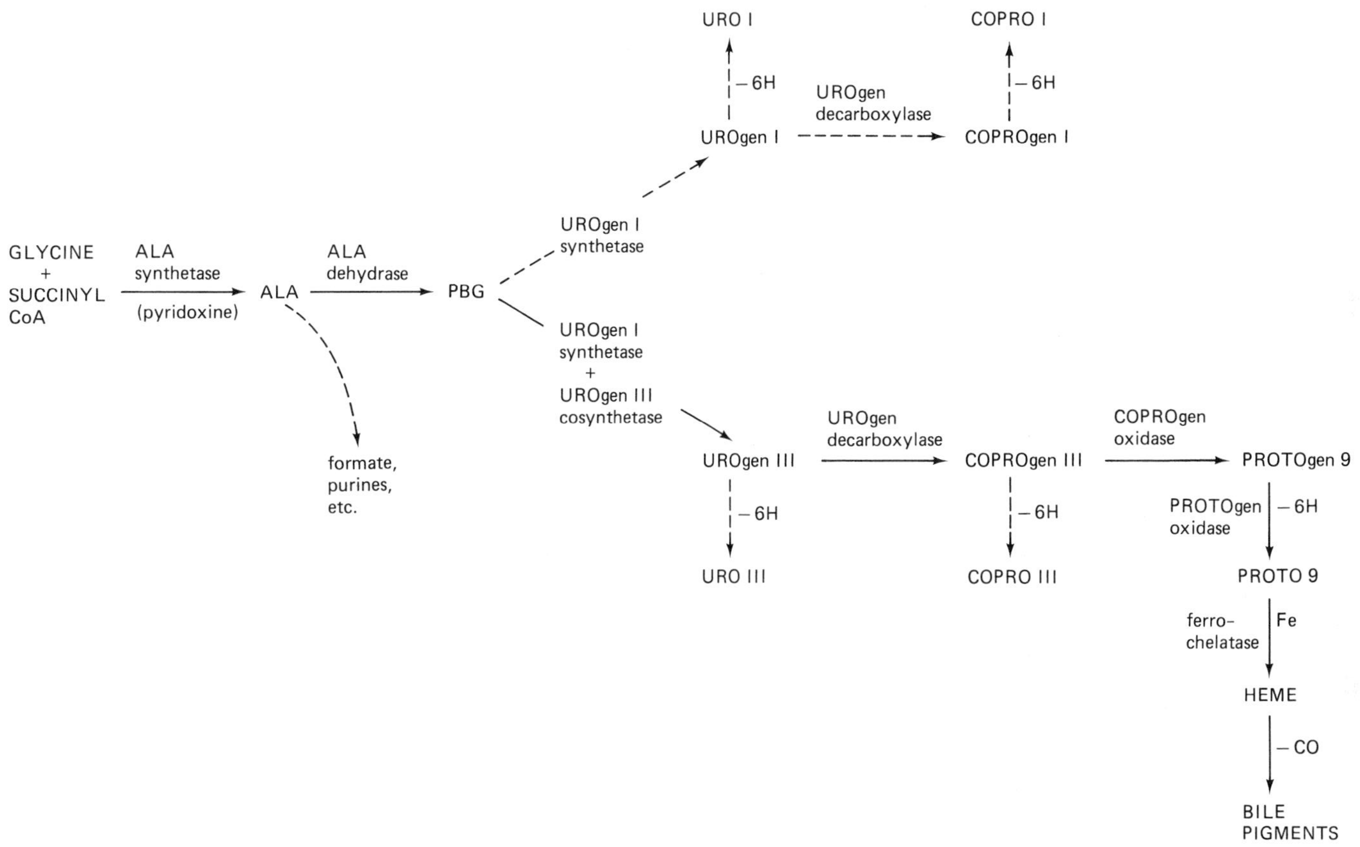

Fig. 7.2
Pathway of heme biosynthesis. Heavy lines refer to the main biosynthetic pathway. Dashed lines refer to potential detours or blind alleys from this route.

sis. Heme is the prosthetic group of hemoglobin, myoglobins, catalase, the cytochromes, and certain other enzymes.

B. Defects in heme biosynthesis

1. Hypochromic anemias

These anemias, resulting from impaired synthesis of heme or hemoglobin, are discussed in lecture 6. In the light of the foregoing discussion concerning the major locus of heme synthesis, it is of interest that iron-laden mitochondria are the basis of the ring sideroblast of sideroblastic anemia.

2. Porphyrias

a. Pathophysiology

Porphyrias are characterized not by decreased heme synthesis or hypochromia but by *overproduction of prophyrins* and/or the porphyrin precursors ALA and PGB (see table 7.1). These disorders are due to partial blocks at one or another step in the biosynthetic pathway. Heme synthesis remains normal either because these steps are not rate limiting or because of a negative feedback loop that involves heme and ALA synthetase. Excessive production of porphyrin or porphyrin precursor originates in either the *bone marrow* (erythropoietic porphyria) or the *liver* (hepatic porphyria), the two major sites of heme biosynthesis. Many patients with different types of porphyria have the biochemical abnormalities unaccompanied by clinical symptoms. These are considered to have "latent" porphyria.

Increased activity of the rate-controlling enzyme ALA synthetase has been found in many forms of *hepatic porphyria*. In *acute intermittent porphyria* (AIP), this is due to a decrease in UROgen synthetase, which potentially limits heme synthesis. In this disorder and in *coproporphyria* and *variegate porphyria*, the enzyme deficiencies are not truly limiting (see table 7.1), and ALA synthetase activity is normal but "sensitized" to induction by drugs, glucose deprivation, or other factors. The resulting increase in ALA synthetase activity accounts for the excessive production of ALA and PBG that is characteristic of acute attacks of hepatic porphyria, which has been termed the "precursor syndrome."

b. Relation to drugs

Barbiturates, griseofulvin, sulfonamides, stilbestrol, and many other agents may precipitate attacks of AIP in persons with latent AIP, variegate porphyria, or coproporphyria, or they may exacerbate the disorder in symptomatic patients with these disorders. Most of these drugs act by increasing the activity of hepatic ALA synthetase, which is already enhanced or sensitized because of an underlying defect in heme synthesis. Hexachlorobenzene has caused *porphyria cutanea tarda* in normal subjects by inhibiting UROgen decarboxylase activity in the liver.

c. Glucose effect

Glucose blocks the induction of ALA synthetase in the liver. A high carbohydrate diet prevents the chemical induction of hepatic porphyria in experimental animals and is used with partial success in the treatment of patients with acute hepatic porphyrias. Conversely starvation, as with intercurrent illness, may precipitate clinical attacks.

d. Clinical features

There are two general forms of porphyria. In *true porphyrias,* excessive production of porphyrins is associated with photosensitivity and dermatitis. These symptoms result from the fluorescence of porphyrins in skin, which leads to photooxidative and photocatalytic effects. Hemolytic anemia in congenital erythropoietic porphyria is presumably related to fluorescence of porphyrins in and around erythrocytes. Urine is red if there is an excess of uroporphyrin.

In *precursor syndromes* (e.g., acute intermittent porphyria) excessive production of the porphyrin precursors ALA and PBG, as the result of increased ALA synthetase activity, is associated with bizarre neurologic and endocrinologic abnormalities. The pathophysiology is still unclear, although excess ALA may be toxic to nerve tissue. There is no photosensitivity or red urine in the absence of an excess of true porphyrins.

e. Genetics

Most porphyrias are inherited abnormalities. However, the following acquired forms occur: (1) Lead intoxication is associated with excessive production of ALA and coproporphyrin, of unknown significance in the genesis of clinical symptoms that may resemble those of AIP (abdominal colic, neuropathy, encephalopathy, etc.). (2) Porphyria cutanea tarda apparently develops as the result of alcoholic liver disease (with iron loading) or in response to certain drugs (e.g., estrogens). However, it now appears that many of these patients have a latent genetic defect (decreased UROgen decarboxylase activity), which is made overt by the liver dysfunction or the drug. (3) Hexachlorobenzene can cause a true acquired form of porphyria cutanea tarda, as demonstrated in a famous outbreak in the 1950s in Turkey, where this drug was being used as a fungicide in grain.

II. HEME DEGRADATION AND BILE PIGMENT PRODUCTION

A. Normal pathways

Bile pigments include biliverdin, bilirubin, urobilinogen, urobilin, and related compounds. Bile pigment is formed by enzymatic cleavage of the α-methene bridge of heme, with release of the linear tetrapyrrole biliverdin and carbon monoxide. Biliverdin is then enzymatically reduced to bilirubin within the same cell. This

Table 7.1
Types of Human Porphyria[a]

Type (synonyms)	Clinical manifestations	Chemical findings
I. Erythropoietic		
A. Congenital erythropoietic porphyria; Gunther's disease[t]	Severe photosensitivity and dermatitis; erythrodontia (stained teeth); hemolytic anemia with splenomegaly	Large amounts or URO and COPRO I in bone marrow, red cells, urine; COPRO I in stool; urine red, fluoresces red in UV light
B. Congenital erythropoietic protoporphyria[t]	Mild photosensitivity and dermatitis ("solar urticaria"), hemolytic anemia rarely	Increased PROTO 9 (and some COPRO III) in bone marrow, red cells, plasma, and stool; urine normal (URO not increased)
C. Chronic lead toxicity[a]	Photodermatitis absent; abdominal colic, neuropathy, encephalopathy; hypochromic anemia with stippled red cells, some hemolysis	Increased urinary ALA (not PBG) and COPRO III; increased red cell COPRO and PROTO
II. Hepatic		
A. Acute intermittent porphyria; porphyria hepatica; "pyrrolia"; Swedish porphyria[p]	Acute attacks of abdominal colic, CNS and peripheral nerve involvement, psychic changes, hypertension, constipation; photosensitivity and dermatitis absent	ALA and PBG (pyrrole) in liver and urine; fresh urine usually has normal color (porphyrins not increased); urine becomes dark on standing
B. Variegate porphyria; mixed hepatic porphyria; South African porphyria[t,p]	Moderate (or absent) photodermatitis; in some cases acute attacks of abdominal pain and neurologic disorder as in AIP, usually precipitated by drugs	Increased COPRO, PROTO, and "X-porphyrin" in liver, stool; increased COPRO in urine; ALA and PBG in urine during acute attacks
C. Coproporphyria[t,p]	Photodermatitis mild or absent; acute attacks may be induced by drugs	Increased COPRO in stool, urine; ALA and PBG in urine during acute attacks
D. Porphyria cutanea tarda; symptomatic porphyria[t]	Photodermatitis	Increased URO in liver, urine; urine may be red
E. Hexachlorobenzene toxicity[t]	Photodermatitis	Increased URO in liver, urine; urine may be red

Note: *t* = true porphyria (photosensitivity, excretion of true porphyrins);
p = precursor syndrome (neuropsychiatric disorder, excretion of ALA, PBG).
a. Lead intoxication is listed because of its resemblances to porphyria.

Inheritance	Biochemical defect
Homozygous for abnormal gene (recessive)	Decreased UROgen cosynthetase in developing red cells, causing abnormal production of type I isomers
Heterozygous for abnormal gene (dominant); latent cases frequent	Defect in developing red cells, causing overproduction of PROTO 9; decreased ferrochelatase activity (? unstable enzyme molecule)
None (acquired)	Complex defect in developing red cells: decreased ALA dehydrase, ferrochelatase, COPROgen oxidase, and possibly ALA synthetase; decreased intracellular iron transport; depressed globin synthesis; abnormal mitochondria and ribosomes. Relation of symptoms to excess ALA production is unclear
Heterozygous for abnormal gene (dominant); latent cases frequent	Defect in liver: decrease in UROgen synthetase with secondary increase in ALA synthetase in patients with active disease, causing increased ALA and PBG production; basis of abdominal and CNS symptoms unclear (possibly related to excess ALA or PBG)
Heterozygous for abnormal gene (dominant); latent cases frequent	Defect in liver; decrease in PROTOgen oxidase (or possibly ferrochelatase) with secondary "sensitization" of ALA synthetase
Heterozygous for abnormal gene (dominant); latent cases very frequent	Defect in liver: decreased COPROgen oxidase with secondary sensitization of ALA synthetase
In some cases latent genetic defect (dominant) brought out by liver disease or drugs, e.g., estrogens; ? an entirely acquired defect in other cases	Defect in liver: decrease in UROgen decarboxylase; ALA synthetase probably not increased. Typically associated with iron overload in the liver; may be ameliorated by phlebotomies
None	Hexachlorobenzene inhibits UROgen decarboxylase in liver

two-step conversion occurs in RES cells in spleen, liver, and elsewhere (figure 7.3). Bilirubin is rapidly excreted into bile by the liver. Bile pigments are excretory products that cannot be reconverted to porphyrinogens or heme. Urobilinogen is a bile pigment (i.e., it is a product of heme catabolism); uroporphyrin is a cyclic (ring) tetrapyrrole that is a by-product of heme synthesis (i.e., it is related to the anabolic pathway).

1. Sources of bile pigment

Most bile pigment is normally derived from hemoglobin at the end of the red cell life span. In addition, an "early-labeled" fraction of bile pigment is observed within the first few days after administration of a labeled heme precursor such as ^{14}C-glycine. It normally accounts for about 15% of the total labeled pigment (figure 7.4). This early-labeled fraction originates partly from nonhemoglobin hemes, largely in the liver, but probably also in all tissues in which heme is synthesized. There is also an erythropoietic

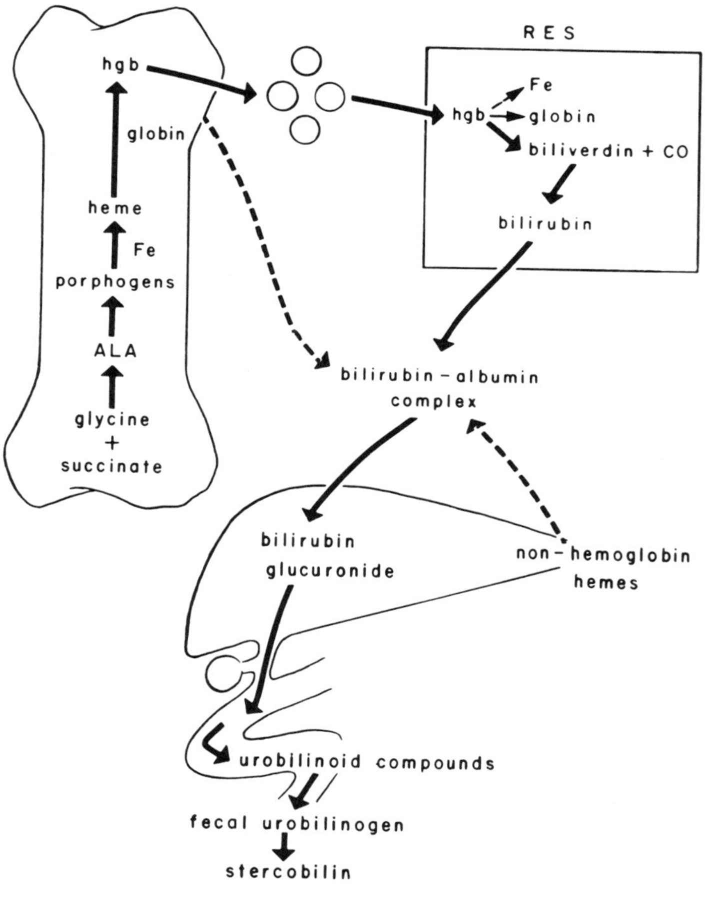

Fig. 7.3
Schematic summary of heme and bilirubin metabolism.

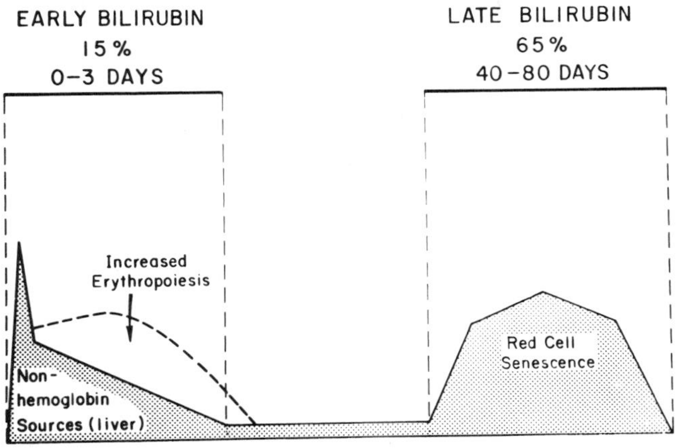

Fig. 7.4
Sources of bile pigments in the rat. This scheme also applies in general to humans, although in them the early-labeled fraction is formed from 0–5 days and the late fraction from 90–150 days. These data were derived from studies employing glycine-2-^{14}C as heme precursor. (From S. H. Robinson, in F. Stohlman, Jr., ed., *Hemopoietic Cellular Proliferation,* New York: Grune & Stratton, 1970)

component that becomes prominent when red cell production in the bone marrow is accelerated or abnormal, especially with ineffective erythropoiesis. This component is presumably derived from the hemoglobin of prematurely destroyed erythroid precursors.

2. Bilirubin excretion

Bilirubin is transported in plasma bound to albumin (figure 7.3). Hepatic excretion occurs in three phases: (1) uptake of unconjugated bilirubin from plasma into liver cell; (2) enzymatic conjugation of bilirubin, primarily with glucuronic acid; and (3) secretion of conjugated bilirubin into the bile canaliculus.

After excretion via bile into the intestine, bilirubin is reduced to a series of urobilinogen compounds by the intestinal bacteria.

B. Overproduction of bile pigment

1. Mechanisms of jaundice

In broad terms, hyperbilirubinemia may be due to increased production of bilirubin (less common) or decreased hepatic excretion (more common). In overproduction states, there is unconjugated ("indirect-reacting") hyperbilirubinemia in which the unconjugated bilirubin does not gain access to the urine. Fecal urobilinogen is increased. Unconjugated hyperbilirubinemia also occurs with defects in the uptake or conjugation phases of hepatic excretion. With impaired hepatic secretion, dysfunction of the bile canaliculi, or extrahepatic biliary obstruction, there is some regurgitation of conjugated ("direct-reacting") bilirubin from the liver into the plasma with some spillover into the urine.

2. Causes of bilirubin overproduction

1. Increased rate of destruction of circulating red cells (hemolytic anemia). This is by far the most common cause of overproduction jaundice (see lecture 11).

2. Abnormal hepatic heme metabolism in liver disorders, with an increase in early-labeled bilirubin production. This has been documented thus far only in experimental liver injury.

3. Ineffective erythropoiesis (i.e., destruction of defective red cell precursors within the marrow or soon after release into the peripheral blood). This occurs in thalassemia, megaloblastic anemia, sideroblastic anemia, erythroleukemia, and a few other disorders. Some hemolysis of circulating red cells usually also occurs in these states. Ineffective erythropoiesis is associated with an increase in early-labeled bilirubin production.

SELECTED REFERENCES

Kappas, A., et al. The porphyrias (Chapter 60). In Stanbury, J. B., Wyngaarden, J. B., and Frederickson, D. S., eds., *Metabolic Basis of Inherited Disease,* 5th ed., New York: McGraw-Hill, 1982, pp. 1301–1384.

Kappas, A., et al. The porphyrias (Chapter 44). In Wintrobe, M. M., Lee, G. R., Boggs, D. R., Bithell, T. C., Forester, J., Athens, J. W., and Lukens, J. N., eds., *Clinical Hematology,* 8th ed., Philadelphia: Lea and Feibiger, 1981, pp. 1021–1042.

Robinson, S. H. Bilirubin metabolism and jaundice. In Joachim, H. I., ed., *Pathobiology Annual,* New York: Appleton-Century-Crofts, 1976, pp. 299–316.

Robinson, S. H., and Glass, J. Disorders of heme metabolism: Sideroblastic anemia and the porphyrias (Chapter 12). In Nathan, D. G., and Oski, F. A., eds., *Hematology of Infancy and Childhood,* 3d ed., Philadelphia: Saunders, 1985, in press.

LECTURE 8 Hemoglobin I. Structure and Function

H. Franklin Bunn

I. HEMOGLOBIN SYNTHESIS

A. Structural genes

Multiple structural genes govern the biosynthesis of globin in maturing human erythroid cells. Each gene results in the formation of a structurally unique polypeptide chain. The resulting gene products have been named α, β, γ, δ, ϵ, and ζ chains. The α and ζ genes are located on chromosome 16; the others are located on chromosome 11. Each newly synthesized globin chain links covalently with heme (ferroprotoporphyrin 9), as described in lectures 6 and 7. Further discussion of the globin genes is given in lecture 10.

B. Combination of chains

Globin chains (or subunits) combine to form tetramers of mol. wt. 64,500. The physiologic function of hemoglobin depends on the presence of two α chains and two non-α chains. For example, normal adult hemoglobin, or *hemoglobin A,* is $\alpha_2\beta_2$. Normal fetal hemoglobin, or *hemoglobin F,* is $\alpha_2\gamma_2$.

C. Synthetic rates of globin chains

Globin chain synthesis is discussed in detail in lecture 10. The synthetic rates of the five globin chains vary during the transition from embryonic and fetal life to neonatal life, as shown in figure 8.1.

D. Chains in normal hemoglobin

Table 8.1 summarizes the nomenclature and chain composition of the several hemoglobins found in normal subjects at various stages of life. The most abundant minor hemoglobin component in

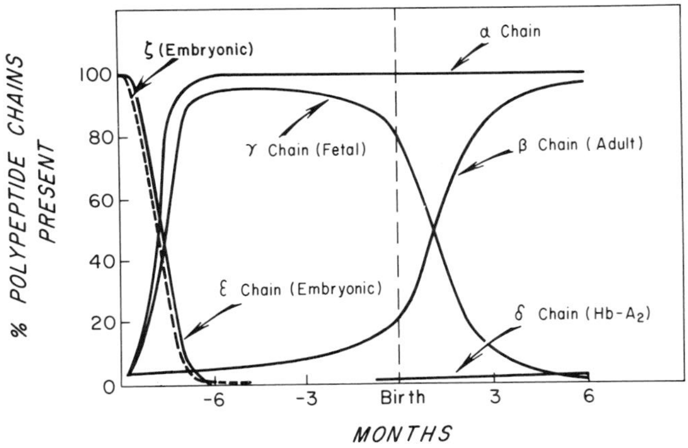

Fig. 8.1
Relative rates of synthesis of different globin chains during embryonic and neonatal life. (From D. L. Rucknagel, *Clin. Obst. Gynec.* 12(1969): 49).

Table 8.1
Structure of Normal Hemoglobins

Hemoglobin	Structure	Comments
A	$\alpha_2\beta_2$	Comprises 92% of adult hemoglobin
A_{1c}	α_2 (β-NH-glucose)$_2$	Comprises 3% of adult hemoglobin. Increased in patients with diabetes
A_2	$\alpha_2\delta_2$	Comprises about 2% of adult hemoglobin. Elevated in β thalassemia
F	$\alpha_2\gamma_2$	Predominant hemoglobin in fetus from the 3d through 9th month of gestation. Facilitates transfer of oxygen across placenta. Increased in β thalassemia and other disorders
Gower 1	$\zeta_2\epsilon_2$	Present in early embryo. Facilitates transfer of oxygen to embryo.
Gower 2	$\alpha_2\epsilon_2$	
Portland	$\zeta_2\gamma_2$	
H	β_4	Found in α thalassemia (α-/--). Low solubility. Nonfunctional
Barts	γ_4	Trace present in newborns. May comprise 100% of hemoglobin in homozygous α thalassemia (--/--). Nonfunctional

adult red cells is hemoglobin A_{1c}, which is a posttranslational modification of glucose with the N-terminal amino of the β chain according to the reaction scheme in diagram 8.1. This minor component is elevated 2–3-fold in red cells of diabetics and provides a useful measurement of the adequacy of diabetic control. Furthermore, this chemical modification occurs in other tissues and may contribute to the long-term complications of diabetes.

II. HEMOGLOBIN STRUCTURE

A. Primary and secondary

The primary amino acid sequences of the normal human hemoglobins, and nearly 400 genetic variants, have been established by chemical methods (primarily "finger-printing" and peptide analyses). The normal α chain contains 141 amino acid residues in linear sequence; the β chain has 146 residues. The δ and γ chains differ from the β chain by 10 and 39 amino acids, respectively. Analysis of hemoglobin F shows it can contain two structurally distinct chains that differ by a single amino acid at position 136. In some chains (termed G_γ), glycine occupies this position; in others (A_γ), alanine does. As described in lecture 10, different structural genes specify G_γ and A_γ.

About 80% of native hemoglobin is in the α helical form. Many amino acid residues are homologous in comparable helices of the α and β chains of human and animal hemoglobins. These are

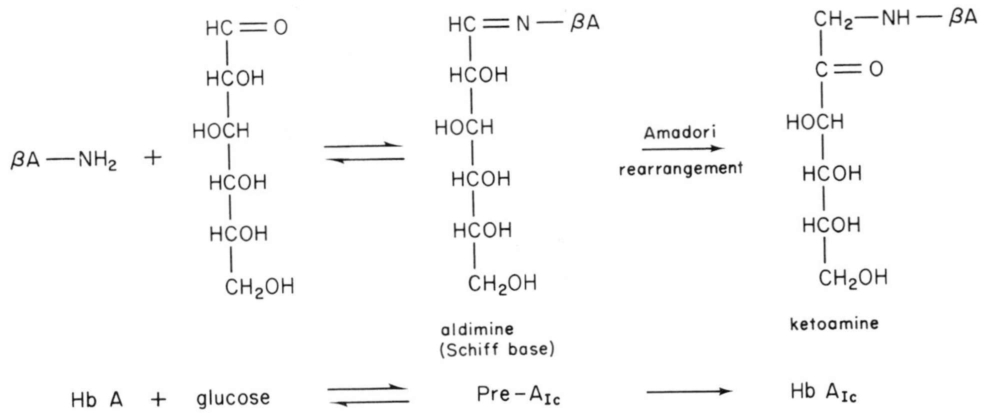

Diagram 8.1

termed *invariant residues*. An example is the histidine at F8 (β92, α87), the imidazole moiety of which is bonded covalently to heme iron. The primary structure of the normal human β chain is shown diagrammatically in figure 8.2.

B. Tertiary and quarternary

From x-ray analyses of hemoglobin crystals, Perutz and associates have worked out the three-dimensional structure of human hemoglobin. This remarkable achievement has facilitated progress in relating structure to function. The tetramer was shown to be a spheroid with a diameter of about 55 Å and a single axis of symmetry. The four hemes lie in clefts situated equidistantly on the surface of the molecule. Upon deoxygenation all four chains undergo conformational changes (figure 8.3), the distance between β chain hemes increasing by 7 Å. X-ray data indicate that the deoxy conformation is stabilized by intra- and interchain salt bonds, including some dependent on proton binding and others on the presence of 2,3-disphosphoglycerate (2,3-DPG; see below). These are sequentially broken upon addition of oxygen. The primary physiologic properties of the molecule, namely, heme-heme interaction and the Bohr effect, have recently been explained in terms of such stereochemical transitions. Some of these oxygen-linked salt bonds are shown diagrammatically in figure 8.4. At specific sites, protons are bound preferentially to deoxyhemoglobin. This is the structural basis of the Bohr effect, which is discussed below. The binding of 2,3-DPG to deoxyhemoglobin is shown in figure 8.4A.

III. HEMOGLOBIN FUNCTION

A. Heme-heme interaction

The familiar sigmoid shape of the oxygen-hemoglobin dissociation curve (figure 8.5) is of great physiologic importance for it permits a considerable transfer of oxygen from hemoglobin to tissues with

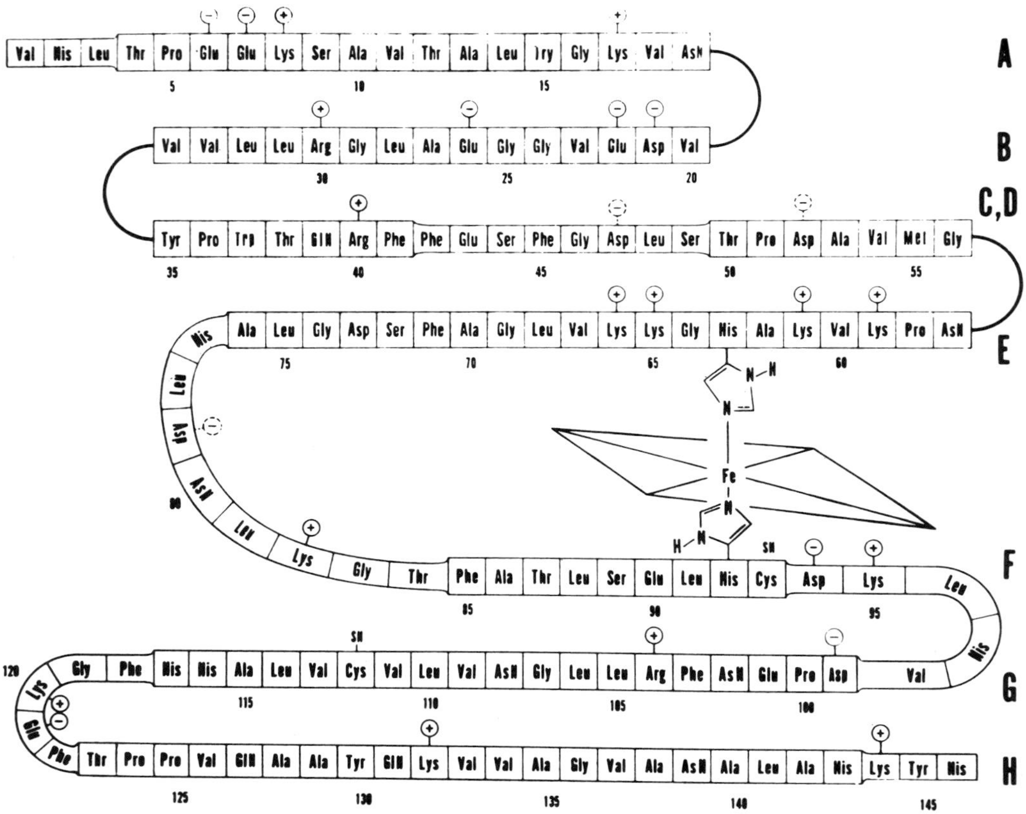

Fig. 8.2
Normal human β chain. Diagrammatic scheme shows the sequence of 146 amino acids from the N-terminal end above to the C-terminal end below. Helical regions are designated by single letters (A, B, E, etc.). Amino acid residues within helical regions are in squares. Nonhelical regions are represented by two letters (CD, EF, etc.) and nonhelical residues by rectangles. (From M. Murayama, in R. Nalbandian, ed., *Molecular Aspects of Sickle Cell Hemoglobin,* Springfield: Charles C Thomas, 1971)

only a small drop in oxygen tension. In contrast, myoglobin and single α and β chains lack heme-heme interaction and therefore have hyperbolic (non-sigmoid) oxygen dissociation curves. Thus, heme-heme interaction, a critical function of hemoglobin (i.e., $\alpha_2\beta_2$), depends on the interaction of pairs of unlike chains.

B. Bohr effect

The oxygen affinity of hemoglobin is directly related to pH over the pH range 6.0–8.5. A corollary to that statement is that oxyhemoglobin is a stronger acid than deoxyhemoglobin. The conversion from deoxy to oxy conformation decreases the pKs of acid groups of certain specific (and invariant) amino acid residues.

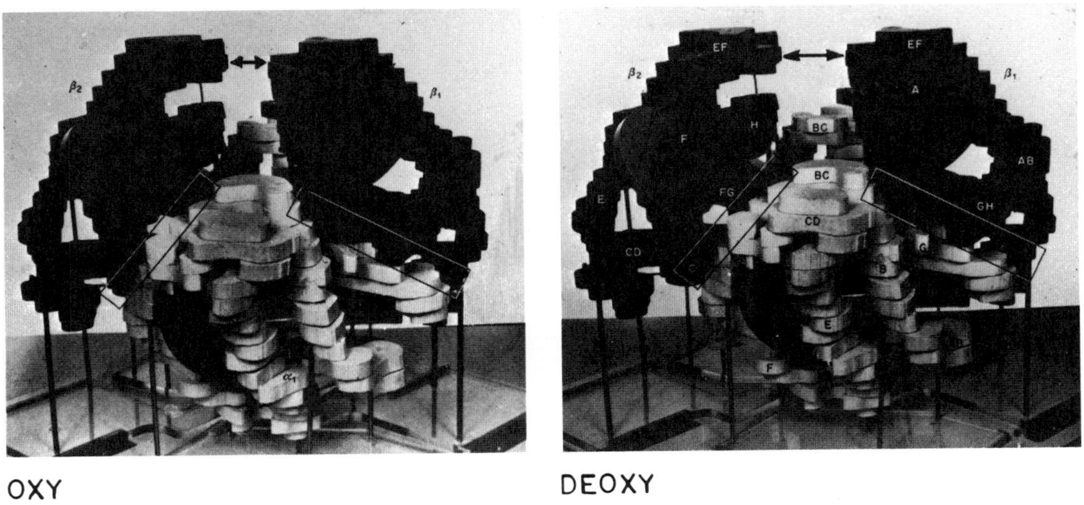

Fig. 8.3
Three-dimensional model of hemoglobin. The β chains are shown in black, the α chains in white. (One α chain is largely hidden from view.) Note the change in the distance between β chains on oxygenation. (From M. F. Perutz, *Nature* 228(1970): 726)

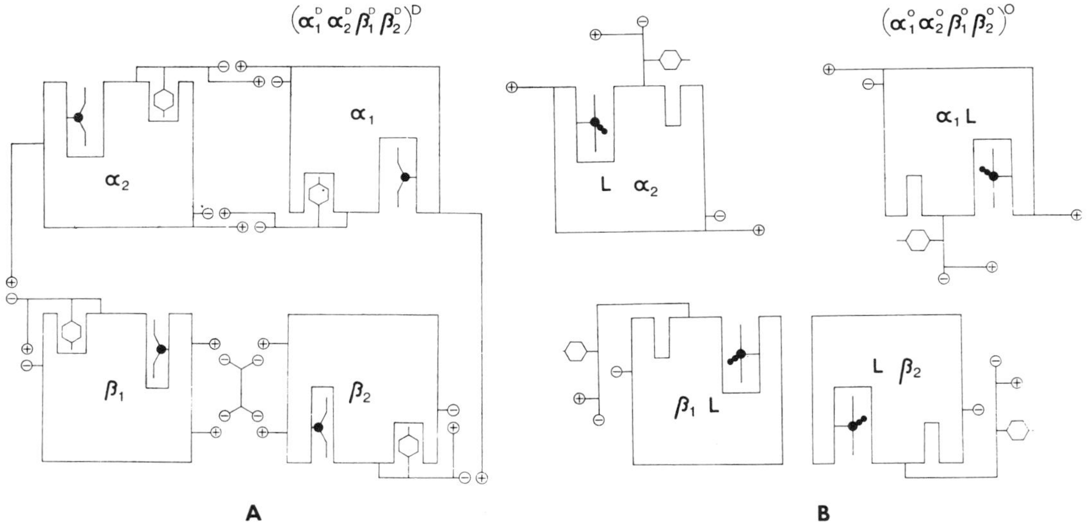

Fig. 8.4
Diagrammatic representation of the quaternary configurations of deoxyhemoglobin (*A*) and oxyhemoglobin (*B*). The salt bonds that stabilize the deoxy conformation are broken when the molecule is oxygenated. The binding of the negatively charged 2,3-DPG to the β chains of deoxyhemoglobin is shown (above *A*). (From M. F. Perutz, *Nature* 228(1979): 726)

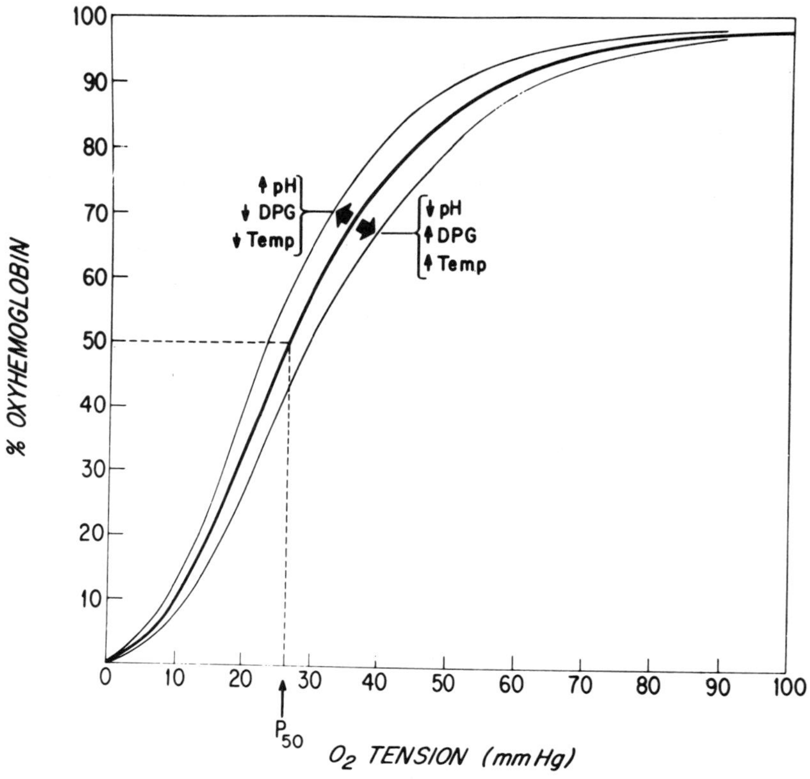

Fig. 8.5
Normal oxygen-hemoglobin dissociation curve and the effects on oxygen affinity of changes in pH, temperature, and red cell 2,3-DPG level.

Under physiologic conditions, oxygenation releases about 2.8 protons:

$$HbH + 4O_2 \rightleftharpoons Hb(O_2)_4 + 2.8H^+$$

The Bohr effect is physiologically advantageous (1) in *tissues,* where the decrease in pH due to CO_2 uptake lowers oxygen affinity and thereby enhances oxygen release; and (2) in *lungs,* where expulsion of CO_2 raises pH and thereby increases oxygen affinity and uptake.

C. Role of 2,3-DPG

1. Binding to hemoglobin

Unlike other tissues, red cells contain a high concentration of the organic phosphate ester *2,3-diphosphoglycerate* (2,3-DPG), which is a glycolytic intermediate. Its concentration in normal red cells equals that of hemoglobin tetramer (about 5mM). It is a highly charged anion, which is partially protonated at physiologic pH:

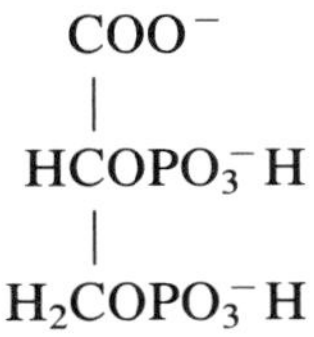

When it is added to hemoglobin, 2,3-DPG sharply lowers oxygen affinity without disturbing heme-heme interaction or the Bohr effect. 2,3-DPG has been shown to bind at a specific site to deoxyhemoglobin (more avidly than to oxyhemoglobin) in a 1:1 molar ratio. Thus, the reaction can be written as follows:

$$\text{HbDPG} + 4O_2 \rightleftharpoons \text{Hb}(O_2)_4 + \text{DPG}.$$

This equation should be compared to that given above for the Bohr effect.

2. Adaptation to hypoxia

An increased concentration of 2,3-DPG within the red cell favors the lowering of the oxygen affinity of blood in two ways: *direct* binding to deoxyhemoglobin as described above; and *indirectly* by lowering the pH within the red cell relative to plasma pH.

The position on the oxygen-hemoglobin dissociation curve is an important determinant of oxygen delivery to tissues. As diagrammed in figure 8.6, oxygen delivery to an organ or tissue is directly proportional to blood flow, hemoglobin concentration, and the difference in oxygen saturation of arterial and venous blood. Patients with various types of hypoxia may compensate in the following ways: (1) total cardiac output increases when hypoxia is severe and the distribution of blood flow may be altered so as to maintain the oxygenation of vital organs; (2) erythropoiesis increases as a result of increased erythropoietin production; (3) oxygen unloading ($A_{SAT} - V_{SAT}$) is enhanced by a shift to the right in the oxygen-hemoglobin dissociation curve (with resulting decrease in oxygen affinity) that is mediated by increasing 2,3-DPG in the red cell. The extent to which oxygen unloading can be enhanced is illustrated in figure 8.7.

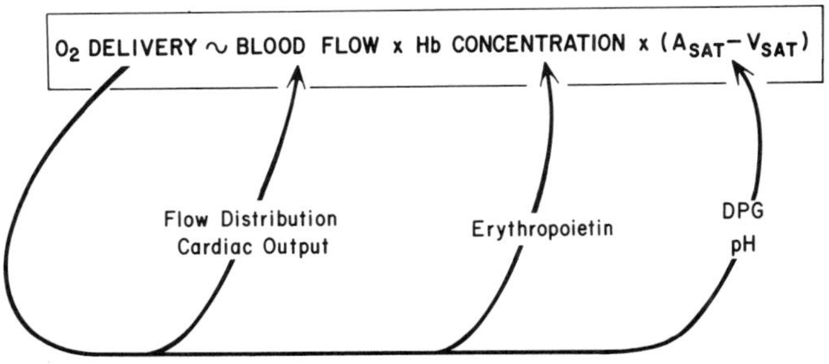

Fig. 8.6
Diagram of factors regulating oxygen delivery to tissues.

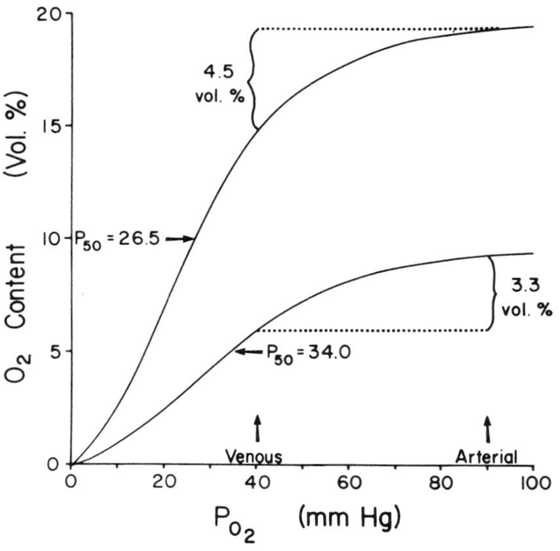

Fig. 8.7
Enhancement of oxygen unloading by decreased red cell oxygen affinity in a patient with anemia. Anemic patient with a 50 per cent reduction in hemoglobin concentration has only a 27 per cent reduction in oxygen unloading. (From Klocke, R. A.: *Chest 69*(1972): 795)

The mechanism by which red cell 2,3-DPG is elevated in hypoxic states is not well understood. Red cell pH is probably the most important determinant of 2,3-DPG levels. Alkalosis causes an increase in 2,3-DPG, and acidosis causes a decrease. The direct effect of pH on red cell oxygen affinity (Bohr effect) is opposite to the indirect effect of pH on the 2,3-DPG level.

A "shift to the right" occurs in the various clinical types of hypoxia, among them (1) high-altitude effects; (2) pulmonary insufficiency; (3) cardiac right-to-left shunt; (4) congestive heart failure; and (5) severe anemia of any type.

3. Shifts to the left

A "shift to the left" of the oxygen-hemoglobin dissociation curve impairs oxygen release to the tissues. The following conditions can cause such a shift: (1) multiple transfusions with blood that has been stored more than 5 days in acid-citrate-dextrose solution and has become depleted of 2,3-DPG; (2) rapid correction of metabolic acidosis; (3) the presence of hemoglobin F (as in fetal blood), which contains γ chains instead of β chains and thus interacts only weakly with 2,3-DPG, thereby facilitating the transport of oxygen from mother to fetus; and (4) the presence of a chemically altered hemoglobin such as methemoglobin, carboxyhemoglobin (to be discussed below), or certain of the hemoglobin variants to be discussed in lecture 9.

IV. ACQUIRED ABNORMALITIES

A. Carbon monoxide poisoning

Carbon monoxide (CO) arises from combustion of organic material, particularly hydrocarbons such as petroleum and tobacco tar. It is an important toxic component of tobacco smoke. It is produced endogenously in the catabolism of heme, which results in formation of 1 mole each of CO and bilirubin per mole of heme (see lecture 7).

1. Toxicology

The hazards of CO intoxication are evident in its frequent use in suicide attempts and its seriousness as an industrial toxin. The mechanism of toxicity depends on the fact that CO and oxygen compete for the same binding site in heme, but CO is bound 210 times more firmly than oxygen. Thus, carbonmonoxyhemoglobin (also called carboxyhemoglobin, abbreviated HbCO), unlike oxyhemoglobin, dissociates with difficulty. These relations may be summarized as follows:

$$\frac{[\mathrm{HbCO}]}{[\mathrm{HbO_2}]} = 210\,\frac{p\mathrm{CO}}{p\mathrm{O_2}}.$$

The binding of CO to hemoglobin prevents the molecule from assuming the deoxy conformation. As a result, remaining heme groups that have not bound CO have an increased affinity for oxygen. Thus, increasing concentrations of HbCO in blood cause a progressive "shift to the left" and loss of sigmoidicity of the oxygen dissociation curve. This results in decreased release of oxygen to tissues. Figure 8.8 compares oxygen dissociation curves in an anemic patient in whom half of the hemoglobin is missing, with a patient having a normal total hemoglobin level but in whom half the hemoglobin is in the form of HbCO. In terms of tissue oxy-

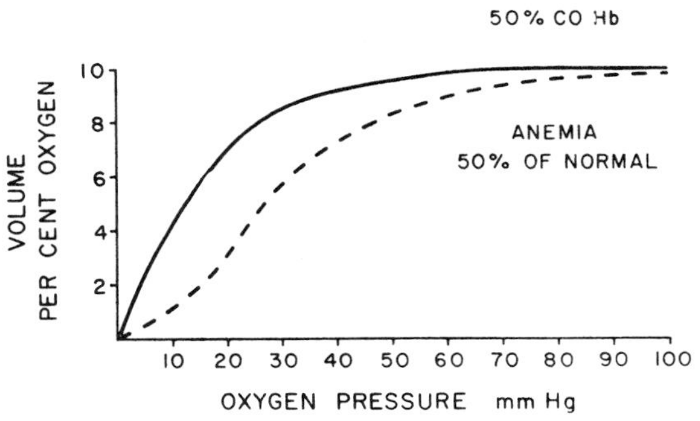

Fig. 8.8
Demonstration that oxygen release to tissues, as determined by shape and position of the oxygen-hemoglobin dissociation curve, is less abnormal in anemia than in CO poisoning.

genation, loss of hemoglobin is a less serious hazard than conversion of hemoglobin to HbCO.

2. Clinical features

In normal subjects, the maximum level of HbCO is 2% of total hemoglobin. Symptoms of acute poisoning vary with the level of HbCO. At 6–10%, vision and time discrimination are impaired. Unconsciousness followed by death occurs at 40–60%. There are no proven effects of chronic intoxication. Some workers have postulated a relation between chronic CO poisoning and coronary artery disease.

HbCO is a cherry-red pigment. When CO poisoning is suspected because of known exposure or symptoms of anoxia in the absence of cyanosis, the presence of HbCO can be established by studies of the visible absorption spectrum. The intoxicated victim should be immediately removed from exposure to carbon monoxide. Oxygen should be administered, and when necessary ventilation should be supported.

B. Methemoglobinemia

1. Pathophysiology

Methemoglobin is the form of hemoglobin in which the iron has been oxidized. It is sometimes called ferr*i*hemoglobin or hem*i*globin in contrast to reduced hemoglobin, which has been termed ferr*o*hemoglobin or hem*o*globin. Methemoglobin is continually being formed in normal red cells (in the absence of exogenous oxidant drugs or toxins) and is continually being reduced to hemoglobin. In normal red cells under steady-state conditions, the methemoglobin level does not exceed 1% of the total hemoglobin.

Two enzymatic reduction mechanisms are found in red cells. An enzyme called *cytochrome b_5 reductase* or *NADH diaphorase* catalyzes the reduction of methemoglobin in a reaction that is coupled with the oxidation of NADH to NAD.

Methemoglobinemia may develop when (1) normal red cells are exposed to excess oxidant drugs or toxins or (2) red cells are congenitally deficient in cytochrome b_5 reductase.

Red cells also contain an *NADPH-dependent methemoglobin reductase* system that requires the presence of an exogenous electron carrier such as methylene blue (MB) and thus does not function physiologically. MB accepts electrons from NADPH (with formation of NADP and MBH) and transfer them to Fe^{+++}-heme to form Fe^{++}-heme. When MB is present, NADPH-dependent reductase is more active than NADH-cytochrome b_5 reductase. (See diagram 8.2.) The significance of methemoglobin ies in the fact that Fe^{+++}-heme cannot bind oxygen. As in the presence of CO-hemoglobin, an increasing concentration of methemoglobin causes a progressive increase in oxygen affinity of the remaining functioning hemes on the hemoglobin tetramer (see figure 8.8). The result is decreased oxygen release to tissues.

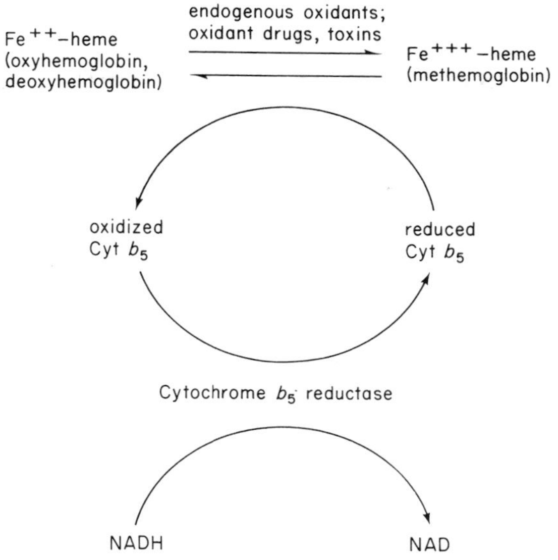

Diagram 8.2

2. Etiology

a. Congenital — Causes of congenital methemoglobinemia include (1) deficiency of cytochrome b_5 reductase and (2) presence of a hemoglobin M (see lecture 9).

b. Acquired — Causes of acquired methemoglobin include (1) exposure to oxidant drugs or toxins that act directly such as nitrates from well water (that are reduced to nitrites by intestinal flora), chlorates, and quinones, and (2) agents that act indirectly such as aniline, acetanilid, and sulfonamides. Persons heterozygous for cytochrome b_5 reductase deficiency are more susceptible to oxidant agents than normal subjects.

3. Clinical features — A methemoglobin level in excess of 1.5 gm/100 ml (10% of total hemoglobin) leads to visible cyanosis. (In contrast, cyanosis does not become visible until the level of reduced hemoglobin reaches 5.0 gm/100 ml.) If methemoglobin exceeds 35% of total hemoglobin, headache and dyspnea may result. Levels over 70% are lethal. In some patients with congenital methemoglobinemia, mild polycythemia may result from chronic anoxia (see lecture 20).

4. Treatment — In mild cases, intravenous methylene blue administration activates NADPH-dependent methemoglobin reductase and readily corrects methemoglobinemia. In severe cases involving oxidant toxins, renal dialysis and exchange transfusion with fresh blood may be necessary. Orally administered methylene blue or ascorbic acid is a useful maintenance therapy in congenital methemoglobinemia.

C. Sulfhemoglobinemia

Sulfhemoglobinemia is associated with the presence in blood of a poorly characterized hemoglobin derivative with a characteristic absorption spectrum that distinguishes it from methemoglobin. It can be produced in vivo by various oxidant drugs including sulfonamides, phenacetin, and acetanilid. Unlike methemoglobin, sulfhemoglobin cannot be converted back to hemoglobin. When sulfhemoglobinemia occurs, it persists until the red cells containing the abnormal pigment are destroyed.

SELECTED REFERENCES

Adamson, J. W., and Finch, C. A. — Hemoglobin function, oxygen affinity and erythropoietin. *Ann. Rev. Physiol.* 37(1975): 351.

Baldwin, J. — Structure and cooperativity of haemoglobin. *Trends in Biochem. Sci.* 5(1980): 224.

Bunn, H. F., and Forget, B. F. — *Hemoglobin: Molecular, Genetic and Clinical Aspects,* Philadelphia: W. B. Saunders, 1984.

Bunn, H. F., et al. — The glycosylation of hemoglobin: Relevance to diabetes mellitus. *Science* 200(1978): 21.

Nienhuis, A. W., and Benz, E. J. — Regulation of hemoglobin synthesis during the development of the red cell. *New Eng. J. Med.* 197(1977): 1318, 1371, 1430.

Perutz, M. F. — Hemoglobin structure and respiratory transport. *Sci. Am.* 239(1978): 92.

Schwartz, J. M., et al. — Hereditary methemoglobinemia with deficiency of NADH cytochrome b5 reductase (Chapter 75). In Stanbury, J. B., Wyngaarden, J. B., and Frederickson, D. S., eds., *Metabolic Basis of Inherited Diseases,* 5th ed., New York, McGraw-Hill, 1983, pp. 1654–1665.

LECTURE 9 Hemoglobin II. Sickle Cell Anemia and Other Hemoglobinopathies

H. Franklin Bunn

I. HEMOGLOBIN VARIANTS

Nearly 400 human hemoglobin *variants* of known structure have been reported to date. The majority were discovered incidentally in the course of population surveys and are not associated with clinical manifestations.

A. Genetic basis

Over 90% of the human hemoglobin variants are single amino acid substitutions in the α, β, γ, or δ subunits. These can all be explained by single base substitutions in the corresponding triplet codon. As shown in table 9.1, other molecular mechanisms must be invoked to explain the structure of a minority of the known hemoglobin variants.

A hemoglobin variant is inherited as an autosomal codominant trait. A pedigree of a family having genes for hemoglobin S and hemoglobin C is shown in figure 9.1 (right). Statistically, one-quarter of the offspring will be normal (AA), one-quarter will be SA heterozygotes, one-quarter will be CA heterozygotes, and one-quarter will be SC double heterozygotes.

B. Detection

Abnormal hemoglobins are usually detected by electrophoresis of red cell hemolysate. If the substituted amino acid alters the net charge, the isoelectric point and electrophoretic mobility of the variant hemoglobin will differ from those of hemoglobin A. The effects of amino acid substitutions at β6 on the isoelectric point are illustrated in table 9.2 and figure 9.2.

C. Clinical classification

The common clinically significant human hemoglobin variants can be classified as follows:

1. Sickle syndromes
    a. Sickle cell trait (AS)
    b. Sickle cell anemia (SS)
    c. Double-heterozygous states (sickle-β thalassemia; SC disease; SD disease)
2. Unstable hemoglobin variants (congenital Heinz body hemolytic anemias)
3. Variants with high oxygen affinity (familial erythrocytosis)
4. The M hemoglobins (familial cyanosis)

The sickle syndromes to be described below are clinical problems only in homozygotes or double heterozygotes. In contrast, unstable variants, high-oxygen-affinity variants, and M hemoglobins are

Table 9.1
Molecular Bases of Human Hemoglobin Variants

Basic mechanism	Chain	Examples
A. Amino acid substitution(s) (with nucleotide base substitution(s) in codon)		
1. One substitution	α	I, Memphis, M Boston [120]
	β	S, C, D, E, Seattle [270]
	γ	F Texas I, F Hull [20]
	δ	A_2 Sphakiá, A_2 Flatbush [10]
2. Two substitutions	α	J Singapore
	β	C Harlem
	β	Arlington Park
	β	C Ziguinchor
	β	S Travis
B. Amino acid deletions (with deletion of corresponding codon(s) or nonhomologous crossing-over)	β	Gun Hill (5)
	β	Tochigi (4)
	β	Niteroi (3)
	β	St. Antoine (2)
	β	Lyon (2)
	β	Tours (1)
	β	Leiden (1)
	β	Freiburg (1)
	β	Leslie (Deaconness) (1)
	β	Coventry (1)
C. Fusion hemoglobins (with nonhomologous crossing-over between genes coding for two different subunits)	δβ	The Lepores
	βδ	Miyada, P Congo, P Nilotic
	γβ	Kenya
D. Elongated subunits		
1. Base substitution in termination codon	α	Constant Spring
	α	Icaria
	α	Koya Dora
	α	Seal Rock
2. Frame shift	α	Wayne
	β	Tak
	β	Cranston

Note: Number of variants known signified by brackets; number of amino acid residues deleted signified by parentheses.

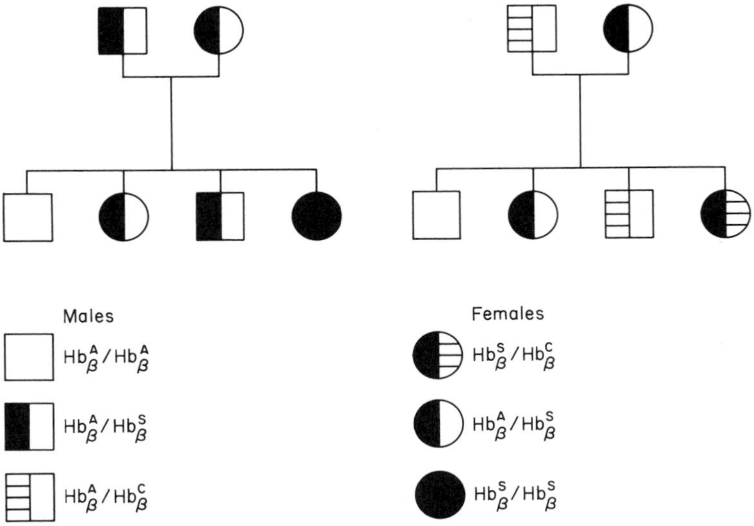

Fig. 9.1
Pedigrees of families with genes for hemoglobin S and A (left) and hemoglobin S, C, and A (right).

encountered only in heterozygotes. In these states, homozygosity would be lethal.

II. SICKLE SYNDROMES

In 1910, Herrick described a black student with a hemolytic anemia and peculiar elongated or "sickled" red cell on the blood smear. The subsequent elaboration of the molecular and genetic basis of sickle cell disease is one of the most absorbing chapters in the history of molecular biology. The various states associated with the presence of hemoglobin S ($\alpha_2\beta_2^{6Glu\rightarrow Val}$) are listed in table 9.3, in order of clinical severity.

A. Sickle cell trait

About 8% of black Americans are heterozygous for hemoglobin S. Thus their red cells contain hemoglobin S and A. In parts of central Africa where malaria is endemic, nearly 25% of the population has the sickle trait. The gene has persisted because of balanced polymorphism, whereby heterozygotes are slightly protected against falciparum malaria.

Table 9.2
Effect of Substitution at β6 on Isoelectric Point

Hemoglobin	β chain sequence	Isoelectric point
A	H_2N-Val-His-Leu-Thr-Pro-*Glu*-Glu . . .	7.0
S	H_2N-Val-His-Leu-Thr-Pro-*Val*-Glu . . .	7.2
C	H_2N-Val-His-Leu-Thr-Pro-*Lys*-Glu . . .	7.4

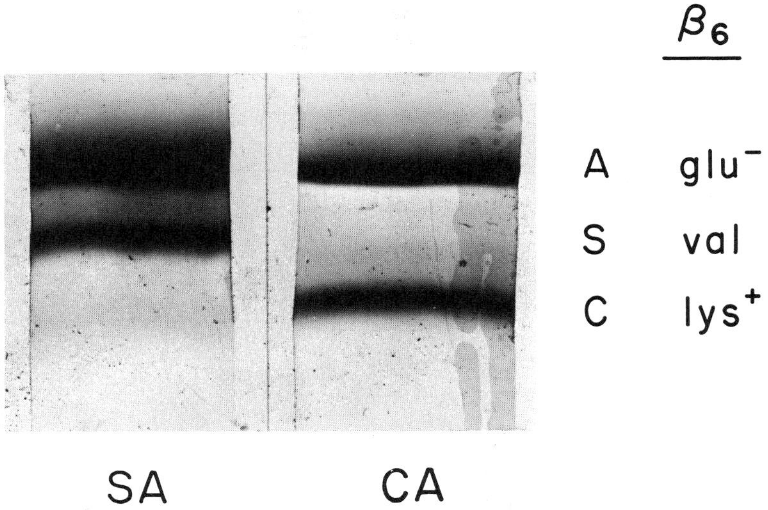

Fig. 9.2
Electrophoresis of hemolysates of individuals with sickle trait (SA) and hemoglobin C trait (CA).

Table 9.3
Varying Clinical Severity of the Different Sickle Syndromes

Genotype	% of hemoglobin S	% of non-S hemoglobin	Clinical severity
SS	80–90	5–15 (F)	+ +/+ + + +
SO, SD	30–40	60–70 (O,D)	+ +/+ + + +
S-β thalassemia	80	20 (A + F)	+/+ + +
SC	50	50 (C)	+/+ + +
S-HPFH[a]	70	30 (F)	0
AS	30–40	60–70 (A)	0

a. Double heterozygous state for hemoglobin S and hereditary persistence of fetal hemoglobin (see lecture 10).

1. Clinical features

Life expectancy and morbidity of individuals with sickle trait resemble those of a comparable group with hemoglobin A. SA red cells sickle far less readily than SS red cells. (See Table 9.4.) Accordingly, SA heterozygotes develop sickling crises rarely and only when severely hypoxic. Splenic infarction occurs only occasionally. Since the renal medulla is unusually susceptible to

Table 9.4
Comparison of Intracellular Sickling and Solubility in the Sickling Disorders

Genotype	pO_2-50% sickled cells (mm Hg)	Solubility (g/100 ml)
SS	30–50	19
S-β thalassemia	22–32	variable
SC	10–20	26
S-HPFH	~10	24
AS	2–7	28

sickling, these patients often display an impaired ability to concentrate urine and rarely have recurrent episodes of painless hematuria due to medullary infarction. Individuals with the sickle cell trait should not be placed in high-risk categories by employers or insurers.

2. Diagnosis

The diagnosis rests upon the following laboratory tests:

1. Sickling preparation. A blood sample mixed with an oxygen-consuming reagent such as metabisulfite is examined under the microscope for sickled cells.

2. Solubility tests (e.g., dithionite tube test). These tests depend on the fact that deoxyhemoglobin S has low solubility at high ionic strength.

3. Mechanical precipitation tests. Hemoglobin S has an increased rate of surface denaturation and forms a precipitate when a dilute solution is shaken vigorously.

4. Hemoglobin electrophoresis (figure 9.2). Individuals with the sickle cell trait have about 35% hemoglobin S and 60% hemoglobin A.

B. Sickle cell anemia

The clinical manifestations of sickle cell anemia are all attributable to a specific molecular lesion: the substitution of valine for glutamic acid at the 6th residue of the β chain.

1. Molecular basis of sickling

Upon deoxygenation, a red cell containing hemoglobin S acquires an elongated crescent shape or sickle shape. Electron micrographs reveal bundles of fibers each with a diameter of 180 Å, running parallel to the long axis of sickling (figure 9.3). Each fiber consists of a 14-strand helical polymer having an inner core of 4 strands and an outer layer of 10 strands (see figure 9.3). Both hydrophobic and electrostatic bonds contribute to the stabilization of the helical polymers. In addition, there are interactions between neighboring fibers. The mechanism of sickling can be studied in vitro by determination of the hemoglobin concentration at which polymerization occurs, i.e., the solubility. As shown in table 9.4, this concentration is relatively low for deoxyhemoglobin S.

Sickling, both within the red cell and in a hemoglobin solution, is greatly affected by the presence of non-S hemoglobin. This can be confirmed by solubility measurements (table 9.4). Hemoglobin F appears to inhibit gelation. These experimentral results agree with well-known differences in clinical severity of the various sickle syndromes: SS, SF, and SA. Other uncommon hemoglobin variants also interact with hemoglobin S. Such information has been valuable in localizing the sites on the hemoglobin molecule responsible for the interaction of neighboring tetramers in the polymer. In order for hemoglobin S to form a sickle polymer (or fiber), it must be in the deoxy form.

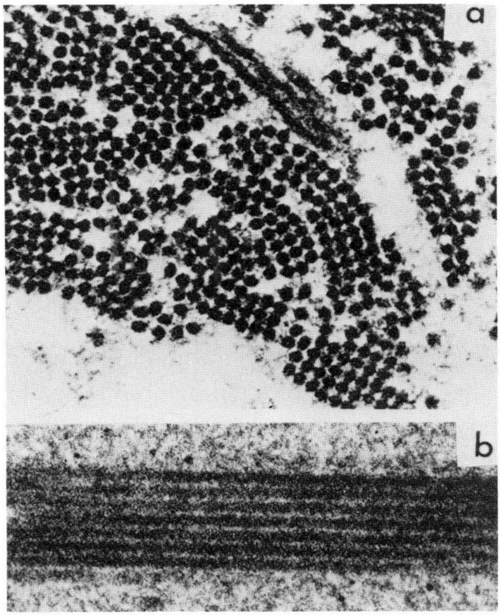

Fig. 9.3A
Electron micrographs of concentrated solution of deoxygenated hemoglobin S (×57,500): *a*, transverse section; *b*, longitudinal section showing parallel fibers.

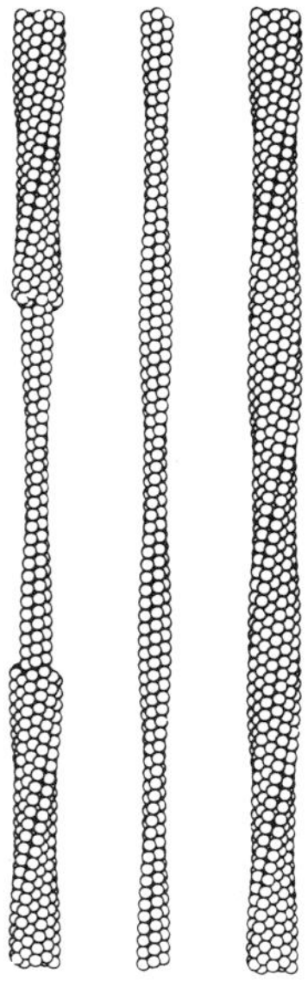

Fig. 9.3B
Model of sickle fiber showing an inner core and outer layer. Each deoxyhemoglobin S tetramer is represented as a sphere. (From Dykes et al., *J. Mol. Biol.* 130(1978): 451)

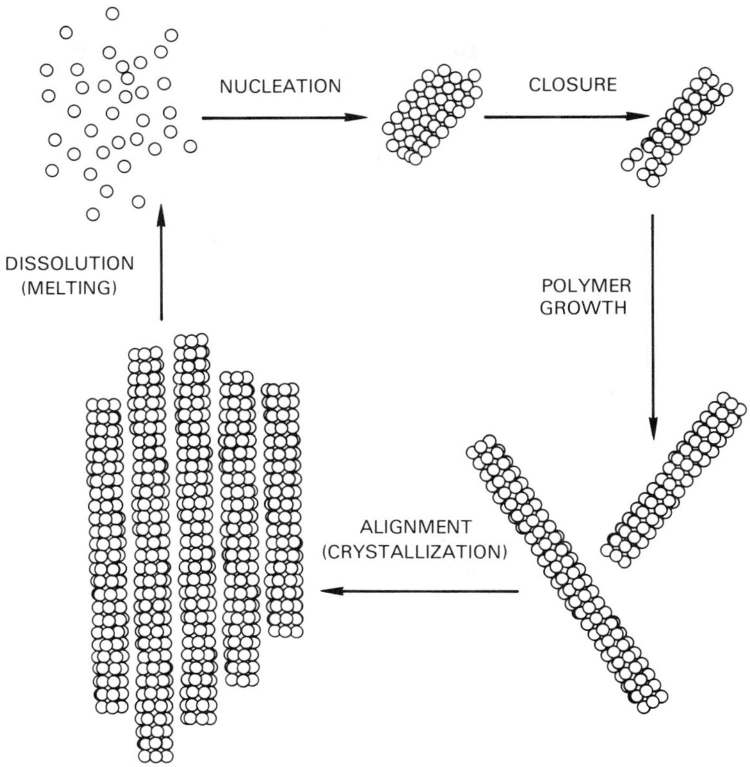

Fig. 9.4
Model of the polymerization of deoxyhemoglobin S. Monomeric hemoglobin aggregates in supersaturated solutions to form the compact nucleus for a single fiber. The fibers grow and then align into an ordered structure (tactoid or nematic crystal). (Courtesy of Dr. J. Hofrichter and Dr. W. Eaton)

Kinetic considerations are of importance in determining to what extent sickling occurs in solution or in the red cell. The initial and rate-limiting step is nucleation, that is, aggregation of individual hemoglobin tetramers into helical fibers (figure 9.4). This process is markedly concentration dependent. Once formed, the fibers undergo a phase transition from a random orientation to parallel alignment. This alignment of fibers is responsible for the distortion of the red cell into an elongated sickled form. Upon oxygenation or cooling, the polymers dissolve and the gel readily liquefies or melts (see figure 9.4).

2. Events at the cellular level

As sickle polymer forms, red cells become rigid and may further obstruct capillary blood flow. Obstruction of flow leads to local tissue hypoxia, further deoxygenation of hemoglobin, and therefore further intracellular polymerization. This vicious cycle may amplify microscopic obstruction into macroscopic infarction.

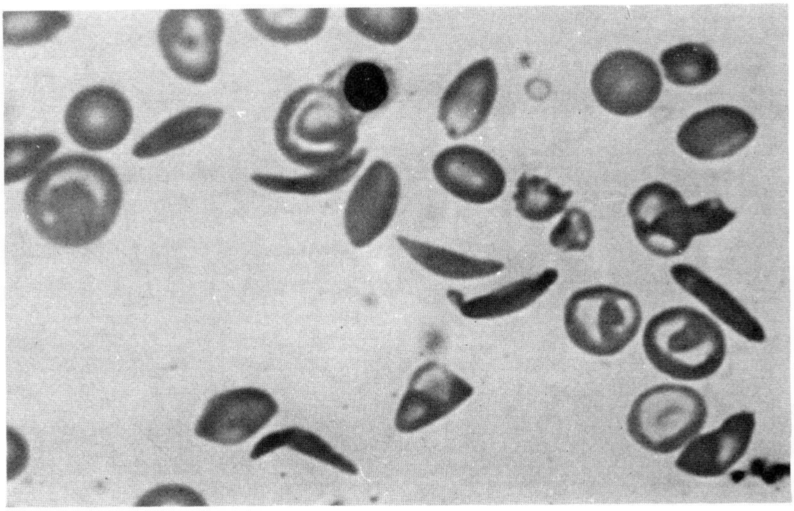

Fig. 9.5
Blood smear of patient with sickle cell anemia showing irreversibly sickled cells. (Photomicrograph by C. von Kapff)

Ordinarily, the sickled cell resumes a normal shape upon reoxygenation. However, the membrane of SS red cells may become damaged with resulting formation of *irreversibly sickled cells* (ISC; figure 9.5). Continuous formation and destruction of ISCs probably contributes to the severe hemolytic anemia occurring in sickle cell anemia. Furthermore, these rigid cells may initiate small vessel occlusion.

Several independent factors promote intracellular polymerization of Hb S. Increased corpuscular hemoglobin concentration is the most important since the rate of polymerization is so concentration dependent. The rate and extent of deoxygenation is another critical factor. Finally, both acidosis and increased red cell 2,3-DPG promote polymerization of sickle hemoglobin by lowering oxygen affinity (lecture 8) and therefore increasing levels of deoxyhemoglobin S.

3. Clinical features

a. Constitutional signs

Children with SS disease have impaired growth and development; general failure to thrive; and increased tendency to develop serious infections (especially with pneumococcus). These patients have marked impairment of splenic function (see lecture 2) with inadequate clearance of blood-borne bacteria. The spleen develops recurrent infarcts and in time becomes a nubbin of fibrous tissue. Infection is a common complication owing in part to the absence of splenic function. Infection frequently triggers the development of painful crises.

b. Anemia

SS homozygotes have a severe hemolytic anemia, hematocrit values ranging between 18 and 30%. Those red cells with relatively low hemoglobin F levels are likely to become ISCs and therefore have the shortest life spans. Anemia becomes increasingly severe if erythropoiesis is also suppressed. The two main causes of such suppression are aplastic crises due to infection and megaloblastosis due to folic acid deficiency. A decrease in red cell production, however transient, can rapidly depress the hematocrit.

c. Vasoocclusive phenomena

As noted, the morbidity and mortality of sickle cell disease is due primarily to recurrent vasoocclusive phenomena. These can be divided into two groups: painful crises and chronic organ damage.

Painful crises may appear suddenly in any part of the body. The common sites are abdomen, chest, and joints. About a third of painful crises are preceded by a viral or bacterial infection. The frequency and severity of painful crises is highly variable. It may be difficult to distinguish between painful sickle crises and another acute process. Abdominal crisis may mimic biliary colic, appendicitis, or perforated viscus. A sickle crisis in the extremities may mimic osteomyelitis or an acute arthritis such as gout or rheumatoid arthritis. The incidence, severity, and duration of pain crises vary markedly among patients and even in a given patient.

Chronic organ damage consisting of anatomical or functional damage to various tissues is due to the cumulative effect of recurrent vasoocclusive episodes. Any organ or system may be involved, but the following are most commonly encountered:

Cardiopulmonary system. Impairment of pulmonary function is common. Patients have hypoxemia due in part to intrapulmonary arterial-venous shunting. Congestive heart failure develops frequently owing to the burdens of chronic severe anemia and hypoxemia. Although more oxygen is extracted by the myocardium than any other tissue, myocardial infarction is rare.

Hepatobiliary system. Icterus and increased tendency to form gallstones commonly results from chronic hemolysis and impaired liver function. Hepatic infarction may occur.

Genitourinary system. The hypertonic and acidic environment in the renal medulla promotes sickling with resulting microinfarcts. Virtually all patients have isosthenuria. Like those with sickle trait or SC disease, SS homozygotes may develop significant and prolonged painless hematuria as a result of papillary infarcts. Male patients with sickle cell disease occasionally develop priapism (spontaneous, painful, and continued engorgement of the penis).

Skeletal system. The development of bone infarcts produces characteristic x-ray abnormalities. Biconcave "fish-mouth" vertebrae are pathognomonic of sickle cell disease (figure 9.6). Aseptic necrosis of the femoral head is common and can lead to disability.

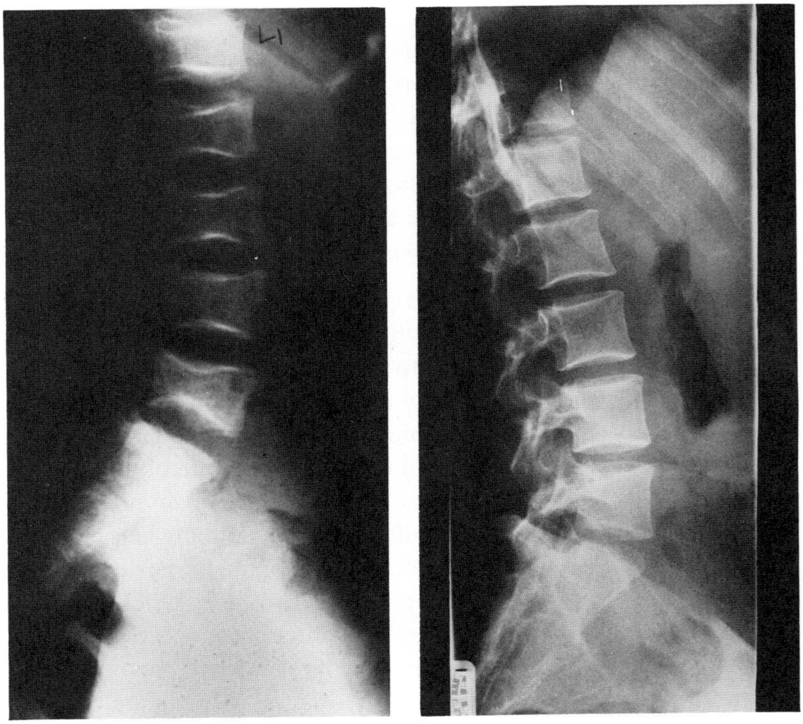

A B

Fig. 9.6
A, lateral view of lumbar spine of patient with sickle cell anemia. Note biconcave fish-mouth vertebrae. *B,* comparable view of a normal lumbar spine.

Like infarcts in other organs, bony infarctions often become infected. Osteomyelitis is frequently due to salmonella.

Eye. Ocular complications include retinal infarcts, peripheral vascular disease, arteriovenous anomalies, vitreous hemorrhage, retinitis proliferans, and retinal detachment. Major ocular complications are more common in SC disease than in SS homozygotes.

Skin. Chronic skin ulcers often occur in the distal lower extremities, particularly in severely anemic patients and in tropical areas.

Nervous system. A quarter of all patients with SS disease eventually develop some type of neurological complication. Hemiplegia is the most frequent. Coma, convulsions, or visual disturbances also occur. Patients generally recover from these episodes.

4. Diagnosis

The diagnosis is usually suspected from the clinical appearance of the patient and the appearance of the blood smear (figure 9.5). Hemoglobin electrophoresis shows 80–95% hemoglobin S, 0–20% hemoglobin F, and a normal amount of hemoglobin A_2. The diagnostic tests for sickling described above are positive.

5. Therapy

Many antisickling regimens have been proposed to date, but none has stood the test of time. Currently accepted management of sickle cell anemia is primarily supportive and conservative. Since these patients risk developing infections, which may trigger painful and aplastic crises, it is important to detect infection early and treat promptly with antibiotics. Pneumococcal vaccination may prevent the development of meningitis. Anemia increases markedly if the patient becomes folic acid deficient. Since these patients have an increased folic acid requirement, they should be given a daily supplement.

Painful crises should be treated promptly with analgesia and hydration. Since crises may be aborted if treated early, it is advisable to give patients a supply of analgesics (e.g., codeine) that can be self-administered.

Blood transfusions have a limited role in the management of sickle cell anemia. Between crises, patients usually tolerate anemia well and do not derive much subjective benefit from transfusions. Replacement of 70% of the patient's SS red cells with normal AA red cells (hypertransfusion) reduces the recurrence rate of strokes in children. Furthermore, hypertransfusion may be a useful way of getting a patient through a limited period of risk such as pregnancy or surgery. However, the risks of isoimmunization, iron overload, and hepatitis are sufficient reasons to minimize transfusion.

Currently a number of investigators are attempting to treat sickle cell disease by inducing an increase in Hb F. This can be accomplished by the administration of certain antineoplastic agents such as 5-azacytidine and hydroxyurea. The mechanism underlying the increase in the Hb F synthesis is unclear.

6. Prevention

Genetic counseling may be useful in the prevention of sickle cell anemia. If both marital partners are SA heterozygotes, they may decide not to have children, knowing that there is a 25% chance that an offspring will be an SS homozygote.

The antenatal diagnosis of sickle cell anemia can now be made early in the 18th to 20th week of pregnancy by the testing of a small sample of amniotic fluid. There are endonucleases that can distinguish between the normal β globin gene and the β^S gene at the site of base substitution. If it is established that a fetus is an SS homozygote, the parents may elect to interrupt a pregnancy.

7. Prognosis

The clinical course of homozygous SS disease is highly variable. Most published assessments of prognosis have been unduly pessimistic. In the United States, an increasing number of patients are surviving into adulthood and bearing offspring. Although patients who have relatively high hemoglobin F levels tend to have milder clinical manifestations, this relation is of little prognostic value in a given patient.

C. Other sickle syndromes

1. Sickle-β thalassemia

β thalassemia, a disorder characterized by absent or diminished β chain synthesis, is fully discussed in lecture 10. In sickle-β thalassemia, both β-globin genes are defective, one producing an abnormal β chain and the other affecting the rate of β chain synthesis. The disease is variable in its clinical manifestations. It occurs primarily in Mediterranean people. Like homozygous β thalassemia, sickle-β thalassemia is milder in blacks than in Mediterranean people. Patients have moderately severe hemolytic anemia (hematocrit 25–35). Splenomegaly occurs in 70% of the cases. Various vasoocclusive phenomena may occur, but painful crises are less frequent and severe than in homozygous sickle cell anemia.

2. Diagnosis

The blood smear reveals hypochromic microcytic red cells with polychromatophilia, target cells, stippling, and rare ISCs (figure 9.7).

Hemoglobin electrophoresis reveals that 60–90% of the hemoglobin is S and 10–30% is F. Hemoglobin A is about 10–30% if the patient is capable of producing some β^A chains (see β^+ thalassemia in lecture 10). Hemoglobin A_2 is moderately elevated in sickle-β thalassemia.

3. Prognosis and therapy

Most patients require little specific therapy. If the spleen is sequestering red cells in significant amounts, splenectomy may be beneficial.

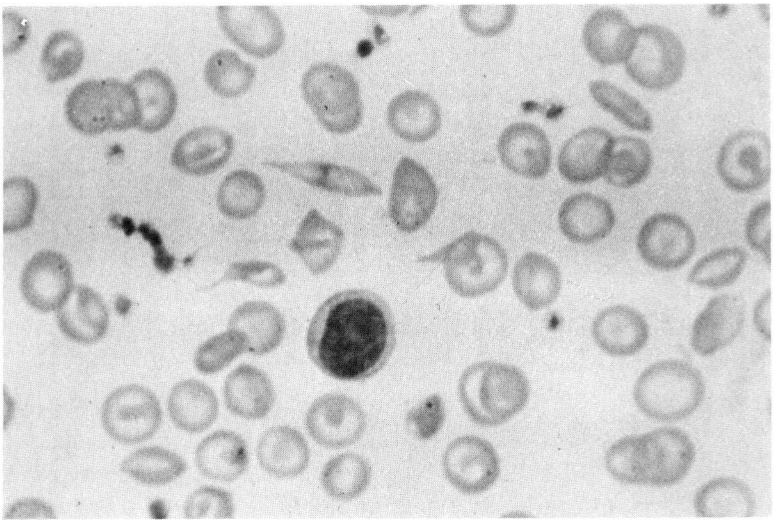

Fig. 9.7
Blood smear of patient with sickle-β thalassemia. (Photomicrograph by C. von Kapff)

D. Sickle-C disease

The gene frequency for hemoglobin C ($\alpha_2\beta_2^{6Glu\rightarrow Lys}$) is a quarter of that for hemoglobin S. Nevertheless, SC disease is almost as common among adults as SS disease since life expectancy in SC disease is nearly normal. There are two reasons why SC is a disease whereas AS is benign. First, intracellular hemoglobin concentration is significantly higher in SC red cells owing to the presence of Hb C (see below). Second, SC red cells have at least 10% higher level of hemoglobin S than have AS red cells. Patients have a

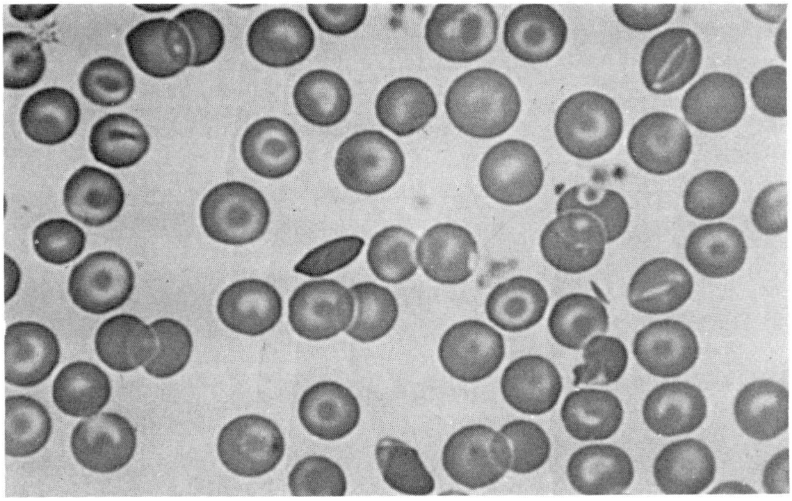

Fig. 9.8
Blood smear of patient with sickle-C disease. (Photomicrograph by C. von Kapff)

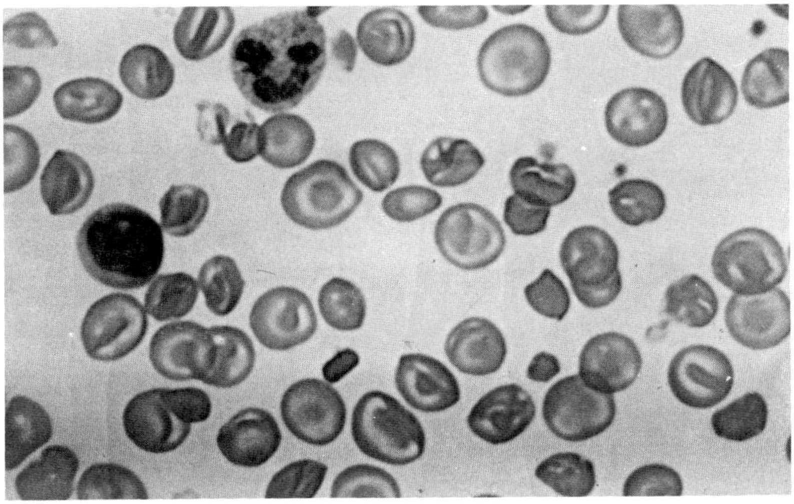

Fig. 9.9
Blood smear of patient with homozygous hemoglobin C disease. (Photomicrograph by C. von Kapff)

mild to moderate hemolytic anemia and usually have splenomegaly. The blood smear shows target cells and occasional plump sickled forms (figure 9.8). Painful crises or organ infarcts occur occasionally. Ocular complications are common, as are hematuria from renal medullary infarcts, aseptic necrosis of the femoral head, and various complications during pregnancy.

E. Homozygous C disease

Homozygous hemoglobin C disease produces a mild congenital hemolytic anemia with splenomegaly. Hemoglobin C is less soluble than hemoglobin A, and it tends to form intracellular crystals, particularly if red cells are suspended in a hypertonic medium. CC red cells are dehydrated. The blood smear reveals striking target cells (figure 9.9). Red cell osmotic fragility is decreased. Significant complications are rare, and no specific therapy is required.

III. UNSTABLE HEMOGLOBINS

Over 60 unstable hemoglobin variants are known. These hemoglobins cause hemolysis in heterozygous subjects. In many instances, the homozygous state would be lethal. The molecular abnormality is often an amino acid substitution in the heme pocket of the β chain (figure 9.10). In comparison to hemoglobin A, such hemoglobins readily autooxidize to methemoglobin, whereupon the heme becomes detached and residual relatively insoluble globin forms an intracellular precipitate, or *Heinz body*. Some unstable hemoglobins result from an amino acid subtitution that distorts or interrupts the helical structure of the involved chain, for example, hemoglobin Bibba ($\alpha_2^{136Leu \rightarrow Pro}\beta_2$). The abnormal subunits of a few unstable variants have deletions of 1–5 amino acid residues (table

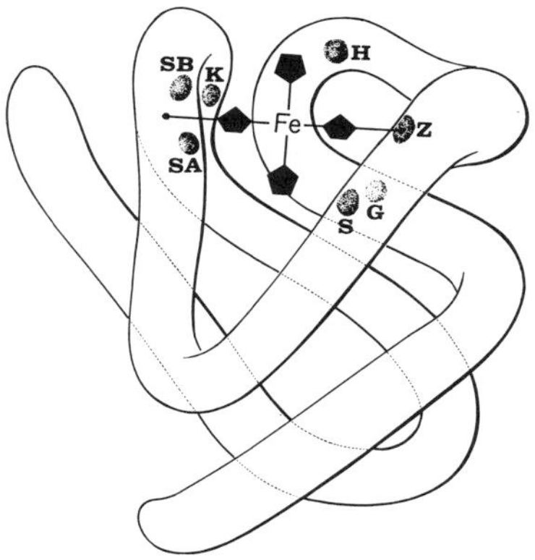

Fig. 9.10
Unstable hemoglobins. The diagram depicts a three-dimensional representation of a β chain. Sites of amino acid substitutions of some of the unstable hemoglobin variants are designated with letters. Note their proximity to the heme group: K = Köln, β98 Val→Met; H = Hammersmith, β42 Phe→Ser; Z = Zurich, β63 His→Arg; G = Genova, β28 Val→Ala; SA = Santa Ana, β88 Leu→Pro. (From H. Jacob and K. Winterhalter, *Proc. Nat. Acad. Sci. USA* 65(1970): 697)

9.1). The precipitated inclusions impair red cell deformability, and the cell becomes trapped in the RES. The inclusions may be "pitted" from the red cell (see lecture 2) or the entire cell may be destroyed (see lecture 11). The heme may be catabolized aberrantly to form *dipyrroles*, which cause the excretion of dark-colored urine. Unstable hemoglobin should be suspected in any patient with congenital hemolytic anemia. Its presence is confirmed by supravital Heinz body stains, hemoglobin electrophoresis, and the heat stability test, in which hemolysate is heated to 50°C. Unstable hemoglobins form a precipitate; normal hemoglobins do not.

IV. HEMOGLOBINS WITH ABNORMAL OXYGEN AFFINITY

A. High-oxygen-affinity variants

Familial erythrocytosis may be due to the inheritance of a stable hemoglobin variant having increased oxygen affinity. Over 20 different *high-oxygen-affinity hemoglobin variants* have been discovered to date. Like unstable hemoglobins, they are found only in heterozygotes. The amino acid substitution is likely to be in the $\alpha_1\beta_2$ contact area, or at the C-terminus of the β chain. Interference in the normal conformational isomerization between deoxyhemoglobin and oxyhemoglobin leads to altered oxygen affinity and decreased heme-heme interaction.

The major pathophysiologic consequences of the presence of a high-oxygen-affinity hemoglobin are (1) decreased unloading of oxygen in tissues; (2) increased erythropoietin production; and (3) familial erythrocytosis.

B. Low-oxygen-affinity variant

Pathologic consequences of the presence of a *low-oxygen-affinity hemoglobin variant* differ depending on which hemoglobin is present. Hemoglobins Kansas, Beth Israel, and St. Mandé cause cyanosis because the amino acid substitution affects one of the $\alpha_1\beta_2$ interface residues. Oxygen affinity is decreased and the hemoglobin tends to dissociate into subunits. The lower affinity for oxygen of few variants increases the availability of oxygen in the tissues.

Table 9.5
The M Hemoglobins

Amino acid substitution	Name of hemoglobin (location of propositus)
$\alpha_2^{58His\rightarrow Tyr}\beta_2$	Boston, Osaka, Gothenburg
$\alpha_2^{87His\rightarrow Tyr}\beta_2$	Iwate, Kankakee, Oldenburg
$\alpha_2\beta_2^{63His\rightarrow Tyr}$	Saskatoon, Chicago, Emory, Kurme, Radom
$\alpha_2\beta_2^{92His\rightarrow Tyr}$	Hyde Park
$\alpha_2\beta_2^{67Val\rightarrow Glu}$	Milwaukee

As a result, erythropoietin secretion decreases and the hematocrit drops. Despite their rarity, these hemoglobins are important in probing the chemistry and physiology of hemoglobin function.

V. HEMOGLOBINS M

As noted in lecture 8, familial cyanosis may be due to inheritance of one of the M hemoglobins. This group includes five variants. In four, tyrosine is substituted for the invariant distal (E7) or proximal (F8) heme-linked histidine of the α or β chain (see fiure 8.2). The fifth variant (M Milwaukee) involves substitution of glutamic acid for valine at the β^{67} locus. These changes stabilize the hemes of the abnormal globin chains in the ferric form. This alters the absorption spectrum and gives the hemoglobin a brown color. It also alters the oxygenation of the normal (nonmutant) chains.

Families with the same hemoglobin M have been discovered in many widely separated areas (table 9.5). Variants have been designated by the place of origin, sometimes with competing names. Homozygosity for hemoglobin M would probably be lethal. Heterozygotes are usually asymptomatic except for cyanosis, though hemoglobins M Saskatoon and M Hyde Park are also unstable and may cause mild hemolysis.

SELECTED REFERENCES

Bunn, H. F., and Forget, B. G. — *Hemoglobin: Molecular, Genetic, and Clinical Aspects,* Philadelphia: W. B. Saunders, 1984.

Bunn, H. F., et al. — Molecular and cellular pathogenesis of hemoglobin SC disease. *Proc. Natl. Acad. Sci., U.S.A.* 79(1982): 7527.

Castle, W. B. — From man to molecule and back to mankind. *Semin. Hematol.* 13(1976): 159.

Charache, S. — Treatment of sickle cell anemia. *Ann. Rev. Med.* 32(1981): 195.

Dean, J., and Schechter, A. N. — Sickle cell anemia: Molecular and cellular bases of therapeutic approaches. *New Eng. J. Med.* 299(1978): 752, 804, 863.

Eaton, W. A., et al. — Delay time of gelation: A possible determinant of clinical severity in sickle cell disease. *Blood* 47(1976): 621.

Ley, T. J., et al. — 5-Azacytidine increases γ-globin synthesis and reduces the proportion of dense cells in patients with sickle cell anemia. *Blood* 62(1983): 370.

Noguchi, C. T., and Schechter, A. N. — The intracellular polymerization of sickle hemoglobin and its relevance to sickle cell disease. *Blood* 58(1981): 1057.

Orkin, S. H., et al. — Improved detection of the sickle mutation by DNA analysis. *New Eng. J. Med.* 307(1982): 32.

Powars, D. R. — Natural history of sickle cell disease: The first ten years. *Semin. Hematol.* 12(1975): 267.

LECTURE 10 The Thalassemias

David G. Nathan

I. INTRODUCTION

A. Definitions

The thalassemias (named from the Greek word for sea) are a heterogeneous group of inherited disorders of hemoglobin synthesis characterized by absent or diminished synthesis of one or the other of the globin chains of hemoglobin A. In the *α-thalassemias,* α chain synthesis is absent or diminished; in the *β-thalassemias,* β chain synthesis is absent or diminished. Diverse molecular mechanisms account for the various thalassemias. Clinical manifestations vary with the nature and severity of the defect.

The terms *Mediterranean anemia* and *Cooley's anemia* were used in the older literature to denote β thalassemia. The term *thalassemia major* has also been used to refer to the homozygous state and *thalassemia minor* and *thalassemia intermedia* to heterozygous states of various degrees of severity.

B. Geographic distribution

Although the thalassemias are found all over the world, specific forms occur with high frequency in certain populations—notably in Mediterranean populations (i.e., from southern Italy and Greece) and Oriental populations (i.e., from Thailand, China, and the Philippines). β-thalassemia is more common in Mediterranean populations; α-thalassemia is prevalent in Oriental populations. In Italy and Greece, 5–10% of the population are heterozygous for β-thalassemia. In Thailand, the gene frequency for the various forms of heterozygous α-thalassemia reaches 25%. Sporadic cases of thalassemia are common among Africans and American blacks. Generally, the distribution of thalassemia follows the malaria belt (figure 10.1). The high frequency of thalassemia in these areas may be attributable to the fact that the heterozygous thalassemias enhance resistance to malaria.

C. Pathophysiology

1. Basic mechanisms

A unifying concept underlies our understanding of the pathophysiology of all the thalassemias: Deficient or absent synthesis of a specific globin chain leads to unbalanced chain synthesis. This has two effects: (1) inadequate hemoglobinization of developing erythroid cells with resulting hypochromia; and (2) more important, various specific sequelae of unbalanced globin chain synthesis. For example, chains present in relative excess, particularly when of the α type, precipitate in the developing erythroid cell. This damages surface membrances in both developing and mature cells. Cells thus handicapped either die in the bone marrow (thus causing ineffective erythropoiesis) or, if released from the mar-

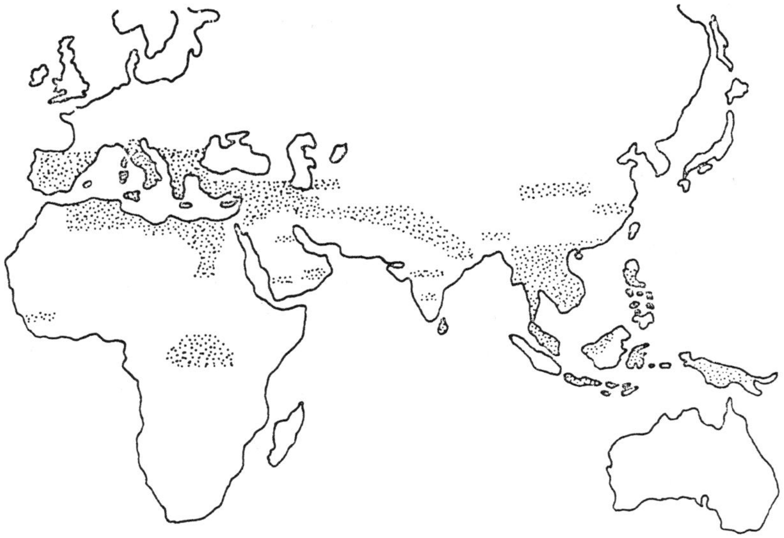

Fig. 10.1
Geographical distribution of the thalassemias, indicated by speckled regions.

row, are promptly removed by the RES (thus causing hemolysis). Both phenomena compound the anemia and lead to compensatory erythropoietin-induced marrow hypertrophy. This in turn leads to a hypermetabolic state, skeletal changes, and increased intestinal absorption of iron and iron overload. This web of causes and effects in homozygous β-thalassemia is diagrammed in figure 10.2.

2. Clinical implications

Clinical severity varies broadly, ranging from benign to lethal. The severity of a particular thalassemia is related to (1) patterns of inheritance, that is, heterozygosity or homozygosity; (2) severity of the particular thalassemia defect; (3) degree of compensation, especially with respect to γ globin chain production (see below and figure 10.2); (4) presence of interacting thalassemia defects (e.g., simultaneous inheritance of α- and β-thalassemia defects, presence of β^S, β^E); and (5) presence of interacting factors of unknown character.

D. Molecular biology of globin genes

1. Hemoglobin structure

Molecular structure of various normal hemoglobins (summarized in table 8.1) should be reviewed because it is essential to an understanding of the basis of thalassemia. It also permits a classification of these disorders on the basis of primary defect rather than by overlapping and somewhat confusing clinical descriptions. It will be recalled that all normal hemoglobins are formed at tetramers of two α (or α-like) chains and two non-α globin chains.

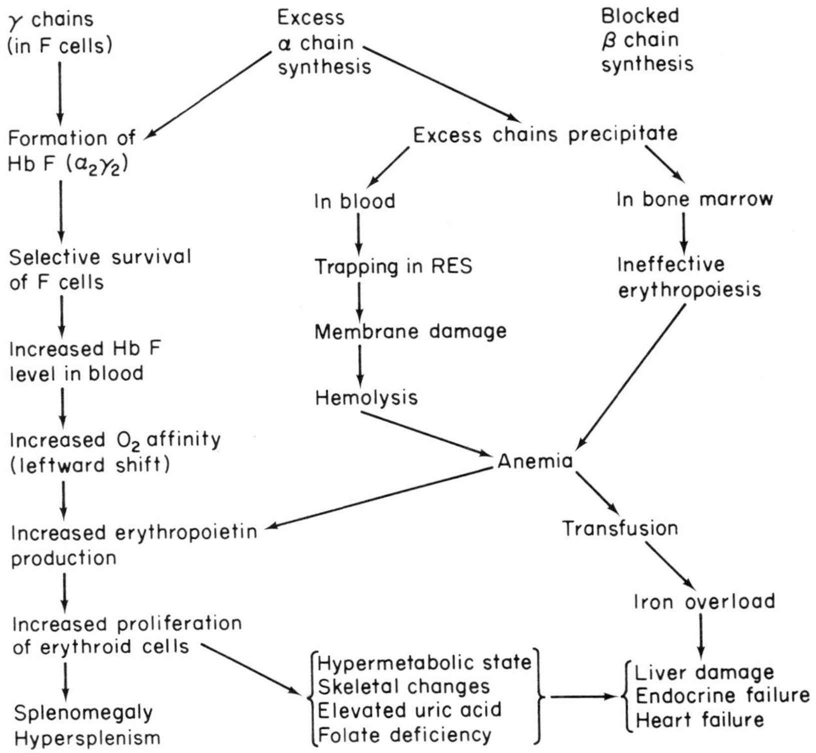

Fig. 10.2
Pathophysiology of homozygous β-thalassemia.

Hemoglobin A is a $\alpha_2\beta_2$. Hemoglobin A_2, $\alpha_2\delta_2$, comprises about 2% of adult hemoglobin, and hemoglobin F, $\alpha_2\gamma_2$, is predominant in fetal life and is only 1–2% in normal adults.

2. Reactivation of hemoglobin F

The time sequence of hemoglobins present in fetal and adult life is shown in figure 8.1. This evidence of hemoglobin "switching" reflects a changing pattern of erythroid progenitors, each expressing different programs of gene expression in the differentiated erythroid cells to which they give rise. The substantial disappearance of hemoglobin F in the first 6 months of neonatal life reflects the cessation of γ chain synthesis. Reactivation of hemoglobin F synthesis often occurs in normal pregnancy and in severe disorders of erythropoiesis, including hemolytic anemias such as thalassemia and sickle cell anemia and leukemia. This occurs in a restricted subset of red cells (F cells), which increase in number in anemia. They produce an amount of hemoglobin F that rarely exceeds 20% of the total. In contrast, all of the red cells in a fetus produce hemoglobin F, so that the amount of hemoglobin F is a substantial percentage of the total.

3. Organization of globin genes

The α chain genes are on a different chromosome from the non-α chain genes (figure 10.3). Ordinarily, the α chain gene is dupli-

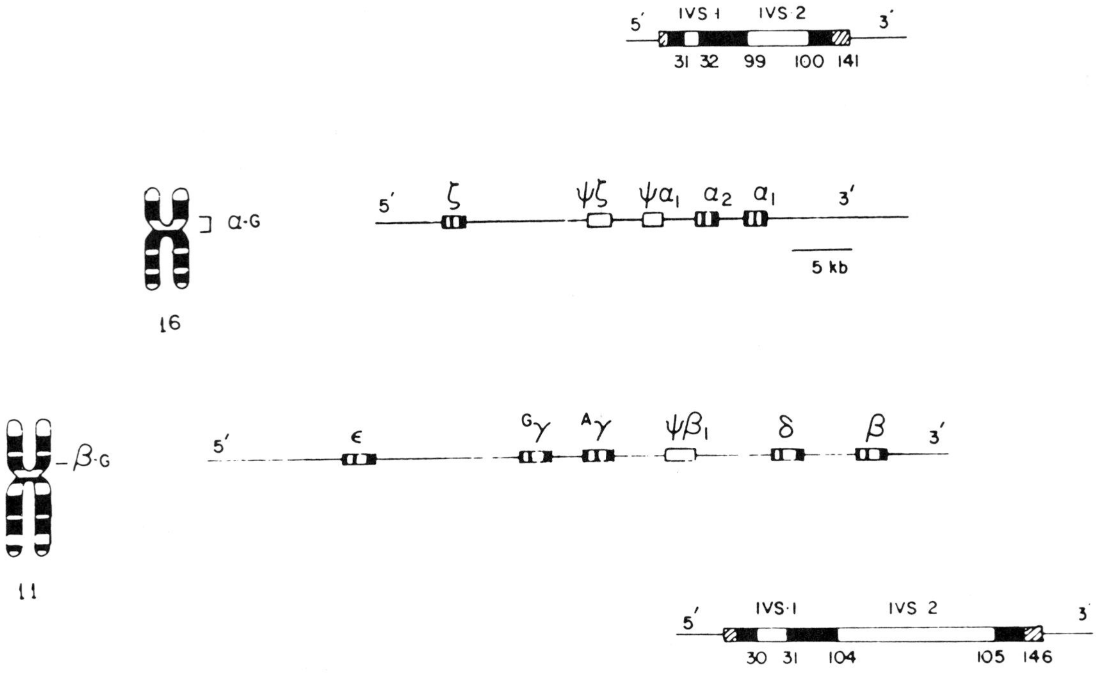

Fig. 10.3
The chromosomal localization and genomic organization of the human globin genes. To the left, the α- and β-globin gene complexes are positioned on chromosomes 16 and 11, respectively. In the center, the arrangement of genes in the two complexes is depicted. The general structures of the genes are shown at the top and bottom with the location of the IVS shown by the codon numbers below the schematics. Coding regions are shown by closed boxes and IVS by open boxes.

cated—that is, there are two α genes per haploid set of chromosomes. Recent work employing restriction endonuclease techniques of gene mapping and gene cloning has revealed many details of globin gene arrangements in DNA.

The α *genes* are on chromosome 16:

	5′ α_2	α_1 3′
nucleotide distance	3,700	

The β *genes* (and the γ and δ genes which are linked to the β genes) are on the short arm of chromosome 11:

	G_γ	A_γ	δ	β
nucleotide distances	3,500	14,000	5,500	

The difference between G_γ and A_γ is explained in lecture 8.

In sum, there are per diploid cell

α genes	4
β genes	2
δ genes	2
γ genes	4

The extensive homology of duplicated α and γ genes can lead to a high potential rate of deletion due to unequal crossing over. The δβ area is at lower risk because homology is less and intergenic distance greater. Like other eukaryotic genes, globin genes are discontinuous or split—that is, coding sequences (exons) are interrupted by sequences of DNA that do not encode globin chains (introns or intervening sequences). The intervening sequences, larger in δ, γ, and β genes than in α genes, are transcribed into a primary transcript RNA or pre-mRNA in erythroid cell nuclei. Then in a maturation process these sequences are removed in precise splicing reactions to yield mature mRNA.

The molecular basis of thalassemia is discussed below.

II. CLINICAL ASPECTS

As noted the thalassemias are named for the affected chain(s). Due to hemoglobin switching, β-thalassemias are usually not clinically apparent until the age of about 6 months.

A. Classification

The following (diagram 10.1) is a simple, broad classification:

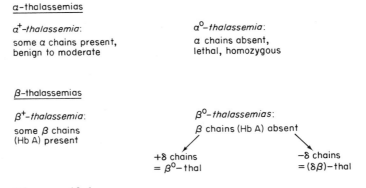

α-thalassemias

α^+-thalassemia:
some α chains present,
benign to moderate

α^0-thalassemia:
α chains absent,
lethal, homozygous

β-thalassemias

β^+-thalassemia:
some β chains
(Hb A) present

β^0-thalassemias:
β chains (Hb A) absent

+δ chains
= β^0–thal

–δ chains
= (δβ)–thal

Diagram 10.1

B. The α-thalassemias

1. Clinical states

The α-thalassemias have been studied extensively in Asian populations. Four principal clinical states are encountered that differ in clinical severity. Each is associated with a different number of deletions of functional α genes. These may be summarized as follows:

Diagnosis	Common name	α globin output (%)	Number of functional α genes	Gene configuration
Normal	Normal	100	4	αα/αα
1 α-thal	Silent carrier	75	3	-α/αα
2 α-thal	α-thal trait	50	2	-α/-α or --/αα
3 α-thal	Hb H disease	25	1	--/-α
4 α-thal	Hydrops fetalis	0	0	--/--

Clinical and genetic features of these syndromes are given in table 10.1. Note that hemoglobin H is β_4. Hemoglobin Bart's is γ_4.

2. Patterns of inheritance

The following matings produce the indicated progeny:

silent carrier × normal → normal (50%) and silent carrier (50%);

silent carrier × trait → trait (25%), normal (25%), Hb H (25%), silent carrier (25%);

trait × trait → hydrops fetalis (25%), normal (25%), trait (50%).

3. Distribution of α genes

Deletion of α genes, often a result of unequal crossing over between two chromosomes, can cause different gene distributions and different risks. For example, blacks with so-called 2 α-thal (see above) usually have a single α gene deleted on each chromosome 16 rather than deletions of both α genes on a single chromosome 16. Therefore blacks with the phenotype 2 α-thal have two deletions in *trans* (i.e., on different chromosomes) rather than two deletions in *cis* (i.e., on the same chromosome). This explains the absence in blacks of homozygous α-thalassemia with hydrops fetalis due to total α gene deletion. The frequency in blacks of chromosomes with two α genes deleted is so low and of chromosomes with single α genes so high that homozygosity for no α genes is very rare. In contrast it is common among the Chinese. In some individuals unequal crossing over can lead to three α genes on one chromosome. This leads to genetic interchange among three types of chromosomes. Duplication of α genes and their flanking regions increases the likelihood of genetic recombination and heterogeneity.

C. The β-thalassemias

The β-thalassemias are characterized by deficient synthesis of β chains and persistent synthesis of γ chains. This results in variable elevations of Hb F. However, γ chain production is usually inadequate to compensate fully for the β chain deficiency. The combination of hemoglobins present in the blood reflects the genotype. It also reflects the selection of the hardiest cells (i.e., usually those with Hb F). Nevertheless, a rough categorization of

Table 10.1
Clinical Aspects of α-Thalassemias

Condition	Parental genotypes	Risk	Hemoglobin pattern	Severity	α mRNA	Genes
Silent carrier (1 α-thal)	Silent carrier, normal	½	Approximately 1–2% Hb Bart's in cord blood	0	Presumed slight deficiency	1 of 4 α genes deleted
Heterozygous α-thalassemia (α-thal trait) (2 α-thal)	α-thalassemia trait, normal	½	Approximately 5% Hb Bart's in cord blood	Mild; very mild in blacks	Presumed deficiency	2 of 4 α genes deleted; ? 1 of 3 deleted in blacks
Hb H disease (3 α-thal)	(i) α-thalassemia trait, silent carrier (ii) α-thalassemia trait, Hb CS heterozygote	¼ ¼	4–30% Hb H in adults: approximately 25% Hb Bart's in cord blood; when Hb CS gene present, 2–3% Hb CS	Variable, usually thalassemia intermedia	Marked deficiency	(i) 3 of 4 α genes deleted (ii) 2 of 4 deleted; 1 normal; 1 Hb CS gene
Homozygous α-thalassemia (hydrops fetalis with Hb Bart's) (4 α-thal)	Both α-thalassemia trait	¼	80% Hb Bart's; remainder, Hb H and Hb Portland[a]	Lethal	Absent	All α genes deleted
Heterozygous Hb Constant Spring (CS)	Hb CS heterozygote, normal	½	Approximately 1% Hb CS	0	Presumed deficiency	3 of 4 α genes present; 1 Hb CS gene

a. Hb Portland ($\zeta_2\gamma_2$) is derived from the product of the embryonic α-like gene called zeta (ζ) and the product of the gamma genes.

"homozygous" β-thalassemias may be based on hemoglobin patterns, as follows:

	β^+-thal	β^0-thal	δβ-thal	Normal
Hb A	Present (↓)	Absent	Absent	Normal
Hb A_2	Increased	Increased	Absent	Normal
Hb F	Increased (but <100%)	Increased (nearly 100%)	Increased (100%)	Low

Patients with "homozygous" β- or β^0-thalassemia usually have lower *total* hemoglobin levels than those with "homozygous" δβ-thalassemia.

1. Clinical states

As noted, β-thalassemia can be divided into two general types, β^+-thal and β^0-thal. As shown in table 10.2, the clinically severe thalassemias may not in fact be homozygous. In addition, there is considerable mechanistic heterogeneity at the molecular level. This may also lead to clinical heterogeneity. Clinical features of the β-thalassemias are summarized in table 10.3.

D. Therapy

Definitive treatment is not yet available. Therapy is entirely supportive. Carrier states do not require treatment. The following remarks concern management of the β-thalassemias.

1. Transfusion

When untreated, patients with homozygous β-thalassemia may die by the age of 2 or 3 with hematocrits as low as 5–6%. Blood transfusions prevent this outcome. Patients maintained by frequent transfusions from an early age avoid many complications. If hemoglobin levels are kept between 10 and 12 g/100 ml by repeated transfusions, marrow hyperplasia is repressed. Bones do not become demineralized and weakened, and facial changes do not develop. There is less cardiomegaly and hepatosplenomegaly,

Table 10.2
Characteristics of the "Homozygous" β-Thalassemias

	Hemoglobin patterns			
Genotype	Hb A ($\alpha_2\beta_2$)	Hb A_2 ($\alpha_2\delta_2$)	Hb F ($\alpha_2\gamma_2$)	Clinical severity
β^+/β^+	Variable	Variable	↑	Depends upon severity of β gene impairment and extent of γ gene compensation
β^+/β^0	Usually low	Variable	↑	Usually more severe than β^+/β^+
β^0/β^0	Absent	Variable	↑	Very severe unless γ gene compensation is unusually high
$\beta\delta/\beta^+$	Low	Low	↑ ↑	Relatively mild due to increased γ chain production
$\beta\delta/\beta^0$	Absent	Low	↑ ↑	Somewhat more severe than $\beta\delta/\beta^+$ due to absent β chain production
βδ/βδ	Absent	Low	↑ ↑ ↑	Mild due to increased γ chain production

Note: The term *homozygous* is misleading when applied to patients who have inherited two different kinds of thalassemic genes.

Table 10.3
Clinical Aspects of β-Thalassemias

Condition	Parental genotypes	Risk	Hemoglobin pattern	Severity	β mRNA	Genes
Homozygous states						
β^+-thalassemia	Both β^+/β	¼	↓ Hb A, ↑ Hb F, variable Hb A_2	Variable; usually Cooley's anemia	Marked deficiency of β mRNA	β genes present
β^0-thalassemia	Both β^0/β	¼	0 Hb A, variable Hb A_2, residual Hb F	Cooley's anemia	(i) absent β mRNA (ii) mutant, nonfunctional β mRNA present in rare Oriental cases	β genes present
$\delta\beta^0$-thalassemia	Both $\delta\beta^0/\delta\beta$	¼	0 Hb A, Hb A_2; 100% Hb F	Thalassemia intermedia	δ and β mRNAs absent	β genes deleted; probable δ gene deletion
Hb Lepore	Both Hb Lepore/β	¼	0 Hb A, Hb A_2; 75% Hb F, 25% Hb Lepore	Cooley's anemia	β-like mRNA present in reduced amount	β-δ fusion genes present; no normal β and δ genes
Heterozygous states						
β^+-thalassemia	β^+/β, normal	½	↑ Hb A_2, slight ↑ Hb F	Thalassemia minor	Deficient β mRNA	β genes present
β^0-thalassemia	β^0/β, normal	½	↑ Hb A_2, slight ↑ Hb F	Thalassemia minor	Deficient β mRNA, or rarely nonfunctional β mRNA present	β genes present
$\delta\beta^0$-thalassemia	$\delta\beta^0/\delta\beta$, normal	½	5–20% Hb F	Thalassemia minor	Presumed deficiency of β and δ mRNAs	β and probable δ gene deletion on 1 homologous chromosome
Hb Lepore	Hb Lepore/β, normal	½	↑ Hb F, ↓ Hb A_2, 5–15% Hb Lepore	Thalassemia minor	β-like mRNA present	Hb Lepore gene replaces normal β and δ genes on 1 chromosome

better growth and development, and better quality of life. Frequent transfusions, however, inevitably lead to iron overload and its serious complications, including intractable congestive heart failure. Transfusion with young red cells ("neocytes") increases the interval between transfusions. These patients, incidentally, have increased folic acid requirements and require regular supplements.

2. Splenectomy

Splenectomy is often needed to reduce blood volume and red cell pooling. Splenomegaly often causes a gradual increase in the transfusion requirement. Splenectomy reverses this trend. If possible, splenectomy should be deferred until age 5–6, after which there is a lessened risk of overwhelming infection (usually pneumococcal septicemia).

3. Iron-chelating agents

As discussed in lecture 6, the iron-chelating agent desferrioxamine is used successfully in the treatment of acute iron poisoning. However, until recently the effectiveness of such therapy in removing iron accumulations from heart, liver, and endocrine organs has been disappointing. The drug must be given parenterally. Recent work shows that continuous subcutaneous infusion (under the control of a portable infusion pump) for 12 hr each day leads to significant negative iron balance. It is not yet known whether chronic desferrioxamine therapy will prolong survival in patients on frequent transfusion regimens.

E. Prevention

The severity of the thalassemias has prompted serious efforts at prevention. Current methods involve genetic counseling and prenatal diagnosis.

1. Genetic counseling

In principle, genetic counseling of patients with various heterozygous β-thalassemia syndromes should reduce the number of pregnancies for which homozygous β-thalassemia is a risk. Once the type of thalassemia is established, advice concerning the probability of its occurrence among offspring can usually be offered. In practice, it has not yet been established that extensive population surveys and genetic counseling can actually achieve this goal.

2. Prenatal diagnosis

Prenatal diagnosis of the α-thalassemias is of little importance since infants with Hb Bart's and hydrops fetalis usually die in utero and Hb H is compatible with a normal life expectancy. However, a method for the prenatal diagnosis of β-thalassemia would be of great value. Two approaches have been used.

a. Phenotypic method

In the first trimester of normal fetal development, β chain synthesis is at a low level. The actual level can be accurately quantified by appropriate biosynthetic studies on fetal blood cells. Thus, even if the β chain gene is only minimally expressed in fetal development, it is possible to diagnose qualitative and quantitative abnormalities of β chain synthesis in the first 18–20 weeks. By various techniques (e.g., placental aspiration or fetoscopy, which permits needle aspiration under direct visualization of blood vessels on the placental surface), it is usually possible without harming the fetus to obtain relatively pure samples of fetal blood, which can then be subjected to isotopic analysis of the rates of α, γ, and β chain synthesis. This procedure is capable of diagnosing all forms of thalassemia and hemoglobinopathy. Risk to the fetus is about 5%.

b. Genetic method

This procedure analyzes the DNA of amniotic cells or chorionic villi for primary defects or associated plymorphisms. The techniques involve direct restriction enzyme analysis of deletions or single mutations that produce restriction enzyme pattern shifts or application of oligonucleotide hybridization to detect single base alterations. It permits diagnosis of all deletion syndromes, all cases of sickle cell anemia, and most cases of thalassemia. The risk is associated with accrual of sufficient numbers of amniotic or chorionic cells.

III. MECHANISMS IN THALASSEMIA

A. Genetic defects

The central problem is, Why in thalassemia are specific hemoglobin chains not synthesized effectively? It will be recalled that normal synthesis of a protein involves (1) the presence of a normal structural gene in the DNA; (2) transcription of the DNA into a primary RNA product; (3) processing of the initial RNA product to a mature mRNA; (4) transport of mature globin mRNA to cytoplasm, where it associates with ribosomes; (5) translation of mRNA on ribosomes into the amino acid sequence of protein; and (6) structural changes that enhance the stability of the protein products. The first three steps occur in the nucleus of developing erythroid cells

B. Specific defects

Defects have been demonstrated in the thalassemias at almost every level of this process. Genetically, all lesions act in *cis* as regards their linkage to the globin gene. Defects can always be ultimately traced to the mRNA for a specific globin chain that is quantitatively or qualitatively abnormal. The following are examples of specific defects.

1. Deletion of globin structural genes

An *entire gene* may be missing. This is the case in most α-thalassemia mutations. The β gene may be deleted in rare types of δβ thalassemia and HPFH (see below). There may also be deletions of both β and δ genes (figure 10.4).

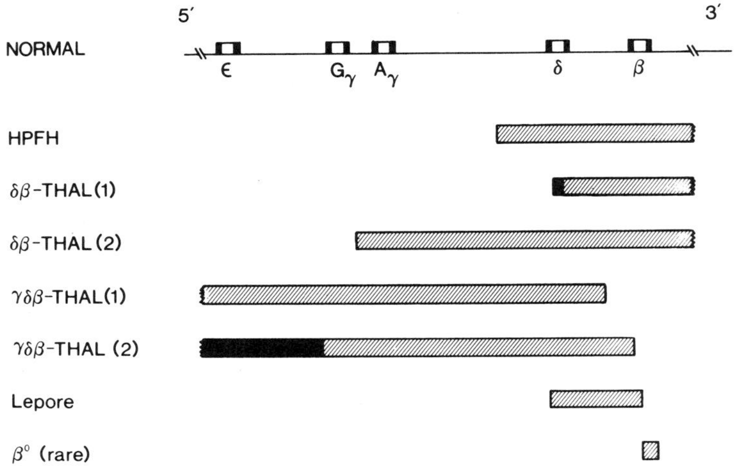

Fig. 10.4
Gene map of the various forms of hereditary persistence of fetal hemoglobin. Bars denote deleted portions.

2. Partial gene deletion

Partial gene deletions account for rare types of β^0-thal and α-thal. Varying degrees of deletion appear to be associated with different clinical syndromes in which Hb F expression is markedly increased. This leads to the syndrome termed *hereditary persistence of fetal hemoglobin,* or HPFH (figure 10.4).

3. Fused globin chains

Nonhomologous crossing over may lead to fused or "hybrid" hemoglobin chains in which a non-α chain contains amino acid sequences corresponding in two different non-α chains. In the Lepore hemoglobins (figure 10.5), a portion of the δ chain and a portion of the β chain have been lost in the process of crossing over. The resulting non-α chain has the character of a δ chain at its N-terminal end and of a β chain at its C-terminal end. The point of fusion is variable. At least three different Lepore hemoglobins are known that differ in the locus of this point. Hemoglobin Lepores have an electrophoretic mobility similar to that of hemoglobin S. Hemoglobin Kenya contains a fused γβ chain.

4. Production of nonfunctional mRNA

Point mutations within the β gene may lead to production of defective mRNA. The mRNA is present, but it cannot be translated into globin. This is the case in about 50% of β^0-thalassemias in which there is a nonsense point mutation that halts translation of β globin early in its synthesis.

5. Abnormal gene transcription

Other point mutations occur that affect the processing of globin pre-mRNA. Aberrant processing with the resulting unstable mRNA product probably explains the majority of β^+-thalassemias and perhaps some α-thalassemias. An example of a common processing defect is shown in figure 10.6.

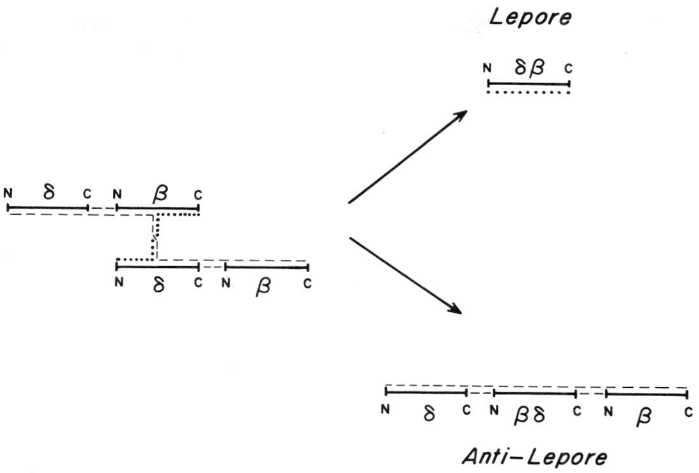

Fig. 10.5
Diagram of nonhomologous crossing-over between δ and β globin genes with resulting formation of Lepore and anti-Lepore globin genes. (From D. G. Nathan and F. A. Oski, eds., *Hematology of Infancy and Childhood*, Philadelphia: Saunders, 1974)

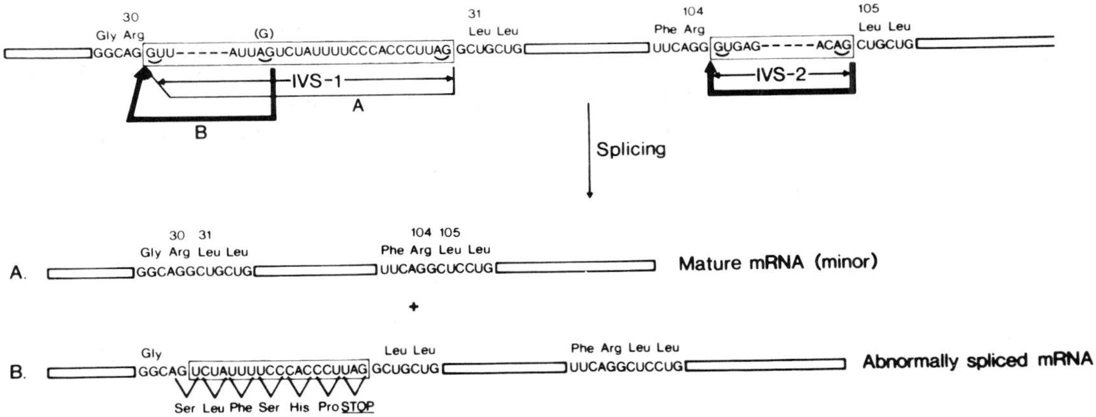

Fig. 10.6
Abnormal processing of β-mRNA precursor in one type of β-thalassemia. A section of transcribed mRNA precursor in the most common type of β^+ thalassemia is shown above. Note that the first intron contains a substitution of an A for G that creates a new 3′ splice acceptor (AG) that resembles the normal splice acceptor just 5′ to the codon for amino acid 31. This new 3′ splice acceptor combines with the splice donor GU (just 3′ to the codon for amino acid 30) at a rate 10 faster than the normal splice acceptor (indicated by the heavy arrow). Therefore 2 mature mRNA's are formed. One, a minor component, is normal. The other, 90% of the total, retains a segment of intron 1 that contains a stop codon. It cannot produce globin chains. Hence severe thalassemia with some hemoglobin A is produced.

6. Production of elongated chain

Globin chains (when present) are usually structurally normal in the thalassemias. An exception occurs in five known α chain variants characterized by the presence of additional amino acid residues at the C-terminal end of the α chain. The prototype example is hemoglobin Constant Spring, in which the α chain is elongated due to a mutation in the codon that normally terminates translation. For unknown reasons, the abnormal α chain is synthesized at a low rate. Therefore, the clinical picture (phenotype) mimics α-thalassemia (see table 10.1).

7. Production of highly unstable globin

In the rare case in which a mutation leads to the production of an unusually unstable hemoglobin, degradation may occur almost immediately after synthesis. This leads to the clinical picture of thalassemia. Hb Indianapolis, a β chain mutant, is an example of such a hemoglobin. The clinical picture resembles β-thalassemia.

8. Molecular polymorphisms

Abnormalities of the gene map (as determined by restriction enzyme techniques) are found in certain populations. These consist of DNA sequence differences (polymorphisms) in regions flanking the structural genes. Demonstration of these polymorphic DNA sequences permits detection of abnormal globin genes that are closely linked to them. This approach is currently in clinical use in the prenatal diagnosis of sickle cell anemia and thalassemia (see lecture 9).

9. Summary of point mutations

As a result of molecular cloning and sequencing studies, over 30 point mutations causing β-thalassemia have been detected. Some affect transcription and clearly demonstrate the importance of 5′ promoter sequences. Other cause nonsense mutations or splicing defects. A summary of the defects and their locations is set out in figure 10.7.

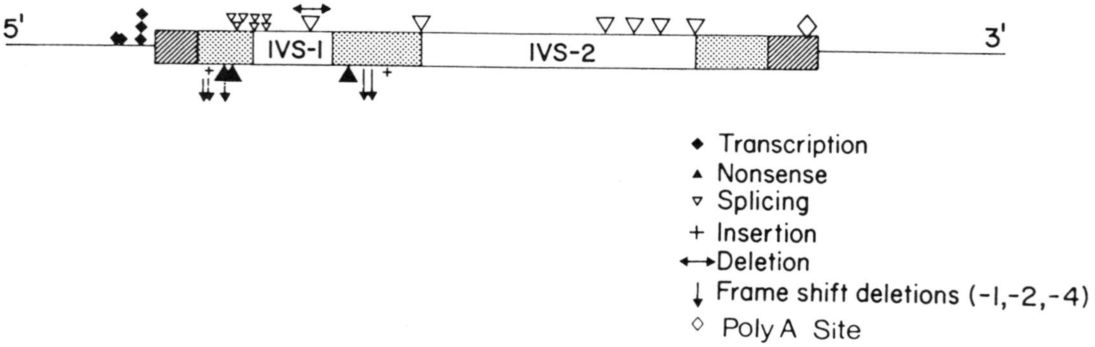

Fig. 10.7
A summary of β thalassemia point mutations.

C. Future possibilities

Recombinant DNA technology now permits isolation of abnormal genes and the characterization of their structure and function. Thalassemia research is currently at the forefront of molecular biology, and it is reasonable to expect in the near future (1) elucidation of specific defects in various thalassemias including those affecting gene transcription or RNA processing; (2) in vitro gene replacement in bone marrow cells using pure genes; (2) improved understanding of gene function and application of this knowledge to other human disorders; and (4) possible reversal by molecular or cellular approaches of the fetal hemoglobin switching mechanism. This would ameliorate the severity of all forms of β-thalassemia.

SELECTED REFERENCES

Alter, B. P. — Prenatal diagnosis of haemoglobinopathies: A status report. *Lancet* 2(1981): 1152.

Chang, J. C., and Kan, Y. W. — β^0-thalassemia, a nonsense mutation in man. *Proc. Nat. Acad. Sci. USA* 76(1979): 2886.

Kan, Y. W., and Dozy, A. M. — Polymorphism of DNA sequence adjacent to the human β-globin structural gene: Relationship to sickle mutation. *Proc. Nat. Acad. Sci. USA* 75(1978): 5631.

Leder, P. — Discontinuous genes. *New Eng. J. Med.* 208(1978): 1079.

Modell, B. — Total management of thalassemia major. *Arch. Dis. Child.* 52(1977): 489.

Nathan, D. G., and Gunn, R. B. — Thalassemia: The consequences of unbalanced synthesis. *Am. J. Med.* 41(2966): 815.

Orkin, S. H., et al. — Application of endonuclease mapping to the analysis and prenatal diagnosis of thalassemias caused by globin-gene deletion. *New Eng. J. Med.* 299(1978): 166.

Orkin, S. H., et al. — Direct detection of the common Mediterranean β-thalassemia gene with synthetic DNA probes: An alternative approach for prenatal diagnosis. *J. Clin. Invest.* 71(1983): 775.

Orkin, S. H., et al. — Linkage of β-thalassemia mutations and β-globin gene polymorphisms with DNA polymorphisms in the human β-globin gene cluster. *Nature* 296(1982): 296.

Orkin, S. H., et al. — Polymorphism and molecular pathology of human beta-globin gene. In *Progress in Hematology,* Brown, E. B. (ed.), New York, Grune & Stratton, 1983, vol. 13, pp. 49–74.

Weatherall, D. J., and Clegg, J. B. — Thalassemia revisited. *Cell* 29(1982): 7.

LECTURE 11 Hemolytic Anemias I. Introduction

James H. Jandl

I. RED CELL LIFE SPAN AND SURVIVAL

A. Determining factors

Red cells have a life span of about 120 days. As the cells age, glycolysis slows, enzyme activity diminishes, and the content of ATP, potassium, and membrane lipids declines. How these and other age-dependent changes lead to removal of senescent red cells from the circulation is uncertain. The *life span* of the red cells—their potential longevity—must be distinguished from their actual *survival*, which encompasses all factors, including premature aging, that may cause their untimely destruction.

B. Measurement

Measurement of red cell survival requires use of a label. Labeled cells may be of *mixed ages* or they may constitute a *cohort*—a group of cells of identical age.

1. Mixed-age labeling

a. Differential agglutination (Ashby technique)

The normal red cell life span was first determined by the Ashby technique, which now is used only in a research setting. The technique utilizes antigenic differences between the red cells of a donor and the cells of the recipient. Usually type O donor red cells lacking the M antigen are given to a recipient whose cells possess the antigen. Thereafter, the recipient's blood is sampled periodically, and antibodies that agglutinate type M cells are added. Survival of donor cells is calculated from the declining number of inagglutinable cells.

The technique has two disadvantages: (1) it does not measure survival of an individual's own red cells; and (2) transfusion of another individual's cells incurs risk of sensitization to minor blood group antigens and premature destruction of donor cells.

b. Diisopropyl fluorophosphate (DFP)

An alternative technique employs diisopropyl fluorophosphate (DFP) labeled with ^{3}H. DFP binds covalently to a serine residue in the cholinesterase of cell membranes. This permits study of the life span of autologous cells. A disadvantage is the loss during the first several days of cells injured by the labeling process. Consequently this technique is not useful in patients with brisk hemolysis.

c. Pathophysiology

Normally both the Ashby and DFP techniques measure the fate of red cells that are evenly distributed as to age from 1 to 120 days. Thus labeled cells diminish at a rate of approximately 1/120 of the infused cells daily (figure 11.1, top right). In *premature destruction,* the red cell survival curve has a similar straight-line pattern, but the descent is steeper (figure 11.1, middle right).

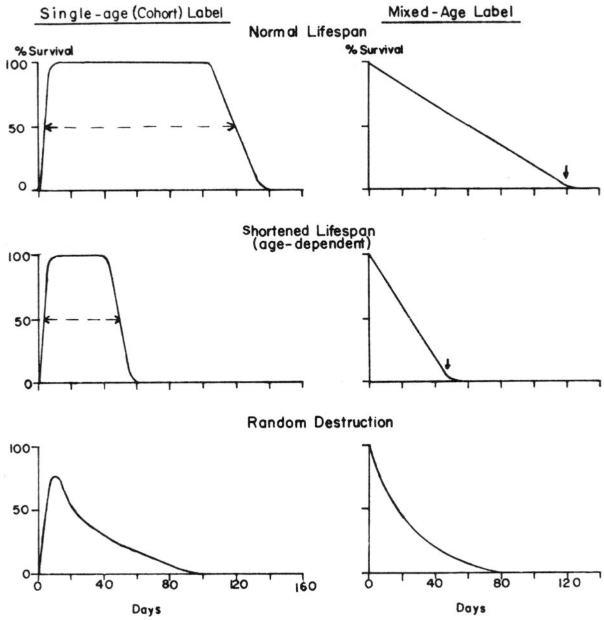

Fig. 11.1
Patterns of red cell survival and life span as revealed by cohort and mixed-age labeling of red cell population. On the left, a single-age cohort of red cells was labeled with the biosynthetic precursor, 2-^{14}C-glycine. Right, a population of cells, evenly distributed as to age, was labeled with ^{3}H-DFP.

In most hemolytic anemias, the labeled red cells are destroyed by a process that is indifferent to cell age. In *random destruction,* a constant fraction of labeled cells is destroyed daily. The rate of this destruction is governed by chance exposure to injury, as by passage through a particular vascular region. When hemolysis is severe, the red cell survival curve usually conforms to a first-order pattern, for the cells do not survive to die a ''natural death'' (figure 11.1, bottom right). In such patients, most red cells are only a few days old, and those surviving 50 to 60 days may be too few to measure.

As the Ashby and DFP methods are unsatisfactory for measuring red cell destruction in hemolytic anemias, where a measurement is most needed, other techniques are employed. The most widely used label is radioactive chromium (^{51}Cr).

2. Cohort labeling

a. Methods

In cohort labeling, a red cell population similar in age is labeled biosynthetically by injecting a radioactive precursor that is incorporated by immature erythroid cells of the bone marrow. Cells so labeled enter the circulation for up to 6 or 7 days, even as some are being destroyed. Some label appears in circulating reticulocytes immediately after injection.

Cohort labeling is unsuitable in studying rapid hemolytic processes and is used primarily in determining red cell life span. During hemoglobin catabolism, the amino acids released are not reutilized; thus 2-^{14}C-glycine provides a good cohort label. On the other hand, ^{59}Fe is not suitable because it is extensively reutilized after lysis of labeled cells (see lecture 6).

b. Pathophysiology

Normally, the percentage of cohort-labeled red cells in the circulation remains constant for about 100 days (figure 11.1, top left). By 120 days radioactivity has declined 50%, and within 140 days it is inappreciable. When red cell life span is shortened, the survival curve has a similar but abbreviated plateau pattern. Cohort labeling is most useful in mild or moderate hemolytic processes. However, the more severe hemolytic anemias associated with random red cell destruction are not accurately characterized by cohort labeling (figure 11.1, bottom left).

3. Measurement of survival in hemolytic anemia: ^{51}Cr method

a. Methods

The only practicable method for studying red cell survival in hemolytic anemias involves labeling a sample of the patient's red cells with ^{51}Cr in its stable form as a chromate anion ($^{51}CrO_4^{=}$). Chromate rapidly permeates red cells, wherein it is trapped by reduction to the nearly impermeant $^{51}Cr^{+++}$ ion. In small amounts, chromate is harmless to red cells. After reinfusion of ^{51}Cr-labeled red cells, total red cell mass can be determined, for red cells remain confined to the vascular compartment. By periodically assaying blood samples for radioactivity, one can ascertain the red cell survival pattern. However, correction must be made for the fact that about 1% of intracellular ^{51}Cr is eluted daily and excreted in the urine.

The ^{51}Cr method also permits determinations of (1) the *site* at which red cells are destroyed (figure 11.2); (2) *vascular pooling* of red cells within organs; (3) *kinetics of mixing* of ^{51}C-labeled red cells in the spleen; and (4) extent of *gastrointestinal blood loss,* for neither Cr^{+++} nor $CrO_4^{=}$ is excreted via the normal GI tract.

b. Patterns

^{51}Cr elution has a marked effect on the shape of the survival curve of normal red cells, transforming it from a rectilinear to a curvilinear pattern. The Ashby and DFP techniques yield a normal half-survival of about 60 days. The half-survival time for ^{51}Cr-labeled normal red cells, however, is about 30 days owing to ^{51}Cr elution. The error introduced by ^{51}Cr elution is minimal in severe hemolytic anemias, in which red cell survival studies are most needed. Figure 11.2 depicts the effects of elution and tissue ex-

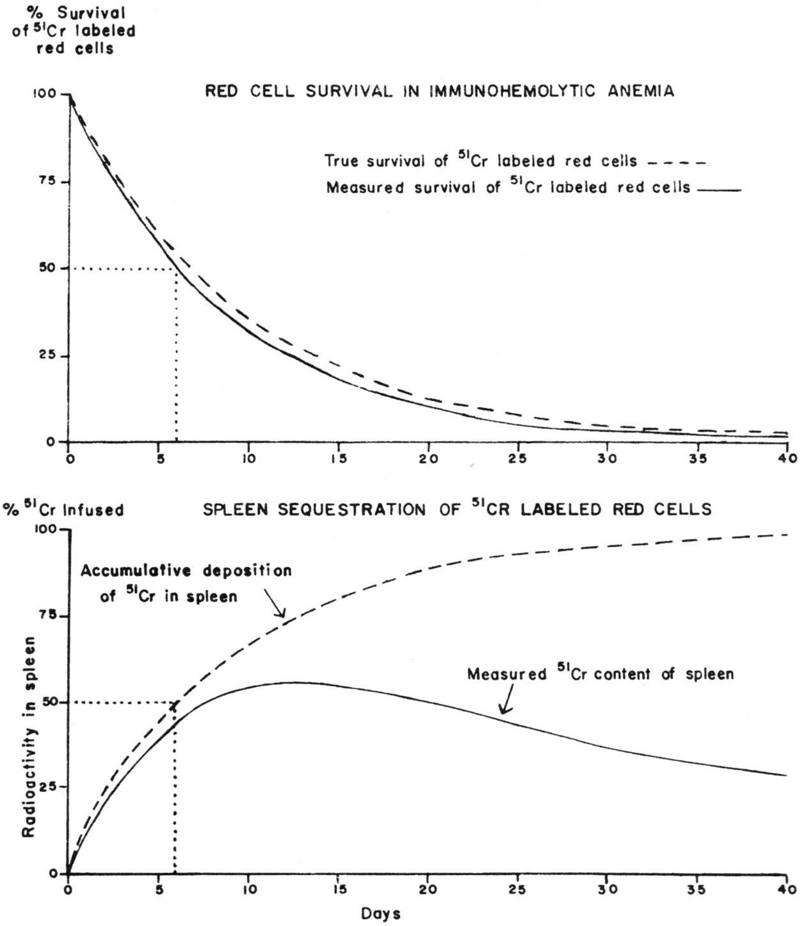

Fig. 11.2
Use of ^{51}Cr method in a patient with immunohemolytic anemia associated with random destruction of 10% of the red cells daily. Top, red cell survival studies show that the "true" half-survival time is 6.9 days and the measured half-survival time, diminished by ^{51}Cr elution, is 6.0 days, a difference having no practical significance. Bottom, spleen sequestration studies show the effect of tissue excretion of ^{51}Cr on the measured ^{51}Cr deposition in the spleen. The accumulated radioactivity would be as shown by the dashed line if all ^{51}Cr deposited in the spleen remained there. Spleen excretes 2½–3% of its ^{51}Cr daily, and accumulation is diminished accordingly (solid line). Half of injected ^{51}Cr was deposited in the spleen by day 6 (dashed line), but half of the radioactivity was not measurable in the spleen until day 7.5. ^{51}Cr localization is best determined during period in which about 3/4 of labeled cells are hemolyzed.

cretion of ^{51}Cr upon measurements of red cell survival and of splenic sequestration.

II. HEMOLYSIS

A. Types

As a clinical term, *hemolysis* means premature red cell destruction, whether due to reduction in red cell life span or to random cell destruction.

1. Extravascular and intravascular sites

In most cases, hemolysis involves the trapping of red cells in spleen or liver sinuses; the cells are then lysed and most of the hemoglobin is catabolized within the sequestering organ. This process is termed *extravascular hemolysis*. Less often, red cells are destroyed within the systemic circulation, and hemoglobin is released into plasma and catabolized only when it is taken up by the liver or lost through the kidneys. This is termed *intravascular hemolysis*.

2. Extracorpuscular and intracorpuscular defects

Hemolytic anemias can also be classified according to whether the initiating event is extrinsic (an *extracorpuscular defect*) or intrinsic (an *intracorpuscular defect*) to the red cell.

3. Hereditary and acquired disorders

A third basis for cataloging hemolytic disorders differentiates those that are *hereditary* from those that are *acquired*.

B. Clinical features

Hemolytic disorders are marked by signs of increased hemoglobin catabolism combined with signs of increased erythropoiesis.

1. Accelerated hemoglobin catabolism

The principal indicators of accelerated catabolism of hemoglobin are (1) jaundice; (2) hemoglobinemia and decreased plasma haptoglobin; (3) hemoglobinuria and hemosiderinuria; and (4) methemalbuminemia.

a. Jaundice

In extravascular hemolysis, macrophages (RES cells) convert most of the hemoglobin from destroyed red cells to bilirubin. As described in lecture 7, this process liberates 1 mole each of iron, carbon monoxide, and bilirubin per mole of heme catabolized. The indirect-reacting (or unconjugated) serum bilirubin is elevated. In brisk hemolysis, direct-reacting (or conjugated) serum bilirubin may also rise.

b. Hemoglobinemia and decreased plasma haptoglobin

Severe hemolysis of any sort elevates the plasma hemoglobin concentration (normal level, <1 mg/100 ml). During intravascular hemolysis, the plasma hemoglobin is high enough to be visible. Levels of 10–20 mg/100 ml give plasma an amber coloration; at 50–100 mg/100 ml, it is reddish.

Plasma *haptoglobin* is an α_2 globulin that binds free hemoglobin and so prevents leakage of hemoglobin from the vascular compartment and excretion into the urine. Haptoglobin and hemoglobin form a complex that is rapidly cleared by the liver. Thus hemoglobinemia diminishes the level of haptoglobin. Plasma normally possesses sufficient haptoglobin to bind 100–150 mg/100 ml of hemoglobin. During hemoglobinemia, haptoglobin is depleted and the level of unbound or free hemoglobin increases. Free hemoglobin is oxidized rapidly to methemoglobin, which lends a mahogany red-brown color to the plasma. A significant portion (40–50%) of circulating free hemoglobin (or methemoglobin) is cleared by the kidneys.

c. Hemoglobinuria and hemosiderinuria

The rapidity with which hemoglobin, despite its molecular weight of 64,500, is filtered by the glomeruli is attributable to its dissociation in dilute solution into half-molecules, pairs of peptide chains, termed *dimers* or αβ *dimers,* having molecular weight of about 32,000 (figure 11.3). Proximal tubule cells reabsorb and catabolize most of the filtered hemoglobin, preventing it from appearing in urine. At normal perfusion pressures, plasma hemoglobin concentrations must exceed 30 mg/100 ml before hemoglobinuria ensues. The renal threshold of about 150 mg/100 ml for plasma hemoglobin therefore reflects two conserving mechanisms: (1) binding of hemoglobin by haptoglobin and (2) absorption of hemoglobin by proximal tubule cells.

After filtration by the glomerulus, hemoglobin tetramers and dimers reequilibrate within the renal tubule (figure 11.3). Organic components of hemoglobin are catabolized rapidly in the proximal tubule cells. Although half the globin and porphyrin are degraded in <30 min, iron atoms are handled differently. Iron released from hemoglobin stimulates synthesis of apoferritin, and ferritin iron soon appears within the tubule cells (see lecture 6). The iron of ferritin and hemosiderin leaves the kidney slowly ($T_{1/2}$ = >30–40 days) both by excretion into the urine and by absorption from tubules into the blood. When hemoglobin uptake and iron accumulation by proximal tubule cells is extensive, the cells exfoliate into

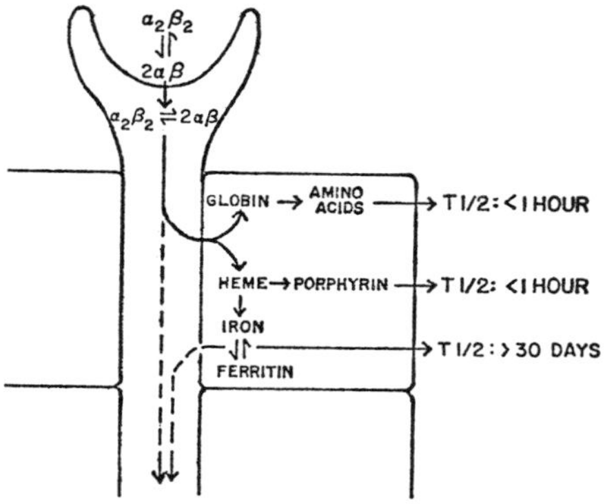

Fig. 11.3
Renal catabolism and excretion of hemoglobin. (From H. F. Bunn and J. H. Jandl, *J. Exp. Med.* 129(1969): 925)

the urine, where they can be detected by the Prussian blue reaction. Hemoglobinuria imparts a red-brown color to urine, reflecting the admixture of hemoglobin and methemoglobin. Hemoglobin may be distinguished from myoglobin in the urine spectroscopically or spectrophotometrically, but only with some difficulty. Table 11.1 lists several simpler means for differentiating hemoglobinuria and myoglobinuria.

d. Methemalbuminemia

When hemoglobinemia persists for an hour or more and the free hemoglobin undergoes oxidation to methemoglobin, *methemalbumin* accumulates. This brown pigment, a hallmark of intravascular hemolysis, forms because of the affinity of albumin for oxidized heme (ferriheme) groups. Plasma albumin possesses two sites that selectively bind ferriheme but not methemoglobin (ferrihemoglobin). The ferriheme is in an exchange equilibrium with the heme of other molecules of free methemoglobin and with heme bound to plasma albumin. Although the affinity of globin for ferriheme far exceeds that of albumin, the concentration of albumin vastly exceeds that of free hemoglobin. Consequently, most of the ferriheme of methemoglobin is shifted onto the albumin, and the level of plasma methemalbumin (ferriheme-albumin) rises disproportionately due to its longer retention in the circulation. (Unlike hemoglobin, methemalbumin is not filtered by the normal glomerulus.) Thus, the plasma becomes brown rather than red, while fresh voided urine shows the reddish color of hemoglobin or red-brown of methemoglobin.

Table 11.1
Differential Diagnosis of Hemoglobinuria and Myoglobinuria

Observation	Hemoglobinuria	Myoglobinuria
Appearance of plasma	Amber to red-brown	Normal[a]
Bilirubin level	Slightly to moderately elevated	Normal
Effect of 80% saturation with ammonium sulfate	Precipitates hemoglobin	Does not precipitate myoglobin (in fresh specimen containing undenatured myoglobin)
Agarose electrophoresis of plasma at pH 8.6	Free plasma hemoglobin migrates near transferrin in β_1-globulin region; addition of haptoglobin[b] moves it into α_2 region. Albumin band may appear yellow or brown due to methemalbumin	Myoglobin migrates near C3. Addition of haptoglobin[b] has no effect

a. Except when associated with renal failure.
b. By addition of normal serum to sample prior to electrophoresis.

Hemopexin, a plasma glycoprotein having the electrophoretic mobility of β_{1B} globulin, also binds ferriheme, and does so with a greater affinity than albumin. Like albumin, it does not bind intact hemoglobin. The hemopexin concentration in normal plasma is 50–100 mg/100 ml. The heme-hemopexin complex is removed from the circulation during hemolysis; thus its level declines.

2. Increased erythropoiesis

The acceleration of erythropoiesis that occurs in hemolytic anemia in response to diminished oxygen transport (see lecture 1) induces intramedullary erythroid hyperplasia. When severe and extended over a long period the following may be observed: (1) intramedullary erythroid hyperplasia; (2) extramedullary erythropoiesis; (3) skeletal deformities; (4) bile pigment gallstones; and (5) nucleated red cells in the blood.

a. Intramedullary erythroid hyperplasia

In acute hemolytic anemia, a sharp increase in iron utilization by the bone marrow occurs within 12–24 hr. Within 2 days, the bone marrow manifests erythroid hyperplasia; and on the 3rd day, barring factors that inhibit the marrow's proliferative response, the reticulocyte count increases (see lecture 1). Erythroid hyperplasia at first occurs only in regions of bone marrow that are normally hematopoietic, the rate of erythropoiesis rising about 3-fold. If hemolytic anemia persists, erythroid hyperplasia spreads throughout the marrow cavity. Should anemia continue, the entire marrow cavity becomes occupied by hematopoietic cells, the rate of erythropoiesis increasing as much as 10-fold.

b. Extramedullary erythropoiesis

In some patients, particularly those with congenital hemolytic anemias (e.g., hereditary spherocytosis and thalassemia), tumor-like erythropoietic masses may appear outside the marrow cavity, often adjacent to the spine. The masses are smoothly rounded or lobulated, often multiple, and when seen in chest films may resemble large encapsulated neoplasms. At autopsy, it is usually possible to demonstrate connections, often by narrow stalks, to the marrow of the vertebral bodies, for they are extrusions from the marrow cavity. Small, and from an erythropoietic standpoint, insignificant, colonies of erythropoietic cells may be found in the spleen, liver, lymph nodes, and perinephric tissues.

c. Skeletal deformities

Severe chronic hemolytic anemia beginning in infancy or early childhood may expand the marrow space sufficiently to deform the patient's appearance. Children with thalassemia or other severe forms of chronic hemolytic anemia often develop *hemolytic facies* with broad cheekbones and protruding maxillae resulting from expansion of marrow space in these bones. This may create severe dental malocclusion and a chipmunk appearance. X-rays show broadening of the medullary cavity throughout most of the skeleton. In the skull, this leads to wide separation of the two tables of the calvarium and eventual demineralization of the outer table. The thin trabecular extensions radiating from the inner table create a "hair-on-end" appearance. During growth, vertebrae become broadened, demineralized, and coarsely trabecular with small radiolucent lakes resembling osteolytic lesions of malignancy. Intervertebral disks are commonly pressed into the thinned-out centers of softened adjacent vertebrae, and intervertebral spaces develop a fish-mouth appearance.

d. Bile pigment gallstones

Gallstones containing bile pigments are common in patients with congenital hemolytic disorders, whether or not there is frank anemia, but are uncommon in patients with acquired hemolytic disorders. They are usually small, numerous, and multifaceted.

e. Nucleated red cells and other abnormalities in blood

Nucleated red cells commonly enter the circulation within several days of the onset of a severe, acute hemolytic anemia. In sustained and severe hemolytic anemia, nucleated red cells may be a persistent feature of the blood. The majority are late normoblasts. Many show the nuclear deformities of normal karyorrhexis, such as lobulation, clover-like deformities, and nuclear fragmentation. Nuclear fragments that are 1 or 2 μm in diameter are known as *Howell-Jolly bodies*.

C. Classification according to mechanisms

Types of hemolytic anemias were categorized above from three broad viewpoints: site of hemolysis, locus of defect, and genetic mechanism. In reality, no simplified classification is fully adequate because categories often overlap. In almost all instances, hemolytic anemias caused by extrinsic or extracorpuscular factors are acquired. In some cases, an intrinsic defect may render the red cell abnormally susceptible to environmental factors that cause little damage to normal red cells. Excepting paroxysmal nocturnal hemoglobinuria, virtually all intrinsic red cell defects are hereditary. The following list is a working classification of the major hemolytic anemias based on the fundamental underlying abnormality.

1. Extracorpuscular defects

1. Immunohemolytic anemias (see lecture 12)

2. Microangiopathic and other hemolytic anemias caused by physical or thermal injury to red cells (see lecture 13).

3. Oxidative hemolysis (Heinz body anemias) caused by exposure to exogenous chemicals or drugs that promote oxidation of red cell constituents (see lecture 14).

4. Hemolysis caused by splenic enlargment: the splenomegaly syndrome or "hypersplenism" (see lecture 2).

5. Hemolysis caused by alteration of red cell membrane lipids, spur cell anemia; hemolysis caused by bacterial phospholipases; etc. (lecture 13).

2. Intracorpuscular defects

1. Defects of the red cell membrane: hereditary spherocytosis; hereditary elliptocytosis (see lecture 13).

2. Metabolic defects due to hereditary deficiencies of red cell enzymes: glucose-6-phosphate dehydrogenase deficiency; pyruvate kinase deficiency; deficiencies of other enzymes of the Embden-Meyerhof glycolytic pathway and hexose monophosphate shunt (see lecture 14).

3. Hemoglobinopathic defects associated with hereditary abnormalities in hemoglobin structure: sickle cell anemia; hemoglobin C disease; hemoglobins unstable to oxidation; others (see lecture 9).

4. Hereditary impairment in rate of synthesis of a hemoglobin polypeptide chain: the thalassemias (see lecture 10).

3. Combined defects

1. Megaloblastic anemia (see lectures 4 and 5).
2. Hypochromic anemias (see lecture 6).
3. Most disorders of the erythron if very severe.

SELECTED REFERENCES

Berlin, N. I. The biological life of the red cell (Chapter 24). In Surgenor, D. MacN., ed., *The Red Blood Cell,* 2d ed., New York: Academic Press, 1975, pp. 957–1019.

Cooper, R. A., and Bunn, H. F. Hemolytic anemias (section 329). In Petersdorf, R. G., Adams, R. D., Braunwald, E., Isselbacher, K. J., Martin, J. B., and Wilson, J. D., eds., Harrison's *Principles of Internal Medicine,* 10th ed., New York, McGraw-Hill Book Company, 1983, pp. 1862–1875.

Cooper, R. A., and Jandl, J. H. Destruction of erythrocytes (Chapter 39). In Williams, W. J., Beutler, E., Erslev, A. J., and Lichtman, M. A., eds., *Hematolgy,* 3d ed., New York, McGraw-Hill Book Company, 1983, pp. 377–388.

Jandl, J. H. Symposium on disorders of the red cell: The pathophysiology of hemolytic anemias: A foreword, *Am. J. Med.* 41(1966): 657.

LECTURE 12 Hemolytic Anemias II. Immunohemolytic Anemias

James H. Jandl

I. INTRODUCTION

A. Definition

Immunohemolytic anemias (also termed autoimmune hemolytic anemias) are acquired disorders in which premature red cell destruction is mediated by an immunologic process. Diagnosis is based on evidence that autogenous *antibodies* (usually IgG) or one or more components of *serum complement* (primarily C3d and some C4) are attached to the patient's red cells.

B. Detection

1. Direct Coombs test

The use of animal antibody reactive with human immunoglobulin to detect a human antibody coating on red cell surfaces constitutes the *direct Coombs test* (or *antiglobulin test*). Red cells with IgG or other protein on their surfaces fail to agglutinate until appropriate Coombs serum is added—hence, the offending immunoglobulin represents an *incomplete antibody*. In the direct Coombs tests, a patient's red cells, washed free of plasma proteins, are mixed with Coombs serum. If immunoglobulin is attached to the cells, Coombs serum causes macroscopic or microscopic agglutination. Because of the diagnostic importance of a positive Coombs test, Coombs-positive hemolytic anemia is a synonym for immunohemolytic anemia.

2. Indirect Coombs test

Serum antibody of the incomplete type is detectable with the *indirect Coombs test*. Antibody in serum in the absence of antibody on the red cell surface indicates isoimmunization (see lecture 15).

3. Other methods

Pretreatment of normal red cells with certain proteolytic enzymes renders them agglutinable by patient's 7S IgG antibodies, a finding equivalent to a positive indirect Coombs test. Cell-bound incomplete antibodies are also detectable by suspending the coated red cells in solutions of linear macromolecules, particularly polyvinylpyrrolidone, dextran, fibrinogen, and—less satisfactorily—concentrated albumin. Subsequent dilution in saline disperses aggregates or rouleaux of normal, uncoated red cells, whereas antibody-coated cells remain clumped (see lecture 16). This is a useful screening test, but it does not identify the protein on the red cell surface as does a monospecific Coombs serum.

C. Classification

Classification of the immunohemolytic anemias can be based on (1) whether antibody attaches to cells at body temperature (*warm-active antibody*) or is active primarily at cooler temperatures (*cold-active antibody*); (2) whether it is IgG or IgM, and whether it activates complement; and (3) whether the hemolytic antibody reacts with an antigenic constituent of the cell. As less than half the cases are associated with defined causative agents or disorders, the best initial approach is to determine the kind of protein present in a given Coombs-positive patient. The immunologic process responsible for hemolytic anemia in most patients is unknown. The expression "autoimmune hemolytic anemia," however convenient, is inadvisable in cases such as drug-induced immunohemolytic anemia for which the etiologic agent is known and the process reversible.

II. MECHANISMS OF RED CELL INJURY

The following discussion considers mechanisms of immune hemolysis that are mediated by IgG warm-active antibodies and IgM or IgG cold-active antibodies (once known in the jargon as cold agglutinins and cold hemolysins).

A. Warm-active antibodies

1. Properties

Characteristics of warm-active antibodies are summarized in table 12.1. Although the thermal range may vary, maximum antibody activity is almost always about 37°C. Most severely affected patients have a strongly positive test when Coombs antiserum is directed against IgG. In some patients, appropriate Coombs antisera reveal that the red cell is also coated with a fragment of inactivated C3. Warm antibodies in immunohemolytic anemias usually possess high effective affinity for the red cell surface and react similarly with red cells from all normal individuals possessing the Rh locus. In two-thirds of patients, the antibody fails to react with red cells that lack the Rh locus, that is, Rh null cells (see lecture 15), and reacts weakly with cells with partly deleted Rh loci.

2. Factors determining hemolytic potency

Warm-active 7S IgG antibodies that are profoundly hemolytic in vivo cause no injury to red cells in vitro, irrespective of the amount of antibody or the presence or absence of complement; there is no change in appearance, metabolism, viscosity, rigidity, or ability to pass through capillary-sized filters. In contrast, infused plasma containing incomplete antibodies induces spherocytosis, increases osmotic fragility of the patient's red cells, and causes hemolysis in vivo.

a. Studies of erythrophagocytosis

Insight into the difference between the in vitro and in vivo effects of incomplete antibodies emerged from studies of antibody-induced *erythrophagocytosis,* that is, ingestion of red cells by fixed or circulating phagocytes.

An antibody that activates "hemolytic complement" while reacting with red cell antigens typically causes abrupt and extensive erythrophagocytosis, provided that fresh serum complement (at physiological pH) and phagocytic cells are present. In the

Table 12.1
Antibodies Associated with Immunohemolytic Anemia

Properties	Warm-active antibodies	Cold-active antibodies
Immunoglobulin class[a]	Usually IgG	Usually IgM
Heavy chain subclass[a]	IgG1 and IgG3	
Sedimentation coefficient	7S	19S
Mol. wt.	160,000	~1,000,000
Temperature optimum	37°C	4°C (0–10°C)
Activation of complement	None or little	Yes, but sequence seldom completed
Agglutination of normal red cells	None or little	Yes (titer >1:300)
Direct Coombs test with		
Antihuman serum	+ + +/+ + + +	+/+ +
Anti-IgG	+ + +/+ + + +	0/+ +
Anti-IgM	0	0
Anti-C3	0/+ +	+ +/+ + +
Anti-C4	0/+	+/+ +
Indirect Coombs test with		
Antihuman serum	0/+ + +	0/+ +[b]
Anti-IgG	0/+ + +	0
Anti-IgM	0	0
Anti-C3	0	0/+ + +[b]
Effective affinity	+ +/+ + + +	tr/+ (at >30°C)
Antigenic specificity	Nonspecific (but often requires Rh locus)[c]	I, i (also H, M, N)
Number of antibody molecules per red cell	10^3–10^5	10^5 or more
Frequency of etiologies		
Idiopathic	55–60%	30–40%
Drug-induced	25–30%	1–5%
Lymphoproliferative disorder	10–15%	15–20%
Mycoplasma infection	0%	25–35%
Other	5–10%	5–10%

a. See lecture 24.
b. Test negative unless fresh, complement-replete serum incubated with cells at cold temperatures.
c. See lecture 15.

blood, most erythrophagocytosis involves granulocytes. Virtually all granulocytes can engage in erythrophagocytosis, many gorging themselves to the point of rupture. Aggregation of numerous red cells with two or more granulocytes leads to characteristic ragged mixed agglutinates (figure 12.1A). Monocytes also engage in complement-mediated erythrophagocytosis, although a smaller percentage of them actually ingests red cells and does so more slowly than granulocytes. In severe cases, pronounced erythrophagocytosis can be observed in the Kupffer cells lining the live sinuses, in the splenic macrophages, and to a smaller extent in macrophages of other tissues.

b. Actions of warm-active antibodies in vivo: receptors for IgG1 and IgG3

The actions of warm-active antibodies are unlike those of complement-activating antibodies. Usually warm-active IgG antibodies mediate cell destruction by causing red cells to be removed in the spleen and, when the spleen is saturated, in the sinuses of the liver (see lecture 2). The physical attributes of red cells coated with IgG antibody are not sufficiently altered to prevent them from percolating through the marginal zone and narrow apertures connecting the cordal and sinus pathways of the spleen. However, they are trapped in the proximal (and later the entire) red pulp as a result of their exposure to surface *receptors,* strong binding sites on macrophages and lining cells of cords and sinuses (figure 12.2). These receptors react specifically with exposed heavy chains, mainly with certain regions of the Fc fragments of the heavy chain subclasses IgG1 and IgG3. (Details of immunogloblin structure are discussed in lecture 24.)

c. Mechanism of spherocytosis

Variable numbers of red cells may become bound to activated lining cells, undergo membrane contraction (and thus become spherocytic), and still escape back into the circulation for a time (figure 12.3). It is emphasized that immunohemolytic anemia secondary to IgG warm antibodies is uncommonly associated with erythrophagocytosis. The injury to IgG-coated red cells trapped by the arborizing processes of macrophages ordinarily occurs on the external surface of the macrophage. It is probable that the trapped red cells are damaged by piecemeal loss of membrane and metabolic deprivation.

d. Factors determining rate and locus of hemolysis

Immune hemolysis by warm-active IgG antibodies in humans is influenced by the three major factors.

First, the *number and distribution of antigens on the red cell surface* determine the spacing of the antibodies. The D antigen and other antigens of the Rh locus—typical of antigens interacting with warm-active antibodies—are widely spaced on the red cell surface (about 1.5 μm apart, a distance over 10 times the span of an IgG molecule). This explains why antibody, even when in excess, fails to induce agglutination. A sparsity of antigenic sites also may render IgM antibodies weak inducers of agglutination.

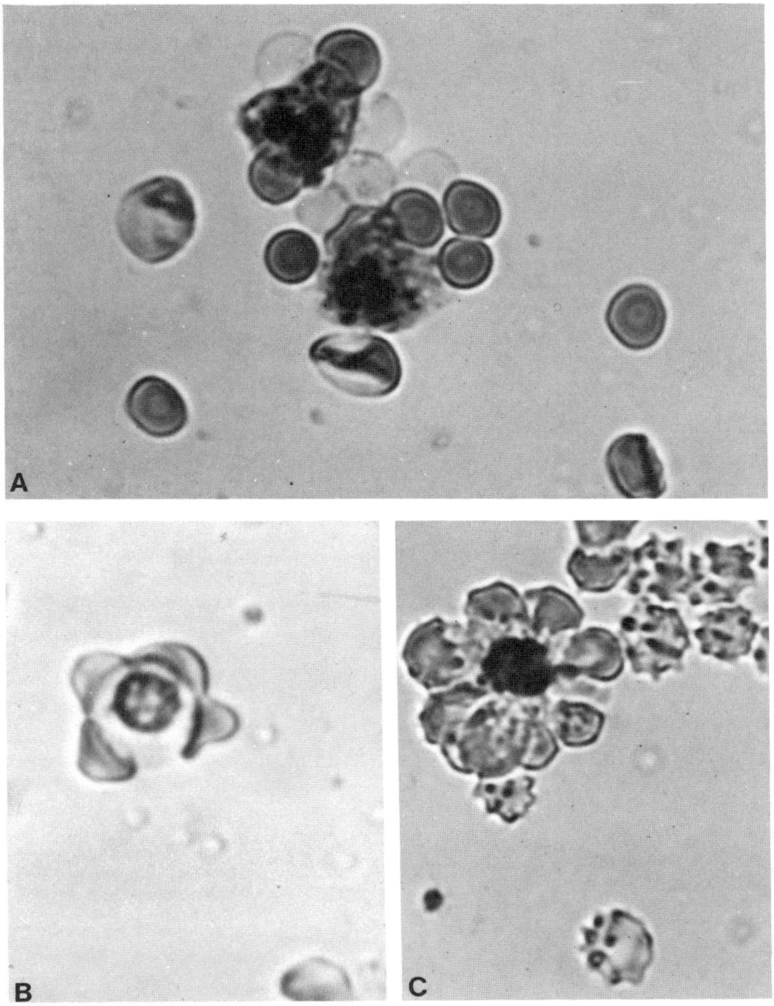

Fig. 12.1
Photomicrographs comparing interactions of red cells with granulocytes (mediated by complement-activating antibodies) and with lymphocytes and monocytes (mediated by Rh antibodies) (×425): *A,* mixed agglutination, showing red cell-granulocyte aggregation, involving several cell types, induced by complement-activating antibodies; *B,* attachment of several anti-D coated red cells to a lymphocyte, showing that characteristic red cell deformation induced by stubby lymphocytic processes; *C,* rosette, in which monocyte is surrounded by numerous adherent anti-D coated red cells, showing severe red cell deformation by long, grasping monocytic processes. (In *A*, cells are suspended in fresh, complement-replete serum; in *B* and *C*, cells are suspended in saline.)

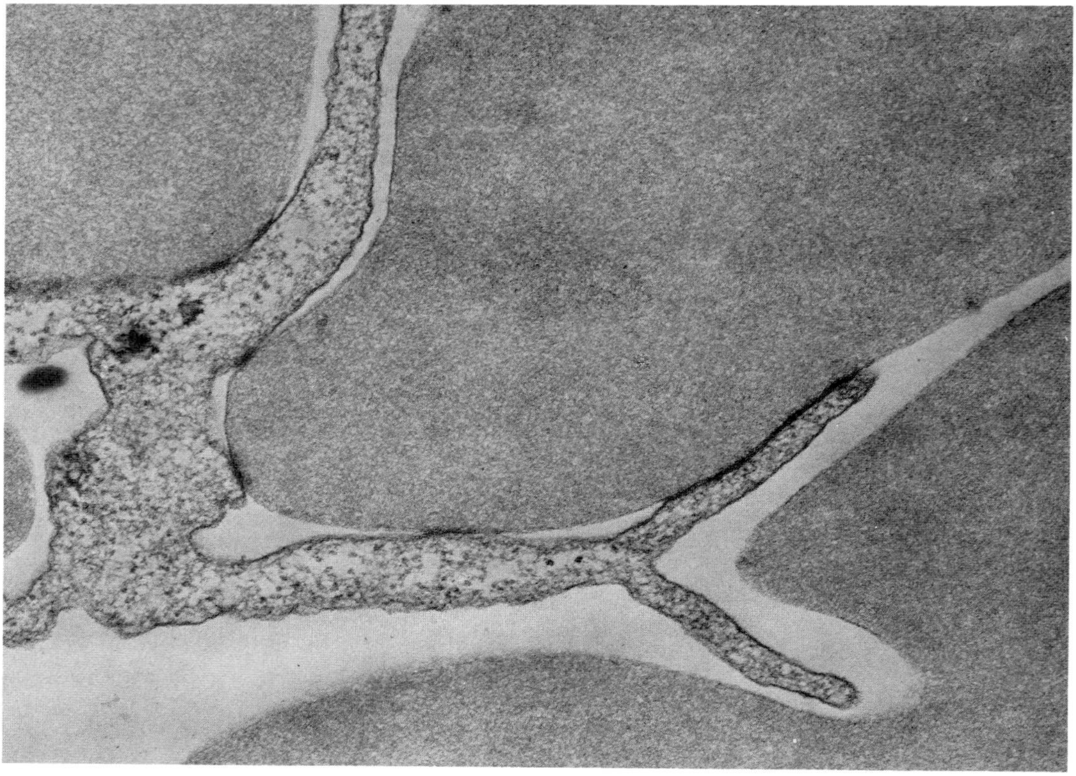

A

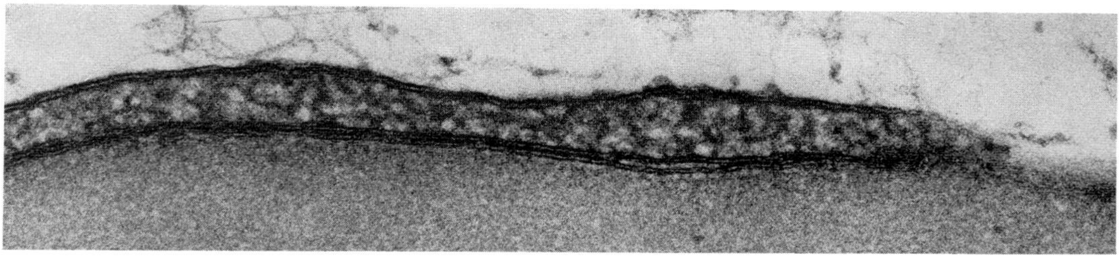

B

Fig. 12.2
Binding of red cells to monocytes. *A,* electron micrograph demonstrating complex, long, branching processes extending around and enmeshing red cells coated with IgG (×21,300). Processes at right (particularly thin end-processes with a diameter of 0.1 μm) adhere to red cells and form the trilaminar pattern characteristic of cell-cell fusion. *B,* detail of fusion pattern (×42,600). Complex arborizing and adherent processes of monocytes (and macrophages) are capable of extending around two or even three "orbitals" of attached red cells. Those few lymphocytes that form incomplete rosettes with IgG-coated red cells appear incapable of extending cytoplasmic processes beyond about 1.5 μm. (From N. Abramson, R. Cotran, and J. H. Jandl, *J. Exp. Med.* 132(1970): 1191)

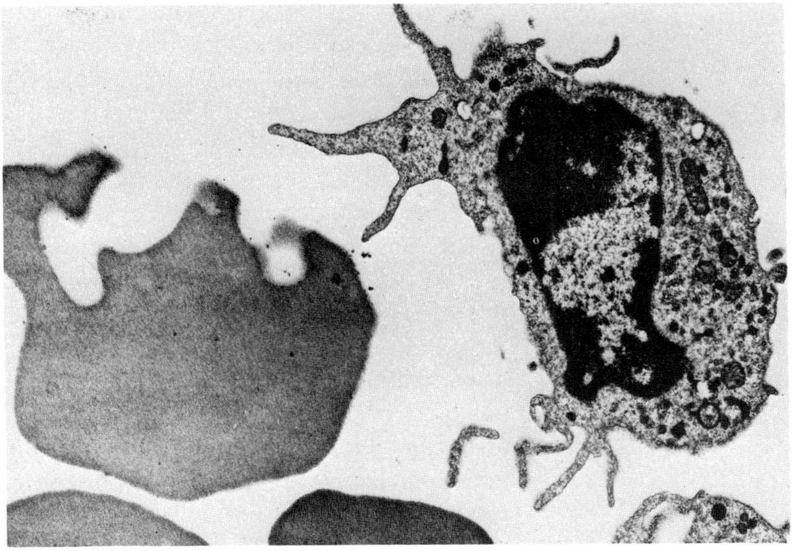

Fig. 12.3
Mechanism of spherocytosis. Electron micrograph (×4,400) of red cell (left) and monocyte (right) 15 min after addition of papain (and cysteine) to a suspension of IgG-mediated rosettes (such as those in figure 12.1C). The released red cell is intact. It is osmotically fragile and would appear as a spherocyte by light microscopy. However, electron microscopy reveals the persisting deformities induced by the monocyte. (From N. Abramson, R. Cotran, and J. H. Jandl, *J. Exp. Med.* 132(1970): 1191)

By clinging to single determinants on each of two cells, several IgM molecules may induce weak agglutination that is easily disrupted, particularly at body temperature.

A second determinant is the *heavy chain subclass* of the IgG antibody. As noted above, heavy chains of subclasses IgG1 or IgG3 bind firmly to Fe receptors on mononuclear cells, although the initial binding is subject to competition by other IgG-coated cells and by free (unbound) IgG1 or IgG3.

A third determinant is the *functional capacity of the RES*. As discussed in lecture 2, the capacity of RES cells (macrophages, monocytes, activated endothelial lining cells, etc.) for destroying antibody-coated red cells depends on (1) the number of cells that are phagocytic or are capable of binding the Fc portion of IgG molecules; (2) the number of antibody-coated cells circulating through these organs; and (3) the regional blood flow to major organs of the RES.

These factors influence the sites of red cell clearance. Small quantities of IgG-coated red cells are cleared almost exclusively by the spleen. Splenic blood flow per minute is normally 3–5% of cardiac output. The rate of clearance of anti-D-coated red cells infused into the circulation is approximately 3%/min with a $T_{1/2}$ of clearance of about 20 min. Thus, when the number of antibody-coated red cells is small relative to the mass of available RES cells, all or most of the splenic arterial blood is cleared of the antibody-coated cells. In contrast, when an immunohemolytic anemia is associated with intravascular agglutination, agglutinated red cells are cleared from the blood at a rate approximating the rate of blood flow through the entire RES, the bulk of which is in the liver. In this instance, the rate of clearance would approximate hepatic blood flow—about 37% of cardiac output.

The rate of red cell destruction in warm antibody immunohemolytic anemia is determined by saturation kinetics. At a given level of antibody per red cell, $T_{1/2}$ for red cell clearance may be several days. However, as splenic proliferation occurs in response to the sequestration workload, all splenic components increase in number by 5- or 10-fold. Consequently, splenic blood flow and clearance capability increase proportionately. In severe immunohemolytic anemia primarily involving splenic sequestration, $T_{1/2}$ of red cell clearance is rarely less than 2 days. The proliferative response of the spleen to trapped red cell debris accounts for most of the splenic enlargement.

B. Cold-active antibodies

1. Properties

Most cold-active antibodies are 19S IgM immunoglobulins. The temperature optimum for these antibodies is 2–4°C. Above 10°C, effective affinity of antibody for red cell antigen diminishes; above 30°C, attached antibodies dissociate rapidly from the cells. On electron microscopy, cell-bound IgM appears as a strand positioned so as to bridge the 200–300-Å gap that normally separates blood cells. By bridging cells and forming a lattice structure, IgM antibodies cause agglutination. As most IgM antibodies bind red cell antigens primarily at low temperatures, agglutination in vivo is restricted to blood perfusing superficial vessels subject to environmental cooling. However, as cool blood is returned to the warm central circulation, antibody is released quickly and agglutinates disperse.

2. Cold agglutinin titer

In order to quantify antibodies that agglutinate red cells in the cold, serial dilutions of patient's serum are mixed with a 1% suspension of normal type O red cells. The highest dilution (often expressed as its reciprocal) at which visible agglutination occurs denotes the *cold agglutinin titer.* Patients may have cold agglutinin titers in excess of $1:10^6$.

3. Antigen specificity: the I-i system

The *I-i system* of red cell antigens is related to the ABO(H) system, which will be discussed in lecture 15. The I antigen is present in the red cells of most adults, and a low concentration of cold-active IgM with anti-I specificity is present in healthy individuals. In early infancy, I antigenicity replaces the allelic i antigenicity that typifies fetal and cord red blood cells. Consequently, a cold-active antibody may be identified as anti-I if it strongly agglutinates normal adult red cells and fails to agglutinate cord blood cells in comparable fashion. Some anomalous cold-active antibodies possess *anti-i* specificity. Others react with antigens in combination (e.g., the antibody agglutinates cells only if both A and I antigens are present), and some are multispecific for M and N determinants.

4. Factors determining hemolytic potency

These include (1) effects of mechanical trauma on circulating agglutinates; (2) participation of the complement system; (3) thermal range of the antibodies; and (4) the presence of anti-I IgG.

a. Mechanical factors

Mechanical trauma to circulating agglutinates is probably not an important cause of hemolysis unless severe cold exposure is accompanied by muscular exertion.

b. Serum complement

If IgM antibody binds to red cells long enough to activate the complement sequence (several seconds at most), "hemolytic complement" is generated and hemolysis occurs. When activation is sustained, severe intravascular hemolysis ensues. Activation of the complement pathway is usually interrupted midway in the response, with deposition on the red cell of fragmented and inactivated complement components (primarily from C3 and C4). Inactivated C3 is incapable of generating "hemolytic complement"; therefore, a strongly positive anti-C3 Coombs reaction in patients with cold antibodies does not usually signify extensive hemolysis. Often there is no hemolysis, for blocking of the antigens with C3d fragments prevents antibody from binding.

c. Temperature

The striking thermal dependence of cold-active antibodies is determined mainly by effects of temperature on the distribution and reactivity of antigen on the red cell membrane.

d. Antigen density

There are roughly 1 million I antigens per red cell—a density comparable to that of blood group antigens A_1 and B. The close proximity of I-combining sites permits some anti-I IgG to bind to red cells in the steric arrangement required for activation of complement. Red cells of patients with high titers of cold-active antibodies often are agglutinated by both anti-C3 and anti-IgG Coombs sera.

C. Activation of complement

When antibodies reacting with red cell antigens cause all complement components to be sequentially converted to their active forms, "hemolytic complement" is generated and the red cell undergoes hemolysis.

1. Mechanism of complement-mediated hemolysis

Lysis of red cells by "hemolytic complement" is due to profound alteration in membrane permeability. Although "hemolytic complement" does not produce actual holes in cell membranes, it does create large (80–100 Å) circular depressions that are visible on electron microscopy. In cross-section, these defects are imperforate craters in which the bilaminar membrane structure is thinned out to a single layer.

2. Pathways of complement activation

In reacting with red cell antigens, IgM activates the first complement (C1) and launches the "classical pathway" of the complement cascade. The C1q subunit of C1 bears a combining site for the exposed Fc portion of IgM. Its addition to the antibody-antigen complex activates C1r, which then converts C1s to an esterase reactive with C4. This step leads to the generation of large amounts of the complex C4b2a (the C3 convertase), which activates hundreds of C3 molecules. This key amplification step liberates split products of C3, including a major fragment, C3b, that adheres to nearby cell surfaces and facilitates their phagocytosis by neutrophils and macrophages equipped with C3b receptors. In the "alternative pathway" for activating C3, the properdin system bypasses the first three complement components.

3. Noncompletion of complement sequence

The complement system is governed by checks and balances. If the pathway is stalled or if C3b-coated cells are not phagocytized, plasma C3b inactivator splits each adsorbed molecule into two small fragments: C3c, which leaves the scene, and C3d, which cannot bind to macrophage receptors. Coating of red cells with functionless C3d blocks the antigenic determinants and confers protection during subsequent encounters with the IgM antibody. Coating of red cells with C3d accounts for their agglutination by anticomplement sera and for the benign course of most patients with cold-active IgM autoantibodies. Fortunately extensive formation of hemolytic complement and severe intravascular hemolysis is rare, being limited primarily to a minority of patients with anti-I in high titer, patients with the rare episodic disorder paroxysmal cold hemoglobinuria, and recipients of mismatched blood transfusions.

III. CLINICAL DISORDERS

A. With warm-active antibodies

Immunohemolytic anemias associated with warm-active antibodies are idiopathic in almost 60% of the patients (see table 12.1). They are drug induced in 15–30%, associated with lymphoproliferative disorders in 10–15%, and with other disorders in 5–10%.

1. Idiopathic type

a. Clinical features

Idiopathic immunohemolytic anemia occurs in both sexes at all ages. Hemolysis may be acute and occasionally explosive in onset, severe anemia occurring within several days. In most patients, the disorder is self-limited, duration varying from 2–3 weeks to several years. One or more relapses may occur over a period of years. In some, hemolysis is chronic and unremitting. The early symptoms are those of acute anemia (see lecture 1)—dyspnea, weakness, dizziness upon rising, pounding in the ears, pallor, etc. Mild icterus is common. Symptoms of the initial severe phase often disappear as the patient establishes a compensatory erythropoietic response. Splenomegaly, with some tenderness, initially occurs within a few days of the onset. If the hemolytic process continues and reaches a steady state, the spleen may enlarge to 10–12 times its normal weight, extending 2–6 cm below the left costal margin. Massive splenomegaly is not encountered unless the spleen is affected by an associated disease (e.g., chronic lymphocytic leukemia). Hepatomegaly may result from congestive heart failure induced by anemia. Reduction in red cell mass is usually not offset by an increase in plasma volume, and blood volume may be diminished by 1–2 liters.

b. Laboratory findings

The direct anti-IgG Coombs test is typically positive, but occasionally it is initially negative or doubtful. When this occurs, antisera from several sources should be tried, and the test should be performed at several dilutions; a prozone may be caused by an excess of antiglobulin relative to its antigen (IgG). Hemolysis may precede the appearance of detectable antibody. Other early findings in severe cases may include hemoglobinemia, methemalbuminemia, hemosiderinuria, and hemoglobinuria.

When anemia enters a steady state 2–3 weeks after onset, hematologic examination may reveal a hematocrit of about 20%; a reticulocyte count of 10–30% (with large reticulocytes); nucleated red cells; spherocytosis affecting 10–60% of the red cells; normal or slightly elevated white count; and a normal platelet count. In a few patients, platelet levels decline sharply, inducing thrombocytopenic purpura (Evans's syndrome). In most cases, a patient's ^{51}Cr-labeled red cells are sequestered entirely, or primarily, in the spleen (see figure 11.2). When confined to the spleen, the rate of red cell destruction gradually becomes equilibrated by increased red cell formation as the marrow response is established. When hepatic red cell destruction is appreciable, the hemolytic rate may exceed the proliferative capacity of the marrow. Factors that commonly interfere with the compensatory response of marrow include folic acid deficiency and infection. In chronic hemolysis, the nutritional requirement for folic acid, which is needed in DNA synthesis (lecture 5), may increase 2- to 3-fold. Administration of folic acid is advisable in such cases. Infection, such as "parvo-like" viral infections, may dangerously suppress cell proliferation in the bone marrow. Less frequent causes of relative marrow failure include exposure to myelosuppressive drugs (e.g., chloramphenicol, various cytotoxic drugs) and uremia.

2. Drug-induced immunohemolytic anemias

Many drugs and chemicals have been found to induce Coombs-positive hemolytic anemia. A summarized listing of offending compounds, grouped according to the four different mechanisms of action, is presented in table 12.2.

a. Hapten-type mechanism (stibophen model)

Stibophen is the archetypical drug of this class. Other drugs that may act similarly include quinine, quinidine, sulfonamide and sulfanilylurea derivatives, five or six congeners of phenacetin, and PAS. These drugs induce Coombs-positive hemolytic anemia by binding to a plasma protein. The *drug-protein complex* is antigenic, the drug serving as a hapten. Antibodies form to the drug-protein complex, and antigen-antibody complexes formed in the plasma are deposited on red cell surfaces. Cell-bound *immune complexes* tend to activate the complement system; additionally, the complexes may activate complement in the serum, in which case complement fragments are deposited on circulating red cells (which are "innocent bystanders"). The cells become agglutinable by anti-C3 Coombs antiserum. When the elicited antibody is IgM, it is seldom demonstrable on washed red cells because most IgM

Table 12.2
Drug-Induced Immunohemolysis: Proposed Mechanisms

Features	Hapten type: Binding of drug to protein	Hapten type: Binding of drug to red cell	Unknown
Representative drug	Stibophen	Penicillin	Aldomet®
Positive Coombs test	Rare	Uncommon (only at high doses)	Common (varies with dose)
Hemolysis in those with positive Coombs test (and severity)	Usual (occ. severe)	Frequent (mild to moderate)	Uncommon (occ. severe)
Effect of drug withdrawal:			
On Coombs test	Negative in few weeks	Negative in 2–3 months	Negative in 3–18 months
On hemolysis	Rapid, complete improvement	Rapid, complete improvement	Improvement in several weeks; recovery in several months
Direct Coombs test	C3 (occ. IgG)	IgG (occ. C3)	IgG
Antibody causing positive Coombs test and hemolysis	IgM (occ. IgG)	IgG (occ. IgM)	IgG
Antibody (from red cell eluate or serum):			
Binds to red cells only if drug present	Yes	Yes	No
Causes red cells to adhere to mononuclear cells:			
Drug present	No	Yes	Yes
Drug absent	No	No	Yes

antibodies dissociate readily at ambient temperatures. As with cold antibodies, evidence for an immune reaction is inferred from finding complement components (primarily inactivated C3b and C3d) on the red cells. In some patients, the antibody elicited by the drug-protein complex is IgG; complement components and IgG are both detected on the red cell in such cases.

b. Hapten-type mechanism (penicillin model)

An analogous but sequentially different mechanism for drug-induced Coombs-positive hemolytic anemia occurs in patients receiving large doses of penicillin intravenously. Penicillin also acts as a hapten, but in a different manner. When added to red cells suspended in saline, or in greater amounts to whole blood, penicillin binds covalently to proteins in the red cell membrane. The *cell-drug complex* is antigenic, eliciting IgG antibodies directed against "penicillinized" red cells. The IgG Coombs tests is positive; the C3 Coombs test is usually negative. In some cases, IgM may also participate, although this antibody to penicillin is ordinarily harmless.

Immune hemolysis induced by hapten-type mechanisms occurs only when all three reactants—drug, protein (or red cells), and antibody—are present. In both hapten-type mechanisms, the hematologic picture resembles idiopathic immunohemolytic anemia. The term *autoimmunity* is inappropriate since antibody is specific for an exogenous compound. Cases now considered idiopathic may later be attributable to exogenous compounds in the environment. Therapy consists of withdrawing the causative agent. Hemolysis ceases when drug elutes from the cells or drug-coated red cells are removed.

c. Unknown mechanism (Aldomet® model)

Doubt as to whether exogenous drugs or chemicals commonly cause Coombs-positive hemolytic anemia was dispelled when it was recognized that the anti-hypertensive drug α-methyl DOPA or Aldomet® (α-methyl-3,4-dihydroxy-L-phenylalanine) often causes a typical positive IgG Coombs test. Complement is not activated. The frequency of this reaction in patients receiving Aldomet® for >3 months is dose related, ranging from about 10% at a daily dose of 0.75 g to almost 40% at 2.0 g. The IgG Aldomet® antibody is similar in different patients. It appears to react with the Rh locus, showing little or no reaction with Rh null red cells or with red cells of species lacking the Rh locus. Affinity of the Aldomet® antibody for red cells is less than that of warm isoantibodies of the anti-D type (see lecture 16). Consequently, fewer than 1% of those who develop a positive Coombs test during Aldomet® therapy have significant hemolytic anemia. In Coombs-positive but nonanemic patients, the Coombs test is usually 1–2+; on withdrawal of drug, it becomes negative in 3–4 months. In patients with hemolytic anemia, the Coombs test is 3–4+; on withdrawal it becomes negative in 6–24 months.

Aldomet®, its congeners, and degradation products cannot be shown to affect or participate in the interaction between eluted antibody and normal red cells. Proof that the antibody is drug induced is entirely epidemiologic—that is, a positive Coombs test is rare in normal individuals and in hypertensive patients not receiving Aldomet®. The only other medication known to cause Aldomet®-like Coombs-positive hemolytic anemia is the anti-inflammatory drug mefenamic acid. L-DOPA, which is administered to patients with Parkinson's disease, causes a positive Coombs test in 5% to 8% of patients. Unlike α-methyl DOPA (a synthetic analogue), L-DOPA (a physiologic compound) does not cause hemolytic anemia. Presumably, other medications or chemical agents may cause immunohemolytic anemia of the Aldomet® type.

3. Therapy

Therapy of immunohemolytic anemia induced by warm-active antibodies, whether the antibodies are idiopathic or drug induced, varies with the clinical situation.

a. Transfusion

Catastrophic hemolysis with severe anemia requires prompt infusion of fluids and red cells. Normal ABO-compatible red cells will survive at least as long as the patient's red cells, and usually longer. Cross-matching (discussed in lecture 16) may be difficult in some patients but should not deter administration of life-saving transfusion of ABO-compatible blood or packed cells.

b. Corticosteroids

Most patients (80%) respond to corticosteroids, which suppress hemolysis by inhibiting RES activity and antibody synthesis. The reticulocyte count begins to rise in 48 hr. The indirect Coombs test, if positive, soon becomes negative, and in a few weeks the direct Coombs test usually weakens and may disappear. About one-third of patients relapse unless large doses of corticosteroids are continued. Continuation of steroid therapy beyond 2–3 months poses serious risks.

c. Splenectomy

Patients who do not respond to corticosteroids within several weeks of therapy are candidates for splenectomy. Those nonresponders with moderate or severe hemolysis who neither develop splenomegaly nor accumulate ^{51}Cr-labeled red cells in their spleens rarely benefit from splenectomy. Those with splenomegaly (which is invariably present when splenic sequestration is extensive) and striking ^{51}Cr uptake should undergo splenectomy, provided the patient is an acceptable candidate for surgery. Splenectomy removes the filter of antibody-coated red cells but does not alter antibody levels. The Coombs test may remain positive or become even more strongly positive despite a good remission after splenectomy.

d. Immunosuppressive drugs

Occasional patients partially benefit from therapy with immunosuppressive cytotoxic drugs; these agents depress the entire im-

Table 12.3
Characteristics of Various Cold Agglutinins

Clinical setting	Antigenic specificity	Usual titer[a]	Clonal characteristics	Associated hemolysis
Normal	Anti-I Anti-i Anti-H	<50	Polyclonal	None
Postinfection	Anti-I Anti-i	10^2–10^4	Polyclonal	None to severe
Lymphoproliferative disorders	Anti-I	10^2–10^6	Often monoclonal	Mild to severe
Idiopathic cold agglutinin disease	Anti-I	10^2–10^6	Often monoclonal	Mild to severe

a. Expressed as reciprocal of titer.

mune system, but in some cases disproportionately affect the vigorous immunohemolytic process.

e. Treatment of associated diseases

As indicated in table 12.1, Coombs-positive hemolytic anemia is common in patients with lymphoproliferative disorders, particularly chronic lymphocytic leukemia and certain lymphomas. It may also be associated with teratomas, dermoid cysts, carcinoma, SLE, and ulcerative colitis. Successful treatment of the underlying disorders usually improves the hemolytic process.

B. With cold-active antibodies

1. Classification

Most normal serum contains low concentrations of IgM anti-I that causes red cells to agglutinate in the cold.

Elevated titers of cold-active antibodies occur in three clinical circumstances (table 12.3): (1) during recovery phase of *Mycoplasma pneumoniae* and, less often, of infectious mononucleosis (the former has anti-I specificity, the latter anti-i); (2) in association with lymphoproliferative disease; and (3) in idiopathic cold agglutinin disease.

2. Clinical features

Symptoms are due to vasoocclusion in regions of the circulation exposed to cooling and may include painful stiff fingers and toes; blanching or stagnant cyanosis of the skin overlying affected joints; urticaria, generalized or restricted to exposed areas; mottled cyanosis and painful blanching of skin; and local dry gangrene in acrocyanotic regions.

Affected patients are generally older than those with warm-active antibodies. Overt hemolytic anemia develops in a minority of patients. Hemolysis, when it occurs, is usually mild, but it may be severe. in patients with cold-active antibody hemolysis, ^{51}Cr-labeled red cells are usually sequestered in the liver. Splenomegaly is uncommon.

3. Therapy

Antibody titers may be brought down by therapy with an alkylating agent such as chlorambucil. Splenectomy is not usually indicated, and corticosteroid therapy is of little benefit. As IgM is largely intravascular, plasmapheresis has been used to reduce antibody levels in some acute cases. The best therapy is preventive: avoidance of cold exposure and use of measures such as mittens and long underwear. When the cold agglutinin syndrome is associated with lymphoproliferative disorder, improvement may follow antileukemic or antilymphoma therapy (see lectures 21–22).

4. Paroxysmal cold hemoglobinuria

Paroxysmal cold hemoglobinuria (PCH) is a rare, potentially life-threatening, episodic disorder caused by acquisition of the *Donath-Landsteiner (D-L) antibody,* a cold-active complement-fixing antibody. More common at the turn of the century, PCH is usually associated with syphilis, particularly congenital syphilis, or various viral infections.

A paroxysm of hemolysis begins with the binding of D-L antibody to red cells at or below 20–25°C. When blood temperature rises several degress, complement is rapidly and fully activated. The resulting lysis of circulating red cells is accompanied by pronounced erythrophagocytosis and abrupt granulocytopenia. A weakly positive anti-C3 or anti-IgG Coombs test may appear and persist for a day or two. D-L antibody reacts with two of the P system's blood group antigens, usually P_1 and P_2 (see lecture 15). If antibody persists, recurrence is prevented simply by avoidance of cold.

SELECTED REFERENCES

Abramson, N., and Lee, D. P. Immune hemolytic anemias. *D.M.* (April 1974): 1–35.

Bowdler, A. J. The role of the spleen and splenectomy in autoimmune hemolytic disease. *Semin. Hematol.* 13(1976): 335.

Dacie, J. V. Autoimmune hemolytic anemia. *Arch. Intern. Med.* 135(1975): 1293.

Ferrant, A., et al. Assessment of the sites of red cell destruction using quantitative measurements of splenic and hepatic red cell destruction. *Br. J. Haematol.* 50(1982): 591.

Murphy, S., and LoBuglio, A. F. Drug therapy of autoimmune hemolytic anemia. *Semin. Hematol.* 13(1976): 323.

Petz, L. D. Autoimmune hemolytic anemia. *Hum. Pathol.* 14(1983): 251.

Rosse, W. F. Interaction of complement with the red-cell membrane. *Semin. Hematol.* 16(1979): 128.

LECTURE 13 Hemolytic Anemias III: Membrane Disorders

Samuel E. Lux

I. NORMAL RED CELL MEMBRANE

When red cells are hemolyzed in hypotonic media, a membranous residue, the red cell *ghost,* remains.

A. Structure

1. Membrane lipids

The primary membrane structure is a bilayer of *phospholipids* intercalated with molecules of *unesterified cholesterol* and *glycolipids*. The average ghost is half-lipid and half-protein by weight. This amounts (per cell) to about 2.4×10^8 phospholipid molecules, 1.9×10^8 cholesterol molecules, 1.2×10^7 glycolipid molecules, and 4.5×10^8 protein molecules in a total surface area of about 140 μm^2. The lipids are asymmetrically organized. Choline phospholipids (phosphatidyl choline and sphingomyelin) are primarily on the outside half of the bilayer, and amino phospholipids (phosphatidyl ethanolamine and phosphatidyl serine) are on the inside half. Cholesterol is approximately equally distributed. The forces that maintain this asymmetry are not well understood, although there is some evidence that the membrane skeleton (see below) is involved in this process.

The lipids are mobile in the plane of the membrane. This gives the membrane the properties of a viscous, two-dimensional fluid.

2. Membrane proteins

The membrane contains 10 major and perhaps as many as 200 minor proteins (figure 13.1). These are also asymmetrically organized. All the glycoproteins are exposed on the outer membrane surface. Most are proteins carrying red cell antigens (see lecture 15) and/or receptors (e.g., glycophorins A and B) or transport proteins (e.g., protein 3, the anion exchange channel). These *integral membrane proteins* penetrate or span the lipid bilayer, interact with the hydrophobic lipid core, and are tightly bound to the membrane.

Membrane proteins that lack carbohydrate are confined to the cytoplasmic membrane surface. They include certain enzymes (e.g., band 6, glyceraldehyde-3-phosphate dehydrogenase), structural proteins such as spectrin and actin, and hemoglobin. These *peripheral membrane proteins* are external to the lipid bilayer and bind to each other or to anchoring sites on integral membrane proteins.

3. Membrane skeleton

The major peripheral membrane proteins are organized into a two-dimensional protein network that laminates the inner membrane surface (see figure 13.1). The principal components of this *mem-*

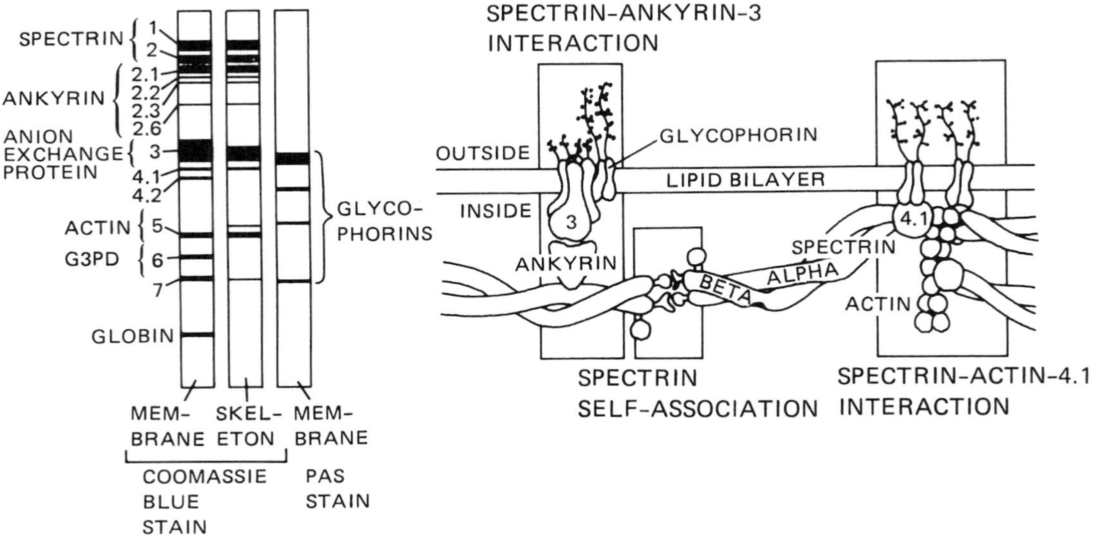

Fig. 13.1
Composition and arrangement of red cell membrane proteins. *Left,* SDS-polyacrylamide gel patterns of the major proteins (stained with Coomassie blue) and sialoglycoproteins (stained with periodic acid Schiff, PAS) of the red cell membrane and membrane skeleton. *Right,* schematic illustration of the organization of the major proteins and sialoglycoproteins. The major integral proteins, protein 3 and the glycophorins, traverse the lipid bilayer. The major peripheral membrane proteins, spectrin, actin, ankyrin, and protein 4.1 form a protein meshwork (the membrane skeleton) that is attached to the inner membrane surface. Like ankyrin, proteins 4.2 and 6 (not shown) bind to the cytoplasmic portion of protein 3. The location of protein 7 is unknown.

brane skeleton are spectrin, actin, protein 4.1, and ankyrin (which includes proteins 2.1, 2.2, 2.3, and 2.6). The skeleton can be isolated by extracting intact red cells or ghosts with nonionic detergents. *Spectrin,* the major skeletal protein, is a dimer composed of two long, flexible chains (α and β subunits or proteins 1 and 2) aligned in parallel and variably twisted around each other. Spectrin dimers interact at their head to form tetramers or higher-order oligomers (spectrin self-association). At their tail end spectrin molecules bind to *short filaments of actin.* This binding is greatly strengthened by *protein 4.1,* which binds to spectrin near the actin binding site. Because multiple spectrins can bind to each actin filament, this interaction serves as a molecular junction, which allows the spectrin to branch and form a two-dimensional network. The skeleton is anchored to the overlying lipid bilayer by *ankyrin,* which binds to spectrin near its head end and links it to the cytoplasmic pole of protein 3. Interactions between spectrin and some of the inner membrane lipids and between protein 4.1 and some of the glycophorins probably also occur but are less well understood.

B. Major functions

1. Membrane skeletal functions

The membrane skeleton is a major determinant of red cell membrane shape, flexibility, and durability. Selective extraction of spectrin and actin or heat denaturation of spectrin (at 49°C) produces spontaneous membrane vesiculation. Mice with hereditary deficiencies of spectrin have extremely fragile red cells that spontaneously lose membrane fragments in the circulation, leading to marked spherocytosis and severe hemolysis. As noted, the skeleton helps to stabilize the asymmetric organization of membrane phospholipids. It also interacts with and immobilizes most of the membrane spanning (integral) proteins and thus determines at least in part, the arrangement of these proteins on the external membrane surface. Because membrane fusion, endocytosis, and certain cell-to-cell interactions require rearrangement of integral membrane proteins, these processes are also influenced by the organizational state of the membrane skeleton.

2. Maintenance of cell volume

The red cell controls its volume and water content primarily through control of its Na^+ and K^+ content. The cell membrane is relatively impermeable to cations. Small, passive cation leaks are normally balanced by the active outward transport of Na^+ (3 mEq/liter of red cells/hr) and inward transport of K^+ (2 mEq/liter/hr). These cation pumps are linked, require ATP, and are dependent on the membrane enzyme *Na-K ATPase*. This enzyme is specifically inhibited by cardiac glycosides such as ouabain. A remarkably small number of pumps (estimated to be 300 per cell) suffices to maintain a high-K^+ (100 mEq/liter red cells) and low-Na^+ (10 mEq/liter red cells) concentration inside the cell. If cation leakage increases, cation pumps have limited compensatory ability. If this capacity is exceeded, red cell volume changes in parallel with the total cation change. Red cells swell when (Na^+ leak in) > (K^+ leak out) and shrink when (Na^+ leak in) < (K^+ leak out).

3. Ca^{++} homeostasis

Excessive intracellular Ca^{++} is deleterious to the red cell, and the cell actively extrudes Ca^{++} from its interior with an efficient ATP-dependent calcium pump (*Ca-ATPase*). Intracellular Ca^{++} is normally almost undetectable (around 0.1 to 1 μM). If ATP levels fall (to below 20% of normal) or if Ca^{++} leakage exceeds the capacity of the calcium pump, intracellular Ca^{++} accumulates and changes the red cell from a biconcave disk to an *echinocyte*—a spiculated sphere with many short, regular projections. Elevated intracellular Ca^{++} also causes a selective loss of K^+ and H_2O (*Gardos effect*). The result is a crenated, dehydrated, almost indeformable cell that is highly susceptible to splenic sequestration and destruction. Recent studies have shown that the calcium pump is modulated by a cytoplasmic calcium-binding protein called *calmodulin*. When intracellular Ca^{++} concentrations rise, Ca-calmodulin combines with and activates the Ca-ATPase, accelerating Ca^{++} egress.

4. Anion exchange

Physiologically, the red cell is a critical component of CO_2 transport. HCO_3^- ions are carried by red cells to the lungs, where they are exchanged for Cl^-. The exchange process is massive ($\sim 7 \times 10^{10}$ anions/RBC/sec) and requires a large number of exchange channels ($\sim 5 \times 10^5$). Recent studies have shown that the channel is formed by protein 3, the major red cell membrane component.

II. INTERACTIONS BETWEEN RED CELLS AND SPLEEN

A. Structure

Circulating red cells must repeatedly squeeze their 7-μm-diameter bodies through the narrow, elliptical fenestrations that separate the splenic cords and sinuses (figure 13.2; also see figure 2.5). The normal red cell is diverted through the spleen about 120 times per day and completes the journey in approximately 30 sec, but ab-

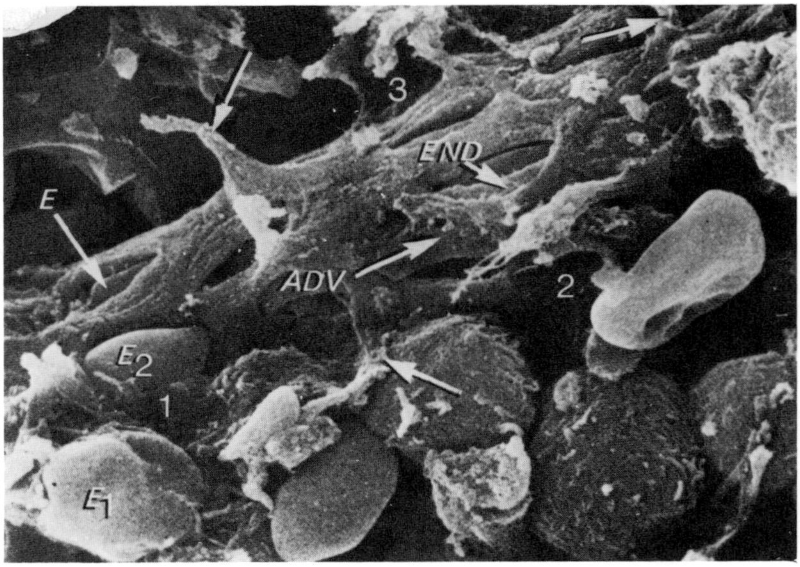

Fig. 13.2
Scanning electron micrograph of a splenic sinus wall viewed from a splenic cord. A portion of the overlying cordal structure has been removed. The narrow transmural slits between the endothelial (END) cells of the sinus wall are easily seen. It is likely that these cells are normally opposed and that the slits are potential structures rather than fixed pores. They are evident here because of a drying artifact. Note that the adjacent erythrocytes (E) are considerably larger than the slits and hence must be flexible to pass into the splenic sinuses. ADV = adventitial cell.

normal red cells may be detained for periods of minutes to hours in the stagnant, acidic, hypoxic, hypoglycemic environment of the splenic cords. This is an exacting test and is often fatal for old or defective red cells.

B. Red cell deformability

Red cells are detained in the splenic cords if they are poorly deformable or if they bear proteins (e.g., IgG1, IgG3, or C3b) that are bound to receptors on splenic phagocytes (see lecture 12). Probably other, still undefined, alterations in the topography of the external membrane surface also attract the attention of phagocytes and lead to red cell demise. Decreased red cell deformability may result from (1) an increase in cytoplasmic viscosity (e.g., sickled cells, dehydrated red cells); (2) intracellular rubbish (e.g., Heinz bodies); (3) membrane rigidity (e.g., secondary to oxidant-induced cross-linking of the membrane skeleton); or (4) a decrease in red cell surface-to-volume ratio.

C. Surface-to-volume ratio

1. Spherocytosis

Spherocytosis occurs as the surface-to-volume ratio declines. This may occur because of loss of membrane surface (microspherocytosis) or gain in volume (macrospherocytosis). Because the red cell membrane is flexible but not stretchable, the red cell becomes progressively less deformable as its spheroidicity increases. This impairment has been likened to an obese man attempting to bend at the waist, but a more useful analogy is the plastic sandwich bag. This bag is flexible but not elastic—similar to the red cell membrane. A simple test will convince the reader that the inflated bag, like the spherocyte, is almost indeformable.

2. Target cells

Increases in the surface-to-volume ratio may be due to an increase in membrane surface area or a decrease in cell volume. The resulting flattened cells appear in blood smears as target cells.

3. Osmotic fragility

The *osmotic fragility test* measures the ability of red cells to swell in hypotonic media and is a useful indirect measure of the surface-to-volume ratio (figure 13.3).

Spherocytes, with a decreased surface-to-volume ratio, are highly fragile; that is, they can tolerate less osmotic swelling than normal red cells before they burst. Target cells, in contrast, are relatively osmotically resistant.

III. PATHOPHYSIOLOGY OF RED CELL SHAPE CHANGES

Because the etiology and pathogenesis of many of the membrane disorders are still unknown, it is most useful to classify these diseases by the changes in shape they produce. Red cell shape may be considered in terms of the corresponding changes in membrane

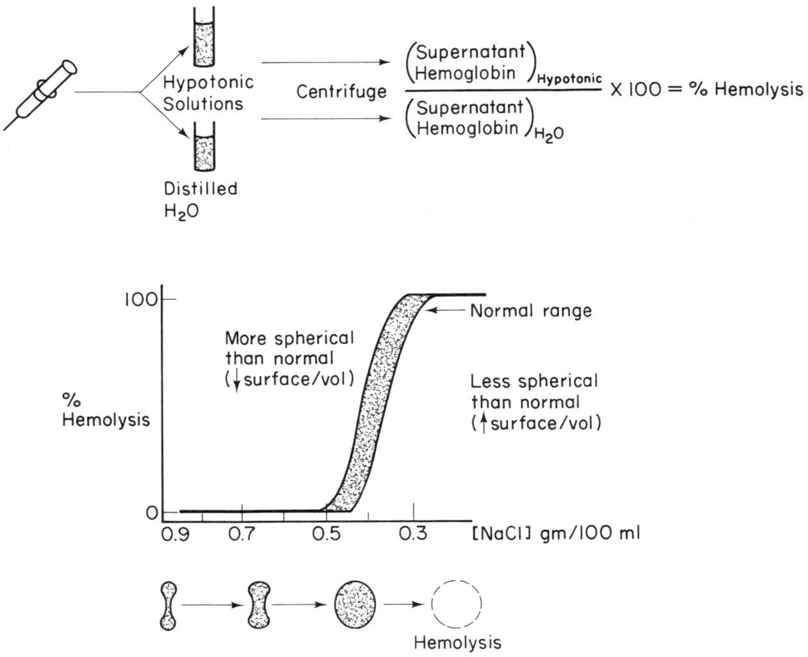

Fig. 13.3
Schematic illustration of the osmotic fragility test. Equal aliquots of blood are placed in equal volumes of buffered salt solutions of varying osmolarity or in distilled water. After a brief incubation, the unhemolyzed red cells are removed by centrifugation and the supernatant hemoglobin released at each salt concentration is compared to the distilled water sample (100% lysis) to determine the percentage hemolysis. The osmotic fragility (OF) curve is a plot of the percentage hemolysis vs. the sodium chloride concentration (conventionally plotted as decreasing from left to right on the X-axis).

surface and intracellular volume (see diagram 13.1). An expanded form of this concept is presented in figure 13.4.

A. Hereditary spherocytosis (HS)

Hereditary spherocytosis (HS) is a relatively common hemolytic anemia that affects about 1 of every 5,000 individuals in the United States. It is usually inherited as an autosomal dominant, but in approximately 25% of the cases neither parent is affected. Whether this is due to decreased penetrance, spontaneous mutation, or a subclass of patients with autosomal recessive inheritance is still unresolved.

1. Pathogenesis

The underlying defect is in the red cells. This is shown by the shortened survival of HS red cells that have been transfused into normal subjects and the normal survival of normal red cells that have been transfused into HS patients.

Pathophysiologically the primary defect appears to be membrane instability. Biomechanical measurements indicate that red

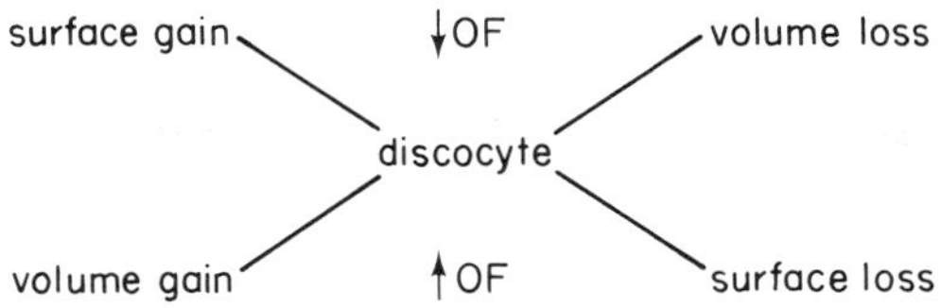

Diagram 13.1

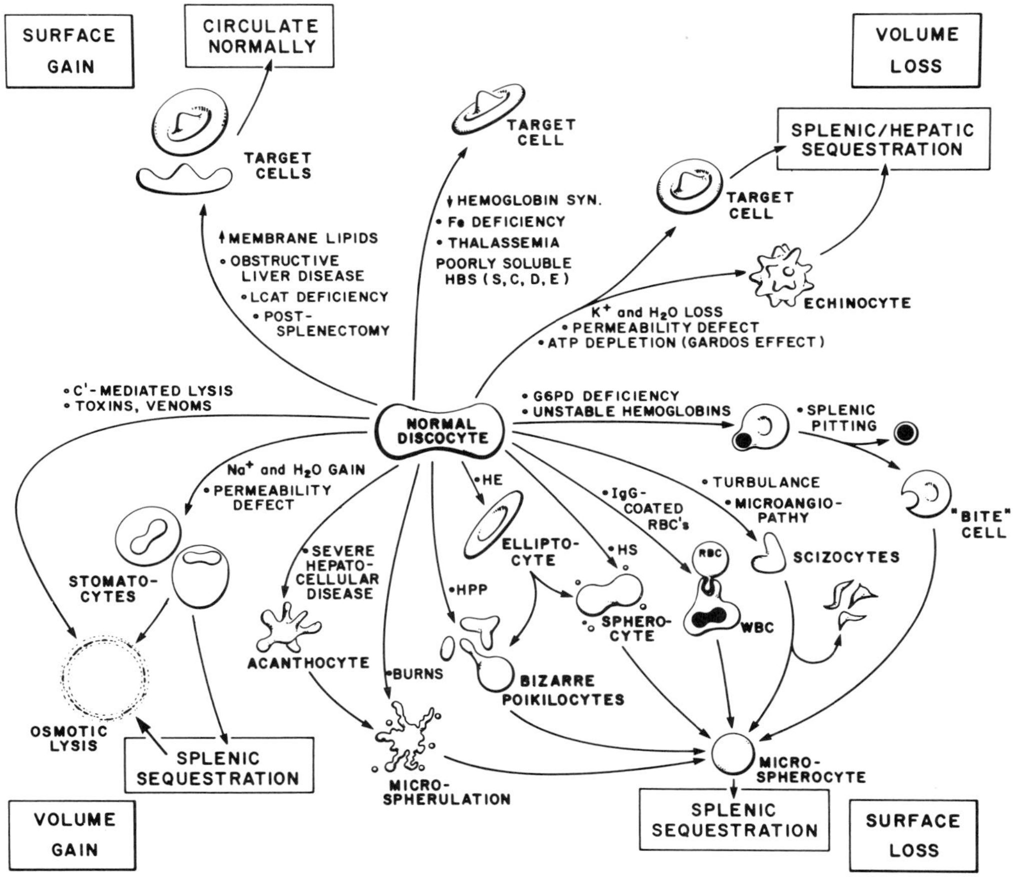

Fig. 13.4
Summary of the major abnormalities of red cell surface area, volume, and shape.

cell membranes from some HS patients fragment more easily than normal membranes when suction stress is applied to local areas of the membrane. This weakness suggests a defect of the membrane skeleton.

Recent studies have identified quantitative and qualitative defects in spectrin, the major skeletal protein. Careful measurements show that HS red cells are *spectrin deficient* and that the degree of spectrin deficiency correlates with the degree of spherocytosis and with clinical severity. Most HS patients have only mild deficiency (spectrin content 75–90% of normal), but in rare, apparently homozygous patients, spectrin content may be as low as 30–50% of normal. These individuals have very severe, transfusion-dependent hemolysis.

In a subset of HS patients (~5–15%) a qualitative defect in spectrin in also present. Approximately half of the spectrin molecules *lack the ability to bind protein 4.1*. (This is the expected proportion in a dominant disease like HS since only one of the two presumed spectrin genes will be abnormal.) As a consequence the defective spectrins bind poorly to actin, weakening the skeleton. Presumably in these patients spectrin deficiency is secondary to the 4.1-binding defect. It remains to be determined whether the spectrin deficiency observed in other HS patients is due to similar, unidentified structural defects or is caused by a primary abnormality in spectrin synthesis.

As shown in figure 13.5, it is believed that the membrane weakness leads to repeated loss of membrane fragments as the HS red cell circulates and a gradual decrease in surface-to-volume ratio (or increase in spheroidicity). For the reasons discussed earlier, this process eventually causes the HS red cell to become detained in the splenic cords, where, for unknown reasons, membrane surface loss is augmented by the toxic cordal environment. This pro-

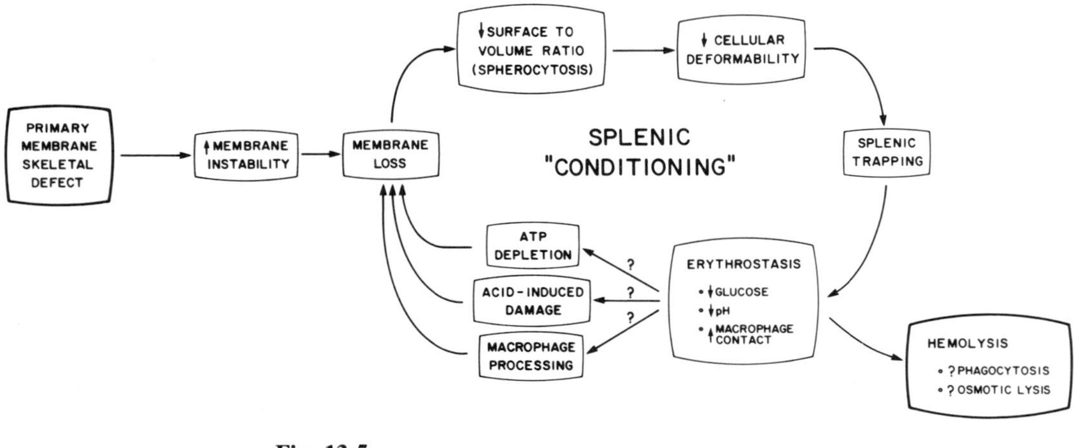

Fig. 13.5
Currently popular (but unproved) model for the pathophysiology of HS.

cess of "*splenic conditioning*" can be partially simulated by incubating red cells in the absence of glucose for 24 hr. Under these conditions, HS red cells lose membrane fragments more rapidly than normal, a phenomenon that forms the basis of the *incubated osmotic fragility test*. In vivo, conditioned red cells are prevalent in the splenic pulp as expected, but some escape into the peripheral circulation. They are detectable as a hyperspherical "tail" on osmotic fragility curves and form the dense, hyperchromic microspherocytes characteristically seen on peripheral blood smears of HS patients. It is likely that many HS red cells never escape the conditioning process. Those that do are especially susceptible to recapture by the spleen and eventual destruction.

2. Clinical features

Neonatal jaundice is frequent and may occasionally require exchange transfusion (see lecture 16). After the neonatal period, most patients develop a partially compensated hemolytic state with mild-to-moderate anemia, intermittent mild jaundice especially during viral infections, and splenomegaly. However, it is important to realize that clinical severity can vary widely, even within the same family. Approximately one-quarter of the patients are entirely compensated and have no anemia, little or no jaundice, and only slight splenomegaly. In contrast, a small proportion are severely anemic and transfusion dependent. Untreated older children and adults usually develop pigment gallstones secondary to increased bilirubin production, and concern about complications of gallstones, such as cholecystitis and biliary obstruction, is the major impetus for splenectomy (see below) in most patients.

The blood smear shows variable numbers of spherocytes and polychromatophilia. The reticulocyte count is usually >8% and is almost always abnormal. The bone marrow shows normoblastic erythroid hyperplasia.

3. Crises

The clinical course is interrupted in most patients by periodic crises characterized by worsening anemia. Three types of crises occur: hemolytic, aplastic, and megaloblastic (table 13.1). Mild *hemolytic* crises are probably the most frequent, but usually are clinically insignificant. They are presumably secondary to the reticuloendothelial hyperplasia that accompanies many infections. *Aplastic* crises, due to viral suppression of erythropoiesis, are less frequent but are often severe enough to require transfusion. Recent studies indicate that many of these are caused by a human parvovirus-like agent. *Megaloblastic* crises occur when dietary intake of folic acid is inadequate for the increased needs of the erythroid HS bone marrow (see lecture 5). These may be prevented by administration of folic acid supplements.

Table 13.1
Types of Crises Seen in Patients with Hemolysis

Type of crisis	Anemia	Reticulocytes	Jaundice	Cause	Comment
Hemolytic	↑	↑	↑	Infection	Frequent, mild
Aplastic	↑	↓	↓	Infection	Infrequent, severe
Megaloblastic	↑	↓	↑	Relative folate deficiency	Infrequent

4. Diagnosis

Spherocytosis, the hallmark of the disease, is always present, but in 20–25% of patients, typical microspherocytes are sparse and spherocytosis is difficult to recognize on the blood smear. In these patients, the unincubated osmotic fragility test will often be normal or only slightly abnormal since it simply quantifies what is visible on the smear. The incubated OF, however, is almost always abnormal and is the most reliable simple diagnostic test available.

5. Therapy

Splenectomy dependably halts both red cell conditioning and hemolysis in the usual types of HS and is the recommended therapy. Following splenectomy, spherocytosis persists (because the basic red cell defect is unchanged), but conditioned microspherocytes disappear and changes typical of the postsplenectomy state (Howell-Jolly bodies, target cells, siderocytes, and acanthocytes) become evident in the blood smear.

Since splenectomy increases susceptibility to sepsis from pneumococci and certain other encapsulated bacteria, especially during infancy and early childhood (see lecture 2), it is usually delayed until age 5 or 6. The risk of postsplenectomy sepsis can be further reduced with *pneumococcal vaccine;* however, the predicted risk of fatal sepsis in HS patients (~1/100–1/400) is still 25–100 times the estimated risk in the general population. The major controversies at the present time are whether this risk warrants withholding splenectomy in patients with mild HS and whether splenectomized patients should be maintained on prophylactic antibiotics.

B. Hereditary elliptocytosis (HE)

Hereditary elliptocytosis is also inherited as an autosomal dominant and is relatively common (~1:2,500), particularly the mild form (see below). The disease is due to defects in the membrane skeleton since ghosts and isolated skeletons retain the elliptical shape. The precise molecular abnormalities in the membrane skeleton responsible for HE are currently the subject of active investigation. Some examples are discussed in the following sections.

1. Mild HE

This is the common form of HE (~90% of cases). It is often, though not always, caused by structural defects in the head end of spectrin, which interfere with spectrin self-association. Practically it is little more than a morphologic curiosity. Most patients have no anemia or splenomegaly and only mild hemolysis (reticulocyte count 1–4%). The blood smear shows prominent elliptocytosis (usually > 40%, normal < 15%). A minority (10–20%) has moderate hemolysis and is classified as a sporadic hemolytic variant. The reason(s) for this variation is unknown. In general patients with mild HE require no therapy; however, it is important to remember that they may develop significant hemolysis if the spleen hypertrophies in response to various stimuli (e.g., infectious mononucleosis, cirrhosis). In addition the physician must be alert for *transient neonatal hemolysis*. Neonates in some HE families (particularly black families) have a moderately severe hemolytic anemia with red cell budding, fragmentation, and poikilocytosis. The relative paucity of elliptocytes may create diagnostic confusion; however, the diagnosis is easily made from family studies since one of the parents will have typical mild HE. During the first year or so of life hemolysis gradually declines in these infants, and the disorder evolves into typical mild HE. This curious phenomenon is unexplained. Presumably it reflects a difference in the fetal red cell or the circulatory system of the newborn that augments the primary defect in spectrin self-association.

2. Hereditary pyropoikilocytosis (HPP)

This rare autosomal recessive disorder is characterized by moderately severe hemolytic anemia, marked red cell fragmentation, and bizarre poikilocytosis. It is most common in blacks. When heated for short periods, HPP red cells fragment (and their isolated spectrin denatures) at 45–46°C instead of the normal 49°C. This *exceptional heat sensitivity* constitutes the primary test for the disease. Hemolysis decreases after splenectomy, but the bizarre red cell morphology and heat sensitivity are unchanged. The following recent evidence suggests that HPP is related to mild HE: (1) all patients have a defect in spectrin self-association that is qualitatively similar to the defect in mild HE but more severe; (2) patients with HPP often have relatives with mild HE. A current explanation is that HPP patients are either homozygous for mild HE, homozygous for a related "silent" mutation, or doubly heterozygous for mild HE and the putative silent gene defect.

3. Spherocytic HE

This variant (~10% of cases) is clinically and pathophysiologically similar to hereditary spherocytosis. Patients typically have moderate hemolysis, mild anemia, and splenomegaly. Elliptocytes are less prominent and more rounded than in typical mild HE. Spherocytes are usually evident and may predominate in some individuals; however, at least one family member will have clear-cut elliptocytosis. Patients with this form of HE, like those with HS, have osmotically fragile red cells and respond well to splenectomy. A deficiency of protein 4.1 occurs in some but not all families with this disorder.

It is still uncertain how the various membrane skeletal defects relate to the abnormal red cell shapes and the presence or absence of hemolysis in the elliptocytosis syndromes. One unproved hypothesis is that HE skeletal defects, such as weakened spectrin self-association, alter the material properties of the membrane and increase its propensity to develop a permanent, plastic deformation. HE red cells are disc shaped, as are reticulocytes, and acquire their elliptical shape in the circulation. Since normal red cells undergo elliptical deformation in the capillaries, it is possible that HE red cells, with their weakened skeletons, simply rearrange to adopt this configuration on repeated passage through the microcirculation. When the skeletal defect is severe, as in HPP, the red cells cannot withstand circulatory shear stresses and fragment in the circulation. In these disorders the compliant skeletons are easily deformed, and bizarre poikilocytes result.

IV. MEMBRANE SURFACE LOSS DUE TO OTHER CAUSES

A. Immunohemolytic anemia

As discussed in lecture 12, phagocytes bearing receptors for IgG1, IgG3, and C3b can bind and detain red cells coated with these substances, remove portions of their membranes, or, in some cases, phagocytize them completely. Escaped red cells return to the circulation as spherocytes, destined for splenic detention and recapture by phagocytes.

B. Heinz body hemolytic anemias

The intracellular precipitation of hemoglobin to form Heinz bodies occurs in unstable hemoglobinopathies (lecture 9) and in oxidant hemolysis (e.g., G-6-PD deficiency). As discussed in lecture 2, splenic "pitting" of Heinz bodies may lead to the appearance of "bite cells" and occasionally to spherocytes.

C. Mechanical injury

The most important hemolytic anemias in this class result from mechanical damage to red cells produced in the high-pressure arterial or arteriolar circulation by pathological blood vessels. These processes all cause red cell fragmentation (helmet cells, triangular fragments, and other schizocytes) and intravascular hemolysis (see lecture 11). The presence of such cells should suggest a number of specific causes. Hemolysis due to mechanical injury in the arterial circulation usually results from excessive turbulence around an *artificial heart valve* (especially the aortic valve) or other intraventricular prosthesis. The shear stress produced literally tears the red cells apart. Hence it has been called the *Waring blender syndrome*. It is also termed *macroangiopathic* hemolytic anemia. Hemolysis in the arteriolar circulation, *microangiopathic* hemolytic anemia, may result from damage to arteriolar endothelium or from fibrin deposition within the vessel. Microangiopathic hemolytic anemias are caused by: disseminated intravascular coagulation (DIC; see lecture 28); localized intravascular coagulation (e.g., in cavernous hemangiomas); certain renal vascular disorders (malignant hypertension, severe glomerulonephritis, transplant rejection) and other forms of vasculitis; diffuse carcinomatosis; thrombotic thrombocytopenic purpura (TTP), a rare, often fatal, disorder displaying hemolytic anemia with red cell fragmentation, thrombocytopenia, renal disease, neurologic abnormalities, and fever (see lecture 27); and hemolytic-uremic syndrome, a disorder of childhood that resembles TTP but is more common and less often fatal.

D. Thermal injury

Spherocytes appear when blood is heated to temperatures above 49°C, due to damage to spectin, which is denatured at that temperature. The spherocytes result from marked membrane fragmentation (microspherulation). Spherocytic hemolytic anemia may result from third-degree burns covering more than 20% of the body surface.

E. Toxins

Various chemicals, bacterial toxins and venoms (e.g., of snakes, brown spiders) can cause membrane injury and spherocytosis. *Clostridium welchii* septicemia is a clinically important example of this process. Severe, rapidly progressive, intravascular hemolysis and microspherocytosis is common in this condition and may be fatal.

F. Spiculated red cells

1. Acanthocytes

Acanthocytes are rounded red cells with *irregular* thorny projections. They occur in some patients with severe hepatocellular disease (where they are often called spur cells) and in a variety of other rare conditions.

a. Liver disease

In patients with severe liver disease, acanthocytosis occurs in two stages: *cholesterol loading* and *splenic remodeling* (figure 13.6). In the first stage, abnormal cholesterol-laden lipoproteins, produced by the diseased liver, transfer their excess cholesterol to circulating red cells and increase membrane cholesterol, the cholesterol/phospholipid ratio, and the membrane surface area. This is an acquired process and can be mimicked in vitro by incubating normal red cells in spur cell plasma or in artificial media containing cholesterol-rich lipid dispersions. Microscopically, these cholesterol-laden red cells are flattened (leptocytes) with a scalloped pe-

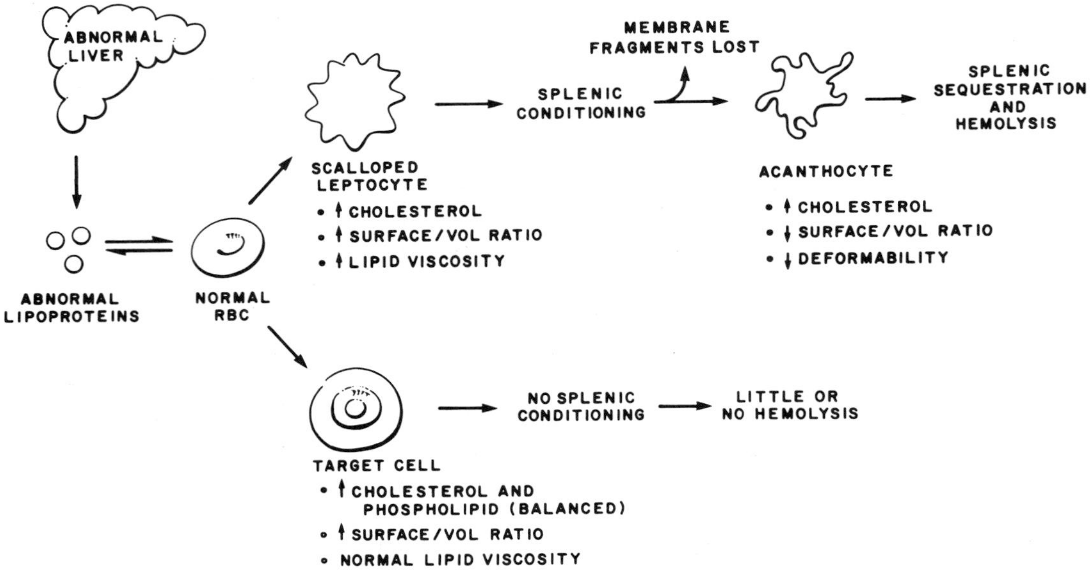

Fig. 13.6
Schematic illustration of the pathophysiology of acanthocyte (spur cell) and target cell formation in liver disease.

riphery. In vivo, these cells are converted into spur cells by a poorly defined process of splenic conditioning. Over a period of days membrane lipids and surface area are lost, cellular rigidity increases, and the cells assume a typical acanthocytic form (figure 13.6). Splenectomy prevents the formation of spur cells and their premature destruction, but it is a high-risk procedure in these very ill patients and is seldom indicated.

b. Other causes

Acanthocytes are also prominent in patients with a rare anomaly of the Kell blood group antigens (McLeod phenotype), in the rare disease abetalipoproteinemia, in the poorly defined disorder infantile pyknocytosis, and in some patients with anorexia nervosa.

2. *Echinocytes*

Unlike the irregularly spiculated acanthocyte, echinocytes (crenated cells, burr cells) are covered with short, uniform spicules arranged in a *regular* array. This difference is easily appreciated in scanning electron micrographs but is difficult to discern in blood smears. Echinocytes are common in patients with severe *uremia* and occur in small numbers in normal newborns, in splenectomized patients, and in various hemolytic anemias. They have a nearly normal survival. Less viable echinocytes occur in conditions associated with *cell dehydration* and decreased intracellular volume (to be discussed) and occasionally are observed in patients with disseminated carcinoma or microangiopathic hemolytic anemia.

V. DISEASES ASSOCIATED WITH INCREASED MEMBRANE SURFACE

A. Biliary obstruction

As noted earlier, *target cells* form when the red cell surface-to-volume ratio rises. Patients with liver disease associated with *biliary obstruction* often develop target cells. The pathogenesis of this shape change is analogous to that discussed earlier for spur cells (i.e., the red cells acquire excess lipids from abnormal lipoproteins), except that the lipid transfer involves *both cholesterol and phospholipids* in a ratio similar to that which exists normally in red cell membranes (figure 13.6). As a consequence, membrane surface area expands, but the cholesterol/phospholipid ratio is nearly normal. Because cellular deformability is unimpaired, these cells survive well, and the abnormality, while morphologically interesting, produces no clinical morbidity.

B. Other causes

The spleen normally removes some membrane lipid and protein components from reticulocytes soon after their release into the circulation. This poorly understood process is referred to as surface remodeling or splenic "polishing." In splenectomized patients, this excess membrane material expands membrane surface area, and small numbers of target cells appear on the blood smear. Finally, excess membrane surface and targeting is a prominent feature in the rare patients who are deficient in the plasma enzyme lecithin:cholesterol acyltransferase (LCAT).

VI. DISEASES ASSOCIATED WITH VOLUME LOSS

A. Hemoglobin abnormalities

Target cells are also common in patients with abnormal hemoglobin synthesis (i.e., iron deficiency, lecture 6; and thalassemia, lecture 10) and in patients with certain abnormal hemoglobins (e.g., hemoglobins S, C, D, and E; see lecture 9).

B. Cations

Loss of intracellular water leads to red cell dehydration or *xerocytosis*. As noted, cell water is regulated by intracellular monovalent cation content. If red cell membrane permeability is altered so that loss of K^+ (the predominant intracellular cation) exceeds gain of Na^+ (the predominant extracellular cation), total cation content and cell water decline. This occurs as a primary disorder in the rare disease *hereditary xerocytosis* and as a secondary event in disorders associated with intracellular Ca^{++} *accumulation* (e.g., sickle cell anemia; see lecture 9) or *ATP depletion* (e.g., pyruvate kinase deficiency; see lecture 14). Morphologically, dehydrated red cells are typically either targeted or contracted and spiculated. Because dehydration elevates intracellular viscosity, these cells are relatively rigid and risk splenic sequestration and hemolysis.

VII. DISEASES ASSOCIATED WITH VOLUME GAIN

A. Water volume

The analogous but opposite disorder to hereditary xerocytosis is *hereditary hydrocytosis*. In this rare condition, an inherited defect in Na^+ permeability causes *massive Na^+ influx,* which overwhelms the Na-K pump and leads to an increase in intracellular cations and water. Severe hemolysis results. The partially swollen blood cell appear on blood smears as *stomatocytes* (i.e., red cells with a mouthlike band of pallor across the center of the stained cell).

B. Other causes

Stomatocytes are also seen as an acquired defect, not associated with hydrocytosis or cation changes—particularly in patients with acute *alcoholism* and in various types of liver disease. Little hemolysis is present.

C. C′-mediated intravascular hemolysis

Complement-mediated hemolysis may be considered a form of volume gain since red cell destruction occurs by rapid osmotic swelling (colloid osmotic hemolysis). Practically, however, conplement lysis is so rapid that swollen macrospherocytes, which must occur as intermediates in this process, are not seen. Clinically, complement-mediated hemolysis occurs in some immunohemolytic anemias (e.g., PCH), in some transfusion reactions (e.g., ABO blood group incompatibility), and in *paroxysmal nocturnal hemoglobinuria* (*PNH*).

1. PNH

a. Pathophysiology

PNH is an *acquired* membrane disorder that results from population of the bone marrow by *clones of abnormal stem cells* (figure 13.7). Most often these abnormal clones arise from a mutagenic event occurring in the course of *marrow hypoplasia,* but sometimes they occur without hypoplasia. There is no extracorpuscular defect. Normal red cells survive normally in patients with PNH. The basic membrane defect is unknown, but its functional consequence is an *increased sensitivity to activated complement* due to an increased ability of PNH membranes to fix C3 and to more efficient penetration of the PNH membrane by the terminal lytic sequence of complement. All three cell lines are affected. The de-

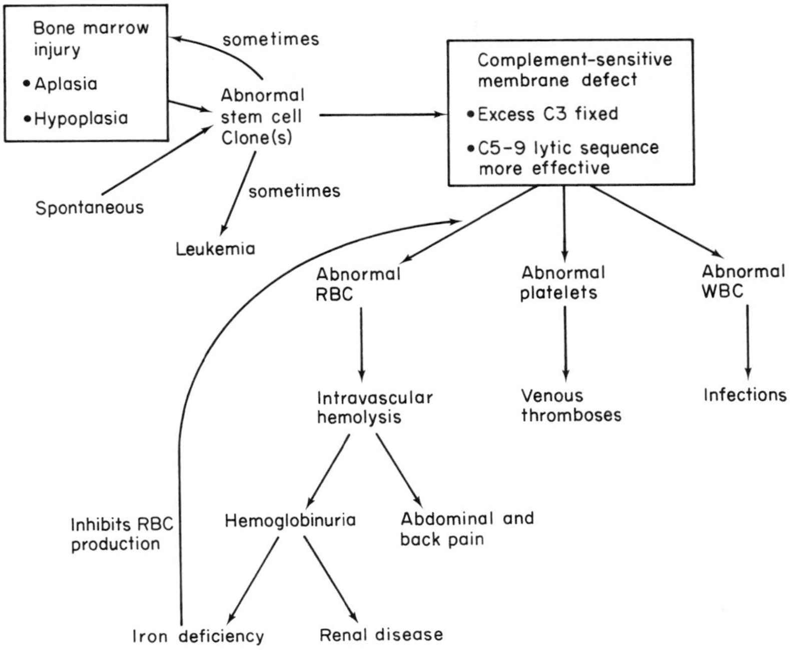

Fig. 13.7
Pathophysiology of PNH.

gree of complement sensitivity (and symptoms) varies widely, due, in part, to variability in the proportion of stem cells in the abnormal clones and, in part, to the degree of complement sensitivity of each of the clones. In addition to complement sensitivity, there is *diminished acetylcholinesterase* activity in PNH red cells, increased susceptibility to hemolysis by hydrogen peroxide, and diminished leukocyte alkaline phosphatase.

b. Clinical features

Classically, as the name implies, PNH patients present with hemoglobinuria that, for unknown reasons, is worse at night and remits during the day. However, nocturnal hemoglobinuria is not evident in many patients, and some have chronic hemolysis with no obvious hemoglobinuria at all. Most patients have chronic *hemosiderinuria,* however, and many eventually develop *iron deficiency* or renal damage due to chronic iron deposition. Iron therapy is sometimes necessary, but it may be hazardous since iron-induced reticulocytosis produces new complement-sensitive cells and may exacerbate hemolysis. During hemolytic episodes, patients may experience severe abdominal or back pain that may resemble the so-called surgical abdomen. Some patients develop (or revert to) aplastic anemia, and many develop isolated leukopenia and/or thrombocytopenia during the course of the disease. Others suffer from recurrent venous thromboses, especially of the portal venous system. These are thought to be due to activation of the complement-sensitive platelets by C3. Infections due to leukopenia and/or abnormal function of the PNH phagocytes may also be a problem. Occasionally, the PNH clone becomes more abnormal and evolves into acute myelocytic leukemia.

c. Diagnosis

It is evident from this litany of symptoms and complications that PNH may present in many guises and is frequently considered in differential diagnoses. The diagnosis depends on detection of complement-sensitive red cells. In humans complement fixes to red cells at a slightly acid pH. PNH red cells lyse under these conditions even in the absence of antibody. The *acid-serum lysis test* or Ham test is a measure of this property. In the *sucrose hemolysis test* (or *sugar water test*), a medium of low ionic strength (i.e., isotonic sucrose) is used to aggregate serum globulins onto the red cell surface. This activates complement and promotes hemolysis of PNH red cells. In general, the sugar water test is slightly more sensitive and the Ham test is slightly more specific in detecting the disease.

d. Therapy

There is no specific therapy for PNH. Symptomatic treatment is employed as needed for anemia (washed red cell transfusions), iron deficiency ($FeSO_4$ therapy), thrombocytopenia (platelet transfusions), and thromboses (anticoagulation). In some patients, androgens are useful because of their ability to stimulate erythropoiesis. Corticosteroids are effective in blunting acute episodes of hemolysis, but the doses required are too high for chronic use. As expected in a disease characterized by intravascular hemolysis, splenectomy produces little improvement. In patients with severe PNH-induced marrow aphasia, bone marrow transplantation may be life saving.

SELECTED REFERENCES

Cohen, C. M. — The molecular organization of the red cell membrane skeleton. *Semin. Hematol.* 20(1983): 141.

Cooper, R. A. — Hemolytic syndromes and red cell memrane abnormalities in liver disease. *Semin. Hematol.* 17(1980): 103.

Knowles, W., et al. — Spectrin: Structure, function and abnormalities. *Semin. Hematol.* 20(1983): 159.

Lux, S. E. — Disorders of the red cell membrane skeleton: Hereditary spherocytosis and hereditary elliptocytosis (chapter 72). In Stanbury, J. B., et al., eds., *The Metabolic Basis of Inherited Disease,* 5th ed., New York, McGraw-Hill, 1983, pp. 1573–1605.

Lux, S. E. — Disorders of the red cell membrane. In Nathan, D. G., and Oski, F. A., eds., *Hematology of Infancy and Childhood,* 3d ed., Philadelphia, W. B. Saunders, in press.

Palek, J., and Lux, S. E. — Red cell membrane skeletal defects in hereditary and acquired hemolytic anemias. *Semin. Hematol.* 20(1983): 189.

Singer, D. B. — Postsplenectomy sepsis. In Rosenberg, H. S., and Bolande, R. P., eds., *Perspectives in Pediatric Pathology,* Chicago: Yearbook Medical Publishers, 1973, 1:285–311.

LECTURE 14 Hemolytic Anemias IV. Metabolic Disorders

Samuel E. Lux

I. NORMAL RED CELL METABOLISM

A. Embden-Meyerhof pathway

Mitochondria and microsomes are lost as reticulocytes mature into adult red cells; consequently, mature red cells consume little oxygen and do not synthesize protein. Glucose, the main metabolic substrate of red cells, is metabolized via two major pathways: (1) the *Embden-Meyerhof* or *glycolytic pathway*; and (2) the *hexosemonophosphate (HMP) shunt pathway* (figure 14.1).

Glucose enters red cells by a carrier-mediated process that is independent of insulin. Approximately 90–95% of glucose is metabolized to lactate via the glycolytic pathway.

1. Production and function of ATP

This is the only pathway capable of ATP synthesis in mature red cells, 2 moles of ATP being generated per mole of glucose consumed. Compared to other cells that possess mitochondria and an active Krebs cycle (that generates 38 moles ATP per mole of glucose consumed), ATP production from glycolysis is highly inefficient. Nevertheless, the meager ATP production (2–3 mmoles/liter of red cells/hr) permits renewal of 150–200% of total red cell ATP (1.0–1.5 mmole/liter red cells/hr) every hour. Important functions of red cell ATP include active transport of Na and K, maintenance of low intracellular calcium levels, phosphorylation of membrane proteins, and sustenance of glycolysis itself.

2. Production and function of NADH

Glycolysis is the major source of red cell NADH, an essential cofactor in a variety of oxidation-reduction reactions. One such reaction is the maintenance of heme iron in the reduced state, an enzymatic process that is mediated by *NADH-methemoglobin reductase (diaphorase)*. Oxidation of heme iron to Fe^{+++} produces methemoglobin, which does not transport oxygen (see lecture 8).

3. Metabolism and function of 2,3-DPG

As noted in lecture 8, red cells have a uniquely high concentration of 2,3-DPG (approximately 5 mmoles/liter of red cells). Only traces of this metabolic intermediate are present in other cells. This compound is formed by the *Rapaport-Luebering shunt*, a pathway that branches from the main glycolytic pathway at 1,3-DPG. The fraction of glucose diverted through this pathway is not precisely known, but it is enhanced when intracellular ATP levels are elevated. For years, the function of 2,3-DPG was enigmatic since glucose metabolism through 2,3-DPG is energetically uneconomical. Glucose degradation to 2,3-DPG utilizes 2 ATPs, while further conversion of 2,3-DPG to lactate produces 2 ATPs (one for each 2,3-DPG metabolized). Since red cells do not have glycogen stores, this 2,3-DPG reserve is a potential ATP source in times of substrate deprivation. Subsequent work revealed the in-

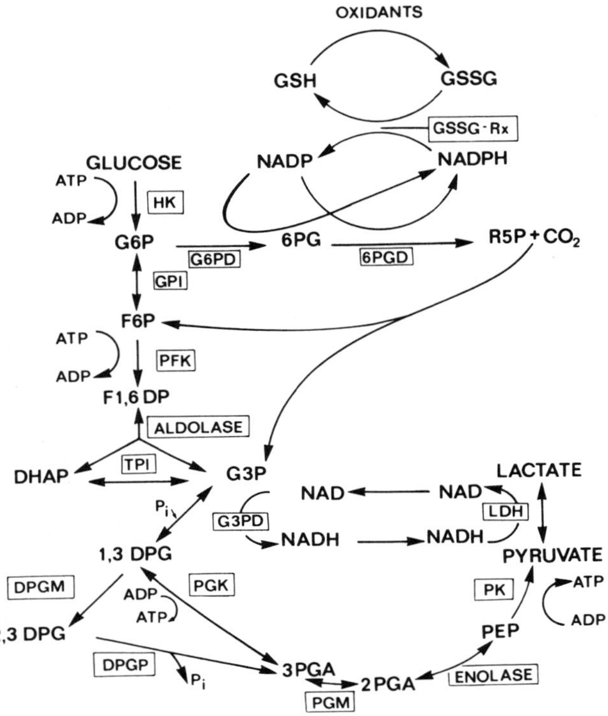

Fig. 14.1
Erythrocyte glucose metabolism. *Abbreviations of enzymes (boxed)*: HK, hexokinase; GPI, glucose-phosphate isomerase; PFK, phosphofructokinase; TPI, triose-phosphate isomerase; G3PD, glyceraldehyde-3-phosphate dehydrogenase; PGK, phosphoglycerate kinase; DPGM, diphosphoglyceromutase; DPGP, diphosphoglycerophosphatase; PGM, phosphoglyceromutase; PK; pyruvate kinase; LDH, lactic dehydrogenase; G6PD, glucose-6-phosphate dehydrogenase; 6GPD, 6-phosphogluconate dehydrogenase; GSSG-Rx, glutathione reductase. *Abbreviations of substrates*: G6P, glucose 6-phosphate; F6P, fructose 6-phosphate; F1,6DP, fructose-1,6-diphosphate; DHAP, dihydroxyacetone phosphate; G3P, glyceraldehyde-3-phosphate; 1,3DPG, 1,3-diphosphoglyceric acid; 2,3DPG, 2,3-diphosphoglyceric acid; 3PGA, 3-phosphoglyceric acid; 2PGA, 2-phosphoglyceric acid; PEP, phosphoenolpyruvate; 6PG, 6-phosphogluconate; R5P, ribulose-5-phosphate; GSH, reduced glutathione; GSSG, oxidized glutathione. Cofactors are given standard abbreviations: NAD, NADP, NADH, NADPH, and Pi (inorganic phosphate).

traerythrocytic role of 2,3-DPG as a *modulator of oxygen transport* by hemoglobin.

B. HMP shunt

Approximately 5–10% of utilized glucose is normally metabolized through the HMP shunt.

1. Production of NADPH

The HMP shunt is the *major source of NADPH* in human red cells (2 moles of NADPH being produced for each mole of glucose metabolized). Under conditions in which NADPH oxidation is accelerated, glucose metabolism through the shunt is enhanced. The most important reactions associated with NADPH oxidation are those related to glutathione metabolism.

2. Glutathione

Red cells contain relatively high concentrations (2 mM) of reduced glutathione (GSH), a tripeptide (γ-glutamylcysteinylglycine) that is synthesized de novo by mature red cells. Its $T_{1/2}$ is 4 days. GSH is an intracellular buffer that protects red cells against injury by exogenous and endogenous oxidants. Oxidants such as superoxide anion (O_2^-) and hydrogen peroxide (H_2O_2) are produced by macrophages in association with infection and by red cells in the presence of certain drugs (see lecture 18). Injury to cell proteins occurs if these agents accumulate. Normally, this is prevented by *GSH*, which inactivates such oxidants. This detoxification can occur spontaneously, but it is enhanced by *glutathione peroxidase*. Catalase also degrades peroxides, but under physiologic conditions it is less important. In the process of reducing hydrogen peroxide, GSH is itself converted to oxidized glutathione (GSSG) and mixed disulfides with protein-thiols (GS-S-protein).

3. Relation between HMP shunt and glutathione metabolism

GSH levels must be maintained in order to maintain protection against oxidant injury. This is accomplished by *glutathione reductase*, which catalyzes the NADPH-mediated reduction of GSSG and mixed disulfides to GSH. Oxidation of NADPH stimulates HMP shunt activity, which regenerates NADPH. Thus, it is the tight coupling of HMP shunt and glutathione metabolism that normally protects red cells from oxidant injury.

II. HEMOLYSIS DUE TO DEFECTS IN HMP SHUNT OR GLUTATHIONE METABOLISM

A. Introduction

HMP shunt defects are common, but glycolytic pathway defects are relatively rare. Almost all shunt defects are due to *glucose-6-phosphate dehydrogenase* (G-6-PD) deficiency. This is the most common enzyme abnormality associated with hemolytic anemia and one of the most common disorders in humans. It affects millions of people throughout the world. In contrast, *pyruvate kinase* (*PK*) deficiency, the most common glycolytic abnormality, affects only hundreds or a few thousands of patients.

B. G-6-PD deficiency

1. Pathophysiology

Defects in the HMP shunt or glutathione metabolic pathways impair the ability of red cells to defend themselves against oxidative assault. The probable pathophysiologic sequence is shown in figure 14.2. Oxidants produced by infections or oxidant drugs are normally detoxified by GSH; but GSH levels are not maintained in G-6-PD deficiency because of the diminished ability to generate NADPH. As a consequence, the oxidants are free to damage vital cellular constituents. Oxidation of hemoglobin leads to the formation of functionless *methemoglobin* and intracellular precipitation of damaged hemoglobin as *Heinz bodies*. Heinz bodies are not visible in ordinary Wright's stained blood smears but are demonstrable with supravital stains such as *methyl violet*. Heinz bodies attach to the red cell membrane by unknown mechanisms. In vitro, this causes increased membrane leakiness to cations, increased osmotic fragility, and decreased deformability. In vivo, Heinz bodies are "pitted" from circulating red cells by the spleen (see lecture 2) and thus are more plentiful in splenectomized patients. "Bite cells," that is, hyperchromic red cells with a localized invagination, presumably at the site of Heinz body removal, appear in the circulation during acute hemolytic episodes. Red cells with a submembraneous hemoglobin-free area (blister cells) may also be seen. Small numbers of spherocytes are also observed. They are thought to arise from repetitive loss of

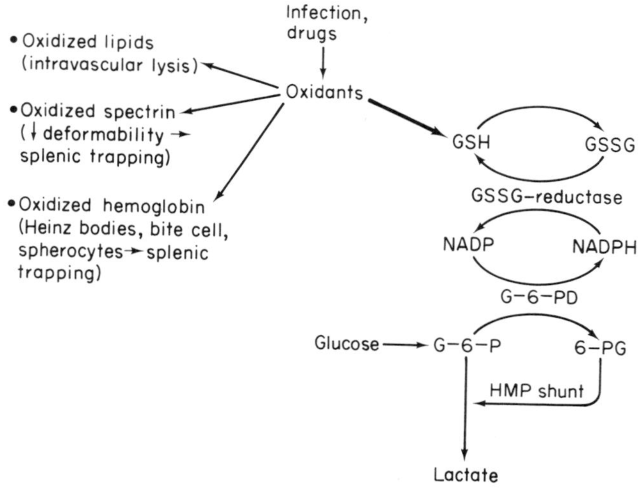

Fig. 14.2
Pathophysiology of hemolysis associated with G-6-PD deficiency.

small amounts of membrane surface during the pitting of Heinz bodies. Membrane damage occurs due to oxidative cross-linking of spectrin and lipid peroxidation. The damage inflicted on hemoglobin and the membrane skeleton leads to diminished red cell deformability and splenic trapping. Lipid damage probably produces direct intravascular hemolysis.

2. G-6-PD variants

Over 150 G-6-PD variants are now known. Fortunately (for physicians and students), only a few of these are clinically important. The normal enzyme is termed *G-6-PD*^{B} or *Gd*^{B}. It is present in about 70% of American blacks and in more than 99% of whites. *Gd*$^{A+}$ is a normal variant that is present in about 20% of American blacks. Its electrophoretic mobility is greater than Gd^{B}'s due to substitution of an asparagine for aspartic acid in the amino acid sequence. *Gd*$^{A-}$, the most common variant associated with hemolysis, is found in about 10% of American blacks and in many African black populations. Its electrophoretic mobility is identical to Gd^{A+}'s, but its catalytic activity is decreased. *Gd*^{Med} is the second most common abnormal variant. It is found in peoples of the Mediterranean area (Italians, Greeks, Sardinians, Sephardic Jews, Arabs, etc.), in India, and in SE Asia. Its electrophoretic mobility is normal, but its catalytic activity is markedly reduced. *Gd*^{Canton} is a relatively common variant in Oriental populations that produces a clinical syndrome similar to that associated with Gd^{A-}.

3. Relation between abnormal enzyme and hemolysis

As normal red cells age in vivo, the activity of intracellular Gd^{B} decays slowly with a $T_{1/2}$ of about 60 days (figure 14.3). Despite this loss of active enzyme, older red cells retain enough activity to produce NADPH and maintain glutathione as GSH in the face of oxidant stress.

The defect in Gd^{A-} results in a *labile enzyme* that disappears

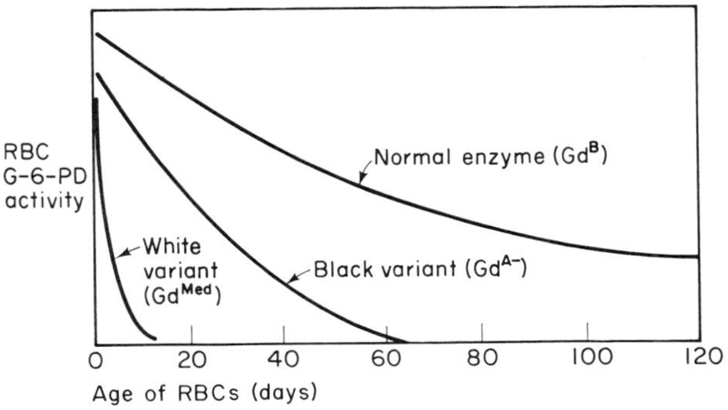

Fig. 14.3
Intracellular decay of red cell G-6-PD as a function of cell age. G-6-PD normally decays as red cells age. The top curve shows the decay rate for Gd^{B}, the normal enzyme. The middle and lower curves show the greater than normal decay rates for Gd^{A-} and Gd^{Med} variants.

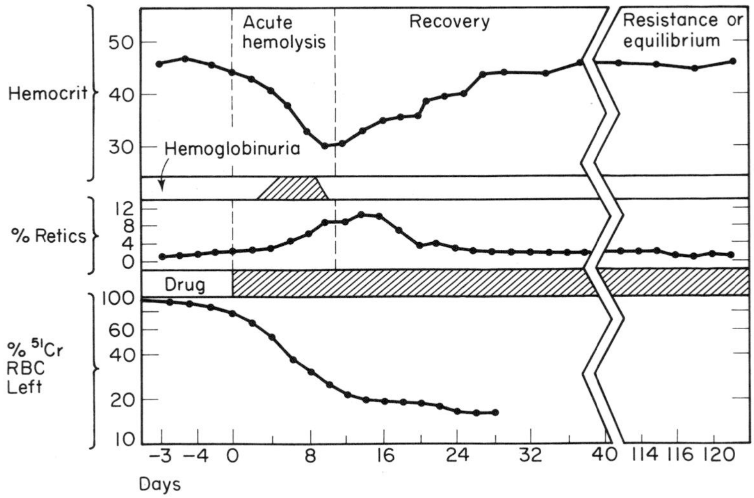

Fig. 14.4
Course of drug-induced hemolysis in an individual with Gd^{A-}. Note that hemolysis abates, and apparent resistance to the drug develops after the initial hemolytic episode due to repopulation with young red cells. (From A. S. Alving et al. *Bull. World Health Organ.* 22(1960): 621)

with a $T_{1/2}$ of about 13 days. *Young red cells* thus have *normal* enzyme activity, while *older red cells* are grossly *deficient*. A consequence of this heterogeneity is that hemolysis is self-limited in individuals with Gd^{A-}. This is shown graphically in figure 14.4, which depicts the course of primaquine-induced hemolysis in individuals with Gd^{A-}.

Acute hemolysis with hemoglobinuria and decreased ^{51}Cr red cell survival develops when the drug is first administered, but this is followed by a recovery phase in which anemia and reticulocytosis abate and red cell survival improves despite continued administration of the drug. The explanation is that once the oxidant-sensitive older red cells are destroyed, the remaining young cells are oxidant resistant. Since only about 50% of the cells are oxidant sensitive in Gd^{A-}, the bone marrow can compensate by simply doubling its output. This apparent drug resistance persists as long as the drug is continuously administered. Note, however, that if the drug is stopped for 2–3 months, older red cells will survive and accumulate and the patient will again become drug sensitive.

Gd^{Med} is considerably more unstable than Gd^{A-} (figure 14.3). Very little activity is present in mature red cells. Despite this, chronic hemolysis does not occur, which must indicate that endogenous oxidant stress is normally very low. When threatened by oxidant drugs or infections, however, these patients are at much greater risk because virtually their entire red cell population can be destroyed.

4. Clinical features

The clinical features of Gd^{A-} and Gd^{Med} are compared in table 14.1. The most dramatic clinical presentation is acute intravascular hemolysis. These patients typically develop hemoglobinemia (pink to brown plasma), hemoglobinuria (dark or even black urine), and jaundice acutely with an infection or within 1–3 days of exposure to the offending drug. In severe cases, abdominal or back pain may be prominent. Symptoms of acute anemia (dizziness, palpitations, dyspnea) may also develop. Heinz bodies appear in the red cells, and some bite cells, blister cells, and/or spherocytes may be seen on the blood smear. In many cases, however, red cell morphology is relatively normal. More often, hemolysis is less dramatic, and a modest decline of hemoglobin (3 or 4 mg/dl) occurs without hemoglobinuria or prominent symptoms. These episodes are easily overlooked unless the physician is alert.

The discovery of G-6-PD deficiency followed the observation that black soldiers developed hemolysis after receiving primaquine for malaria. Subsequently, numerous other oxidant drugs have been implicated as causative agents (table 14.2). The most common cause of hemolysis, however, is *infection*. Virtually every type of infection has been implicated. The source of the oxidant stress in infections is unknown.

a. Favism

Severe hemolytic episodes occasionally follow exposure to *fava beans* or their pollen. This rare phenomenon occurs mainly in individuals with Gd^{Med}; it is not seen in Gd^{A-}. Not all patients with Gd^{Med} are susceptible; hence other factors must be involved. So far, however, these have not been identified.

b. Chronic nonspherocytic hemolytic anemia (CNSHA)

In some patients with rare variants of G-6-PD, chronic hemolysis occurs in the absence of obvious oxidants. These cases are characterized by an enzyme that is unable to maintain basal NADPH production. Variants generally have either a high K_m for NADP or a low K_i for NADPH. Consequently, enzyme activity measured under ideal conditions in vitro (high [NADP], low [NADPH]) may be nearly normal, while the activity of the enzyme under physio-

Table 4.1
Clinical Comparison of the Two Common Forms of G-6-PD Deficiency

	Gd^{A-}	Gd^{Med}
Frequency	Common in black populations	Common in Mediterranean populations
Degree of hemolysis	Moderate	Severe
G-6-PD defect	Old red cells	All red cells
Hemolysis with:		
Drugs	Unusual	Common
Infection	Common	Common
Need for transfusions	No	Sometimes
Chronic hemolysis	No	No

Table 14.2
Drugs Commonly Leading to Hemolysis in G-6-PD Deficiency

Antimalarials	**Analgesics**
Primaquine	Acetanilid
Quinacrine (Atabrine®)	Acetylsalicylic acid[a]
	Acetophenetidin (Phenacetin®)[a]
Sulfonamides	**Sulfones**
Sulfanilamide	Diaminodiphenyl sulfone (Dapsone®)
Salicylazosulfapyridine (Azulfidine®)	
Sulfisoxazole (Gantrisin®)[a]	
Other Antibacterials	**Miscellaneous**
Nitrofurantoin (Furadantin®)	Dimercaprol (BAL)
Nitrofurazone (Furacin®)	Napthalene (moth balls)
Chloramphenicol[a]	Methylene blue[a]
Para-aminosalicylic acid	Vitamin K (water-soluble analogues)[a]
Nalidixic acid	Ascorbic acid[a]

Note: A more comprehensive list of drugs that have been implicated in oxidant-induced hemolysis appears in E. Beutler, *Pharmacol. Rev.* 21(1969): 73.
a. Hemolysis is infrequent and generally requires high concentrations of the drug. Probably a risk in Gd^{Med} but not in Gd^{A-} or Gd^{Canton}.

logical conditions in vivo (low [NADP], high [NADPH]) may be markedly depressed.

5. Genetics

The gene for G-6-PD is located on the X-chromosome. Thus, inheritance of G-6-PD is sex linked. Males have one type of G-6-PD; females can have two types. For example, 70% of black males have Gd^B, 20% have Gd^{A+}, and 10% have Gd^{A-}. Black females, however, can be heterozygous for any two of these enzymes. According to the *Lyon hypothesis* (the validity of which is strongly supported by data of G-6-PD genetics), only one X-chromosome is active in any somatic cell; thus, individual red cells of females contain only one G-6-PD type. In view of the Lyon hypothesis, any given red cell in heterozygous-deficient females is either normal or deficient. The implication that these women have a double population is confirmed by cytochemical red cell stains. (This phenomenon has permitted useful studies of the cellular origin of tumors. Isolation of enzyme from tumor cells in women heterozygous for Gd^B and Gd^A has demonstrated that tumors may be of either unicentric or multicentric origin.)

Mean enzyme activity in females who carry a gene for G-6-PD deficiency may be normal, moderately reduced (usual), or grossly deficient, depending on the degree of "Lyonization." Deficient cells in females are just as susceptible to oxidant injury as enzyme-deficient cells in males. The overall magnitude of hemolysis, however, is less because of the smaller population of vulnerable cells.

Despite the disadvantage of a gene for G-6-PD deficiency, it remains common in many geographic areas. Its prevalence has been attributed to a selective advantage it is believed to provide against malaria caused by *Plasmodium falciparum*. This proposal is supported, though not proved, by epidemiologic studies and by observations in heterozygous females demonstrating the resistance of cells containing deficient enzyme to malarial involvement. However, the prevalence of Gd^{A+} in blacks is unexplained in terms of genetic polymorphism.

6. Diagnosis

Several tests for the diagnosis of G-6-PD deficiency are currently available. Their sensitivity is variable and their usefulness is determined by the clinical situation (sex of patient, ethnic background, and proximity to hemolytic episode).

Commonly used *screening tests* are based on NADPH-mediated dye decolorization or the reduction of methemoglobin in the presence of methylene blue. This test is of limited sensitivity since 30–40% of the cells must be abnormal if deficiency is to be detected.

Definitive assay of the enzyme depends on direct spectrophotometric measurement of NADPH production. This test is more sensitive than the screening test but still requires 20–30% deficient cells for an abnormal result. The sensitivity can be enhanced by comparing the level of G-6-PD to other age-dependent enzymes. With this modification, diagnosis of G-6-PD can be made even after a hemolytic episode.

The cyanide-ascorbate test measures the ability of red cells to prevent ascorbate-induced oxidation of hemoglobin. One of the unique aspects of this test is that intact red cells are used instead of hemolysate. Thus each red cell serves as its own cuvette. As a consequence, as few as 10–15% enzyme-deficient cells can be detected. This sensitivity makes the test useful in the diagnosis of G-6-PD deficiency in female heterozygotes and in males following a hemolytic episode. In addition, this test can detect other abnormalities of the HMP shunt or glutathione metabolism (to be discussed).

Cytochemical estimation of G-6-PD activity in individual red cells can be performed with the aid of tetrazolium dyes. This test can detect the presence of less than 5% G-6-PD-deficient cells and is particularly useful for identifying female heterozygotes.

C. Other abnormalities of GSH metabolism

Abnormalities of GSH metabolism, the first line of defense against oxidants, can also be associated with hemolysis.

1. Decreased GSH synthesis

Defects in the enzymes responsible for GSH synthesis have been reported in rare patients. Erythrocytes lacking these enzymes have very low levels of GSH. Clinically, the disorders are similar to G-6-PD deficiency—that is, a mild-to-moderate hemolytic anemia that is sensitive to oxidant drugs.

2. GSSG reductase deficiency

In early reports, deficiency of GSSG reductase had been associated with a variety of other hematologic abnormalities. It is now known that flavin adenine dinucleotide (FAD) is a cofactor of GSSG reductase. Many apparent enzyme deficiencies have been shown to be related to abnormalities of riboflavin metabolism. Actual inherited deficiencies of GSSG reductase are thought to exist, but they are rare, and no case of hemolysis due to this deficiency has ever been proved.

3. GSH peroxidase deficiency

Many individuals (including all newborn infants) are relatively deficient in this enzyme, but this deficiency does not appear to produce significant hemolysis. This may, in part, reflect the fact that nonenzymatic reduction of peroxide by GSH occurs at a significant rate.

III. HEMOLYSIS DUE TO DEFECTS IN GLYCOLYSIS

A. General features

Abnormalities in virtually every glycolytic enzyme have been described, but pyruvate kinase (PK) deficiency accounts for about 90% of all cases associated with hemolysis.

1. Genetics

Glycolytic enzymopathies display an autosomal recessive pattern of inheritance. Hemolysis is seen in the homozygous state. Heterozygotes are normal although their red cells contain less than normal levels of enzyme activity. Phosphoglycerate kinase (PGK) deficiency is an exception since this enzyme appears to be sex linked.

2. Relation between abnormal metabolism and hemolysis

Hemolysis due to glycolytic defects is purportedly due to inhibition of the vital ATP-dependent reactions that control membrane function. However, red cell ATP content is not invariably decreased because (1) the mean cell age is very young (reticulocytes have increased ATP levels); (2) defective cells with low ATP content are promptly removed from the circulation; and (3) ATP may be compartmentalized within red cells, in which case one critical locus may be sufficient to cause cell injury.

3. Clinical features

Hemolysis is chronic and is not affected by drugs. *Splenomegaly* is usually present owing to stagnation of cells in this organ. The acidic, hypoxic, and nutrient-poor environment of the spleen is an added insult to the metabolically abnormal red cells. Thus, the hemolytic rate frequently decreases following splenectomy. The blood smear often contains some *dense spiculated red cells*, particularly after splenectomy, but this is not invariable or unique to these disorders. In most cases, red cell morphology is unremarkable in unsplenectomized patients.

4. Diagnosis

A major problem in the diagnosis of glycolytic enzyme abnormalities is the fact that the most seriously affected cells are removed in vivo and thus are unavailable for analysis in vitro. Definitive diagnosis requires spectrophotometric enzyme assays performed under a variety of conditions (e.g., with varying substrate and cofactor concentrations) in order to detect enzymes with abnormal kinetics. Measurement of glycolytic intermediates may reveal subtle enzyme abnormalities since the concentration of intermediates is usually increased proximal to a defect and decreased distal to it.

B. Pyruvate kinase (PK) deficiency

Since PK catalyzes one of the major reactions responsible for ATP production in glycolysis, it is not surprising that deficiency of this enzyme causes hemolytic anemia. Hemolysis can be mild and compensated or severe enough to require frequent transfusions. The improvement of severe hemolysis following splenectomy is related to the fact that *PK-deficient reticulocytes* depend on mitochondrial oxidative phosphorylation as an ATP source. In vitro incubation of PK-deficient reticulocytes under hypoxic conditions or with inhibitors of oxidative phosphorylation causes ATP levels to fall; cells subsequently gain Ca^{++}, lose K^{+} and water, and become rigid. PK-deficient reticulocytes sequestered in the hypoxic spleen presumably undergo similar degeneration. Although anemia improves following splenectomy, reticulocytes increase to 50–70%. This *paradoxical reticulocytosis* is due to increased reticulocyte survival once the adverse metabolic environment of the spleen is removed. The distal glycolytic block in PK deficiency causes a 2–3 fold increase in red cell 2,3-DPG (to 10–15 mmoles/liter of red cells); this minimizes some adverse effects of the anemia since 2,3-DPG enhances oxygen release from hemoglobin (see lecture 8).

C. Glucose phosphate isomerase deficiency

Glucose phosphate isomerase (GPI) deficiency is the second most common glycolytic disorder that produces hemolysis. Because products of HMP shunt metabolism are recycled through GPI, defects in this enzyme lead to some oxidant sensitivity. The specific cell injury leading to hemolysis is not known.

IV. HEMOLYSIS DUE TO DEFECTS IN RED CELL NUCLEOTIDE METABOLISM

A. Pyrimidine-5′-nucleotidase deficiency

Deficiency of pyrimidine-5′-nucleotidase is the third or fourth most common enzyme deficiency leading to hemolysis. This enzyme functions to degrade pyrimidine nucleotides to cytidine and uridine, which can diffuse out of the cell. Lacking this activity, red cells accumulate partially degraded messenger and ribosomal RNA, which produces prominent *basophilic stippling* of up to 5% of the red cells on blood smears. Interestingly, the basophilic stippling of lead poisoning is apparently produced by a similar mechanism since pyrimidine-5′-nucleotidase is markedly inhibited by lead. Patients with the inherited (autosomal recessive) deficiency of this enzyme have a chronic, moderately severe hemolytic anemia. The mechanism of hemolysis is unknown. Splenomegaly is common, but splenectomy produces little discernible benefit.

SELECTED REFERENCES

Beutler, E. Abnormalities of the hexose monophosphate shunt. *Semin. Hematol.* 8(1971): 311.

Harris, J. W., and Kellermeyer, R. W. Red cell destruction and the hemolytic disorders (Chapter 9). In *The Red Cell—Production, Metabolism, Destruction: Normal and Abnormal*, rev. ed., Cambridge, MA: Harvard University Press, 1970, pp. 517–660.

Luzzatto, L., and Testa, U. Human erythrocyte glucose-6-phosphate dehydrogenase: Structure and function in normal and mutant subjects. *Curr. Topics Hematol.* 1(1978): 1.

Mentzer, W. C., Jr. Pyruvate kinase deficiency and disorder of glycolysis. In Nathan, D. G., and Oski, F. A., eds., *Hematology of Infancy and Childhood*, 3d ed., Philadelphia: W. B. Saunders, in press.

Piomelli, S., and Vera, S. G6PD deficiency and related disorders of the pentose pathway (Chapter 18). In Nathan, D. G., and Oski, F. A., eds., *Hematology of Infancy and Childhood*, 2d ed., Philadelphia: W. B. Saunders, 1981, pp. 608–642.

Valentine, W. N. Hemolytic anemia and inborn errors of metabolism. *Blood* 54(1979): 549.

LECTURE 15 Blood Groups I. Physiology

W. Hallowell Churchill, Jr.

I. INTRODUCTION

Blood group antigens and their associated antibodies are important not only in clinical medicine but also in anthropology, human genetics, and forensic science.

A. Definition

The *blood groups* are determined by antigenic structures on the surface of red cells and are detected by reactions with specific antibodies. The antigenic phenotype is under genetic control and remains relatively constant throughout life. A blood group *system* is defined by antigens that are regulated either by allelic genes or closely linked genes.

B. Known blood groups

The number of red cell blood groups now exceeds 400. Table 15.1 is a simplified listing of some of them with the dates of their discovery. Note that the rate of detection of new blood group systems greatly increased after the development of the Coombs test in 1945.

C. Antibodies: sources and properties

1. Normal humans

Antibodies to some blood group antigens occur in the serum of individuals who lack the antigen and have had no prior exposure to it. Such antibodies are referred to as *natural isohemagglutinins*. The major ones are directed against surface antigens such as the ABO, Ii, and P systems, the specificity of which is controlled by oligosaccharides. It is presumed that these antibodies are elicited by similar sequences on microbial surfaces. These antibodies are usually IgMs. They are effective hemolysins because they fix complement efficiently.

2. Immunized animals

If animals are immunized with *human red cells,* they may form antibodies to certain of the xenogeneic blood group antigens. This is an important source of blood group antisera. Initially these sera are carefully absorbed with human red cells to establish specificity. Recently developed antigen-specific *monoclonal antibodies,* which do not require such absorption, may soon replace the blood group antigens now raised in animals.

3. Immunized humans

The third major source of blood group antibodies are donors who have been allogenically immunized either by (1) prior blood transfusion or (2) previous pregnancies. Such antibodies, sometimes called *immune antibodies,* are elicited by prior exposure to red

Table 15.1
Survey of Major Red Cell Blood Group Systems

System	Important antigens[a]	Year discovered	Discoverer(s)	Antibody source[b]
ABO	A_1, A_2, *B*, *H*, A_3, A_m, A_x	1900–1902	Landsteiner	*1*
MNSs	*M*, *N*, *S*, *s*, U, M^g, Mi^a, Hu, He Mt^a, Vw, M_2, N_2, S_2	1927	Landsteiner and Levine	*2*
P	P_1, p^k, P_2, (Tj^a)	1927	Landsteiner and Levine	*2*
Rh	*D*, *C*, *E*, *c*, *e*, C^w, E^w, ce, Ce, G, CE, cE, D^u, C^u, E^u, LW	1939–1941 1940	Levine Landsteiner and Wiener	*3* *4*
Lutheran	Lu^a, Lu^b	1945	Callender and Race	*5*
Kell	*K*, *k*, Kp^a, Kp^b, Js^a, Js^b	1946	Coombs et al.	*3*
Lewis	Le^a, Le^b	1946	Mourant	*1*
Duffy	Fy^a, Fy^b, Fy3, Fy4, Fy5	1950	Cutbush and Mollison	*5*
Kidd	Jk^a, Jk^b	1951	Allen and Diamond	*3*
Wright	Wr^a, Wr^b	1953	Holman	*3*
Diego	Di^a, Di^b	1955	Layrisse et al.	*3*
Cartwright	Yt^a, Yt^b	1956	Eaton et al.	*5*
Xg	Xg^a	1962	Sanger et al.	*5*
Dombrock	Do^a, Do^b	1965	Swanson et al.	*5*
Colton	Co^a, Co^b	1967	Heisto et al.	*5*

a. The most important antigens in each system are in italics.
b. Numbers refer to source of original antibody, as follows: *1,* naturally occurring isohemagglutinin of normal human serum; *2,* serum from rabbits immunized with human red cells; *3,* serum from mother of baby with erythroblastosis fetalis; *4,* serum from rabbits immunized with rhesus monkey red cells; *5,* serum from subjects given transfusion with incompatible blood.

cell antigens and are commonly IgGs. It is often difficult to provoke an immune response in animals to the particular antigens for which an antibody is desired. Hence antibody is still being harvested from allogeneically immunized humans.

The prevalence in Caucasians of immune red cell antibodies other than the most common one, anti-D, is shown in table 15.2. Together with anti-D, the antibodies shown in table 15.2 are those most likely to cause clinical problems for the transfusionist. The prevalence of these antibodies provides a measure of antigenic potency that is based on comparisons of the frequency of a particular antibody and the calculated frequency of possible immunizations (i.e., the chance of a positive donor as encountering a negative recipient). Thus, for Kell, the probability of an immunizing combination is 3.5 times less than with Duffy (Fy^a), but anti-Kell is 2.5 times more common than anti-Fy^a. Therefore Kell must be 9 times more potent than Fy^a. Similar calculations can be used to rank the other important blood group antigens. However, as yet there is no good structural explanation for the relative antigenic potencies observed. Fortunately many blood group antigens have no opportunity to establish their antigenic potency because

Table 15.2
Prevalence of Immune Red Cell Antibodies Other Than D (or CD or DE)

Antibody	%
E	32.7
K (or k)	28.7
c	19.2
Fy^a or Fy^b	11.2
Jk^a or Jk^b	4.3
Ce	2.5
C (or Ce)	0.7
S (or s)	0.2
Others	0.5

their incidence is so high that the probability of an immunizing event is very low.

D. Methods of detection

1. Agglutination by specific antibody

Under physiologic conditions of pH and ionic strength, normal red cells repel each other owing to their negative surface charge, or *zeta potential.* The charge, which is largely attributable to sialyl residues, serves to keep the cells in suspension with a minimum intercellular distance of about 250Å. Reaction of red cells with antibody causes visible agglutination if the antibody is capable of bridging the distance between adjacent cells. Such antibodies (usually IgM) are termed *complete* or *saline* antibodies or agglutinins. The presence of such antibodies is detected by agglutinations, which are readily observable on glass slides or in small test tubes.

2. Enhancement of agglutination by antibody

a. Reduction of zeta potential

In many cases weak agglutination must be enhanced to be detected. Antibodies that fail to produce agglutination with red cells in saline have been called *incomplete* antibodies. This is a misnomer because lack of agglutination is due to the number of antibodies on the cell surface and to the immunoglobulin class (usually IgG) and not to the fact that the antibodies are incomplete in some sense. In such a situation several techniques are available for enhancing the aggregation by reducing the zeta potential and thus shortening the intercellular distances. Zeta potential can be reduced by the addition of colloid (albumin, polyvinylpyrrolidone, or dextran) to the suspending medium or by removal of the negative charge from the red cell surface by treating cells with neuraminidase or proteolytic enzymes such as papain or ficin. Use of enzyme-treated cells may enhance weak reactions and facilitate identification of antibodies that might otherwise be missed.

b. Insertion of antibody red cell bridges

Agglutination may be produced or enhanced by the addition of Coombs reagent (i.e., antiglobulin antibody) to a suspension of washed red cell antigens. As described in lecture 12, Coombs reagent may have specificity for IgG or complement (usually $C3_b$ and $C3_d$) or any of its components. Coombs reagents do not have specificity against IgM or IgA and hence will not detect antibody of these classes on red cell surfaces.

3. Use of lectins

Antibody-like substances with specificity for red cell surface carbohydrates can be extracted from a variety of plant seeds of mollusks. These reagents are useful in identifying such blood group antigens as A, B, H, M, and N. Two pounds of lima beans could provide enough anti-A lectin for all the blood grouping of an entire year in the United States.

4. Automated techniques

Solid phase antibody immobilization techniques, automated blood grouping, and cross-matching are now being developed. The advantages of these techniques are their sensitivity, objectivity, and speed. At this time, however, blood banking in contrast to chemistry is still lacking in automated techniques.

E. Genetics

Inheritance of blood group antigens is according to Mendelian laws. Heredity is generally autosomal codominant, i.e., there is an expression of both alleles in the heterozygous individual. A notable exception to the usual mode of inheritance is the case of Xg^a, which is X linked. Some systems, notably ABO, Rh, and MNSs, encompass more than two alleles. Most systems, however, involve two common alleles; remaining alleles are usually rare.

1. Linked genes

Owing to the normal crossing over of homologous chromosomes at meiosis, most of the genetic loci—even those on the same chromosome—show independent inheritance. If two loci are near each other, however, crossing over is diminished, and the genes appear to be inherited together through successive generations, or linked. The Rh and MNSs complexes, for example, constitute groups of closely linked loci.

2. Interaction with other genes

The expression of some blood groups depends on the interaction of genes at several different loci. For example, in the Lewis system, expression of Le^b depends on the interaction of the Hh gene and the Se/se system. H is required to produce the substrate for Le^b, and the Se gene is required to make this substrate available. Thus the genotype Le^b cannot be expressed if an individual lacks either the H gene or the Se gene.

3. Loci of blood group genes on chromosomes

Loci of some blood group genes are known. These are summarized in table 15.3. In some cases blood group loci are linked with genetic diseases. For example, the rare nail-patella syndrome is linked to the ABO locus; hereditary elliptocytosis is linked to the Rh locus.

4. Occurrence of blood group antigens

A and B antigens are ubiquitous and are found in animal tissues, plants, and bacteria. Rh antigens are present only on the red cells of primates. In any individual, A, B, H, Le^a, Le^b, P, and I may be present in many tissues, whereas other blood group antigens are probably limited to the red cells (and, in the case of MN, Kell and Diego, to the neutrophils as well).

II. ABO SYSTEM

A. Historical notes

The ABO system, clinically the most important, was the first blood group discovered. In 1900 Landsteiner obtained blood from six colleagues. On mixing serum from one individual with washed red cells from another in all possible combinations, he noted agglutination with some combinations but not with others. He was thus able to classify individuals on the basis of antigens on their red cells and agglutinins in their serum. In subsequent work Landsteiner recognized that the pattern of reactions could be explained by two antigens, which he designated A and B. He also noted a reciprocal relation between the presence of antigen and agglutinin. The Landsteiner scheme is summarized in table 15.4.

Table 15.3
Chromosome Assignments of Blood Group Loci

Locus	Chromosome
ABO	9
Rh	1
Fy	1
Chido, Rogers	6
MNSs	4
Xg	X
Sc	1

Table 15.4
The ABO System Defined by Anti-A and Anti-B

Blood groups	Antigens on red cells	Antibodies in serum
O	None	Anti-A and anti-B
A	A	Anti-B
B	B	Anti-A
AB	A and B	None

B. Subdivisions of A antigen

A antigen and anti-A are complex. Anti-A serum from a group B donor contains two types of antibodies, anti-A and anti-A_1 (see table 15.5). If certain A or AB cells (A_2 or A_2B) are used to absorb such antiserum, reactivity with A_2 or A_2B cells is lost, but the antiserum continues to react with certain other A or AB cells (A_1 or A_1B). On the other hand anti-A absorbed with A_1 or A_1B cells removes all reactivity. Thus all A cells have a common A antigen, but A_1 or A_1B cells have an additional antigen (A_1).

Of all group A bloods 80% are A_1 and 20% are A_2. An A_2 individual may become immunized against A_1, but such antibodies are clinically significant only if they react at 37°C. When a clinically significant anti-A_1 antibody is present, the patient must be transfused with O cells. Other rare subgroups of A and B exist. In general they have less of the antigen on the cell surface, and in some cases there may be qualitative differences. Their main importance is that they can be mistyped as Group O.

C. Genetics

1. Phenotypes and genotypes

A child receives one of four genes from each parent: A_1, A_2, B_1, or O. Six phenotypes are possible because expression of A_2 is masked by A_1; however, there are ten genotypes: Group A_1 individuals may be one of three genotypes: A_1A_1, A_1O, A_1A_2. In Group B individuals, the genotypes correspond to the phenotypes.

2. Determination of genotypes

To determine which of several genotypes is responsible for an ambiguous phenotype, appropriate studies must be performed on members of a family. Figure 15.1 illustrates such studies in two families in which ambiguous ABO phenotypes are resolved by studies of family members.

D. H antigens

As shown below, the H antigen is the precursor of the A and the B antigen. It is converted to A by the addition of N-acetylgalactosamine (GalNac) and to B antigen by the addition of D-galactose (Gal). It follows that O cells, in which conversion to A or B has not occurred, will have the most H antigen. Conversely cells with the largest number of converted sites (A_1 cells) will have the least amount of H antigen. Thus antibodies with H specificity are less likely to react with A and B cells than they are to react with O cells.

Table 15.5
Subdivisions of A Antigen and Anti-A Serum

		Reactions with	
Group	Antigens	Anti-A	Anti-A_1
A_1	AA_1	+	+
A_2	A	+	−

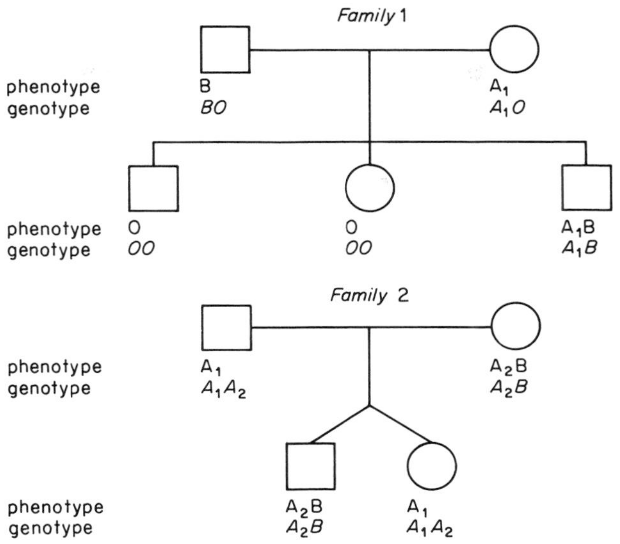

Fig. 15.1
Illustration of the usefulness of family studies in the elucidation of phenotypes. *Family 1* (upper diagram), ambiguous phenotypes of father and mother (B and A_1) are shown to be associated with genotypes BO and A_1O by demonstration of two type O children. *Family 2* (lower diagram), ambiguous phenotypes of father and daughter (A_1) are shown to be associated with genotypes A_1A_2 by demonstration of phenotypes A_2B in mother and twin son. (From R. R. Race and R. Sanger, *Blood Groups in Man*, 6th ed., Oxford: Blackwell, 1975)

In the rare variant called *Bombay*, the H precursor cannot be converted to H antigen. These cells lack H antigen, and hence A or B phenotype cannot be expressed, even if the suitable genotype is present. Despite the lack of A, B, and H groups, these cells survive normally. However, patients with Bombay blood invariably have anti-H and thus can be transfused only with Bombay bloods.

E. Chemistry of antigens

1. Effect of branching in surface carbohydrates

The chemistry of ABOH antigens—and of other blood groups in which specificity is controlled by surface carbohydrates (Lewis, Ii, and P antigens)—was elucidated in studies of soluble blood group substances and, more recently, of red cell glycosphingolipids. There are at least four families of H antigens; they differ in chain length and in complexity of branching of the surface carbohydrates (see figure 15.2). The linear configurations (H_1, H_2) are present on fetal and neonatal cells. After age 2, red cells acquire the adult phenotype, which is much more branched. Differences

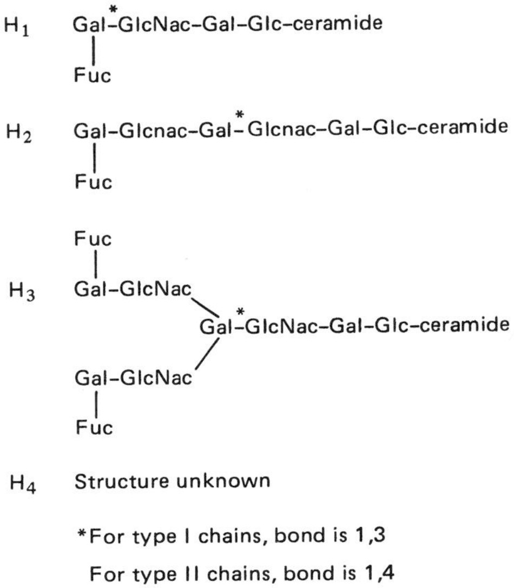

Fig. 15.2
Proposed structure of H antigens. Diagrams show nonreducing ends of the carbohydrates of four H antigens. Abbreviations: GlcNac, N-acetylglucosamine; Gal, D-galactose; Fuc, L-fucose; Glc, D-glucose. Note: asterisk (here and in text) denotes 1,3 bond.

in the distribution of straight and branched chains may explain qualitative differences between A_1 and A_2 cells, the latter having more branched H chains.

The H chain exists as two types. Type II, with a 1,4 bond between the terminal Gal (galactose) and GlcNac (N-acetylglucosamine), is found exclusively on the surface of cells. Type I, with a 1,3 bond between the terminal Gal and GlcNac, is found in the soluble blood group substances but not on the cell surfaces.

The immediate precursor of the H chain lacks the terminal Fuc (fucose). Bombay blood lacks the *glycosyl transferase* needed to convert the H precursor in the H antigen by the addition of Fuc).

2. Role of gene products in determining specificity

Although specificity of these antigens is controlled by the surface carbohydrate oligosaccharide, the gene product in each case is a glycosyl transferase that adds appropriate sugars to the carbohydrate chain. Thus assay of specific glycosyl transferases can establish genotype. In Group O it had been thought that gene product is not expressed; however, recent evidence suggests that a protein antigenically similar to the glycosyl transferase in A and B genotype is present but without function. Rather than lacking a gene, Group O individuals may have an abnormal nonfunctional glycosyl transferase.

III. OTHER CARBOHYDRATE ANTIGENS

A. Lewis system

Lewis antigens derive from the same precursor as the ABOH antigen; however, Lewis antigens are made from Type I precursor oliogosaccharides (Gal*GlcNac–Gal–Glc* with 1,3 bonds from the terminal Gal to GlcNac). Site of synthesis is unknown. Soluble plasma antigens are absorbed after synthesis onto red cell surfaces. These antigens develop in the postnatal period so that the final phenotype is not apparent in the first 2 years. In Caucasians about 72% are Le^{a-b+}, 22% are Le^{a+b-}, and 6% are Le^{a-b-}. In black populations as many as 40% are the double-negative phenotype.

Expression of these antigens depends on the interaction of the H gene, the Se gene, and the Le gene. Individuals with the Le gene make an antigen called Le^a, which resembles H substance, differing only in the position of its Fuc. If an individual lacks the secretor (Se) gene, Le^a is found in body fluids and absorbed onto red cells. If Se is present, H substance is also present in body fluids, and it is converted to Le^b by the adition of a second Fuc, so that all Le^a is converted to Le^b. These individuals characteristically have the phenotype Le^{a-b+}. The following combinations are possible:

Le gene	Se gene	Phenotype
+	+	Le^{a-b+}
+	–	Le^{a+b-}
–	+ or –	Le^{a-b-}

B. P system

These antigens were recognized by antisera developed in rabbits. They are glycosphingolipids and originate on a ceramide dihexose (Gal–Gal–ceramide). In the rare individual unable to add sugars beyond the initial two, a p antigen is said to be present. Addition of another Gal yields an antigen called p^k. Subsequent addition of GlcNac converts p^k to P antigen, which is the antigen against which Donath-Landsteiner antibody is directed (see lecture 12). P_1 antigen is synthesized by a different route in which the type II H-chain precursor is converted to P_1 by addition of Gal. The most common antibody against these antigens is anti-P_1. It is naturally occurring and causes hemolytic reactions only if it is reactive at 37°C. On the other hand individuals with a p or p^k phenotype have antibodies against determinants of most red cells; hence, they are difficult to transfuse.

C. Ii system

Most cold antibodies have specificity against the Ii antigen system (see table 12.3). These antigens are found in red cells and nonhematopoietic tissues. Fetal and red cells and their precursors have i. Red cells do not fully develop I until age 2. The transition from i to I is mediated by an enzyme under the control of a separate gene, tentatively called Z, the absence of which causes persistence of i. Z is responsible for converting straight-chain i sequences to a more complex branched-chain I sequence. Both I and i are made up of either branched- or straight-chain sequences of galactose N-acetylglucosamine (Gal–GlcNac) in recurring sequences. I and i cannot be considered alleles because the transition from i to I is accomplished by the action of a separate enzyme.

Most sera have low titers of clinically insignificant anti-I antibodies. Significant hemolysis is usually due to anti-I antibodies of high titer and wide amplitude. Rarely, anti-i antibodies cause hemolysis. The hemolysis in infectious mononucleosis is an example.

IV. THE SIALOGLYCOPROTEINS: MNSs AND U ANTIGENS

A. Clinical features

These three antigen pairs are controlled by three separate, closely linked genes. M and N antibodies are usually naturally occurring and rarely clinically significant. Unlike most other naturally occurring antibodies, anti-M is usually IgG rather than IgM. Dialysis patients may acquire an anti-N if exposed to dialysis equipment sterilized with formaldehyde. M and S tend to segregate together, as do N and S. U antigen is always present except in S-s- individuals, in whom U is absent about three-quarters of the time. These individuals may acquire an anti-U antibody that can cause transfusion reactions and hemolytic disease of the newborn.

B. Antigen structure and genetics

After SDS polyacylamide gel, electropheresis, staining with PAS stain reveals four sialoglycoproteins, which are called α, β, γ, δ sialoglycoproteins (SGPs). α SGP, also termed glycophorin A, is associated with MN activity, and β SGP, or glycophorin B, is associated with Ss and U activity.

Glycophorin A has been purified and fully sequenced. The mol. wt. is 31,00. About 70 amino acids extend beyond the membrane; 20 are in the lipid bilayer and 40 are in the cell cytoplasm. The N-terminal portion is glycosylated with a tetrasaccharide whose structure is NANA–Gal–GalNac–Ser/Thr, where NA denotes

$$\begin{array}{c}\text{NANA–Gal–GalNac–Ser/Thr}\\ \qquad\;\;|\\ \qquad\;\;\text{NANA}\end{array}$$

neuraminic or sialic acid. These are identical for both M and N; however, amino acid sequencing shows that M activity correlates with serine in position 1 and glycine in position 5. Thus MN antigens are probably the result of differences in interaction of the oligosaccharides with polypeptides that display the genetically controlled differences. Similar studies have associated glycophorin B with Ss and U activity. The genes controlling these antigens are autosomal.

C. Contribution of oligosaccharide on sialoglycoproteins to polyagglutination: T, T^k, and Tn antigens

Removal of terminal sialic acids (NAs) of the major oligosaccharide exposes Gal-GalNac. This disaccharide reacts with most adult sera because of a naturally occurring antibody called anti-T. Hence these cells are called *polyagglutinable*. The most common cause of so-called *T activation* is exposure in vivo or in vitro to bacterial neuraminidase. *T^k activation* occurs when a similar process exposes GlcNac, presumably by the action of another bacterial product, β-endogalactosidase, on ABH and I oligosaccharides. *Tn activation* results from exposure of GalNac through lack of the two terminal sugars. This persistent defect is due to a stem cell mutation. Tn activation has been observed in patients with acute myelocytic leukemia.

V. RH SYSTEM

A. Historical notes

In 1939 Levine and Stetson described an antibody in the serum of a mother of a stillborn fetus and noted that this antibody reacted with the red cells of her husband and about 80% of ABO-compatible donors. Independently Landsteiner and Weiner reported in 1940 that antisera prepared in rabbits against the blood of the rhesus monkey reacted with the red cells of about 85% of Caucasian New Yorkers.

Although initially thought to have the same specificity, which was termed Rh (for rhesus), these antisera were later shown to differ. The rabbit antisera detect a specificity LW that can be separated from the Rh specificity. The complexity of the Rh antigen system was soon demonstrated by the identification of many other related specificities in this system.

B. Nomenclature: relation to genetic models

1. Fisher-Race theory

The nomenclature is confused because two parallel systems are used interchangeably. The Fisher-Race system postulates three closely linked genes designated Cc, Dd, and Ee. In this system the Rh antigen is renamed D; the allele for d has never been identified. However, antisera have been developed against the C, c,

E, and e. The term *Rh positive* refers only to the presence of the D antigen, also called Rh or Rh factor. *Rh negative* denotes absence of D but does not denote absence of other antigens of the Rh system (C, c, E, or e). Studies of families have shown that all possible combinations of these phenotypes can be identified, but some are more common than others (table 15.6). Products of the three closely linked genes segregate together.

2. Weiner system

The Weiner system assumes that there is one gene with multiple specificities and that each of the three-letter complexes in the Fisher-Race system is the product of a single gene symbolized by a single letter and superscript (table 15.6).

In converting from Weiner to Fisher-Race nomenclature, R signifies presence of D and r absence of D, which is symbolized d. Superscript 1 or prime (′) implies presence of C and e; superscript 2 or double prime (″) implies presence of c and E. Thus, R^1 = CDe; R^2 = cDE; r′ = Cde; r″ = cdE, r = cde, etc. Other rules are given in textbooks.

3. Rosenfield system

This system avoids commitment to a specific genetic theory and identifies antigens by number—for example, D = Rh 1, C = Rh 2, E = Rh 3, c = Rh 4, and e = Rh 5.

Each of these systems has some advantages. The Weiner system is convenient shorthand for gene complexes that in the Fisher-Race system would require 3 letters to specify; the Rosenfield system lends itself to computerization.

Recent data on the chemical structure of the Rh antigen suggest that the Weiner model is probably correct. A single protein has been purified to homogeneity that has the appropriate specificities for the gene complex of whole cells and includes the D, C, and E antigens.

Table 15.6
Frequencies of Rh Gene Complexes in England

Gene complex		
Fisher-Race nomenclature	Wiener nomenclature	Frequency
CDe	R^1	0.4076
cde	r	0.3886
cDE	R^2	0.1411
cDe	R^0	0.0257
C^wDe	R^{1w}	0.0129
cdE	r^u	0.0119
Cde	r^1	0.0098
CDE	R^z	0.0024

Source: R. R. Race and R. Sanger, *Blood Groups in Man*, 6th ed., Oxford: Blackwell, 1975.

C. Compound antigens

Some isoantibodies have specificity for what appears to be a combination of two known antigens, such as c and e. Such *compound antigens* can be recognized only if the genes are part of the same haplotype. The main use of these antisera is in genetic studies.

D. Weakened antigens

Some individuals have a weakly reactive D antigen, which is called D^u. Formal terminology would be Rh^+, D^u variant, even though it would appear to be Rh negative without special techniques. For purposes of transfusion, the D^u variant is considered as Rh^+. Genetically Rh^+, D^u variant recipients are Rh^+ and are unlikely to be sensitized by administered Rh^+ blood.

The chemical basis for the weakened D antigen is not understood. One theory postulates that the normal D antigen is made up of four components and that weakened antigen is due to the absence of some of these components. Another theory proposes that the presence of C, d on the haplotype opposite the D causes this effect.

E. Deleted antigens: Rh null cells

Rare individuals lack part or all of the common Rh antigens. In Fisher nomenclature partially deleted cells lack one or more of the antigens (− D −); fully deleted cells (− − −) are called *Rh null cells* and lack all evidence of Cc, D, Ee antigens. Unlike cells lacking ABOH antigens, red cells lacking Rh antigens have many abnormalities, including shortened survival, stomatocytic morphology, and impaired transport of sodium and potassium ions.

The Rh null syndrome is caused either by a gene that blocks conversion of Rh precursor to Rh antigens or, in some cases, to absence of an Rh structural gene. In the latter instance heterozygotes express only a single Rh haplotype.

These partially and fully deleted cells are valuable reagents for studying the specificity of warm-type autoimmune antibodies found in immunohemolytic anemia (see lecture 12).

F. Rh antigen structure

The D antigen depends on membrane phospholipids for expression and is thought to be an integral membrane protein of mol. wt. 7,000–10,000. Partial purification has been achieved by gel electrophoresis and affinity chromatography with Rh immune globulin. The D antigen is a proteolipid because it is extractable in chloroform/methanol and binds to dicyclohexylcarbodiimide. Binding is specific for D, and interaction with other Rh antigens or Fy^a or A antigen cannot be demonstrated. A protein that in addition to D has Cc and Ee specificities has also been purified. These findings tend to validate the Weiner model.

The D antigen of Rh positive red cells is confined to the outer surface of the red cell membrane. Rh negative red cells have an equivalent amount of D antigen on the inner membrane surface, which is decreased by trypsin. In contrast D activity on positive cells is enhanced by trypsin. These findings suggest that D antigen is synthesized but not presented on the outer surface of Rh negative cells.

VI. OTHER CLINICALLY SIGNIFICANT SYSTEMS

A. Kell system

The Kell antigen system rivals the Rh system in its complexity and clinical importance. Appearing in response to prior immunization, anti-Kell antibodies have caused hemolytic transfusion reactions and hemolytic disease in newborns. Anti-kell is a common antibody, but because about 90% of bloods are Kell negative, it is easy to find blood to use in patients with anti-Kell. The main antigen pairs, K-k, Kp^a-Kp^b, and Js^a-Js^b, are controlled by three closely linked loci or three subloci of a single gene. Unlike the situation in the Rh system, not all expected combinations have been found. The incidence of these antigens also varies according to race (table 15.7).

The autosomal loci of these genes are unknown. Little is known of antigen biosynthesis, but investigation of the so-called MacLeod phenotype (k Kp^b Js^b) suggests two steps in the synthetic process of these antigens. Synthesis of precursor of Kell antigen, Kx, is controlled by a locus on the X chromosome. A second autosomal gene, whose location is unknown, then converts this precursor to the normal Kell antigens.

MacLeod cells are acanthocytes with reduced survival in vivo. Normal Kell antigens are present in decreased amounts, and antibody may develop against Kx (the precursor substance) and Km (a high incidence antigen associated with the usual Kell antigens). Leukocytes normally display Kx antigen, but Kx is absent in patients with the X-linked chronic granulomatous disease (see lecture 18). Both MacLeod syndrome and chronic granulomatous

Table 15.7
Racial Distribution of Kell Antigen

Antigen	% of bloods positive	
	Caucasians	Blacks
K	9.0	3.5
k	99.8	>99.9
Kp^a	2.0	< 0.1
Kp^b	99.9	>99.9
Js^a	< 0.1	19.5
Js^b	>99.9	98.9

disease exist separately or together with Kx lacking involved cell lives.

Kell antigens are thought to be glycoproteins, but antigen structure is unknown.

B. Duffy system

Distribution of the relatively simply Duffy phenotypes in Caucasians and blacks is shown in table 15.8. These antigens are degraded by proteolysis, but structural information is unavailable. Double-negative phenotype red cells, Fy (a−b−), are totally resistant to invasion by *Plasmodium vivax*. Hence selective pressures may be responsible for the high incidence of this phenotype in blacks. The genes are located on chromosome 1. Individuals of double-negative phenotype lack Fy3, which travels with Fy^a and Fy^b. They may acquire antibody against Fy3, which reacts with all Fy(a) or Fy(b) positive cells. Transfusion of incompatible blood into Duffy-sensitive individuals can cause severe hemolysis.

C. Kidd system

The Kidd system behaves like a two-allele system with a silent allele of infrequent occurrence. In Caucasians the incidence of Jk^a is 77% and of Jk^b 72%. The double-negative phenotype is rare and occurs mainly in Chinese and South American Indians. Jk^a and Jk^b are always associated with another antigen, Jk^3, which is also lacking on the double-negative phenotype. Hence these individuals may make an antibody against Jk^3.

Immunization to Kidd is caused mainly by transfusions. Kidd antibodies are evanescent warm-active incomplete antibodies that may not be detected in red cell antibody screens. Consequently they often cause delayed transfusion reactions, which may be severe. A reliable transfusion history is the best way to prevent such reactions.

D. Lutheran system

This system parallels the Kidd system. There are two common alleles, Lu^a and Lu^b, and a silent one. Lu^a is found in 8% of Caucasians and Lu^b in more than 99%. The double-negative phenotype is caused by either a dominant inhibitor gene or a recessive silent allele. The phenotype caused by dominant inhibitor displays small amounts of Lu^a and Lu^b and hence does not make antibody

Table 15.8
Racial Distribution of Duffy Antigen

	% of bloods positive	
Phenotypes	Caucasians	Blacks
Fy (a+ b−)	17	9
Fy (a+ b+)	49	1
Fy (a− b+)	34	22
Fy (a− b−)	−	68

against Lu^3, an antigen that travels with Lu^a and Lu^b. On the other hand double negatives with the silent allele do make anti-Lu^3 and thus may become difficult transfusion problems. In addition two other closely liked allelic pairs and several high incidence antigens have been identified. Fortunately the latter are usually of little clinical importance.

The autosomal location of Lu genes has not been identified, but it is closely linked to the Se/se gene of the ABOH system. Antigen structure is unknown.

E. Xg^a blood group

This antigen is controlled by a gene on the X-chromosome. It is not clinically significant but is of interest as a marker for X chromosomes that appear to escape inactivation by the Lyon mechanism. This is in contrast with Xk, which is inactivated. Thus MacLeod females can have a mixture of MacLeod and normal red cells.

VIII. USES OF BLOOD GROUPING DATA

A. In clinical medicine

1. Pretransfusion testing

Prior to transfusion blood is typed and cross-matched (by methods described in lecture 16) to establish ABO and D compatibility. Typing for other antigens is omitted unless the recipient is known to be sensitized to them. Justification of this policy is that it is easier to provide antigen-negative blood for individuals who become sensitized (10–15% of multitransfused patients) than it is to match blood more extensively with the recipient's phenotype prior to sensitization.

2. Hemolytic disease of the newborn

The relationship between blood groups and transplacental hemolytic disease of the newborn and other acquired hemolytic anemias is discussed in lectures 12 and 16.

B. In genetics

Blood groups are important for chromosome mapping because their inheritance can be traced serologically, and sometimes they can be localized quite precisely. For example, the Rh locus is on the short arm of chromosome 1 and is part of the linkage group that can be easily separated from the Duffy locus. Distribution of blood groups of large populations is useful in the study of population movement and origins of different ethnic groups.

C. In forensic medicine

1. Identification studies

Demonstration of blood groups in fresh or even dried blood or other materials (such as semen) is indispensable in establishing the human origin of the specimen and in identifying the individual from whom it came.

2. Paternity testing

In cases of disputed paternity, blood grouping of mother, child, and putative father can either exclude paternity or give a statistical probability that an accused man is the father. It is almost always possible now, by the use of many genetic markers, to establish when a man is not the father of a child.

SELECTED REFERENCES

Anstee, D. J. The blood group MNSs: Active sialoglycoproteins. *Semin. Hematol.* 18(1981): 13.

Hakomori, S. Blood groups ABH and Ii antigens of human erythrocytes: Chemistry, polymorphism and their developmental change. *Semin. Hematol.* 18(1981): 39.

Huestis, D. W., et al. *Practical Blood Transfusion,* 3d ed., Boston: Little, Brown, 1981.

Marcus, D. M. Blood group immunochemistry and genetics. *Semin. Hematol.* 18(1981): 1.

Marcus, D. M., et al. The P blood group system: Recent progress in immunochemistry and genetics. *Semin. Hematol.* 18(1981): 63.

Mollison, P. L. *Blood Transfusion in Clinical Medicine,* 7th ed., Oxford: Blackwell, 1983.

Petz, L. D., and Swisher, S. N. *Clinical Practice of Blood Transfusion,* New York: Churchill Livingston, 1981.

Tippett, P. Chromosomal mapping of blood genes. *Semin. Hematol.* 18(1981): 10.

Yoshida, A., et al. Immunologic homology of human blood group glycosyltransferases and the genetic background of blood group (ABO) determination. *Blood* 54(1979): 344.

LECTURE 16 Blood Groups II. Transfusion Therapy

W. Hallowell Churchill, Jr.

I. HISTORICAL NOTES

Transfusion into human beings of calf blood was first attempted in 1667 by Dennis. The resulting hemolytic transfusion reaction, which was described magnificently, quickly caused this procedure to be banned. No further effort at transfusion therapy was initiated until 1818 when Blondell attempted to transfuse women hemorrhaging during childbirth. Little progress was made until 1900 when recognition of the ABO blood groups permitted matching of major blood groups and 1914 when development of anticoagulants allowed preservation of donated blood in vitro. Since that time transfusion therapy has advanced to the point that each year millions of units of blood are now being drawn and fractionated into components so that products from one unit may be reliably used by more than one recipient.

II. BLOOD COLLECTION

A. General methods

Recruitment of blood donors is carried out by local, regional, and national organizations, all of which face the problem that only about 5% of eligible donors actually donate even though the need for safe blood is widely publicized. Voluntary donors are a safer source of blood than paid donors. Studies suggest that altruism, replacement of blood used by a friend, and peer pressure are all important motivating factors, whereas fear of needles and the overall process of blood donation are important deterrents.

Blood donation is a routine and relatively painless process taking about 45 minutes. Side effects are minimal. Most prospective healthy donors between the ages of 17 and 66 can be accepted. They are rejected only when (1) their blood may be hazardous to a recipient or (2) medical problems might make donation hazardous.

B. Specialized methods

1. Autologous donation

The safest procedure is an *autologous donation* in which the recipient is given his or her own blood. This eliminates the possibility of transfusion reaction or transmission of blood-borne disease. The availability of anticoagulants, which permit a shelf life of up to 49 days, and the preservation of blood by freezing for longer periods make "banking one's own blood" an option for many patients undergoing elective surgery. The main problems are the logistics of storing the blood and returning it to the donor at surgery. Donors with hematocrits as low as 34 can be accepted (ordinary donors have hematocrits of at least 38), but the number of donations may be limited by the donor's marrow response to phlebotomy (bleeding). There may also be added costs, especially if the blood must be frozen. None of these obstacles is significant compared to the cost of blood-transmitted hepatitis and/or acquired immune deficiency syndrome (AIDS), which is a risk with heterologous donations.

2. Apheresis donation

Cell separators now available can, by continuous or discontinuous centrifugation techniques, selectively remove large numbers of platelets or white cells from a single donor in about 2 hours. These components are essential during cancer or leukemia chemotherapy and other disorders. Donors undergoing apheresis suffer no significant side effects.

III. PREPARATION AND STORAGE OF BLOOD

A. Component preparation

A *unit of whole blood* contains 450 ml of blood plus 63 ml of an anticoagulant-preservative. Whole blood can be separated into various components by a series of differential centrifugations. Packed *red cells* with a hematocrit of about 70 (termed *packed cells*) are made by centrifugations of whole blood and removal of platelet-rich plasma. *Platelet concentrate* is then prepared by centrifugation of this fraction and resuspension of the platelets. The remaining platelet-poor plasma, if frozen within 6 hours of collection, is *fresh frozen plasma* (FFP). It contains all the coagulation factors in the initial unit of blood. *Cryoprecipitate* is made by thawing FFP and removing all the thawed plasma with the exception of the cold-precipitated material in the last 10–15 ml. This fraction is rich in factor VIII, fibrinogen, and fibronectin. Plasma that is not used as such can be converted to 5% albumin for use as a blood volume expander. Its advantage is that, after pasteurization, it no longer transmits hepatitis virus. In contrast concentrates of factor VII and factor IX, both of which are prepared from large pools of plasma, are consistently contaminated with hepatitis virus.

B. Blood preservation and storage

Storage conditions are designed to minimize hemolysis, loss of red cell 2,3-DPG and ATP, and accumulation of extracellular K^+ and NH_3, all of which reflect the "storage lesion" of banked blood. Shelf life is determined by assays of in vivo survival. To be acceptable, 70% of red cells must survive at least 24 hours after transfusion. Improved anticoagulant-preservatives, which contain additional adenine, glucose, and mannitol, have increased shelf life from 21 days for ACD (acid citrate dextrose) anticoagulant-preservative or CPD (citrate phosphate dextrose) to 49 days for the latest formulations, which are called *Adsol* or *Nutricel*.

After treatment with a cryoprotective agent such as glycerol, red cells can be preserved indefinitely in the frozen state (at

−80°C). This approach is particularly useful for the preservation of rare blood types and the preparation of red cells with more than 95% of the white cells removed.

IV. PRETRANSFUSION TESTING

A. Of donor unit

After collection the donor unit is typed to determine ABO and Rh and screened for serum antibodies and hepatitis B antigen. This procedure has decreased the incidence of blood-borne hepatitis B; however, it does not detect non-A, non-B hepatitis virus, for which no assay is available. Following testing the unit is released for use in the form of packed cells, platelet concentrates, and fresh frozen plasma.

B. Of recipient

1. Drawing the blood specimen

A blood specimen must be drawn from the intended recipient within 48 hours of transfusion, properly labeled with the patient's name, date, and time, and initialed by the phlebotomist. Mislabeling of patient specimens is the most dangerous error that can occur. Blood banks have no means of detecting the error unless they have the patient's blood type on file.

2. Typing

ABO and Rh group of the recipient is determined by testing both red cells with known antisera (forward typing) and his or her serum with red cells of known ABO phenotype (reverse typing). If forward and reverse typing results do not agree, the discrepancy must be resolved prior to transfusion. Possible explanations include subgroups of A and B, agammaglobulinemia, neonatal sera, laboratory error, cold antibodies, and polyagglutinable cells (see lecture 15). When the type has been established, transfusion of ABO-compatible blood without further testing would bring the risk of incompatibility to less than 3%.

C. Antibody screen

Recipient serum is screened for anti-red cell antibodies by incubation with cells of known phenotype that include the clinically important red cell antigens. These must be present in the homozygous state because occasional antibodies are not detected by heterozygous cells. After incubation, cells are washed and tested for antibody by addition of the Coombs reagent. If this procedure is negative, recipient serum is said to be free of anti-red cell antibodies. Under these circumstances the chance of incompatibility on subsequent cross-match is about 0.5%.

D. Cross-match: the final check

A *major cross-match* is carried out by incubating the recipient's serum with donor red cells and testing for agglutination in both saline and in media designed to enhance agglutination (see lecture 15). Cells are then washed and tested for antibody by the addition of Coombs serum. Occasionally the major cross-match will reveal incompatibility when the antibody screen was negative. Consequently major cross-matching with Coombs reagent is carried out when blood transfusion is planned. In patients with a relatively low likelihood of needing blood during surgery, testing is often limited to a type and screen. If blood is needed urgently, it can be released after an abbreviated cross-match with essentially the same safety as a full Coombs cross-match.

In an emergency type-specific blood can be obtained in about 5 minutes and fully cross-matched blood in about 1 hour. After a negative antibody screen, blood can be released in about 10 minutes. Availability of fresh frozen plasma depends on the time required to thaw the product—about 45 to 60 minutes. Consequently urgent volume expansion must be accomplished with a crystalloid or 5% albumin.

V. TRANSFUSION THERAPY

The major immediate goals of transfusion therapy are (1) maintenance of oxygen transport; (2) maintenance of adequate hemostasis; and (3) volume replacement. Their goals are best achieved by transfusion of the specific components needed to replace particular deficits. At present there is almost no indication for the use of unfractionated whole blood. Whole blood offers no advantage over component therapy in the maintenance of hemostasis.

A new dimension was added to transfusion therapy with the development of mechanical devices capable of separating specific cell components from the blood of a single donor. These instruments utilize the principle of differential centrifugation. Red cells sediment faster than leukocytes, platelets, or plasma. The principle is applied either by *intermittent flow centrifugation* or *continuous flow centrifugation* to collect a therapeutic dose of platelets or leukocytes from a single normal donor. Separators utilize sterile plastic systems that in most cases are completely disposable.

A. Red cell concentrates (packed cells)

Red cell concentrates are useful for the vast majority of red cell transfusions. This product normally has a hematocrit of 70–80% and consequently has a relatively slow flow rate. Preparation removes both the plasma, which during storage has accumulated excess K^+, NH_3, and hemoglobin, and most of the white cells in the buffy coat. Packed cells are the preferred preparation for patients with chronic anemia. These cells can also be used for replacement of acute blood loss in conjunction with appropriate volume expanders.

B. "Leukopoor" blood

Blood may be treated in a variety of ways to reduce the likelihood of immunologic reactions to white cells and plasma. Preparations in common use include *"buffy coat-poor" blood, washed red cells*, and *frozen-deglycerolized cells*. Of these preparations, *frozen-deglycerolized cells* have the least number of contaminating leukocytes due to the loss of leukocytes during the thawing and washing procedures. Frozen-washed cells are the preferred products for patients requiring prolonged or indefinite red blood cell support.

C. Platelets

Platelets for transfusion may be prepared by sedimentation from a unit of fresh whole donor blood. Platelets obtained in this way are first separated by a light centrifugation of the whole blood. In this maneuver, the red cells sediment to the bottom of the blood bag and the platelets remain in the plasma. The plasma is then separated and centrifuged at higher speeds. This concentrates the platelets and separates them from the plasma. This process yields a unit of random donor platelets that contains approximately 5.5×10^{10} platelets. This unit must be pooled with other random donor platelet units to obtain a therapeutic dose. Under optimal conditions, a single unit of platelets (platelets obtained from a single unit of blood) produces an increase of 5–10,000/mm^3 in the platelet count. Ordinarily 8–10 units of platelets per transfusion are used in a severely thrombocytopenic adult patient.

A therapeutic dose of platelets may be obtained from a single donor using a cell separator or manually using a special blood bag. These procedures yield 4–12 units of single-donor platelets (average 5×10^{11} platelets per bag). The principle advantage of single-donor platelets is the diminished number of platelet antigens (HLA antigens) to which the patient is exposed. The reduced exposure to these antigens tends to lengthen the time period during which patients respond to platelet transfusions. Once patients are sensitized to multiple platelet antigens, they become hematologically unresponsive to all but carefully matched transfusions. In addition, single-donor platelets probably reduce somewhat the exposure of patients to hepatitis viruses.

1. Indications

Platelets are indicated in the treatment of thrombocytopenic patients to prevent or control bleeding. Patients with platelet counts of 20,000–100,000 who are bleeding are candidates for platelet therapy. Patients with platelet counts of $<$20,000 may also be considered candidates for prophylactic platelet therapy. Patients with platelet counts of $>$20,000 who are not bleeding do not appear to benefit from preventive platelet therapy. The choice of platelet product as indicated above depends on the patient's diagnosis and prognosis. In general, patients with chronic hematologic or malignant disease benefit from single-donor platelets if they are available. This is because of the diminished exposure to platelet antigens and the consequent delay in the development of immunologic sensitization.

2. Complications

The complications of platelet transfusions are similar to those of red cell products. They include posttransfusion hepatitis, febrile reactions and urticarial reactions, and the development of alloimmunization to platelet antigens. Platelet transfusions do not lead to acute hemolytic reactions.

D. Granulocytes

Leukocyte transfusions have been under investigation for several years. A number of techniques exist whereby a therapeutic dose of granulocytes ($\sim 10^{11}$ white cells) may be obtained from a normal donor. These cells are collected with the aid of mechanical cell separators. In selected patients who are severely leukopenic, septic, and not responding to conventional treatment, granulocyte transfusions have been shown to be of value. The patients that seem to benefit from these transfusions are those with leukemia undergoing aggressive chemotherapy. However, much work remains to be done before granulocyte transfusions can be considered standard therapy for any illness. Granulocyte transfusions may transmit hepatitis, cause febrile and urticarial reactions, and cause acute hemolytic reactions because of the extensive contamination with red cells. They have also been implicated in severe pulmonary reactions, and are particularly hazardous if given in conjunction with amphotericin B.

E. Fresh frozen plasma (FFP)

FFP is plasma frozen within 6 hours after donation. All of the clotting factors maintain their stability in the frozen product. FFP is extremely useful in replacing clotting factors in patients with deficiencies in one or several clotting factors. The principle disadvantage of FFP is the large volume of plasma required to replace the clotting factors. In addition, FFP may transmit hepatitis and cause febrile and urticarial reactions.

F. Cryoprecipitate

Cryoprecipitate is the cold-insoluble material left in the sediment when a unit of FFP thaws. Cryoprecipitate is rich in factor VIII (antihemophilic factor), factor I (fibrinogen) and fibronectin. Using the definition that 1 unit is the amount of factor activity in 1 ml of fresh plasma, a bag of cryoprecipitate contains 80–100 units of factor VIII and 250 mg of fibrinogen. This product may be used to treat hemophilia A or as a source of fibrinogen. The risk of hepatitis is present, but is far less than with factor VIII concentrates prepared from pooled plasma. Fibrinogen concentrates made from pooled plasma are no longer available in the United States because of the enormous hepatitis risk.

G. Albumin

Human serum albumin is fractionated from pooled plasma and serum by the Cohn fractionation procedure (cold alcohol precipitation). The albumin is rendered hepatitis-free by heating to 60°C for 10 hr. Standard terminology notwithstanding, it is not actually salt poor. Albumin is extraordinarily useful as a safe and effective volume expander. Albumin and immune serum globulin are the only blood products that do not transmit viral hepatitis. Albumin may be stored for long periods of time without deterioration.

H. Clotting factor concentrates

Concentrates rich in factor VIII or factor IX may be prepared by precipitation and lyophilization from pooled plasma. Lyophilized factor VIII concentrates have the advantage of being more concentrated than the cryoprecipitated material. However, these concentrates have a much greater hepatitis risk. Factor IX concentrates, also known as prothrombin complex concentrates, contain factors II, IX, and X, and variable amounts of factor VII. These concentrates are useful in the treatment of hemophilia B (factor IX deficiency). Since they contain the vitamin K-dependent factors, they may also be used in life-threatening vitamin K deficiency or warfarin intoxication. However, the enormous hepatitis risk must be considered. For these last two conditions FFP, a far more infrequent cause of hepatitis, is usually sufficient treatment.

VI. HAZARDS

A. Acute hemolytic transfusion reactions

Hemolytic transfusion reactions are the most serious and dreaded complication of transfusion therapy. They are caused by the immunologic destruction of donor red cells by antibody in recipient serum. The antibody-antigen reaction triggers a variety of systems in the plasma proteins that activate a host of vasoactive substances. Symptoms include fever, chills, back pain, chest pain, facial flushing, hypotension, nausea, vomiting, hemoglobinemia, hemoglobinuria, diffuse bleeding, and renal shutdown. Although the reactions may be caused by any red cell blood group, the most serious are due to ABO reactions. The usual cause of these reactions is a clerical error, such as failure to identify adequately the recipient or inaccurate labeling of patient specimens for typing and cross-match.

B. Delayed hemolytic transfusion reactions

These reactions occur 3–14 days following a transfusion and are associated with immunologic destruction of the donor cells by a specific blood group antibody. They occur in patients who have been previously sensitized to a blood group antigen but do not have detectable antibody at the time of compatibility testing. The immune system is stimulated to produce a secondary response resulting in the rapid production of high levels of specific antibody. Clinically, patients have a positive direct antiglobulin test and evidence of hemolysis. The direct antiglobulin test ultimately becomes negative as the incompatible units are hemolyzed and the indirect antiglobulin test becomes positive. These reactions are usually distinguishable from immunohemolytic anemia by serological testing and can best be avoided by a careful transfusion history.

C. Posttransfusion hepatitis

The transmission of hepatitis remains the most common serious hazard of transfusion. The incidence of this disease differs in various regions of the country, but it is roughly slightly less than 1% per unit of blood or equivalent product. The incidence has been reduced by the expansion of the voluntary blood system as opposed to commercial blood and further reduced by the introduction and refinement of hepatitis B surface antigen testing.

Posttransfusion hepatitis is a viral disease caused by more than one virus. *Hepatitis B* is associated with approximately 10% of the cases of posttransfusion hepatitis. As techniques for detection of HBsAg in blood improve, the number of cases of hepatitis B should diminish further. *Non-B hepatitis* includes the remaining 90% of the cases of posttransfusion hepatitis. The virus or viruses responsible for the vast majority of non-B hepatitis have not yet been conclusively identified. A small number of cases are associated with cytomegalovirus or Epstein-Barr virus.

D. AIDS

Recent evidence has suggested that acquired immune deficiency syndrome (AIDS) can be transmitted by blood products. This conclusion is based on the incidence of AIDS in hemophiliacs receiving factor VIII concentrates and the appearance of AIDS in patients with no known risk factors but with a history of having received one or more blood products. In some of these latter cases, review of the donors of these products has identified individuals with clinical and laboratory evidence of AIDS. Although the incidence of such cases is probably less than one in a million transfusions, these findings provide more reason to limit the use of allogeneic blood transfusions.

E. Other complications

Febrile nonhemolytic reactions, usually mediated by leukocyte antibodies, present with fever, malaise, and flulike symptoms in the absence of hemolysis. They may be reliably distinguished from hemolytic reactions by routine serological investigations. *Urticarial reactions*, or hives, are caused by reactions of patients' antibodies with donor plasma proteins. These reactions are easily treated with antihistamines. Severe *anaphylactoid reactions* are very serious and rapidly progressive hypotensive episodes that occur in patients with anti-IgA antibodies. IgA deficiency occurs infrequently (approximately 1 of 600 normal individuals). The usual IgA-deficient subject has a strong anti-IgA antibody in the serum. The antibody reacts with any IgA in the donor unit and a brisk hypotensive reaction ensues. The unit must be stopped quickly or death may occur. Further transfusions are safe only with IgA-deficient blood products.

Other complications of transfusion include posttransfusion purpura, graft-versus-host disease, pulmonary infiltrates, malaria, toxoplasmosis, volume overload, potassium toxicity, and dilutional coagulopathy.

VII. HEMOLYTIC DISEASE OF THE NEWBORN

Hemolytic disease of the newborn (HDN) is a disease in which the life span of a fetus's red cells is diminished by the action of specific antibodies derived from the mother and transferred to the fetus across the placenta. In its most severe form, death may occur in utero. This illness is also known as *erythroblastosis fetalis*, a name that relates to the presence of markedly increased numbers of nucleated red cells in the blood of the fetus. If the infant is born alive, it may suffer from *hydrops fetalis*, an illness characterized by massive edema of the fetus presumed secondary to anemia, hypoalbuminemia, and cardiac failure. Hydropic infants frequently do not survive.

The discovery of the Rh blood group system between 1939 and 1941 led to the identification of the specificity of the antibody responsible for most cases of HDN, that is, anti-D(Rh_o). Less commonly, antibodies against other antigens of the Rh system or other blood groups such as Kell or antigens of the ABO system have been implicated. The common denominator in all cases is presence in the fetus of a red cell antigen that is not part of the mother's phenotype and against which she has become sensitized. Much progress has been made in the diagnosis, treatment, and prevention of HDN in the past 45 years, especially those cases that are due to the D(Rh_o) antigen.

A. Pathophysiology

HDN develops because of the transfer of specific antibody from mother to fetus. Only maternal antibodies of the IgG class are transferred across the placenta. Thus only IgG antibodies mediate the disease. Sensitization to fetal antigens occurs in the mother primarily as a result of *fetomaternal hemorrhage*. Fetal erythrocytes may be detected in the maternal circulation as early as 8 weeks after conception. However, sensitization is most likely to occur at the time of delivery of the infant since that is the time of the largest fetomaternal hemorrhage. Once sensitized, a mother is at risk for the development of hemolytic disease in subsequent pregnancies.

HDN from ABO antigens occurs in group A or group B children of group O mothers. Since group O mothers have anti-A and anti-B of the IgG class without fetomaternal sensitization, this disorder may develop during the first pregnancy.

The disease affects the fetus in several ways. The fetus is *anemic* with varying degrees of complications, the most serious of which is cardiac failure. In its most severe form, hydrops fetalis, the fetus is massively edematous and may succumb rapidly. The fetus compensates for the destruction of red cells by increasing *extramedullary erythropoiesis* that affects vital organs. Thus, the liver, spleen, and marrow enlarge owing to the presence of erythropoietic cells. This may lead to a decrease in liver function. Finally, the destruction of large quantities of red cells leads to *hyperbilirubinemia*. The newborn is not biochemically equipped to handle the excess load of bilirubin, at least in part because of inadequate activity of bilirubin conjugating enzymes at birth. The elevated bilirubin in the postnatal period may then be associated with *kernicterus*. This complication is characterized by brain damage resulting in death of neurological impairment caused by bilirubin toxicity.

B. Prenatal diagnosis

The prenatal diagnosis of HDN is often suggested by the patient's history. A history of previously affected offspring should alert one to the possibility of HDN. However, many severely affected infants are born in the absence of any previous history. Simple Rh typing of mother and father and screening of the mother's serum for atypical red cell antibodies should be helpful in defining potentially affected fetuses. *Amniocentesis* is the procedure by which amniotic fluid is aspirated (see lecture 10) and analyzed for bilirubin pigment. Increased concentrations of bilirubin in the amniotic fluid are correlated with increased red cell destruction of fetal red cells. The concentrations of bilirubin can be correlated with the prognosis of the fetus, and appropriate steps can then be taken to prevent development of severe disease.

C. Treatment

1. Prenatal

Severe disease may be treated by intrauterine transfusion of blood into the fetus between the 20th and 33rd weeks of gestation. Blood compatible with the mother's serum is introduced into the peritoneal cavity of the fetus via injection. The blood is absorbed across the peritoneum and the transfused blood will not be immunologically destroyed by the maternal antibody. This procedure may be repeated if necessary. Premature induction of labor may be contemplated if the fetus is approximately 33 weeks or older. At birth, the transfer of maternal antibody ceases, and soon after birth the hemolytic rate begins to decline.

2. Postnatal

A number of options exist for the postnatal therapy of an infant with HDN. *Exchange transfusion* is the single most effective means of treating both the anemia and the hyperbilirubinemia of the disease. In the usual practice, 2 units of blood compatible with the mother's are slowly exchanged with the infant's blood. This has the effect of raising the hemoglobin, washing out the offending antibody, and washing out the high level of bilirubin. The process may be repeated if necessary.

In less severe cases, infants may be treated with phototherapy, which has the effect of lowering the serum bilirubin. The infusion of albumin (which binds bilirubin) and the treatment of mothers with barbiturates (which induces higher levels of bilirubin-conjugating enzymes) are less commonly employed.

D. Prophylaxis of Rh disease

One of the major achievements of modern medicine is the development of an effective means of prevention of alloimmunization to the $D(Rh_o)$ antigen. Sensitization to the D antigen may be prevented by the passive injection of 300 μg of IgG anti-$D(Rh_o)$, that is, Rh immune globulin (RhoGam®), to an Rh negative mother of an Rh positive infant within 72 hr of delivery. If the mother has not been previously sensitized to the $D(Rh_o)$ antigen, the passive injection of antibody will prevent immunization. Likewise, patients undergoing therapeutic abortions are also at risk for sensitization to the $D(Rh_o)$ antigen. All Rh negative mothers undergoing abortion should receive a dose of Rh immune globulin to prevent sensitization to the $D(Rh_o)$ antigen. The widespread use of this technique has dramatically reduced the incidence of Rh sensitization and Rh HDN in recent years.

SELECTED REFERENCES

Conrad, M. E. Transfusion problems in hematology. *Semin. Hematol.* 18 (1981): 81.

Curran, J. W., et al. Acquired immunodeficiency syndrome (AIDS) associated with transfusions. *New Eng. J. Med.* 310(1984): 69.

Goldfinger, D. Acute hemolytic transfusion reactions: A fresh look at pathogenesis and considerations regarding treatment. *Transfusion* 17(1977): 85.

Huestis, D. W., et al. *Practical Blood Transfusion*, 3d ed., Boston: Little, Brown, 1981.

Miller, W. V., et al. *Technical Manual of the American Association of Blood Banks*, 7th ed., Philadelphia: Lippincott, 1977.

Mollison, P. L. *Blood Transfusion in Clinical Medicine*, 6th ed., Oxford: Blackwell, 1983.

Petz, L. D., and Swisher, S. N. *Clinical Practice of Blood Transfusion*, New York: Churchill Livingstone, 1981.

LECTURE 17 Leukocytes I. Physiology

William S. Beck

I. INTRODUCTION

We use the terms *leukocyte* and *white cell* to refer to any of the nucleated cells normally present in blood, whose major function is defense against foreign invaders. The terms are usually not used to refer to fixed cells of the RES or free tissue macrophages (discussed in lecture 2), though these cells share many properties with circulating blood leukocytes.

A. Types of leukocytes

The different types of leukocytes may be classified in several ways: (1) by the *type of defense function*—phagocytosis in the case of *phagocytes* (i.e., granulocytes and monocytes), antibody production and cellular immunity in the case of *immunocytes* (i.e., lymphocytes and plasma cells); (2) by the *shape of the nucleus* (polymorphonuclear or mononuclear); (3) by the *site of origin* (myeloid or lymphoid); and (4) by the presence or absence of *specific-staining granules* (granulocytes or nongranulocytes). The granulocytes in turn are classified by the nature of their specific-staining granules, which are neutrophilic, eosinophilic, or basophilic.

B. Normal leukocyte count

Table 17.1 summarizes the reported values for the concentration of various leukocyte types in the venous blood of 105 normal male students, according to Boggs. Note that the majority of blood leukocytes are neutrophils in the normal adult. Lymphocytes predominate in infants and young children.

C. Historical notes

The classic staining researches of Paul Ehrlich (1878 et seq.) led to important advances in the knowledge of leukocytes. Prior to Ehrlich's discovery of polychromatic and supravital stains, granulocytes had been observed and counted, and their capacity for motility and phagocytosis had been recognized—but their

Table 17.1
Normal Values of Blood Leukocyte Concentration

Cell type	Mean (cells/mm^3)	Mean (%)	95% confidence limits (cells/mm^3)
Neutrophils	4,300	55.3	1,800–6,700
Lymphocytes	2,710	34.8	1,400–3,930
Monocytes	500	6.4	140–860
Eosinophils	230	3.0	0–570
Basophils	40	0.5	0–120

Source: Modified from D. Boggs, *Semin. Hematol.* 4(1967): 359.

morphology and classification were unexplored. The main elements of our understanding of the maturation sequence came from the work of Pappenheim (1914).

II. GRANULOCYTES

A. Morphologic aspects of granulopoiesis

1. Maturation stages

Figure 17.1 summarizes the highlights of granulopoiesis. Six maturation stages are recognized: myeloblast → promyelocyte → myelocyte → metamyelocyte → band form → mature polymorphonuclear granulocyte. As shown in figure 17.1, the myeloid maturation sequence is characterized by progressive decrease in nuclear size, the early presence of nucleoli and their subsequent disappearance, late nuclear indentation and segmentation, characteristic changes in chromatin character, early appearance of azurophilic granules, and later appearance of specific-staining granules. Myeloblasts are easily recognized but may be difficult to distinguish from lymphoblasts. *Auer rods,* when present, indicate that the cell is a myeloblast or monoblast. They are not seen in

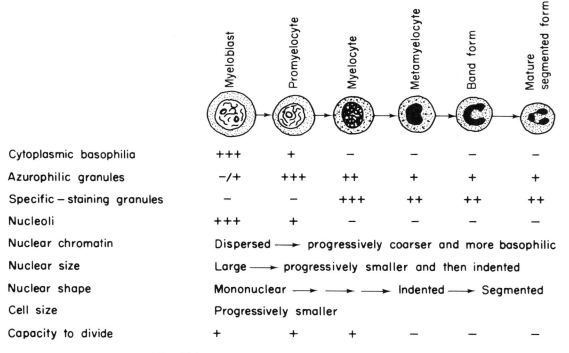

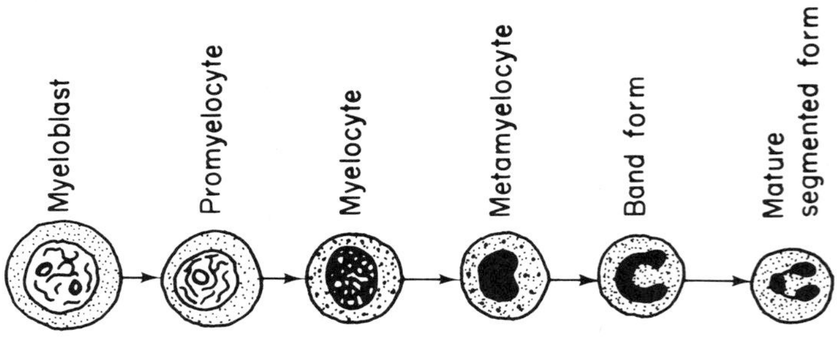

	Myeloblast	Promyelocyte	Myelocyte	Metamyelocyte	Band form	Mature segmented form
Cytoplasmic basophilia	+++	+	–	–	–	–
Azurophilic granules	–/+	+++	++	+	+	+
Specific – staining granules	–	–	+++	++	++	++
Nucleoli	+++	+	–	–	–	–
Nuclear chromatin	Dispersed → progressively coarser and more basophilic					
Nuclear size	Large → progressively smaller and then indented					
Nuclear shape	Mononuclear → → → Indented → Segmented					
Cell size	Progressively smaller					
Capacity to divide	+	+	+	–	–	–

Fig. 17.1
Stages of myeloid cell maturation.

lymphoblasts. These curious structures appear to arise from clumped azurophilic granule material. They are seen only in leukemia (see lecture 21).

2. Granules

The granules visible in stained smears are lysosomes that contain the hydrolytic enzymes and antibacterial agents required for the digestion of phagocytized particles.

Two types of granules are distinguishable: (1) *primary,* or *azurophilic, granules,* coarse reddish-purple granules, 0.8 μm in diameter, that appear first at the promyelocyte stage; and (2) *secondary,* or *specific-staining granules,* neutrophilic, eosinophilic, or basophilic granules, 0.5 μm in diameter, that appear first at the myelocyte stage. Since azurophilic granules are formed only in promyelocytes, their numbers per cell decrease after that stage.

The granules have a distinctive appearance on electron microscopy (figure 17.2). Note in the figure that the Golgi complex is prominent in the promyelocyte. Intense granule synthesis takes place at that stage, and there is evidence that synthesis of both types of granules occurs in the Golgi complex at different stages. The two types of granules appear to come from opposite faces of the Golgi: specific-staining granules from the distal or convex face, azurophilic from the proximal or concave face.

Azurophilic granules contain (in addition to lysosomal hydro-

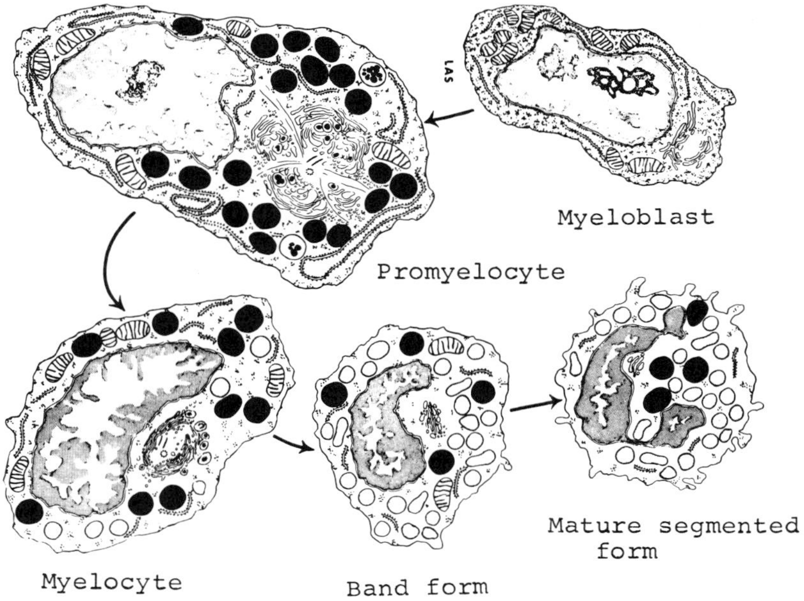

Fig. 17.2
Diagram of maturation stages of granulopoiesis as observed by electron microscopy. Dense lysosomes are primary or azurophilic granules. Lighter lysosomes are secondary or specific-staining granules. Note that both types of granules are found in the mature cell. (From D. F. Bainton and M. G. Farquhar, *J. Cell. Biol.* 28(1966): 277)

lytic enzymes) neutral proteases, myeloperoxidase, glycoaminoglycans, acid phosphatase, cationic bactericidal proteins, and lysozyme. Specific-staining granules contain lysozyme, lactoferrin, and vitamin B_{12}-binding protein. These components are discussed below. Alkaline phosphatase, once thought to be in specific-staining granules, is now localized on the plasma membrane.

3. Acquired and hereditary anomalies

A number of defects of granulocyte morphology are recognized. Although rare, they are interesting for the insight they may give into the mechanisms of maturation.

a. Döhle bodies

Döhle bodies are common and easily recognized abnormalities of neutrophil cytoplasm. They are single or multiple gray-blue cytoplasmic inclusion bodies that are usually seen along the outer edge of mature neutrophils but may occur in earlier forms. They were first described by H. Döhle in 1911 in patients with scarlet fever and were thought by him to be pathognomonic. They were later found in severe infections, pregnancy, burns, cancer, and many other conditions. As noted below, they occur also in certain hereditary anomalies. Döhle bodies are thought to be ribosome-containing remnants of retained promyelocyte cytoplasm.

b. Macropolycytes

Acquired hypersegmented neutrophils occur in megaloblastic anemia (see figure 4.1B). Neutrophil hypersegmentation may also be inherited as a benign autosomal dominant trait.

c. Pelger-Hüet anomaly

This hereditary abnormality is characterized by failure of normal nuclear segmentation. In typical heterozygotes two-lobed nuclei are seen in the majority of mature granulocytes and eosinophils (''pince-nez'' cells). Nuclear chromatin is also condensed. Homozygotes have round nuclei. The disorder, a simple autosomal dominant trait, is benign and occurs in 1 in 6,000 people. A similar acquired disorder, known as pseudo-Pelger-Hüet anomaly, occurs in the course of myeloproliferative conditions and virus infections. It may be due to an abnormality of chromatin synthesis. A similar abnormality occurs in rabbits.

d. Alder-Reilly anomaly

This rare hereditary anomaly is part of a clinical complex arising from disordered polysaccharide metabolism. There results a defect of cytoplasmic maturation. Specific-staining granules fail to develop and coarse azurophilic granules remain. Nuclear maturation and configuration is normal. In some cases all granulocytes (as well as monocytes and lymphocytes) may be affected. In others normal and abnormal cells are present.

e. Chediak-Higashi syndrome (CHS)

This disorder of humans and cattle is associated with hereditary gigantism of specific-staining granules of all cells of the myeloid series, ocular and skin hypopigmentation, and giant melanosomes. Giant lysosomes are present in many body tissues. Granulocyte function is defective, with failure of lysosome fusion in phagocytosis (see lecture 18). Chemotaxis is also impaired. Hence patients suffer severe recurrent infections. Platelets lack dense granules, and platelet function is defective (see lecture 27). Recent data suggest that CHS may be associated with defective microtubular proteins.

f. May-Hegglin anomaly

This is a rare autosomal dominant trait manifested by giant platelets and Döhle bodies in granulocytes. The condition is usually benign, although some patients have a bleeding tendency associated with thrombocytopenia and/or qualitative platelet defect.

B. Physiologic aspects of granulopoiesis

1. Life span

Methods used to determine granulocyte life span employ in vitro or in vivo labeling techniques.

a. In vitro labels

In the in vitro methods, leukocytes are removed from the subject, labeled, and returned to the blood. Thus, only circulating cells are labeled. Diisopropylfluorophosphate-^{32}P (DF^{32}P), once a commonly used label but now commercially unavailable, attaches covalently to a serine residue of a cell protein. Use of this technique revealed two important facts. Upon reinfusion of labeled cells, half of the radioactivity seems to disappear from the blood (figure 17.3A). This observation led to the realization that the total blood granulocyte pool (TBGP) includes two subpools: the circulating granulocyte pool (CGP) and the marginal granulocyte pool (MGP; figure 17.3B). The MGP consists of intravascular cells that have

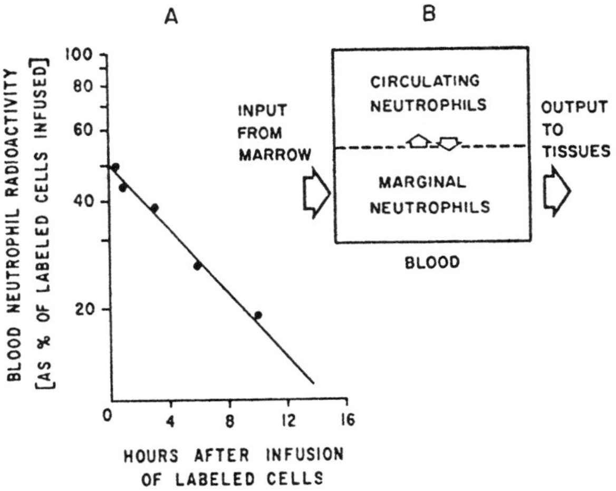

Fig. 17.3
Major conclusions from leukocyte life-span studies employing an in vitro label: *A*, time-course of disappearance of DF^{32}P-labeled neutrophils in a normal subject; *B*, model of blood neutrophil kinetics. (From D. Boggs, in C. E. Mengel, *Hematology: Prnciples and Practice,* Chicago: Year Book, 1972)

marginated along the walls of small capillaries and venules. The leukocyte count, as determined in venous blood samples taken from the axial stream, measures only the CGP. Cells are continually and rapidly exchanged between the two intravascular pools. Certain factors to be described shift cells from one pool to the other. The exponential decline in radioactivity of the CGP (figure 17.3A) indicates that cells are removed from the circulating pool in random fashion with a $T_{1/2}$ of about 6.7 hr (normal range, 4–10 hr). Hence, the CGP turns over 2.5 times per day, and the average time that a cell spends in the blood is about 10 hr. The average number of neutrophils entering and leaving the blood each day in normal adults is 167 $\times$ 10^7/kg body weight. In a 70-kg man, this equals 1.1 $\times$ 10^{11} neutrophils/day. Since 10^{10} neutrophils have a packed volume of 6 ml, volume of the daily output is 66 ml. By use of $DF^{32}P$, Cartwright et al. obtained the results in table 17.2 in normal male volunteers.

New methods for isotopically labeling neutrophils have recently become available. The most promising is indium (^{111}In).

b. In vivo labels

In methods employing in vivo labels, cells take up a systemically administered radioactive substance. Procedures are of two types: (1) those that label early granulocyte precursors and (2) those that label all precursors. Since early presursor cells are actively dividing, DNA labels (inorganic ^{32}P or ^{3}H-dThd) are used to tag them. Labeled DNA provides a stable marker for the studies of granulocyte kinetics.

The time course of radioactivity in blood granulocytes following injection of inorganic ^{32}P (figure 17.4) indicates that a 5–8-day delay occurs before labeled granulocytes enter the blood. Such data also show that the mean age of granulocytes (from myeloblast to death) is 9–10 days and that granulocytes entering the blood quickly move off into the tissues. When $DF^{32}P$ is given systemically, it labels all granulocyte precursors. Thus, for a time, cells emerging from the bone marrow are already labeled. From detailed studies of the time course of radioactivity in blood granulo-

Table 17.2
Blood Neutrophil Values in Normal Subjects

Parameter	Mean	95% confidence limits
Total blood granulocyte pool (TBGP), 10^7 cells/kg	70	14–160
Circulating granulocyte pool (CGP), 10^7 cells/kg	31	11–46
Marginal granulocyte pool (MGP), 10^7 cells/kg	39	0–85
Granulocyte turnover rate (GTR), 10^7 cells/kg/day	163	50–340
Half-disappearance time ($T_{1/2}$), hr	6.7	4–10

Source: From G. E. Cartwright, J. W. Athens, and M. M. Wintrobe, *Blood* 24(1964): 780.

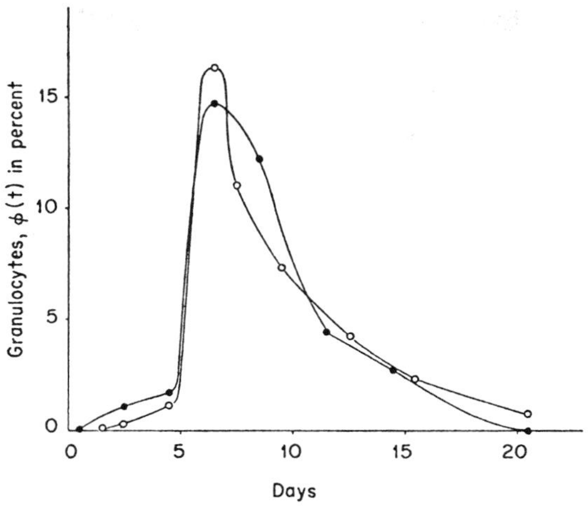

Fig. 17.4
Time course of blood granulocyte radioactivity after in vivo labeling with inorganic ^{32}P in two subjects. (Modified from J. Ottesen, *Acta Physiol. Scand.* 32(1954): 75)

cytes, this methodology provides further confirmation of a $T_{1/2}$ of 7 hr and a 9–10-day interval between early precursor and adult neutrophil.

2. Normal production of granulocytes

One view of granulocyte kinetics postulates a series of concatenated stem cell (i.e., α cell) compartments (figure 17.5). The diagram illustrates two important transitions: the myelocyte → metamyelocyte transition and the marrow granulocyte → blood granulocyte transition, in which labeled marrow cells become labeled blood cells. An earlier transition (initial pluripotential stem cell → maturation series) is equally important, but is less accessible experimentally.

a. Myelocyte → metamyelocyte transition

In the myelocyte → metamyelocyte transition, cells labeled in the proliferating (DNA-synthesizing) compartment move into the nonproliferating compartment as a consequence of serial divisions of myelocytes. Myelocyte divisions are thought to cease after a time, possibly due to accumulation of cytoplasmic inhibitors. There is evidence favoring three models of the myelocyte → metamyelocyte transition: an α → 2α model, an α → 2n model, and an α → α,n model. (These models are explained in lecture 1.) The scheme in figure 17.5A views the transition as an α → α,n model.

Myelocyte production is probably in excess of that represented by the myelocytes entering the metamyelocyte compartment. Excess myelocytes presumably die in the marrow. Hence, a significant amount of ineffective granulopoiesis may occur normally. This model, which remains to be validated, suggests that marrow provides granulocytes quickly on demand, first by dump-

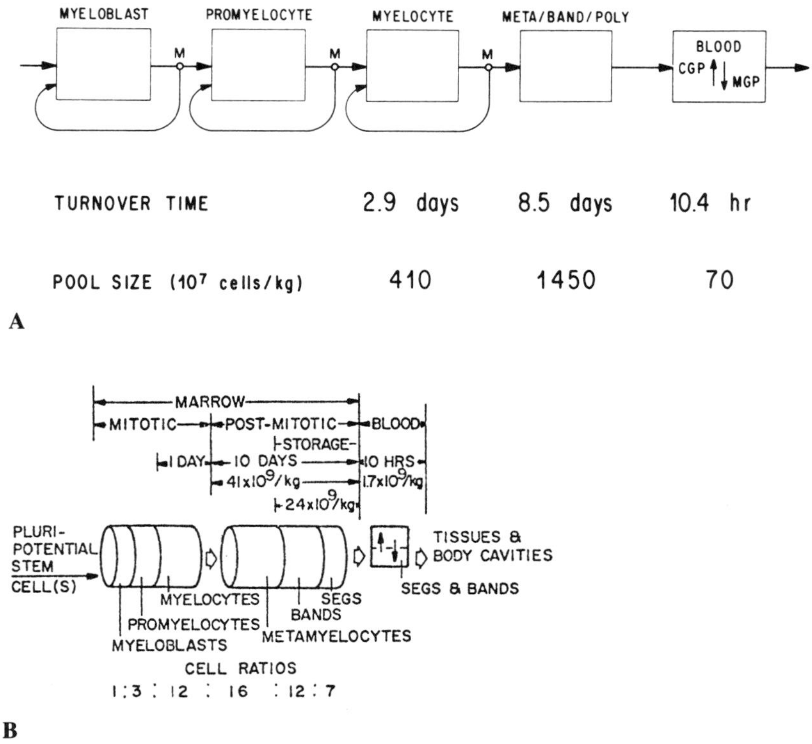

Fig. 17.5
Current models of granulopoiesis: *A,* model according to Cartwright. M denotes a mitotic division. (Modified from G. Cartwright et al., Blood, 24, 780, 1964). *B,* model according to Boggs, (From D. Boggs, *Semin. Hematol.* 4(1976): 359)

ing cells from the marrow granulocyte reserve into the circulation and second by increasing production at the myelocyte level. The latter would have no effect on the blood granulocyte count until after completion of the metamyelocyte and band stages.

b. Marrow granulocyte reserve

The term *marrow granulocyte reserve* was first used to denote the mature granulocytes that were promptly released from marrow in response to *leukapheresis,* an experimental procedure in which massive numbers of circulating granulocytes are removed. In a clinical context, the reserve is the readily mobilizable granulocytes released from marrow in response to an administered test dose of endotoxin. This procedure employs Pyrexal®, a purified pyrogenic lipopolysaccharide from *Salmonella abortus equi.* Following intravenous injection of Pyrexal®, the granulocyte count first drops (in 1–2 hr), then rises by 3,000–5,000 mature cells within 4–5 hr. A smaller response and/or a significant "shift to the left" indicates a decreased granulocyte reserve. The initial drop is due to a shift of CGP cells into the MGP. The rise is due to a reverse shift *and* to an outpouring of marrow reserves. When reserves are depleted, the marrow becomes devoid of mature granulocytes. This marrow pattern is often mistakenly called "maturation arrest."

The reserve, which is shown diagrammatically as the postmyelocyte compartments in figure 17.5, has been estimated to contain 650–1,600 cells $\times$ 10^7/kg. If normal daily granulocyte consumption is 167 cells $\times$ 10^7/kg, the reserve would represent a 4–10-day supply.

c. Release from marrow

The blood granulocyte count is nearly constant in normal subjects. This constancy is achieved in part by two regulatory feedback loops—a slow one that controls entrance of stem cells into the granulopoietic pathway and a fast one that controls release of stored granulocytes from marrow into blood. Cyclic changes in the blood granulocyte count (cyclic neutropenia) may occur when the two loops are operating dyssynchronously.

d. Humoral control revisited

As noted in lecture 1, current evidence suggests that differentiation of pluripotent stem cells into presursor cells committed to granulopoiesis is influenced by humoral agents variously known as *colony-stimulating factor, CSF,* or *leukopoietin,* or *granulopoietin,* a major source of which is a membrane fraction of blood leukocytes or cells of the mononuclear phagocyte series. CSF is also present in modest amounts in serum and urine and various other tissues.

As discussed in lecture 1, granulopoiesis in culture is inhibited by various substances present in normal serum. It should be emphasized that although the CSFs and the other agents just mentioned have interesting in vitro effects, there is still no *direct* evidence on the role of CSF in vivo. Nonetheless, the provocative speculative model in figure 17.6 suggests a scheme for control of both granulocytes and monocytes. It suggests that low CSF levels favor monocyte production and high levels favor granulocyte production. More will be said on monocytes and their production in lecture 18.

e. Fate of granulocytes

The rate of egress of granulocytes from blood into tissues is another factor that determines the granulocyte count. Granulocytes apparently leave the blood on a random basis, though a few may disappear when senescent. The disposition of neutrophils is not known with certainty. In normal subjects, many appear in bronchial and intestinal secretions.

C. Biochemistry

1. Commonplace features

Granulocytes possess most of the major anabolic and catabolic pathways and cell constituents of other body cells, among which are lipids of diverse types, glycogen, sialic acid, amino acids, nucleic acids, trace metals, and other components. They contain the

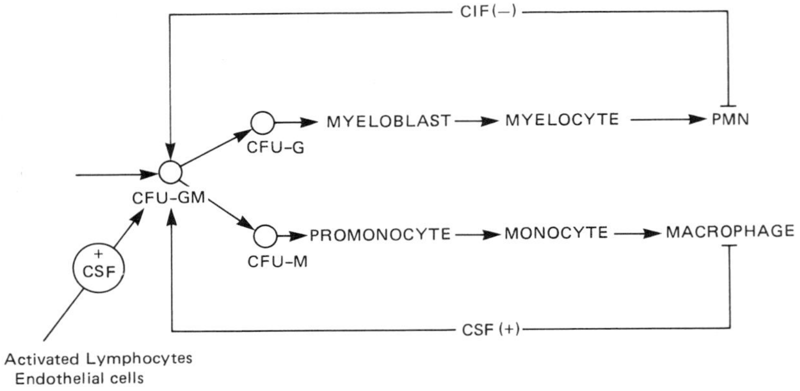

Fig. 17.6
Neutrophils and monocytes are derived from a progenitor cell, which can be identified in culture as a cell that gives rise to colonies containing neutrophils and monocytes or macrophages. This cell, the CFU-GM, differentiates into CFU-G and CFU-M, which give rise to fully differentiated neutrophils and monocytes/macrophages, respectively. Stimulating factors which cause proliferation of these progenitors are referred to as CSF and are elaborated by stimulated lymphocytes, macrophages, and endothelial cells. CIF or colony-inhibiting factors are putative hormones which prevent the proliferation of neutrophil and macrophage progenitors and may be derived from mature neutrophils. The physiologic relevance of these factors is controversial, and their regulation is incompletely understood.

major coenzymes and actively reduce folic acid. As noted in lecture 4, they contain a vitamin B_{12}-binding R-protein. When found in the plasma, it is known as transcobalamin III.

2. Distinctive features

In addition, granulocytes have many unusual biochemical features, among them a rich endowment of lysosomes and associated hydrolytic enzymes, a relatively high content of zinc, and an inability to perform the early steps of de novo purine synthesis. Apolactoferrin, a powerful iron-binding protein in granulocyte lysosomes, may inhibit the growth of iron-requiring bacteria by chelating iron.

Some of the following biochemical features are helpful in clinical diagnosis.

a. Aerobic glycolysis

Granulocytes depend largely on aerobic glycolysis for their energy supply. The tricarboxylic acid cycle occurs in these cells, but, as would be anticipated from the paucity of mitochondria, it is relatively feeble. There is a modest Pasteur effect. These metabolic features became a center of controversy following Warburg's early demonstration that many types of cancer cells possess a higher rate of aerobic glycolysis and a weaker Pasteur effect than normal cells. He concluded that these changes were both diagnostic criteria and causal mechanisms of the neoplastic state. With the discovery of exceptions—normal tissues with similar characteristics (e.g., retina, kidney medulla, jejunal mucosa, and leukocytes) and tumors without them (e.g., minimal deviation hepatomas)—it became clear that the "cancer pattern" of metabolism lacks specificity.

b. HMP shunt pathway

The hexose monophosphate (HMP) shunt pathway is active in circulating leukocytes. As will be discussed in lecture 18, this pathway is stimulated during phagocytosis.

c. Alkaline phosphatase

Leukocyte alkaline phosphatase (LAP), an enzyme closely associated with neutrophilic granules, is readily measured by a quantitative chemical method or a semiquantitative histochemical method. LAP is of interest because activity levels are distinctively altered in disease, as will be discussed later. The leukocytes of chronic myelocytic leukemia are low in LAP. In contrast, those of physiological leukocytosis, myeloid metaplasia, and polycythemia vera are usually high in LAP. LAP levels are increased by pituitary-adrenal activity, the increase appearing only in newly formed cells.

d. Myeloperoxidase

The enzyme, which accounts for the green color of pus and is sometimes called verdoperoxidase, catalyzes the following reactions:

$$H_2O_2 \rightarrow [O] + H_2O, \qquad AH_2 + [O] \rightarrow A + H_2O,$$

where AH_2 is an oxidizable substrate such as benzidine or guaiac. The physiological role of myeloperoxidase will be discussed in lecture 18. Its presence in cells has been used as an indicator that they are members of the myeloid series.

e. Lysozyme (muramidase)

Lysozyme (muramidase) is a powerful hydrolase that is associated with the lysosomes of granulocytes and monocytes. Its level is especially high in leukemic granulocytes and monocytes. When these cells break down in large numbers, serum and urine lysozyme levels become elevated.

f. Cathepsins and plasminogen

Granulocyte cathepsins and other proteases participate in the digestion of fibrin. Granulocyte plasminogen may participate in the initiation of fibrinolysis.

D. Physiologic functions

1. Phagocytosis

The main functions of granulocytes—chemotaxis, phagocytosis, and microbial killing—are discussed in detail in lecture 18.

2. Granulocytes and the plasma kinins

The plasma kinin system consists of a group of polypeptides of low molecular weight (*kinins*). Granulocytes leak a substance that, in the presence of the coagulation factor called Hageman factor (see lecture 26), yields active *kallikrein,* which converts plasma *kininogen* (an α_2 globulin) to one of the prototype kinins, *bradykinin*. Kinins increase vascular permeability, cause local vasodilatation and pain, are chemotactic, and may be responsible for margination of granulocytes along walls of small vessels early in inflammation. This may be one of the several mechanisms for attracting granulocytes to sites of injury or bacterial invasion. Granulocytes are attracted to sites of kinin production, where initially they promote further kinin production. As they accumulate and break down, they eventually destroy kinin. Thus inflammation has two phases: (1) kinin causes local effects (pain, vasodilation, capillary permeability, and chemotaxis); and (2) then granulocytes accumulate as local kinin concentration decreases.

Corticosteroids are believed to exert their anti-inflammatory effect by stabilizing lysosome membranes and preventing release of chemotactic and cytotoxic substances and inhibiting migration of cells to inflammatory sites.

3. Pyrogens and fever

Pyrogen, the fever-producing substance, is believed to be a cationic protein arising from granulocyte and monocyte lysosomes. More of it is present in exudate granulocytes than in circulating granulocytes. Granulocyte pyrogen is probably not the only cause of fever since fever occurs in diseases (like acute lymphocytic leukemia) in which granulocytes are lacking.

E. Antibodies to neutrophils and other granulocytes

1. Heterologous antibodies

Antigens on neutrophils include those shared with other body cells, notably the HLA antigens, and those specific for neutrophils. It has been known since the time of Metchnikoff (1899) that injection of leukocytes into animals of another species elicits antisera that may have relatively little species specificity. For example, guinea pig antiox leukocyte serum may be active as well against rabbit leukocytes. Nevertheless such antibodies appear cell-type specific. Thus, an antineutrophil serum may have little effect on monocytes or basophils. Such results indicate marked antigenic differences among leukocyte types.

2. Alloantibodies

Leukocyte alloantibodies have been described that are related to a system of leukocyte antigens resembling the blood group antigens of erythrocytes (lecture 15). Leukocyte and erythrocyte systems are unrelated, however. Many different leukocyte antigens are now known. Leukocyte alloantibodies are agglutinins. They gain importance because they provide (1) a source of possible severe immune reactions after pregnancy with fetomaternal leukocyte incompatibility (with resulting neonatal alloimmune neutropenia if maternal antibodies elicited by paternal antigens cross the placenta); (2) a cause of the febrile nonhemolytic transfusion reactions occurring after multiple transfusions; and (3) a reason for poor survival of transfused granulocytes.

3. Autoantibodies

Leukoagglutinins are occasionally found in sera of leukopenic subjects who never received a transfusion and who therefore are said to have idiopathic autoimmune neutropenia. They are also found in hematologically normal subjects.

The area is controversial because of the uncertain relation to leukopenia in individual patients and the difficulties of distinguishing autoantibodies and alloantibodies.

4. Antinuclear antibodies

Serum may contain antibodies to nuclear material. A number of antibodies of this type have been found with specificity for DNA, whole nucleoprotein, or other nuclear constituents. Antibody to nucleoprotein is the basis of the *LE (lupus erythematosus) cell test*.

5. Drug-induced antibodies

Although many drugs appear to cause immune neutropenia, the laboratory evidence of an immune mechanism is often sketchy. The famous example of aminopyrine neutropenia is discussed in lecture 19.

F. Eosinophils

Eosinophils are easily recognized by their characteristic staining pattern. Their large granules are rich in a distinctive type of peroxidase. On electron microscopy, they display a crystalloid core that contains the *major basic protein* (MBP) of eosinophils, a functionally important protein of mol. wt. 10,800. When large numbers of eosinophils disintegrate in secretions or exudate, the crystalloids remain intact and may come together to form large particles known as *Charcot-Leyden crystals*.

Until recently, the functions of eosinophils were unknown. There has been a recent upsurge of interest and it is now agreed that the eosinophil is a highly specialized offshoot of the granulocyte series. Eosinophils (and basophils) appear to participate in virtually every form of immunologic tissue injury, yet mechanisms remain unclear.

Two attributes appear to distinguish eosinophils from neutrophils and other leukocytes: (1) an ability to inactivate mediators released from mast cells (see below) and thereby modulate or damp down reactions associated with IgE-mediated degranulation of mast cells, e.g., the anaphylactic reaction and immediate hypersensitivity (in the vicinity of which eosinophils accumulate); and (2) an ability to control parasitic infestations. For example, recent work has shown in vitro that isolated eosinophils, unlike neutrophils, kill schistosomula, the larvae of *Schistosoma mansoni,* in an antibody-dependent, complement-independent process.

This reaction is largely due to the release of MBP onto the surface of the parasite.

The major clinical conditions associated with *eosinophilia* (i.e., elevated eosinophil count) are listed in table 17.3. It is noteworthy that many of them are allergic states (i.e., extrinsic or allergic bronchial asthma, allergic rhinitis, etc.) and parasitic infections. They also accumulate at extravascular sites following multiple antigenic stimulation. Corticosteroids sharply decrease their numbers. This effect was the basis for an early assay of glucocorticoid effects.

G. Basophils

Basophils, the least common blood granulocytes, are members of the *mast cell* family. They contain all of the blood histamine, and they degranulate in allergic reactions in which antigen-antibody reactions of the following type occur (pollen + antipollen IgE). Basophilic granules also contain heparin, hyaluronate, and serotonin. Degranulating mast cells release chemotactic agents (see lecture 18) that attract neutrophils and eosinophils. The latter may then contribute to local control of the disturbance. Basophils also play a role in the deposition of immune complexes in tissues, as well as mediating delayed hypersensitivity reactions. Basophil counts may rise in chronic myelocytic leukemia and other myeloproliferative disorders. They decrease in anaphylactic shock and severe stress. Interestingly, basophils often increase in either bone marrow or blood but not both.

III. MONOCYTES

A. Functions

As discussed briefly in lecture 2, the monocyte is the precursor of fixed and free macrophages in the tissues. Both monocytes and

Table 17.3
Clinical Conditions Often Associated with Eosinophilia

Category	Examples
Drug reactions	Iodide sensitivity, penicillin sensitivity
Allergic reactions	Asthma, angioneurotic edema, hay fever, serum sickness, vasculitis
Parasitic infestations	Amebiases, malaria, hookworm, tapeworm, ascariasis, filariasis, trichinosis
Skin diseases	Exfoliative dermatitis, pemphigus, dermatitis herpetiformis
Neoplasms	Metastatic carcinoma of lung, ovaries, and stomach, Hodgkin's disease, chronic myelocytic leukemia
"Hypereosinophilic" syndromes	Polyarteritis nodosa, eosinophilic granuloma, chronic eosinophilic pneumonia, Loeffler's syndrome
Infections	Brucellosis, tuberculosis, fungus infection, leprosy

tissue macrophages: (1) ingest and degrade dead and dying cells and other foreign particles; (2) secrete substances (i.e., CSF) that stimulate granulocyte production in the marrow; (3) remove substances from the lungs (surfactant) to allow air sacs to open more easily; (4) participate in the killing of neoplastic cells; and (5) produce angiotensin and interferon.

B. Monocytosis

The number of monocytes that can be *counted* in normal blood is given in table 17.1; however, a considerably larger number is in the marginal pool. Also the total monocyte oscillates by about 200 cells/cu mm with a periodicity of 3–6 days. The term *monocytosis* refers to the presence in blood of more than about 800 monocytes/cu mm. Among the disorders often (but not always) associated with monocytosis are: (1) infection (especially tuberculosis, endocarditis, and syphilis); (2) fever of unknown origin; (3) various forms of neoplasia and myeloproliferative disorders; (4) inflammatory disease (especially bowel disease and rheumatoid arthritis); and (5) postsplenectomy state.

IV. LYMPHOCYTES

The lymphocyte, first defined as a morphologic entity by Ehrlich in 1879 and for years neglected by investigators, has recently undergone a renaissance of interest and is now the subject of a large literature. Lymphocytes were discussed in lecture 2 and will be discussed again in lecture 23. We note here only certain highlights in the context of blood leukocytes.

A. Morphology

Lymphocytes are mononuclear cells whose cytoplasm contains no specific-staining granules. They arise from the maturation sequence displayed in figure 23.1. Maturation, as viewed in stained blood smears, consists of progressive intensification of chromatin staining and coarsening of its texture as cell and nucleus become smaller. Mature lymphocytes are rich in free ribosomes and contain a few mitochondria, a small Golgi, and a few lysosomes. Older texts divide lymphocytes into small, medium, and large types, but this is arbitrary since size varies continuously. In living wet preparations, lymphocytes have a characteristic polarized mobility that give them a "hand mirror" appearance.

Lymphocyte maturation occurs mainly in lymph nodes, spleen, and scattered lymphoid tissues throughout the body, some of which are in the marrow. About 5% of the cells in the marrow smear are lymphocytes, and occasional lymphoid nodules are seen in histologic sections of marrow.

B. Functions

An unparalleled burst of scientific progress that began in the 1950s led to important new insights about lymphocytes. Despite the morphologic uniformity long familiar to hematologists, lymphocytes are a heterogeneous population with diverse functions of interest to immunologists. Their main role is in various immunologic reactions.

In summary T lymphocytes are mainly concerned with cellular immunity, immunological memory, and the production of antigen-reaction cells. At least one subpopulation of T cells (*helper cells*) augments antibody production under some circumstances; others (*suppressor cells*) modulate the humoral immune response; still others (*cytotoxic* or *killer cells*) kill specific targets on contact. T lymphocytes are activated by interaction with antigen. They undergo blast transformation, proliferate, and release a variety of nonimmunoglobulin humoral effector substances (called *lymphokines*)—among them *transfer factor, chemotactic factor, migration inhibition factor,* and *lymphotoxin*. These agents mediate immune responses by exerting cytotoxic effects, promoting complement activation, and attracting macrophages.

B lymphocytes mediate humoral immunity. However, most (but not all) antigens cannot stimulate B lymphocytes to proliferate and produce antibody until they have been processed by other cells—neutrophils, monocyte-macrophages, or T lymphocytes themselves acting as helpers.

SELECTED REFERENCES

Bainton, D. F., and Farquhar, M. G. — Origin of granules in polymorphonuclear leukocytes. Two types derived from opposite faces of the Golgi complex in developing granulocytes. *J. Cell. Biol.* 28(1966): 277.

Beck, W. S. — Leukocyte metabolism. *Series Haematologica I* 4(1968): 4.

Beck, W. S. — Biochemical properties of normal and leukemic leukocytes. In Zarafonetis, C. J. D., ed., *Proceedings of the International Symposium on Leukemia-Lymphoma,* Philadelphia: Lea and Febiger, 1968, pp. 245–269.

Blume, R. S., and Wolff, S. M. — The Chediak-Higashi syndrome: Studies in four patients and a review of the literature. *Medicine* 51(1972): 247.

Butterworth, A. E. — Eosinophil function. *New Eng. J. Med.* 304(1981): 154.

Cartwright, G. E., et al. — The kinetics of granulopoiesis in man. *Series Haematologica I* 1(1963): 1.

Golde, D. W. — Neutrophil kinetics (Part V, Section 3). In Williams, W. J., et al., eds., *Hematology,* 3d ed., New York: McGraw-Hill, 1983, pp. 759–769.

Kay, A. B. — Functions of the eosinophil leukocyte. *Brit. J. Haematol.* 33(1976): 313.

Silber, R., and Moldow, C. F. — Composition of granulocytes (Chapter 81). In Williams, W. J., et al., eds., *Hematology,* 3d ed., New York: McGraw-Hill, 1983, pp. 726–734.

Zucker-Franklin, D. — Electron microscopic studies of human granulocytes: Structural variables related to function. *Semin. Hematol.* 5(1968): 109.

LECTURE 18 Leukocytes II. Phagocytosis and its Disorders

Thomas P. Stossel

I. INTRODUCTION

Although leukocytes were discovered late in the eighteenth century, their relevance to human physiology was not appreciated until a century later, when Metchnikoff showed that they are involved in host defense against bacterial infection and in inflammation in general.

The structure, metabolism, and life cycle of neutrophils were discussed in lecture 17. In this lecture, we shall discuss another of the major phagocytic leukocytes, the monocyte, and survey aspects of the physiology of all phagocytic leukocytes that are related to their defensive functions. We shall also review qualitative disorders of these functions.

II. PHAGOCYTIC LEUKOCYTES

A. Neutrophils

As noted in lecture 17, the cytoplasm of neutrophils is filled with glycogen and granules, most of which stain poorly with Wright's stain. The granules are membrane-bound structures that resemble lysosomes. A small fraction of the total granule population contains all of the cell's content of the enzyme, myeloperoxidase, which as discussed below is relevant for its bactericidal activity. It should be noted here that myeloperoxidase-containing granules are synthesized early in neutrophil development—during the promyelocyte stage. Therefore, these granules are counted among the primary or azurophilic granules (see lecture 17). The rest of the granules, synthesized during the myelocyte stage, are the secondary or specific-staining granules.

Only when neutrophils are mature are they capable of directed locomotion and ingesting bacteria. Finding and killing bacteria invading the tissues are the major activities of neutrophils.

B. Monocytes and macrophages

1. Properties of monocytes

This cell has a lobulated nucleus with reticular chromatin strands. The monocyte is sometimes difficult to distinguish from an atypical large lymphocyte. Compared to most lymphocytes, its cytoplasm has a distinct grey hue in Wright's-stained smears, whereas lymphocyte cytoplasm stains various shades of blue. Maroon granules are occasionally present. The monocyte has fewer myeloperoxidase-containing granules than the neutrophil. It subsists primarily on aerobic glycolysis.

2. Life cycle

Monocytes arise in the bone marrow, where they mature more rapidly than neutrophils, the entire maturation process requiring approximately 24–36 hr. The monocyte sojourns in the blood for about 24–36 hr and then enters the tissues, where it may persist for long periods of time. It differentiates throughout its life span; as it does so, its size increases and its properties change. It is now recognized that monocytes are precursors of tissue macrophages, which are differentiated mononuclear phagocytes that reside in the tissues (see lecture 2).

3. Properties of macrophages

The transformation of monocyte to macrophage is accompanied by fundamental changes in cell structure and metabolism. As they become macrophages, the cells increase in size, lose their peroxidase-containing granules, and produce large quantities of lysosomes filled with acid hydrolases. The transformation is also associated wth an increase in mitochondria and an increasing dependence for energy on tricarboxylic acid cycle activity—unlike their monocytic precursors, which depend primarily on glycolysis.

Although macrophages are present in all tissues, they are especially dense in "filter" organs—liver, spleen, lung and lymph nodes—where, perched on endothelial cells and reticulum fibers, they constitute a sentry network (see lecture 2). This network, usually termed the RES, has also been referred to by recent workers as the *mononuclear phagocyte system*. Mononuclear phagocytes (monocytes and macrophages), like neutrophils, can ingest and kill bacteria (particularly pyogenic bacteria) during all phases of their life cycle. Macrophages, especially those previously activated by exposure to products of antigen-primed T lymphocytes, are more efficient in killing and ingesting bacteria than monocytes. However, the mononuclear phagocyte has many other functions. Macrophages, because of their long life, are responsible for the digestion of bacteria killed by neutrophils. They are actively pinocytic and probably play a role in normal serum protein catabolism. They also clear and digest senescent blood cells (see lecture 11). They have biosynthetic capacities and produce enormous quantities of lysozyme as well as proteins of the complement and fibrinolytic systems. Macrophages in various specific locations may have properties unique to their site and as yet undetermined local functions. As noted in lecture 17, macrophages together with lymphocytes are involved in immune responses that include programming lymphocytes for antibody formation and containment, if not killing, of so-called facultative intracellular parasites, viruses, protozoa, certain fungi, and mycobacteria.

III. MOTILE ACTIVITIES

Phagocytes must find and ingest invading microorganizms. Cytoplasmic rearrangements must occur during ingestion. These activities are similar in neutrophils and mononuclear phagocytes and are here described together.

A. Chemotaxis

The interaction between microorganisms and tissues results in the elaboration of many substances that attract phagocytes in the process known as chemotaxis. The best characterized of these are (1) a *low-molecular-weight fragment, C5a,* which is derived from the cleavage of the complement protein C5, the cleavage occurring by activation of the "classical" or "alternative" complement pathways (see lecture 12) or by direct proteolytic attack since bacteria and damaged tissue liberate nonspecific proteases; (2) *bacterial factors,* which are molecules liberated from the bacteria themselves (although not proved, it is suggested that these bacterial factors have structural similarities with synthetic *N-formyl oligopeptides,* which are potent chemotactic factors); and (3) *metabolic products of arachidonic acid,* for example, hydroxyeicosetetraenoic acid (HETE), and leukotriene B_4 (LTB_4), both of which exist in inflammatory fluids. Many other agents can attract phagocytes in vitro. Chemotactic factors must form a gradient in order to be effective. Neutrophils respond more rapidly than monocytes. Phagocytes have surface receptors for C5a and N-formyl oligopeptides, and these receptors appear to be specific and distinct. The dose-response characteristics for chemotactic responses to these agents correlate well with the binding properties of the chemotactic factors to their respective receptors on the phagocyte membranes. The immediate responses activated by the binding are unknown but might include activation of transmembrane calcium fluxes, metabolic phospholipid turnover, and the phosphorylation of intracellular proteins by protein kinases.

Chemotaxis may be assessed semiquantitatively in humans by means of the *Rebuck skin window,* which is prepared by abrading a small skin area on the volar forearm. A clean cover slip is placed over the lesion, covered with cardboard, and taped in place. The cover slip is removed and replaced at 2, 8, and 24 hours. Cover slips stained with Wright's stain show an orderly chemotactic response. The 2-hr slip normally shows mainly neutrophils (about 300); the 8-hr slip shows about 50% monocytes; and the 24-hr slip shows monocytes that have been transformed into macrophages. The skin-window response usually reflects the level of circulating neutrophils.

B. Recognition

Having arrived at the invaded site, the phagocytes must recognize what to ingest. The molecular basis of this recognition is unknown, but it is clear that many microorganisms resist recognition by virtue of their capsules. Serum interacts with these microorganisms to coat them with substances called *opsonins* (from a Greek word meaning "to prepare for dining") that render them attractive to phagocytes. The major opsonins are (1) an antibody of the IgG class that in some instances can coat objects and cause them to be ingested; (2) more commonly a combination of either IgG or IgM antibody plus complement components that causes a large fragment of the third components of complement (C3) to be deposited on the surface of bacteria, which then elicits recognition; and (3) *serum fibronectin* (cold-insoluble globulin), which binds to bacteria and other objects during coagulation of plasma. These opsonins interact with specific receptors on the phagocyte plasma membrane. In the case of IgG, the receptors recognize the Fc portion of the antibody molecule. Fc receptors appear to trigger *ingestion,* whereas C3 and fibronectin receptors are more involved with *binding* of phagocytes to objects.

C. Locomotion and ingestion

The response of phagocytes to chemotactic agents by directed locomotion and to recognizable particles by ingestion results in increased rates of energy metabolism. This fact suggests that energy in the form of ATP is involved in these activities. Also associated with locomotion and ingestion is the formation of large pseudopodia filled with *actin* filaments. These filaments are cross-linked in a gel state by *actin-binding protein* and contracted by *myosin* in the presence of calcium and ATP. Therefore, chemotactic factors and recognition factors activate locomotion and ingestion by influencing the interactions of contractile proteins, probably by altering the concentrations of ionized calcium in the peripheral cytoplasm.

D. Degranulation

During ingestion, pseudopods flow around the bacteria being eaten and encase them within membrane-bound phagocytic vacuoles. The cytoplasmic granules fuse with these vacuoles and secrete their contents into them, simultaneously disappearing from the cytoplasm. Hence, degranulation occurs. The mechanism by which pseudopods fuse at their tips to form the phagocytic vacuole or the fusion mechanism of the granules with the vacuole is unknown.

IV. BACTERICIDAL ACTIVITIES

A. Oxygen-dependent mechanisms

During ingestion neutrophils and mononuclear phagocytes actively metabolize oxygen to produce reactive products that are toxic to ingested bacteria. Recent evidence indicates that the activation of mononuclear phagocytes by products elaborated by lymphoid cells, a consequence of which is heightened ability of macrophages to kill intracellular parasites, may involve the induction of these oxygen-metabolizing mechanisms in the macrophage. The exact nature or location of the oxidase(s) that catalyze this reaction is unknown, but reduced pyridine nucleotides (e.g., NADPH) provide the necessary reducing power. There is evidence that the enzyme contains flavin and a b-type cytochrome. The oxygen metabolites are the following.

1. Superoxide anion

Superoxide anion (O_2^-) is the first reduction product of oxygen. It is a highly reactive substance that is further reduced to hydrogen peroxide, especially at acid pH. It is also available for reoxidation to oxygen in the presence of a suitable agent. Such an agent is nitrobule tetrazolium (NBT), a redox dye that concomitantly becomes reduced to a blue formazan. Measurement of the reduction of NBT to formazan provides a method for detecting activation of oxygen metabolism during ingestion.

2. Hydrogen peroxide

Hydrogen peroxide (H_2O_2) is the product of oxygen metabolism that is probably most important for bactericidal activity by phagocytes. Hydrogen peroxide can react with superoxide to produce the highly reactive *hydroxyl radical* (OH·) as:

$$O_2 + H_2O_2 \rightarrow O_2 + OH^- + OH\cdot$$

The antibacterial action of hydrogen peroxide is potentiated by the enzyme myeloperoxidase, which is delivered into the phagocytic vacuole by degranulation. Halides are cofactors for this potentiation, chloride most likely being the physiologically relevant participant. The reaction of hydrogen peroxide, myeloperoxidase, and chloride produces toxic *hypochlorous acid* (HOCl) and also toxic chloramines. Macrophages lack myeloperoxidase but may have other ways for potentiating the effects of hydrogen peroxide. Lysozyme, also delivered from granules, potentiates the bactericidal action of hydrogen peroxide in the presence of ascorbic acid and certain metals.

B. Detoxification of oxygen metabolites

These highly reactive substances are detrimental to both microbes and animal cells. Control of them is achieved in phagocytes by (1) *localization* of superoxide and hydrogen peroxide to the phagocytic vacuole; (2) the enzyme *superoxide dismutase,* which rapidly converts superoxide diffusing from vacuole to cytoplasm into hydrogen peroxide in the following reaction:

$$O_2^- + O_2^- + 2H^+ \rightarrow H_2O_2 + O_2;$$

(3) the enzyme *catalase,* which destroys hydrogen peroxide in the cytoplasm; and (4) *reduced glutathione* (GSH), which in destroying hydrogen peroxide activates the series of coupled enzymatic reactions shown in diagram 18.1. Note that GSH-mediated hydrogen peroxide catabolism regenerates NADPH, a possible substrate for oxidase-mediated hydrogen peroxide production.

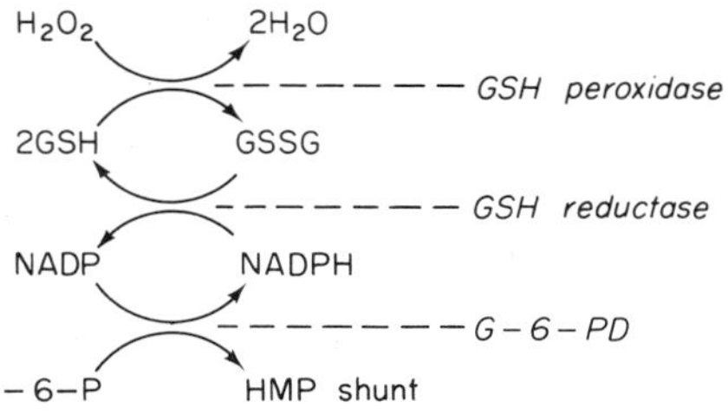

Diagram 18.1

C. Oxygen-independent mechanisms

A number of oxygen-independent factors are damaging to various types of ingested bacteria. One is the *acid pH* of the phagocytic vacuole. Another is *lysozyme,* which hydrolyzes the mucopeptide cell wall of a few microbial species. *Bactericidal proteins* delivered to the phagocytic vacuole during degranulation can kill bacteria by altering the permeability of their membranes.

V. QUALITATIVE DISORDERS OF PHAGOCYTIC FUNCTION

Any of the mechanisms of phagocytic action can go awry, and many examples of such disorders have been reported. When a functional impairment is serious, affected patients suffer from recurrent pyogenic infections. In some instances, the type and severity of infection can be clearly explained by the defect; in others, the correlation is not so clear. A classification of phagocytic disorders is presented in table 18.1.

A. Disorders of chemotaxis and opsonization

Since synergistic activity of antibody and complement components leads to elaboration of chemotactic factors and coating of bacteria with opsonins, it is not surprising that recurrent infections are associated with deficiencies of relevant serum proteins or the presence of agents that prevent complement activation. Thus, patients with antibody deficiency syndromes and complement disorders often have recurrent bacteremias, meningitis, and sinopulmonary infections. The offending organisms are usually high-grade encapsulated pathogens, streptococci, pneumococci, neisseria, *Haemophilus influenzae,* and species of *Pseudomonas.* Specific examples of these deficiency states include (1) congenital agammaglobulinemia; (2) acquired agammaglobulinemia or hypogammaglobulinemia (sometimes associated with multiple myeloma or lymphoproliferative disorders, in which immunoglobulin may be plentiful but useful antibody is depleted); (3) genetic deficiency of C3; and (4) acquired deficiency of C3 and other complement proteins in systemic lupus erythematosus, advanced liver disease, and immune complex diseases.

B. Disorders of locomotion and ingestion

In the following examples, phagocytes are unable to respond to chemotactic factors or opsonins.

Table 18.1
Some Disorders of Phagocytosis

	Cells affected		
Function affected	Neutrophil	Mononuclear phagocytes	Both
Mobilization	Neutropenia		Marrow ablation
Chemotaxis	Neutrophil actin dysfunction; Deficiency of adhesion molecules		Antibody deficiency states; Complement disorders
Opsonization			Antibody deficiency states; Complement disorders
Ingestion	Neutrophil actin dysfunction; Complement receptor deficiency	Macrophage ablation, bypass, diversion	Corticosteroid therapy
Degranulation			Chediak-Higashi syndrome
Oxygen metabolism			Chronic granulomatous disease; Myeloperoxidase deficiency

1. Patients receiving corticosteroids

Neutrophils from patients treated daily with corticosteroids in sufficient doses are impaired in their ability to migrate into inflammatory lesions and to ingest. Monocytes and macrophages from steroid-treated humans or animals also have defective ingestion capacities. The detailed mechanism of steroid action is unknown. These facts are clinically significant because they may explain why (1) steroid-treated patients or patients with Cushing's syndrome are susceptible to pyogenic infection and (2) steroids reduce inflammation and can reduce the clearance of antibody-coated cells as in immunohemolytic anemia (lecture 12) or idiopathic thrombocytopenic purpura (lecture 27).

2. Deficiency of adhesion molecules and of complement receptors

These rare genetic diseases are associated with neutrophils that stick poorly to surfaces or fail to respond to C3-coated bacteria.

3. Neutrophil actin dysfunction

This is a rare congenital disorder in which the patient's neutrophils fail to locomote or ingest because the cytoplasmic actin of neutrophils fails to polymerize into filaments. This entity helps establish a role for contractile proteins in neutrophil functions.

4. Chediak-Higashi syndrome

This rare congenital (autosomal recessive) disorder is associated with (1) neutropenia; (2) giant lysosomal granules in leukocytes (and other cells) that do not fuse normally with phagocytic vacuoles; and (3) defective chemotaxis in neutrophils and monocytes although ingestion is normal. Apparently cells cannot mobilize themselves to respond to a chemotactic gradient. Most patients succumb after entering an accelerated phase, an ill-defined febrile state associated with pancytopenia and massive hepatosplenomegaly. This was also discussed in lecture 17.

5. Macrophage disorders

The infections encountered in the following group of diverse disorders are similar to those seen in patients with humoral disorders.

a. Bypass

Cirrhosis of the liver can produce shunting of portal blood around the macrophage-rich liver. Cirrhosis is also associated wth complement deficiencies. Cardiac shunts may cause systemic venous blood to bypass lung macrophages.

b. Ablation

Splenectomy is associated with a small but finite risk of serious sepsis (see lecture 2).

c. Diversion

Diseases in which macrophages are heavily engaged in ingesting damaged erythrocytes, for example, sickle cell anemia or thalassemia major, are associated with an increased incidence of infection. Adult patients with sickle cell anemia also have asplenia (see lecture 9).

C. Disorders of bactericidal activity

1. Chronic granulomatous disease

This congenital disease is inherited either as an X-linked or autosomal recessive trait. Neutrophils and monocytes do not metabolize oxygen to superoxide or hydrogen peroxide. In most cases, this failure seems to be due to inactivity or lack of the oxidase(s) that metabolizes oxygen. In rare instances, neutrophils totally lacking G-6-PD cannot metabolize oxygen since the reduced pyridine nucleotide substrates of the oxidase(s) are not regenerated.

There are several consequences of the failure of phagocytes to metabolize oxygen. First, affected phagocytes do not kill certain microorganisms that are catalase-positive and thereby capable of destroying hydrogen peroxide produced by their own metabolic processes. Common catalase-positive organisms include *Staphylococcus aureus,* most gram-negative enteric organisms, and many fungi. Catalase-negative organisms, for example, streptococci, pneumonocci, and certain *Haemophilus* species, accumulate hydrogen peroxide in the narrow confines of phagocytic vacuoles that in synergy with granule-derived myeloperoxidase cause their death—in a sense, a form of suicide. Patients with chronic granulomatous disease suffer from recurrent skin, bone, and visceral infections with catalase-positive organisms.

Since affected neutrophils do not metabolize oxygen, metabolic reactions caused by the presence of oxygen metabolites are not activated during ingestion; for example, NBT is not reduced and HMP shunt activity is not increased. The failure to find enhancement of these reactions during ingestion is diagnostic of the disease. Mothers of boys with the X-linked form of the disease have a defective population of cells, in accordance with the Lyon hypothesis.

2. Myeloperoxidase deficiency

This is a rare autosomal recessive disorder in which neutrophils and monocytes (but not eosinophils) totally lack myeloperoxidase. Some patients with myeloproliferative disorders develop an acquired partial myeloperoxidase deficiency. The phagocytes have a bactericidal defect demonstrable in vitro since they lack an agent that potentiates the bactericidal activity of hydrogen peroxide. The defect is less severe than that of chronic granulomatous disease phagocytes. Moreover, most "patients" with myeloperoxidase deficiency are not unduly susceptible to infection. The disorder is important because it provides a model for demonstrating the role of myeloperoxidase in antimicrobial activity.

D. Phagocytes as mediators of inflammation

During ingestion of microbes, phagocytes may spill potent toxins into the surrounding medium. Proteases and the oxygen metabolites, in addition to injuring neighboring cells, can cleave serum proteins to generate chemotactic factors, thereby propagating the reaction. Therefore phagocytes have the capacity to be detrimental as well as helpful to the host. Tissue damage in diverse diseases such as acute glomerulonephritis, rheumatoid arthritis, silicosis, and gout may be phagocyte mediated. It is even possible that the oxidants generated by phagocytes alter genes in normal cells, thus predisposing to mutations and cancer.

E. Clinical approach

1. Diagnosis

The type of disorder can be inferred from the history and documented by (1) measurements of levels of serum immunoglobulins and complement; (2) assay of neutrophil migration and ingestion; and (3) assay of neutrophil oxygen metabolism.

2. Therapy

Therapy occasionally can be specific—for example, gamma globulin in antibody deficiency states. Usually it involves only vigilance and aggressive therapy of specific infections. Granulocyte transfusions are available in some medical centers and may be helpful in extreme cases.

SELECTED REFERENCES

Arnaout, M. A., et al. Deficiency of a granulocyte-membrane glycoprotein (gp 150) in a boy with recurrent infections. *New Eng. J. Med.* 306(1982): 693.

Badwey, J. A., and Karnovsky, M. L. Active oxygen species and the functions of phagocytic leukocytes. *Ann. Rev. Biochem.* 49(1980): 695.

Babior, B. M. The respiratory burst of phagocytes. *J. Clin. Invest.* 73(1984): 599.

Gallin, J. I., et al. Recent advances in chronic granulomatous disease. *Ann. Int. Med.* 99(1983): 657.

Nathan, C. F. Secretion of oxygen intermediates: Role in effector functions of activated macrophages. *Fed. Proc.* 41(1982): 2206.

Southwick, F. S., and Stossel, T. P. Contractile proteins in leukocyte function. *Semin. Hematol.* 20(1983): 305.

Tauber, A. I. Current views of neutrophil dysfunction. *Am. J. Med.* 70(1981): 1237.

Michl, J., et al. Modulation of Fc receptors of mononuclear phagocytes. *J. Exp. Med.* 157(1983): 1746.

Bainton, D. F. Selective abnormalities of azurophil and specific granules of human neutrophilic leukocytes. *Fed. Proc.* 40(1981): 1443.

Ward, P. A., et al. Evidence for role of hydroxyl radical in complement and neutrophil-dependent tissue injury. *J. Clin. Invest.* 72(1983): 789.

Unanue, E. R., et al. Antigen presentation. *J. Immunol.* 132(1984): 1.

Zigmond, S. H., et al. Kinetic analysis of chemotactic peptide receptor modulation. *J. Cell. Biol.* 92(1982): 34.

LECTURE 19 Leukocytes III. Introduction to Pathology

William S. Beck

I. DISEASES OF GRANULOCYTES

A number of themes recur in this necessarily brief survey of the diseases of granulocytes: (1) the fact that a disorder makes a prominent display of an elevated or decreased leukocyte count does not imply that other formed elements are uninvolved; (2) some of the disorders to be discussed closely resemble one another (or evolve into one another), and diagnostic acumen may be needed to sort them out; (3) in general, the disorders to be discussed may be divided into those involving an essentially physiologic response (or reaction) to an outside insult and those involving "spontaneous" abnormal proliferation; and (4) pathophysiological mechanisms of major granulocyte disorders parallel those of red cell and platelet disorders in many cases. We shall begin our review of the several categories of granulocyte disorders at the "reactive" end of the spectrum and work toward the "proliferative" end. (The qualitative granulocyte disorders of phagocytic function were discussed in lecture 18.)

A. Leukocytosis

1. Neutrophilic leukocytosis

Physiologic *leukocytosis* is the classic instance of reactive behavior by leukocytes. It is a normal response to a noxious stimulus. The term is usually applied when the leukocyte count exceeds 10,000/mm^3. *Granulocytosis* refers to an increase in circulating neutrophilis, bands, and, less frequently, metamyelocytes. By common usage, the term does not imply an increase in other granule-containing cells (eosinophils or basophils). The term *neutrophilia* is somewhat less ambiguous, denoting an increase only in neutrophils. Granulocytosis is perhaps the most commonly encountered disorder in clinical medicine. Its principal causes are summarized in table 19.1.

Table 19.1
Common Causes of Physiologic Leukocytosis

Category	Example
Bacterial infections	Especially with pyogenic bacteria, either localized (as in appendiceal abscess) or generalized (as in septicemia)
Inflammation or tissue necrosis	Infarction, myositis, vasculitis
Intoxications	Uremia, eclampsia, acidosis, gout
Neoplasms	Bronchogenic carcinoma, lymphoma, melanoma
Other conditions	Acute hemorrhage or hemolysis, especially in children, postsplenectomy state

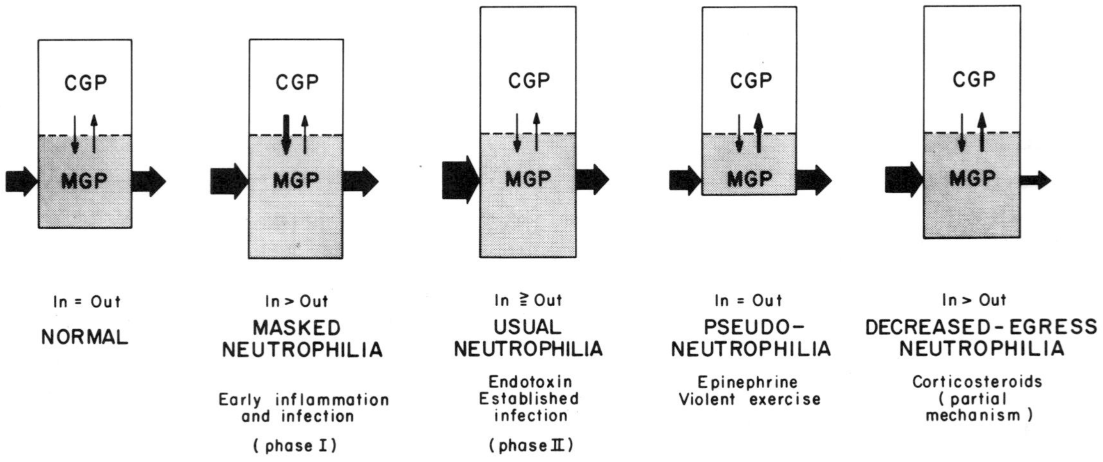

Fig. 19.1
Mechanisms of neutrophilia.

a. Mechanisms

The system of granulocyte production and release, described in lecture 17, is remarkable for its capacity not only to maintain uniformity (despite minor diurnal variations) of the blood granulocyte count in normal subjects but to pour out granulocytes in the presence of infection or stress. A demand for granulocytes imposed by peripheral bacterial invasion is met at first by the egress into the tissue of cells from the MGP. Release of bone marrow reserves is then accelerated. Finally, there is an increased rate of myeloid cell proliferation in the marrow. These additions of new circulating granulocytes are reflected in the blood by a "shift to the left"—that is, a rise in the ratio of nonsegmented to segmented neutrophils. The mechanism of transmission of information to the marrow from the periphery is unknown. It is assumed to involve the feedback loops discussed earlier.

b. Phases

Labeling studies show that leukocytosis of infection or inflammation has at least three phases (figure 19.1). In the *phase of early infection*, (1) release of granulocytes by marrow increases (hence, blood granulocytes "shift to the left"); (2) circulating cells marginate, so that MGP rises before CGP; (3) if egress of cells to tissue exceeds input from marrow, the leukocyte count may decrease (as discussed below under neutropenia); and (4) since circulating cells are marginating, infused cells labeled with $DF^{32}P$ are diluted by newly released unlabeled cells. A $T_{1/2}$ at this time is short, perhaps 2 or 3 hr (normal, 7 hr). Because TBGP is increased in this phase without an increase in leukocyte count, the picture may be termed *masked neutrophilia*.

In the *phase of established infection*, (1) pools equilibrate, so that CGP equals MGP; (2) input from marrow comes to equal output to tissues, though for a time it may exceed output; and (3) the number of granulocyte precursors in marrow increases markedly. During this phase the $T_{1/2}$ of circulating leukocytes is normal.

In the *phase of recovery*, (1) release of cells from marrow decreases sharply; (2) $T_{1/2}$ of circulating granulocytes is prolonged because no new unlabeled cells are being admixed with labeled cells; (3) "shift to the left" disappears; and (4) the leukocyte count subsides to normal. An alternative third phase (to be discussed below) occurs in overwhelming infection. Although the myeloid portion of the marrow has become grossly hyperplastic, reserves are exhausted and neutropenia (i.e., decreased neutrophil count) results. Neutropenia in the course of infection is a poor prognostic sign.

c. Clinical features

Abnormal clinical features associated with leukocytosis include: (1) "shift to the left" in blood leukocytes; (2) toxic granulation and Döhle bodies; (3) fever, due to leukocyte pyrogen; and (4) elevation of LAP (figure 19.2).

2. Other mechanisms of leukocytosis

a. Pseudoneutrophilia

Kinetic studies show that cells from the MGP may reenter the CGP en masse in response to certain vasodynamic states (e.g., violent exercise, epinephrine). The leukocyte count thus may

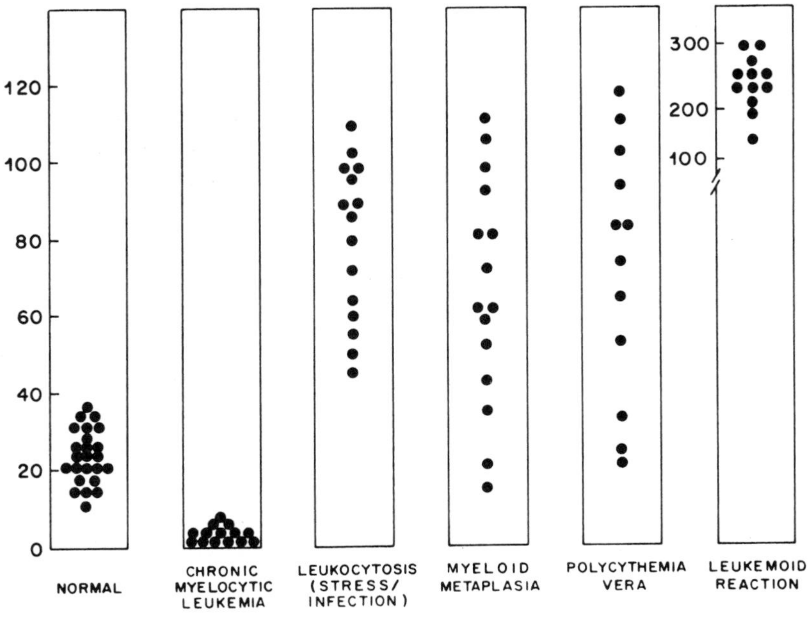

Fig. 19.2
Leukocyte alkaline phosphatase in health and disease. Ordinate, mg P liberated (from β-glycerophosphate) per 10^{10} leukocytes per hour.

be quickly doubled, the rise being independent of increased granulopoiesis as indicated by the fact that it is not prevented by cytotoxic drugs or radiation. The leukocyte count rises by this mechanism in stressful situations (e.g., paroxysmal tachycardia, intense emotion, anesthesia). The pattern is termed *pseudoneutrophilia* because input, output, and TBGP remain normal.

b. Decreased-egress neutrophilia

Administration of pharmacological doses of corticosteroids produces neutrophilia by the following two mechanisms: (1) increasing the release of granulocytes from marrow; and (2) decreasing the egress of granulocytes from blood. Skin-window studies show that in inflammation, corticosteroids decrease the number of leukocytes in inflammatory exudates relative to controls. This partially accounts for the rise in leukocyte count that accompanies stress and steroid administration. These findings also explain in part the seriousness of bacterial infections that accompany steroid therapy in certain patients. Also, it suggests that steroids may be inappropriate therapy in neutropenia simply because they sometimes raise the leukocyte count.

c. Asplenia

Moderate neutrophilia invariably follows loss of the spleen due to surgery or disease. It is presumably the result of persistent circulation of neutrophils that normally are transiently detained in the spleen rather than increased granulopoiesis.

B. "In-between" conditions

1. Leukemoid reaction

A leukemoid reaction is an excessive (but reactive) outpouring of leukocytes with the appearance of immature forms (blasts, myelocytes, metamyelocytes)—hence the term *leukemoid* and the need to distinguish the leukemoid reaction from leukemia. It occurs in response to infectious, toxic, inflammatory, or neoplastic disorders. It may be acute or chronic and rarely lymphocytic. The mechanism is unknown.

Major associated diseases are severe or chronic infection, especially in children; severe hemolysis; and various solid tumors (especially of breast, kidney and lung, and metastatic cancer). The total leukocyte count is typically 50,000–100,000/mm^3. The cells display prominent toxic granulations, and the LAP is extremely high. The high LAP and lack of the so-called Philadelphia (Ph^1) chromosomes are usually adequate to distinguish leukemoid reactions from chronic myelocytic leukemia (CML), as discussed in lecture 21.

Hyperleukocytosis is a variant in which an excessive leukocytosis occurs that is unaccompanied by immature forms. Its causes are similar to those of leukemoid reaction.

2. Leukoerythroblastic reaction

The term *leukoerythroblastic reaction* denotes a blood picture that resembles leukemoid reaction as regards the leukocytes but which includes the presence of substantial numbers of nucleated red cells and abnormalities in the size and shape of mature red cells. It should be noted that one may observe a few nucleated red cells (perhaps 2–3/100 white cells) in any patient with brisk reticulocytosis due, for example, to hemolysis. But patients with leukoerythroblastc reaction may have many nucleated red cells (i.e., 40–80/100 white cells) and relatively few reticulocytes.

The picture most commonly signifies *myelophthisis*, that is, invasion of bone marrow by foreign elements (see lecture 3). Common invaders are metastatic cancer (especially breast cancer), fibrosis, angiitis, granulomas of miliary tuberculosis, and leukemic cells. A leukoerythroblastic-like reaction (in which the blood contains many nucleated red cells and immature leukocytes, albeit with reticulocytosis) may occur in severe hemorrhagic or hemolytic anemias, especially in children. This form of leukoerythroblastosis occurs in the severe hemolytic anemia of the newborn, erythroblastosis fetalis (lecture 16).

C. Neutropenia

1. Definitions

Leukopenia means depression of the leukocyte count. *Neutropenia* (and its near synonym *granulocytopenia*) denotes a total neutrophil (or granulocyte) count of less than 1,500/mm^3. The absolute neutrophil count is the product of total leukocyte count and percentage of neutrophils in the differential count. *Agranulocytosis* means severe granulocytopenia. As noted below, this term has acquired a special connotation.

2. Major causes

Like anemia and thrombocytopenia, neutropenia has many causes. Though it is useful to draw analogies between the causal mechanisms of the three situations, techniques currently available for the routine study of patients with neutropenia are often imprecise or unavailable. For example, one cause of neutropenia is analogous to a cause of immunohemolytic anemia, but procedures for the detection of leukocyte antibodies are not as reliable as the Coombs test. Similarly, we lack a leukokinetic parameter that is comparable in reliability to the reticulocyte count in the area of erythrokinetics. For these reasons, understanding of neutropenia is inferior to that of anemia, and it is often more difficult to elucidate the basis of a given case of neutropenia.

In general, the classifications of anemia and thrombocytopenia are applicable to neutropenia. Neutropenia can arise from decreased production of neutrophils by marrow or accelerated removal from blood. Accelerated removal, in turn, can be due to nonimmune or immune mechanisms. Often neutropenia, anemia,

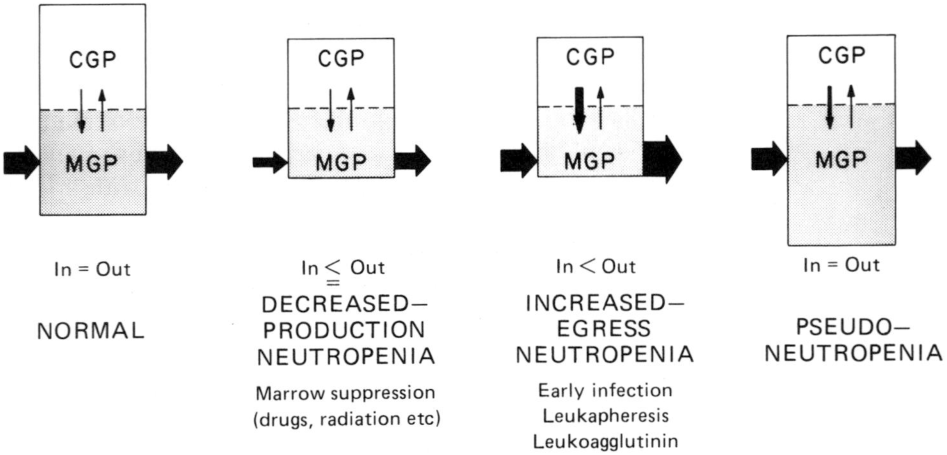

Fig. 19.3
Mechanisms of neutropenia.

and thrombocytopenia occur together (pancytopenia). The following are the major categories of neutropenia.

a. Reduced granulopoiesis

In this broad category, neutropenia is due to diminished neutrophil production in marrow. Granulopoiesis is inadequate to maintain a normal level of neutrophils, which are leaving the blood at a normal rate (figure 19.3). Major underlying causes are (1) the several kinds of aplastic anemia (see lecture 3); (2) myelophthisis from invading cancer cells, fibrosis, granulomas, and so forth (lecture 3); (3) cytotoxic chemotherapeutic agents that by intention or nonintention depress production of granulopoietic cells; and (4) ineffective granulopoiesis, such as occurs in megaloblastic anemia (see lecture 4).

In all of these instances, marrow failure results in decreased inflow of neutrophils. Eventually, there is decreased outflow. Blood neutrophils may show moderate immaturity. Marrow storage and marginal granulocyte pools are decreased, and the mobilization of neutrophils at inflammatory sites is impaired. Neutrophil survival is normal.

The main therapeutic approach to decreased-production neutropenia is to eliminate underlying or causal factors where possible. Lithium carbonate, which stimulates granulopoiesis (and causes neutrophilia in normal subjects), is sometimes used in the treatment of neutropenia and is currently under evaluation.

b. Reduced granulocyte survival

In the second major category of neutropenias, egress of neutrophils to tissues exceeds inflow from marrow (figure 19.3) or, alternatively, abnormal neutrophil destruction is taking place. Major causes are (1) early infection before inflow from marrow increases; (2) leukapheresis; (3) drug-induced leukoagglutinin (agranulocytosis); (4) complement-induced granulocyte aggregation, a recently recognized complication of hemodialysis; and (5) hypersplenism (e.g., in leukemia, lymphoma, Felty's syndrome, and LE, though in these disorders multiple factors may be depressing the leukocyte count). In these situations, increased utilization or destruction of neutrophils in blood results in increased total and effective granulopoiesis in marrow. Some immature neutrophils may enter the blood, with promyelocytes and blasts occasionally being observed. Blood neutrophil survival is short. $T_{1/2}$ after $DF^{32}P$ labeling may be as short as 20–100 min. Thus, this test may help distinguish reduced granulocyte production from reduced survival. The bone marrow contains an increased number of myeloid cells with increased immaturity. Serum leukotoxic substances and leukoagglutinins may be demonstrable. Serum lysozyme may be elevated. Neutrophilia resulting from a drug-induced antibody will be discussed further below.

c. Pseudo-neutropenia

In pseudoneutropenia, circulating (CGP) cells transfer to the MGP. As a result of increased margination—the opposite of epinephrine-induced demargination—neutrophil count decreases although the TBGP is normal. Leukokinetics are otherwise normal. Usually, these are temporary shifts due to hypersensitivity, viremia, hemolysis, or hemodynamic abnormalities. They may also be permanent and may account for some of the constitutional or familial forms of benign neutropenia mentioned in the next section.

3. Other mechanisms of neutropenia

a. Periodic or cyclic neutropenia

This curious genetic disorder (autosomal dominant with variable expression) usually begins in infancy and persists for decades. Neutropenia lasting a few days develops every 21–30 days. During the neutropenic period, fever, stomatitis, vaginitis, proctitis, and skin infections—sometimes severe—may develop, and the total monocyte count often rises. Bone marrow during neutropenia shows myeloid hypoplasia. The cause is unknown, but it is probably related to mild marrow hypoplasia that causes dyssynchrony of the two feedback loops that separately regulate granulocyte production and release (see above). The monocytosis occurring during episodes of neutrophilia may reflect operation of the regulatory system diagrammed in figure 17.6. Many mild cases probably escape detection.

b. Chronic familial neutropenias

A benign autosomal-dominant neutropenia was described by Glänsslen. An autosomal-recessive type associated with consanguinity was described by Kostmann. In this disorder, neutrophil counts are persistently low, and many patients die in early childhood of sepsis. A severe familial neutropenia of infancy was described by Hitzig.

c. Chronic idiopathic neutropenia

An apparently acquired disorder occurs in which patients have low neutrophil counts ($<1{,}000/mm^3$) but few infections. Good exudation ordinarily occurs in skin-window preparations.

d. Other syndromes

Many other neutropenic syndromes have been described, among them neutropenia associated with agammaglobulinemia and dysglobulinemia; neutropenia associated with pancreatic insufficiency; alymphocytic neutropenia; chronic neutropenia with constitutional defects; and the "normal" genetically determined neutropenia of people of African ancestry.

4. Drug-induced neutropenia

We take special notice of drug-induced neutropenia because it is increasing in frequency. Drugs can cause neutropenia by at least two major mechanisms that should be distinguished in a given patient.

a. Drug-induced depression of granulopoiesis

The first mechanism is drug-induced depression of granulopoiesis, which can be caused by (1) cytotoxic radiomimetic agents (e.g., nitrogen mustard) that do irreparable direct damage to marrow; (2) chemotherapeutic antimetabolites (e.g., cytosine arabinoside) that reversibly block cell division; (3) phenothiazine and like drugs that impair DNA synthesis in some patients; and (4) agents like chloramphenicol that idiosyncratically produce marrow aplasia (see lecture 3). The phenothiazines and an ever-growing list of comparable agents (antithyroid drugs, anticonvulsants, antibiotics, etc.) are especially frequent offenders.

When recovery begins, many promyelocytes and early myelocytes may appear, and a brisk monocytosis may herald the return of granulocytes to the blood.

b. Drug-induced leukoagglutinin

In 1922, Schultz drew attention to a syndrome of unknown etiology occurring mainly in middle-aged women in which sepsis and death followed severe sore throat, fever, prostration, and agranulocytosis. The syndrome was shown in 1934 to be associated with ingestion of aminopyrine (Pyramidon®), a widely used aromatic analgesic. About 1% of users developed neutropenia, usually within 7–10 days of the first dose. Sometimes it appeared immediately. When usage of aminopyrine decreased, the disorder became less common.

Aminopyrine-induced neutropenia has been called agranulocytosis, agranulocytic angina, pernicious leukopenia, and Schultz's syndrome. It is usual today to reserve the term *agranulocytosis* for this symptom complex. In this usage, *agranulocytosis* becomes a specific variety of "neutropenia."

The mechanism of aminopyrine-induced agranulocytosis parallels those of quinidine-induced thrombocytopenia (see lecture 27) and certain drug-induced Coombs-positive hemolytic anemias (see lecture 12). A complex between drug and leukocyte protein becomes antigenic. Antibody is elicited that is active only against the complex. In the absence of drug, the antibody remains in the plasma in inactive form. Subsequent administration of drugs to a sensitized individual activates antibody on the neutrophil surface. The result is massive leukoagglutination with pulmonary sequestration and removal of granulocytes from the circulation. Compensatory myeloid hyperplasia then occurs in the marrow. Continued drug administration leads to marrow exhaustion. Peripheral leukocyte destruction accounts for the high fever. In contrast to the situation in marrow-failure neutropenia, bone marrow shows normal erythropoiesis, normal numbers of megakaryocytes, and myeloid hyperplasia, although the more mature forms (myelocytes, metamyelocytes, bands, and polys) are missing. This pattern has been erroneously termed *maturation arrest*. Actually it is a depletion phenomenon resulting from increased peripheral destruction of granulocytes. In only a few cases has a drug-dependent antibody been clearly demonstrated. However, the recently developed staphylococcal slide test for detection of antineutrophil antibodies promises to clarify these cases in the future. This test can demonstrate opsonizing antibodies in the majority of drug-induced immunoneutropenias.

Therapy of aminopyrine neutropenia is unsatisfactory. Some cases are fatal, some become chronic, and some enter remission. The major therapeutic maneuver is withdrawal of the offending drug. Leukocyte transfusion may be helpful in certain cases.

5. Consequences of neutropenia

The major critical consequence of neutropenia is infection. The most dramatic illustration of this tendency is seen in acute drug-induced agranulocytosis. At first, there are few symptoms, but within a day or two patients develop sore throat, chills, fever, necrosis or oral mucous membranes, and bacteremia. When severe neutropenia results from leukocyte destruction, fever is due to pyrogen. Serum muramidase is commonly elevated. However, susceptibility to infection occurs with neutropenia of any cause. Vulnerability to infection becomes serious when the neutrophil count falls below 1,000/mm^3 and very serious when below 500/mm^3. An exception, as noted above, is chronic, idiopathic, benign neutropenia in which neutropenia rarely leads to infection.

D. Myeloproliferative disorders

1. Introduction

We turn now to a group of disorders in which proliferation of blood cells is not a reaction to some external insult, so far as we know. Rather, there is purposeless proliferation by one, several, or all of the marrow cell lines—granulocytes, erythrocytes, and platelets. If it be allowed that fibroblasts (or fibrocytes) are normal marrow elements, these also may proliferate to produce myelofibrosis.

The term *myeloproliferative disorder* was introduced by

Dameshek to designate a group of disorders that had previously been considered separate entities. Although based on meager evidence, the concept gave recognition to certain provocative facts. First, a marrow cell line is almost never singly affected. For example, abnormal erythrocyte proliferation is the most prominent feature of polycythemia vera. However, leukocytes and platelets almost invariably proliferate in this disease. Second, many of these disorders tend to evolve into one ahother. Polycythemia vera may eventually "turn into" myelofibrosis, myeloid metaplasia, or even leukemia. A third justification for the unitary concept of the myeloproliferative disorders is the intimate phylogenetic and embryological relations among the hematopoietic tissues. Since hematopoietic tissues derive from pluripotential cells of mesenchymal origin, it is reasonable to postulate a proliferative or neoplastic abnormality that, once under way, can proceed in one direction or another depending on factors now unknown. Recent work confirms that the myeloproliferative disorders are clonal diseases that are frequently associated with *myelofibrosis*, a reactive process that is not clonal.

Although the concept of myeloproliferative disorders is clinically and heuristically useful, one should remember that until the underlying causes of these disorders are known, the concept is little more than an intellectual convenience.

2. Clinical features

a. General pattern

All of the myeloproliferative disorders can display hyperplasia, dysplasia, or metaplasia of the bone marrow, blood cells, spleen, and other organs. Although the well-known specific disorders, to be discussed briefly below, have characteristic clinical pictures, they all display in some measure (1) signs of hypermetabolism (tissue wasting, intermittent fevers, etc.); (2) hyperuricemia; and (3) little or no tendency for spontaneous remission.

b. Specific disorders

Table 19.2 lists the several disorders that comprise the myeloproliferative syndrome group and indicates the hematopoietic cell lines primarily affected in each. Thus, it is seen that the major

Table 19.2
Cell Lines Involved in Specific Myeloproliferative Disorders

Disorder	Red cells	Granulocytes	Megakaryocytes, platelets	Fibroblasts, reticulum cells
Polycythemia vera	+ + + +	+/+ + +	+ +/+ + +	+ +
Chronic myelocytic leukemia	±	+ + +	+/+ +	−
Myeloid metaplasia	+	+ +/+ + +	+ +	+ +
Thrombocythemia	−	−	+ + + +	−
Erythremic myelosis	+ + + +	−	+	−

manifestation of polycythemia vera (to be discussed in lecture 20) is hyperplasia of red cell elements. However, the other cell lines are also involved. Prominent features of myeloid metaplasia and myelofibrosis (to be discussed below) are hyperplasia of fibroblasts and metaplasia of spleen, liver, and other tissues. In chronic myelocytic leukemia (one of several varieties of leukemia to be discussed in lecture 21), the major manifestation is hyperplasia of granulocytic elements. Hyperplasia of platelet elements predominates in thrombocythemia (to be discussed in lecture 27). In erythremic myelosis (Di Guglielmo's syndrome), the major manifestation is hyperplasia and dysplasia of red cell elements. When leukocyte elements become involved later, the disorder is called *erythroleukemia*.

3. Myeloid metaplasia

a. Introduction

It is appropriate to consider myeloid metaplasia in this lecture because granulocyte proliferation dominates the picture. (The other myeloproliferative disorders will be discussed in later lectures.) The disease complex consists of a leukoerythroblastic blood picture (i.e., immature white cells, marked changes in red cell size and shape, and presence of nucleated red cells), myeloid metaplasia (and thus extramedullary hematopoiesis) in spleen and liver, which may become very large, and variable degrees of myelofibrosis.

b. Significance of myeloid metaplasia

Myeloid metaplasia is a histologic pattern in which an extramedullary tissue comes to resemble bone marrow. Most commonly, the tissue is one that was active in hematopoiesis in embryonic life, that is, spleen, liver, and lymph nodes (see lecture 1). When tissues undergo myeloid metaplasia, they resume hematopoiesis. This occurs in at least two circumstances. One, the most common, is an increased demand for blood cells that cannot be met by marrow hyperplasia alone. This occurs commonly in young children following severe and continuing hemorrhage or hemolysis. It also occurs in certain chronic severe anemias in the adult (e.g., thalassemia). Here myeloid metaplasia is reactive. In the second circumstance, a myeloproliferative disorder is present. This kind of myeloid metaplasia is nonreactive. Its cause is unknown, and for that reason it is sometimes called idiopathic or agnogenic myeloid metaplasia. If often accompanies myelofibrosis. Some workers have held that myeloid metaplasia is a compensatory and reactive consequence of the marrow failure of myelofibrosis. The evidence, however, is against this view. Marrow is often hypercellular (and not fibrotic) in the presence of severe myeloid metaplasia of the spleen and liver. Thus the latter should be viewed as part of a generalized myeloproliferative process. It is more likely that the myelofibrosis (a nonclonal process) is a reaction to the primary myeloid metaplasia.

c. Clinical features

Myeloid metaplasia is a disorder of insidious onset in older patients. Its major features are (1) characteristic red cell changes in blood smears with many "teardrop" forms; (2) splenomegaly that is often massive; (3) anemia; (4) usually elevated platelet and leukocyte counts; (5) immature leukocytes; (6) hyperuricemia (with gout and renal stones); (7) hypermetabolism; (8) high incidence of aneuploidy in involved tissues; and (9) elevated leukocyte alkaline phosphatase (see figure 19.2). The LAP is diagnostically useful because the morphologically similar immature leukocytes of chronic myelocytic leukemia are low in LAP. When there is doubt whether splenomegaly is due to myeloid metaplasia, a scan with ^{59}Fe is useful in demonstrating that erythropoiesis is taking place in the spleen. Needle biopsy of spleen or liver may reveal myeloid metaplasia.

d. Pathology

Two grades of fibrosis are recognized in bone marrow. One is *reticulin* fibrosis. At least in its early stages, it is simply an exaggeration of a pattern present in normal marrow. It occurs in many disorders (benign and malignant) and is of little diagnostic value, though it has been recommended as a prognostic marker in acute leukemia. The other is *collagen* fibrosis, which is also seen in many (though fewer) conditions. They include (1) carcinomatous and lymphomatous marrow infiltration; (2) bone diseases (osteopetrosis, Paget's disease, etc.); (3) various immunological connective tissue disorders; and (4) myeloproliferative disorders.

The myelofibrosis of myeloproliferative disease usually accompanies myeloid metaplasia. Diagnosis requires a marrow biopsy. The process may be patchy or widespread. When widespread, marrow may be unobtainable by aspiration.

e. Therapy

Therapy is palliative and generally unsatisfactory. Nonetheless, the course is relatively prolonged compared to that of the leukemias. Radiation and alkylating agents may diminish the enlarged spleen, leukocytosis, and hypermetabolism. Splenectomy may be indicated if the spleen is massive or if it is causing intolerable red cell sequestration. The anemia is occasionally benefited by androgen therapy.

II. DISEASES OF LYMPHOCYTES

A. Reactive disorders

Lymphocytopenia, though uncommon, is most often associated with corticosteroid therapy, Hodgkin's disease, and various chronic diseases. Little is known of the factors that control the circulating lymphocyte count.

Lymphocytosis can occur as a relative phenomenon in several benign disorders, including pertussis and various virus infections including infectious mononucleosis and acute infectious lymphocytosis.

1. Infectious mononucleosis

Infectious mononucleosis (IM) is a self-limited benign illness that is believed to be caused by Epstein-Barr virus (EBV)—the same agent responsible for Burkitt lymphoma (see lecture 22)—although final proof of the etiological role of EBV is lacking in IM. IM is often communicated by oral contamination (kissing) and is common in young adults. It is associated clinically with (1) a rising titer of heterophile antibody in serum, which is removed by adsorption with beef cells; (2) characteristic atypical lymphocytes in stained blood smears that have been variously known as *virocytes* and *Downey cells*; (3) splenomegaly; (4) lymphadenopathy; (5) pharyngitis; and (6) a propensity for involving diverse organs—liver, myocardium, testes, and so forth.

2. Acute infectious lymphocytosis

This is a benign self-limited disorder that is associated with an increase in circulating small lymphocytes, occurrence in clusters, and diverse symptomatology. A virus similar to Coxsackie A has been suggested as a possible cause.

SELECTED REFERENCES

Adamson, J. W., and Fialkow, P. J. The pathogenesis of myeloproliferative syndromes. *Brit. J. Haematol.* 38(1978): 229.

Burkett, L. L., et al. Leukoerythroblastosis in the adult. *Am. J. Clin. Pathol.* 44(1965): 494.

Greenberg, P. L., et al. The chronic idiopathic neutropenia syndrome: Correlation of clinical features with in vitro parameters of granulocytopoiesis. *Blood* 55(1980): 915.

Harmon, D. C., et al. A staphylococcal slide test for detection of antineutrophil antibodies. *Blood* 56(1980): 64.

Hartl, W. Drug allergic agranulocytosis (Schultz's disease). *Semin. Hematol.* 2(1965): 313.

Joyce, R. A., et al. Neutrophil kinetics in Felty's syndrome. *Am. J. Med.* 69(1980): 695.

King-Smith, E. A., and Morley, A. A. Computer simulation of granulopoiesis: Normal and impaired granulopoiesis. *Blood* 36(1970): 254.

Lichtman, M. A., et al. Neutrophil disorders—general considerations (Part V, Section 4); Neutrophil disorders—benign, quantitative abnormalities of neutrophils (Part V, Section 5). In Williams, W. J., et al., eds., *Hematology*, 3d ed., New York: McGraw-Hill, 1983, pp. 770–772, 773–801.

MacKinney, A. A., and Cline, W. S. Infectious mononucleosis. *Brit. J. Haematol.* 27(1974): 367.

Quesenberry, P. J. Cyclic hematopoiesis: Disorders of primitive hematopoietic stem cells. *Exp. Hematol.* 11(1983): 687.

Silverstein, M. Agnogenic myeloid metaplasia (Chapter 25). In Williams, W. J., et al., eds., *Hematology*, 3d ed., New York: McGraw-Hill, 1983, pp. 214–218.

von Schulthess, G. K., and Mazer, N. A. Cyclic neutropenia (CN): A clue to the control of granulopoiesis. *Blood* 59(1982): 27.

Wang-Peng, J., et al. Cytogenetic studies in patients with myelofibrosis and myeloid metaplasia. *Leukemia Res.* 2(1978): 41.

LECTURE 20 The Polycythemias

William B. Castle

I. INTRODUCTION

A. Terminology

The term *polycythemia* denotes a pattern of blood changes that includes a sustained increase in blood hemoglobin concentration (to about 18 g/100 ml or more), red count (to 6 × 10^6/mm^3 or more), and hematocrit (to 55% or more). The term (and its synonym *erythrocytosis*) is without specific etiologic or diagnostic connotations, polycythemia occurring in a variety of conditions. The increase in red cell and hemoglobin (concentration) may be unaccompanied by an increase in the total red cell mass (volume). Moreover, in mild hypochromic or microcytic anemia, the red count may be somewhat increased while the hemoglobin concentration is less than normal. Thus the proper distinction between polycythemia and anemia is based strictly on the blood's hemoglobin concentration. In this lecture, *polycythemia* and *erythrocytosis* (a term analogous to *leukocytosis*) are used interchangeably to refer to a nonspecific blood picture. *Absolute polycythemia,* or *absolute erythrocytosis,* is polycythemia in which there is an absolute increase in red cell mass (as determined by ^{51}Cr labeling). *Relative erythrocytosis* refers to conditions in which the hemoglobin level, red count, and hematocrit are elevated (owing to decrease of plasma volume) but the red cell mass is normal. *Polycythemia vera,* or *erythremia* (a term analogous to *leukemia*), is a myeloproliferative disease in which increased red cell mass is one of several manifestations of panmyelosis.

B. Historical notes

Paul Bert in 1878 predicted that as a ''harmonious compensation of Nature,'' an increase in red cells and hemoglobin would characterize the blood of humans and animals living at high altitudes. In 1890 Viault supposedly confirmed this hypothesis by finding 16 × 10^6 red blood cells/mm^3 in blood of the Peruvian llama (mountain sheep). He then demonstrated that although their hemoglobin was partially unsaturated, their blood had a relatively normal oxygen content owing to its increased oxygen-carrying capacity. This finding was later confirmed in humans residing at 15,000 feet above sea level near Lima. In 1892 Vaquez described a patient with polycythemia and cyanosis thought to be secondary to arterial hypoxia from an intracardiac septal defect until autopsy disclosed no such lesion. Consequently, he ascribed the polycythemia to overactivity of the blood-forming organs. This early delineation of the primary form (polycythemia vera or erythremia) attracted the attention of Osler at the turn of the century. Another form of polycythemia, sometimes found in association with certain tumors, was first ascribed to humoral agents from a hypernephroma by Forssell in 1946. Familial polycythemia due to an abnormal hemoglobin with increased affinity for oxygen was first reported by Charache and coworkers in 1966.

II. CLASSIFICATION OF THE POLYCYTHEMIAS

In table 20.1, the polycythemias are divided into those associated with relative erythrocytosis (i.e., with normal red cell mass and decreased plasma volume) and those associated with absolute erythrocytosis (i.e., with increased red cell mass). Absolute erythrocytosis is divided into those secondary to variously induced forms of hypoxia with compensatory erythropoietin elaboration (see lecture 1), those secondary to inappropriate erythropoietin activity, and those due to a primary, neoplastic or autonomous increase in erythropoiesis.

III. PATHOPHYSIOLOGY

A. Red cell survival

Whatever the cause, polycythemia is not due to prolonged red cell survival. Erythrokinetic data show that survival is usually normal, though in polycythemia vera a small population of red cells may be short-lived. Increased hemoglobin concentration and red cell mass result from a sustained increase in the level of erythropoiesis in the bone marrow. Although the hematocrit and hemoglobin concentration may be nearly double the normal values, they can be sustained by a doubling of the rate of red cell production. Such an increase in marrow activity is distinctly less than the 6–8-fold increase occurring in various chronic hemolytic anemias with short red cell life spans. Absolute reticulocyte counts in polycythemia are therefore only modestly increased.

B. Blood volume and hematocrit

The major determinants of the blood volume are *red cell mass* and *plasma volume*. Normal values for these in males are, respectively, 28.2 ± 4.7 and 39.7 ± 5.3 ml/kg. Because red cells remain confined in the intravascular compartment, the size of the circulating red cell mass can be altered only by variations in the rate of red cell production as long as red cells are destroyed at a fixed rate. Erythropoietic activity of bone marrow is sensitively regulated by the erythropoietin system, but resulting changes in red cell mass occur slowly. Plasma volume is also regulated by homeostatic mechanisms sensitive to pressure, osmolarity, and flow rate, but plasma volume changes occur rapidly because of the ease with which fluid shifts between the intravascular and extravascular compartments. The *hematocrit* is a measure of the volume of red cells per unit volume of blood. The hematocrit of circulating blood varies in different parts of the vascular tree. Thus, the capillary hematocrit, because of the relatively larger

Table 20.1
Classification of the Polycythemias

Relative polycythemia (decreased plasma volume)	Water deprivation or febrile dehydration
	Loss of water and electrolytes: gastrointestinal disease (vomiting or diarrhea); renal disease; adrenocortical insufficiency; stress (?); Gaisböck's syndrome; vigorous diuretic therapy; etc.
	Loss of plasma: burns; enteropathy; etc.
Absolute polycythemia	
A. Secondary polycythemia	
1. With compensatory erythropoietin elaboration	With low arterial oxygen saturation
	Low pO_2 in inspired air: high altitude
	Low pO_2 in umbilical vein in fetus
	Ventilation-perfusion imbalance and alveolar hypoventilation: insensitivity of respiratory center; restrictive and/or obstructive pulmonary disease; obesity and/or recumbent posture; kyphoscoliosis; sarcoid; pulmonary fibrosis; berylliosis
	V-A shunting: intracardiac septal defects; great vessel anomalies; intrapulmonary A-V aneurysm; hemangiomata
	With normal arterial oxygen saturation
	Decreased oxygen transport by hemoglobin: methemoglobinemia; carboxyhemoglobinemia; M hemoglobins (?)
	Increased affinity for oxygen by abnormal hemoglobins: Chesapeake, Rainier, Little Rock, etc.
	Failure of tissue perfusion: low-output cardiac failure
	Decreased tissue oxygen utilization: $CoCl_2$ administration
2. With inappropriate erythropoietin elaboration	Renal diseases: hydronephrosis, cysts, hypernephroma
	Cerebellar hemangioblastoma (?)
	Hepatoma
	Adrenal virilizing adenoma
	Uterine fibroid (?)
	Thyroid or androgen administration
B. Primary polycythemia	Polycythemia vera (erythremia)

amount of plasma adjacent to the proportionately greater vessel wall surface, is lower than the hematocrit of blood in veins or arteries, which in turn is lower than that of blood in spleen and marrow sinusoids. At a given moment, one-fifth of the blood volume is in the capillaries, the low-hematocrit compartment. Hence, the "total body hematocrit" is lower than the "venous hematocrit." This is confirmed when plasma and red cell volumes are measured simultaneously by isotope dilution techniques, the ratio of body hematocrit to venous hematocrit equaling approximately 0.9. This means that true plasma volume exceeds plasma volume calculated from measurements of red cell mass and venous hematocrit. These considerations imply that elevation of the venous hematocrit can result from an increase in red cell mass or a decrease in plasma volume. The two conditions accounting for absolute and relative polycythemia, respectively, cannot be distinguished unless red cell mass is measured.

C. Homeostasis of oxygen transport

Observations in patients with polycythemia vera and in normovolemic and hypervolemic animals have thrown light on the hemodynamic mechanisms that help to maintain the constancy of the blood hemoglobin level.

1. Viscosity and flow rate

In normal circumstances, hemoglobin leaving the lung is nearly saturated with oxygen. Measured in vitro in capillary tubes, the *viscosity* of such blood increases exponentially with increases in hematocrit (figure 20.1, curve A). When the *flow rate* through the capillary tube is determined (as reciprocal of viscosity) at various hematocrit levels, flow is seen to decrease as an essentially linear function of hematocrit (figure 20.1, curve B). If flow rate is multi-

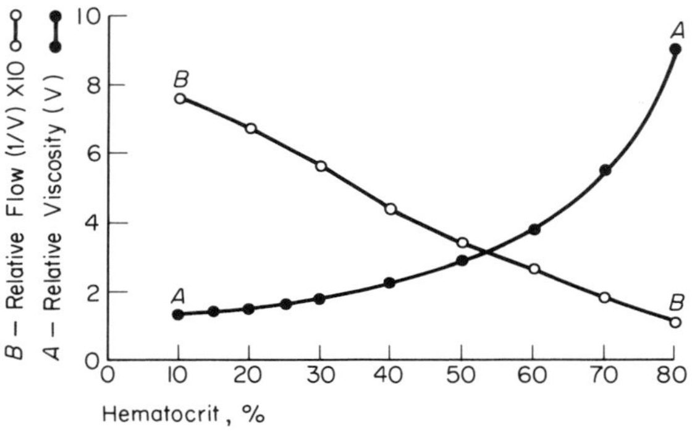

Fig. 20.1
Relation of blood viscosity (curve A) and relative blood flow through a capillary tube (curve B) of human blood of various hematocrits. Curve B is the reciprocal of curve A. In order to employ the same ordinate scale, its values were multiplied by 10. (From W. B. Castle and J. H. Jandl, *Semin. Hematol.* 3(1966): 193, by permission of Grune & Stratton, New York)

plied by oxygen content (a function of hematocrit), the product provides a relative measure of the rate of *oxygen transport* at different hematocrits for this in vitro system. At low hematocrits oxygen content of the blood is small; at high hematocrits flow rate is small. Consequently oxygen transport is maximal in vitro at intermediate hematocrit values of 45–50%. Were this strictly so in vivo, however, if the hematocrit were to increase even slightly, oxygen transport would decrease, tissue hypoxia would occur, and erythropoietin activity would rise. Thus a vicious cycle or positive feedback loop of ever-increasing hypoxia and polycythemia would be established. But these events do not follow a rise in hematocrit in vivo. In 1929 Campbell found in hypertransfused (and presumably hypervolemic and polycythemic) animals that tissue oxygen tension—determined by analysis of peritoneal or subcutaneous gas pockets—increased whenever the hematocrit increased. Modern experiments in animals confirm the appropriate homeostatic responses of tissue pO_2, respectively, to transfusion polycythemia and blood loss anemia (figure 20.2).

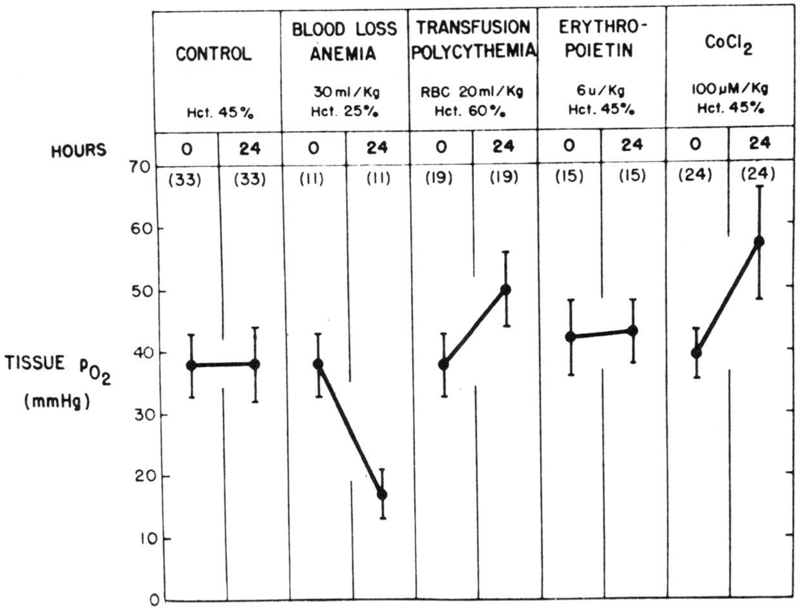

Fig. 20.2
Oxygen tension (mean ± 15.0) of air pockets introduced subcutaneously in rats. The effects of bleeding, transfusion, erythropoietin, and cobalt on the oxygen tension are given. As expected, bleeding causes hypoxia, transfusion causes hyperoxia, and erythropoietin has no immediate effect. Cobalt causes tissue hyperoxia, presumably reflecting reduced oxygen utilization because of inhibited cellular oxidative metabolism. (From A. J. Erslev and T. G. Gabuzda, *Pathophysiology of Blood,* Philadelphia: W. B. Saunders Co., 1975, p. 25, by permission of W. B. Saunders Co., Philadelphia)

2. Blood volume and cardiac output

Despite the increased viscosity of polycythemic blood, polycythemia enhances oxygen transport in vivo. Hence other factors were sought to explain this seeming paradox. These factors were found to be *increased blood volume* and *increased cardiac output*. Blood volume is invariably increased in patients with polycythemia approximately by the amount of the increase of red cell mass. In turn, the venous vascular bed enlarges and peripheral resistance decreases. Since blood pressure remains stable, increased venous return and consequent cardiac output must accompany these peripheral vascular changes. Together the increased cardiac output and the higher hematocrit (oxygen content) result in increased oxygen transport despite the increased viscosity of the blood. Indeed oxygen transport in hypervolemic (polycythemic) dogs is better than in normovolemic dogs, especially at moderately high hematocrits (figure 20.3). This causes an increase in tissue oxygen tension and consequently a decrease in erythropoietin production. On the contrary there is an increase in erythropoietin production in anemic dogs and humans. This occurs because of the decreased tissue oxygen tension that results from the lowered hemoglobin concentration and despite the opposition of lessened blood viscosity and peripheral vascular resistance (hypoxia) that increase cardiac output and despite the rightward shift of the he-

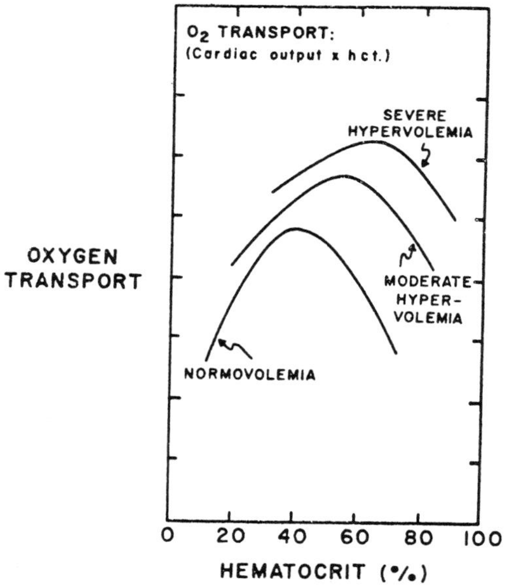

Fig. 20.3
Calculated in vivo oxygen transport in normovolemic and hypervolemic conditions after red cell transfusions in dogs. Oxygen transport increases when red cell mass is increased, because cardiac output and oxygen content of arterial blood are increased. (From J. F. Murray et al., *J. Clin. Invest.* 42(1963): 1150, and E. B. Thorling and A. J. Erslev, *Blood* 31(1968): 332, by permission of Grune & Stratton, New York)

moglobin oxygen dissociation curve due to increased red cell 2,3-DPG (see lecture 8).

In sum the constancy of the normal hemoglobin level, a function of the rate of red cell production, depends on the homeostatic effect of tissue oxygen tension. This implies the existence of tissue oxygen sensors in the negative feedback loop that determines erythropoietin production.

3. Situation in polycythemias

In polycythemia vera the increase in blood oxygen content, blood volume, and cardiac output are not in response to a physiologic need for better tissue oxygenation. Consequently normalization of these is inherently advantageous. In secondary hypoxic polycythemia, however, the arterial blood is unsaturated with oxygen. Nevertheless the rise in cardiac output increases oxygen transport, though to a lesser extent for a given hematocrit. Thus some degree of polycythemia is acceptable provided it can be sustained without cardiac strain.

IV. RELATIVE POLYCYTHEMIA

Two types of fluid shifts account for a high hematocrit in the presence of a normal red cell volume: (1) an absolute decrease in plasma volume and (2) a normal total plasma volume accompanied by an abnormal distribution of blood in the vascular tree such that the fraction in the low-hematocrit (capillary) compartment is relatively increased.

Both may occur acutely, as in dehydration, burns, and after vigorous diuretic therapy, or they may be chronic as in adrenocortical insufficiency. In some cases the condition is chronic and without obvious cause. Such patients are typically florid and tense middle-aged men, sometimes with moderate hypertension, who complain of headaches, dizziness, and increased sweating. Their heavy smoking habits may produce some carboxyhemoglobin. These obese individuals have short necks and hypoventilate in the recumbent position. Both of these traits may produce hypoxic secondary polycythemia. The hematocrit in these patients rarely exceeds 60%. The blood count is otherwise normal. Other frequent laboratory abnormalities are hypercholesterolemia and/or hyperlipemia and modest hyperuricemia. The cases of hypertension and elevated red cell count described by Gaisböck in 1905 as *polycythemia hypertonica* were probably examples of this condition. This picture was later called *stress erythrocytosis,* but this team inappropriately suggests the presence of an elevated red cell mass. Better terms are *relative erythrocytosis* or *spurious erythrocytosis* since they emphasize that hematologic disease is not present. Indeed the venous hematocrit may be elevated in the case of a high normal red cell volume (mass) and a low normal plasma volume (table 20.2). Moreover the estimation of red cell mass is subject to less than precise correlations with body weight and surface area.

Table 20.2
Mean Blood Volume Values in Spurious Polycythemia

Subjects	Venous hematocrits (%)	RBC volume (ml/kg)	Plasma volume (ml/kg)	Hypertension (%)
Normal	47 ± 2.5	28.2 ± 4.1	39.7 ± 5.3	0
Group I	54.2 ± 2.4	32.9 ± 2.2	33.1 ± 3.9	38
Group II	54.6 ± 2.0	27.9 ± 2.4	30.4 ± 5.2	55

Figures are means ±SD. Patients in group I have high normal RBC volumes and slightly low plasma volumes. Patients in group II have low normal RBC volumes and low plasma volumes. Hypertension, more common in group II, probably classifies these as Gaisböck's syndrome or stress polycythemia. (Adapted from N. J. Weinreb and C.-F. Shih, *Semin. Hematol.* 12(1975): 397)

V. ABSOLUTE POLYCYTHEMIA

A. Secondary polycythemia

Cases of secondary or reactive polycythemia are divided into (1) those in which tissues are hypoxic and a compensatory elaboration of erythropoietin occurs and (2) those in which tissue oxygenation is normal but an inappropriate elaboration of erythropoietin takes place. The properties of erythropoietin, its relation with the kidney, and mode of action are described in lecture 1.

1. With compensatory erythropoietin elaboration

a. With low arterial oxygen

The low pO_2 of air at high altitudes decreases arterial oxygen saturation. Partial, temporary compensation is provided the newly arrived lowlander by increases in cardiac output and pulmonary ventilation. The latter elevates alveolar pO_2 but initially causes alkalosis and a leftward shift of the oxygen dissociation curve via the Bohr effect (see figure 8.5). Simultaneously, there begins an increase in red cell 2,3-DPG that causes a rightward shift of the dissociation curve that persists after reestablishment of normal blood pH (see lecture 8). In a few days, the reticulocyte count rises, and over a period of several weeks the hemoglobin concentration increases. However, even in the fully acclimated barrel-chested Andean native, the pO_2 of polycythemic arterial blood remains decreased despite hyperventilation, and there is mild cyanosis. Despite its augmented oxygen content, the oxygen saturation of the arterial blood is always less than the oxygen-carrying capacity (which is proportional to its hemoglobin content), as shown in table 20.3. Despite the lower pO_2 with which arterial blood enters the capillaries, its increased oxygen content helps to maintain a higher average capillary oxygen tension than would have been the case without the increase in hemoglobin and oxygen capacity.

Table 20.3
Arterial Blood in Altitude Polycythemia

		Arterial oxygen		
Altitude (ft × 10^{-3})	Hemoglobin (g/100 ml)	Capacity (vol %)	Content (vol %)	Saturation (%)
0	16.5	21.4	20.6	96.0
4.8	17.1	22.2	20.9	93.8
12.0	19.4	25.2	22.1	87.6
14.7	21.1	27.5	22.3	81.0
17.4	23.2	30.2	23.0	76.2

Source: From A. Hurtado, C. Merino, and E. Delgado, *Arch. Int. Med.* 75(1945): 284.

Most earlier studies were conducted on small groups in high-altitude mining communities (table 20.3). Since many suffered from chronic respiratory disorders including silicosis, results could not be attributed solely to low atmospheric pO_2. Later studies of native Peruvian shepherds and farmers at 14,000 feet above sea level showed mean hemoglobin levels of 17.3 ± 1.5 g/100 ml and mean hematocrits of 51.4 ± 3.9%. These values resemble those found earlier by Hurtado et al. at an altitude of only 4,800 ft (table 20.3). Clearly the striking polycythemia in the industrial Andean group was due to a combination of high altitude and chronic respiratory insufficiency.

Certain animal species may be genetically adapted to low ambient oxygen levels. California ground squirrels living at an altitude of 12,500 ft have a mean hemoglobin of only 14.3 ± 0.8 g/100 ml, whereas laboratory rats born and raised at that altitude have mean levels of 19.3 ± 1.5 g/100 ml. In ground squirrels (and Himalayan sherpas) the leftward shift of the oxygen dissociation curve favors the uptake of oxygen by hemoglobin at high altitude (figure 20.4). Despite the resulting decrease in oxygen unloading in the tissues, the animals were able to perform well at low tissue pO_2 values that killed more than half of the altitude-acclimatized rats in an hour. In both humans and animals such as the Peruvian llama the relatively normal hematocrits at high altitude permit increased oxygen transport without the disadvantage of increased blood viscosity of polycythemia (figure 20.1).

In the other forms of tissue hypoxia—including those induced by cardiopulmonary disease, A-V shunting, or depression of the respiratory center—erythrocytosis likewise results from reduced arterial oxygen content and tissue pO_2 (figure 20.5). Consequently, in these cases determination of arterial pO_2 is a necessary diagnostic procedure. A patient with significant erythrocytosis due to arterial hypoxia is cyanotic even in a warm room, and his or her arterial blood may be unsaturated to a degree corresponding to that of polycythemic subjects residing at high altitude (table 20.3).

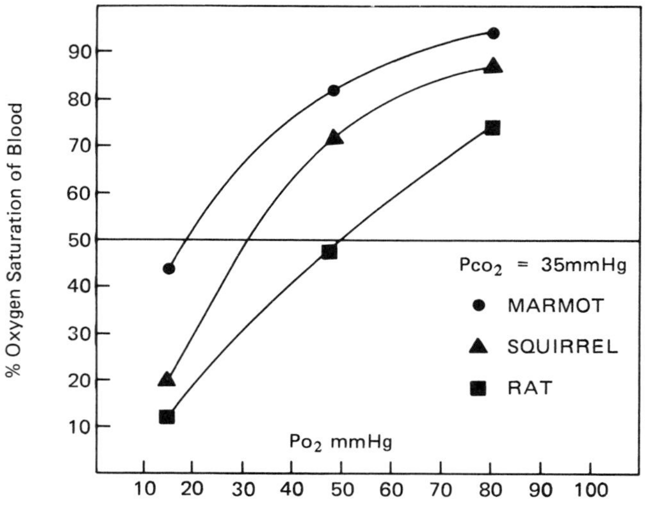

Fig. 20.4
Three-point oxygen-hemoglobin dissociation curves determined for the ground squirrel and marmot native to high altitude and altitude-acclimatized rat. The leftward shift of the native rodent's curves permits higher percentage of oxygen saturation for them at the diminished oxygen tensions of high altitude. (From Bullard, R. W., *J. Applied Physiol.* 20(1966): 997)

In practice, especially in patients with pulmonary disease, the arterial pO_2 level does not always correlate with the degree of erythrocytosis. It may be *high* relative to the hemoglobin concentration because (1) it was determined after therapeutic improvement in respiratory function; (2) the procedure of arterial puncture may briefly stimulate better ventilation via psychological or reflex mechanisms; or (3) respiration during sleep or recumbency, especially in obese subjects, is less effective than during wakefulness, when the determination is made. It may be *low* relative to the hemoglobin concentration because chronic infection accompanying a pulmonary disorder inhibits the erythropoietin response or renders the marrow less responsive to erythropoietin.

b. With normal arterial oxygen

Tissue hypoxia may occur in the presence of normal arterial oxygen saturation in any circumstance that impairs the binding or release of oxygen by hemoglobin. Its well-known association with chronic CO exposure is based on the fact that increasing concentrations of blood carboxyhemoglobin shift the oxygen dissociation curve leftward. Perhaps the heavy cigarette smoking of many patients with "stress polycythemia" produces this effect. According to Astrup, continuous cigarette smoking for 2 hr may result in 15% carboxyhemoglobin. Several hemoglobin variants are described in lecture 9 that cause a leftward shift in the oxygen dissociation curves (obvious at pO_2 50) and erythrocytosis. These

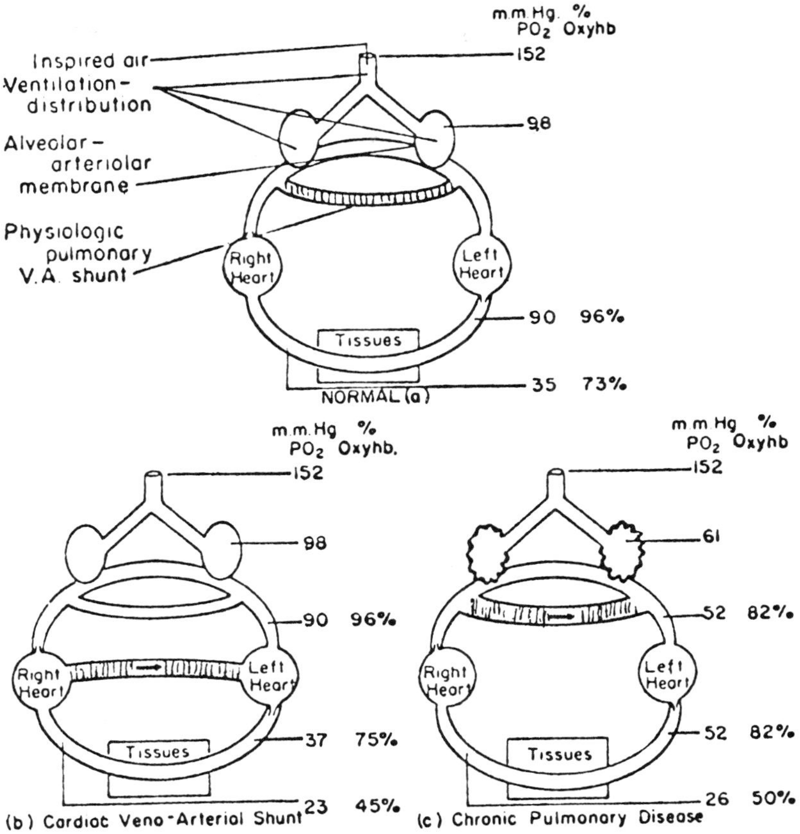

Fig. 20.5
Pathologic physiology of secondary hypoxic polycythemias. In altitude polycythemia, the normal diagram would be modified to show a lower pO_2 in the inspired air with consequent unsaturation of the arterial blood. In hypoventilation polycythemia, as in chronic pulmonary disease, the major abnormality in the transport of oxygen is the lowered pO_2 of the alveolar air. (From M. A. Escobar and F. E. Trobaugh, Jr., *Med. Clin. N. Amer.* 46(1962): 253, by permission of W. B. Saunders, Co., Philadelphia)

genetically determined abnormal hemoglobins cause minimal symptoms. They escaped earlier recognition because most of them are electrophoretically normal and saturate normally a pO_2 of 100. Their high oxygen affinity results from amino acid substitutions that (1) stabilize the oxyhemoglobin form (Chesapeake and Yakima); (2) destabilize the deoxyhemoglobin form (San Diego and Rainier); or (3) inhibit binding of 2,3-DPG (Little Rock). Thus previously reported instances of "benign familial polycythemia" all require reinvestigation as possible manifestations of such hemoglobinopathies. Interestingly polycythemia does not develop in all individuals with these hemoglobin variants, in some instances because the instability of the variant causes an associated hemolysis. Also there are rare instances of benign polycythemia in young persons for which no explanation can be offered for the expanded erythropoietic marrow pool. In others autonomous erythroid colony formation is observed in marrow cultured without added erythropoietin, as in polycythemia vera.

Hemoglobin fails to transport oxygen when its iron is oxidized. This condition (methemoglobinemia) may be acquired (lecture 8) or congenital (lecture 9). Patients with congenital methemoglobinemias rarely display more than slight polycythemia, possibly the result of a mild associated hemolytic process. Finally, tissue hypoxia with normal arterial oxygen saturation may result from substances that cause histotoxic hypoxia. These include cobaltous ion, which binds $-SH$ groups and interferes with tissue oxygen utilization. Thus subcutaneous gas pockets formed in mice injected daily with $CoCl_2$ contain higher oxygen tensions than those of control mice given saline injections (figure 20.2). Sustained sublethal concentrations of cyanide may have a similar effect because of the action of cyanide on tissue cytochromes.

2. With inappropriate erythropoietin elaboration

Appreciation that the effect of hypoxia on erythropoiesis is mediated by a humoral factor, erythropoietin, and development of assay methods for erythropoietin has led to an understanding of many isolated cases of erythrocytosis occurring in the absence of demonstrable tissue hypoxia. The mechanism of erythrocytosis appears to be an exaggeration of erythropoietin production by the tissues that normally produce it or inappropriate secretion by tissues not normally involved in its production.

Renal tissue is involved in the production of erythropoietin, and polycythemia has occurred in association with hydronephrosis and renal cystic disease and in the rejection phase of renal transplants. In these conditions the increased production of erythropoietin is probably analogous to the experimental production of polycythemia in animals by local interference with renal blood or urine flow and consequent stagnant hypoxia of renal tissue. This may also be so with renal tumors.

Polycythemia may also result from an ectopic source of erythropoietin, such as renal or hepatic tumor, cerebellar hemangioblastoma, or large uterine fibroids. During fetal and neonatal life the liver is the primary site of erythropoietin production, but in the adult it contributes only 10%. Renal and hepatic erythropoietins are biologically and antigenically identical. Urinary assays have shown that the increased erythropoietin excretion with tumors is independent of the hematocrit level. Removal of a variety of primary renal tumors has abolished the polycythemia, which has recurred when metastases developed in the opposite kidney (and perhaps elsewhere). The possibility remains that some renal tumors induce increased erythropoietin production by causing local tissue hypoxia and that the subtentorial location of the usual vascular brain tumor associated with polycythemia may allow it to interfere with the respiratory center as in the case of other rare neural lesions. The frequency of the association between hepatic tumors and polycythemia is second only to that of renal tumor. Testosterone and its analogues have a useful therapeutic effect in certain anemias because they increase erythropoietin production or activity. The occasional association of polycythemia with exogenous androgen administration or Cushing's disease and other androgen-secreting tumors probably relates to an effect of androgenic steroids in promoting erythropoietin secretion or activity.

B. Primary polycythemia (polycythemia vera)

An increased red cell mass occurs in both polycythemia vera (erythremia) and the various secondary polycythemias; however, the relatively advanced age of patients with polycythemia vera and the frequent increases in their leukocytes and platelets contrast with secondary polycythemias, which occur at any age and affect only the red cells. Polycythemia vera is one manifestation of the panmyelosis that characterizes the myeloproliferative disorders and is a disease of late middle life and beyond.

As noted in lecture 19, the myeloproliferative disorders are of unknown etiology. There is presumably neoplastic overproduction of one or more of the cell lines arising by differentiation of the marrow stem cell. The underlying defect is probably of the pluripotent stem cell. Consistent with this is the observation that when isoenzymes of G-6 PD were used as cell markers for the study of the cellular mosaicism as determined by the Lyon hypothesis (see lecture 14), it was shown that when females who are Gd^B/Gd^A heterozygotes get polycythemia, all blood cells (red cells, white cells, and platelets) contain one or the other form of G-6-PD. Marrow fibroblasts contain both markers. This implies that the three hematopoietic cell line cells have a clonal origin, as would be expected if initial pathogenesis were due to a rare oncogenic influence (e.g., somatic cell mutation in the hematopoietic stem cell). In addition to occasional chromosomal aberrations, such mutated stem cells have altered proliferative capacities in vitro. Recently stem cells from the marrow of a female G-6-PD heterozygote with polycythemia vera were shown to develop in culture the mutated type of erythroid colonies without the addition of erythropoietin. When erythropoietin was added, however, colonies of the normal erythroid clone appeared, and those of the abnormal clone increased.

1. Clinical features

Clinical symptoms are due to (1) increased red cell mass and blood volume (headache, plethoric appearance, pruritus, dyspnea, and hemorrhage); (2) increased blood viscosity (paresthesias, circulatory stagnation, and thrombosis); and (3) hypermetabolism (night sweats, weight loss, and elevated basal metabolic rate). Hyperuricemia results from the increased nucleoprotein catabolism of hyperactive hematopoiesis. Attacks of gout occur infrequently. Splenomegaly is commonly present. It may not be apparent early but may become massive late in the disease.

Paradoxically hemorrhage and thrombosis are common. Hemorrhage is promoted by (1) increased blood volume that distends veins and capillaries with results similar to the local effects of a venous tourniquet; (2) defective platelet function; and (3) defective clot formation because of masses of red cells entrapped in the clot. Activation of the intrinsic coagulation cascade occurs, but apparently vascular thrombosis is the result of increased blood viscosity with high platelet levels that predispose to platelet aggregation. In addition, the platelets are resistant to PGD_2, a platelet prostaglandin that opposes collagen-induced aggregation in vitro. Blood studies reveal increases of granulocytes and platelets, as well as red cells in many patients with polycythemia vera even in early stages (table 20.4). Some, when first encountered, have only a high platelet count, derived, in contrast to those of reactive thrombocythemia, from strikingly polyploid megakaryocytes. In time they develop erythrocytosis and leukocytosis with a marked shift to the left and elevated LAP. Red cell morphology is normal early in the course unless iron deficiency is present. At this stage the bone marrow is hypercellular with increases of erythroid, granulocyte, and platelet precursors. In time nucleated red cells and irregularities in red cell size and shape ("teardrops") may become prominent in the blood as marrow fibrosis develops in a centrifugal direction. The picture is now that of myeloid metaplasia and myelofibrosis, the latter probably resulting from stimulation of stromal cells by platelet-derived growth factor. This phase in turn may give way to acute myelocytic leukemia, which occurs mainly in patients who have received therapeutic irradiation or myelosuppressive drugs.

Ferrokinetic studies with scanning over the enlarged spleen may

Table 20.4
Features of Primary Polycythemia, Secondary (Hypoxic) Polycythemia, and Relative Erythrocytosis

Manifestations	Primary polycythemia	Secondary polycythemia	Relative erythrocytosis
Clinical features			
Cyanosis (warm)	Absent	Present	May be present
Heart or lung disease	Absent	Present	Absent
Splenomegaly	Present in 75%	Absent	Absent
Hepatomegaly	Present in 35%	Absent	Absent
Laboratory features			
Arterial oxygen saturation	Normal	Decreased	Normal
Red cell mass	Increased	Increased	Normal
White count	Increased in 80%	Normal	Normal
Platelet count	Increased in 50%	Normal	Normal
Nucleated red cells, poikilocytes	Often present	Absent	Absent
LAP	Elevated	Normal	Normal
Bone marrow	Hypercellular; increased erythropoiesis and myelopoiesis; increased megakaryocytes; fibrosis	Increased erythropoiesis	Normal
Erythropoietin	Decreased	Increased	Normal
Serum vitamin B_{12}	Elevated in 75%[a]	Normal	Normal

a. Owing to an increase in transcobalamin III (see lecture 4).

provide an indication of the presence of extramedullary erythropoiesis there. Iron deficiency with microcytosis, hypochromia, and decreased marrow and serum iron develops in some patients as a result of (1) increased utilization of iron stores by excessive hemoglobin synthesis; (2) decreased intestinal iron absorption (in contrast to the increase occurring in anemia); and (3) loss by therapeutic blood removal or gastrointestinal bleeding, especially from peptic ulcer. With appropriate therapy median survival ranges from 10 to 14.5 years.

2. Laboratory features

Blood volume is increased by the amount of increase in red cell mass. Plasma volume remains normal. However, with massive splenomegaly, there may be either an anomalous increase in red cell mass or, more commonly, plasma volume. Blood oxygen saturation is normal. Blood viscosity is increased because of the increased hematocrit. Cardiac output is elevated by the increased venous return due to increased blood volume and lowered peripheral resistance. Clinical and laboratory features of polycythemia vera, secondary hypoxic polycythemia, and relative erythrocytosis are compared in table 20.4.

3. Marrow kinetics

Early in polycythemia vera bone marrow culture reveals normal erythroid and granulocyte/macrophage committed stem cells. The size of the neoplastic stem cell pool is undefined, but with time the percentage of normal committed stem cells declines for both red cells and granulocytes, though at a different rate. Normal CFU-GMs begin to drop out of cycle, and with time normal granulocytes are no longer seen in the blood. Meanwhile an unknown mechanism (independent of erythropoietin) begins inhibiting the development of CFU-Es and BFU-Es so that normal red cells also disappear eventually from the circulation.

4. Therapy

The primary goal of therapy is reduction of blood viscosity. This can be achieved by repeated bleeding and/or by myelosuppressive drugs or radiation.

Bleeding at once reduces blood volume, but it decreases viscosity only after restoration of plasma volume from extravascular sources. It must not be done too rapidly since increased blood volume sustains the increased cardiac output essential for tissue oxygenation with viscous blood. For this reason dehydration is also dangerous, and plasma expanders may be desirable at the time of blood removal. In hypoxic polycythemia phlebotomy is judged beneficial if it increases the oxygen content of the mixed venous blood in the right atrium, which reflects the average tissue pO_2. (Sometimes the patient can guess the value accurately.) Bleeding also leads to iron deficiency, which may further the goal of therapy by lowering the internal red cell viscosity and delaying erythropoiesis. Severe iron deficiency should be avoided. Rapid (or even slow) bleeding may lead to intolerable hemodynamic changes in some patients and unacceptable rises in the platelet count with increased risk of thrombosis.

Radiation, usually with ^{32}P, controls panmyelosis and extends life expectancy but may increase the frequency of late acute leukemia. Myelosuppressive drugs also control panmyelosis but are also leukemogenic in a small percentage of cases. Probably only scheduled phlebotomy should be employed, especially in younger patients, unless it is ineffective alone or too inconvenient. Useful myelosuppressive drugs include melphalan, chlorambucil, and hydroxyurea. Although increased erythropoietic secretion is not responsible for the erythrocytosis of polycythemia vera, it is of interest that erythropoietic secretion does rise in these patients when anemic hypoxia occurs. Thus acute hemolysis or hemorrhage, including excessive therapeutic bleeding, elicits qualitatively normal erythropoietic responses. There is in vitro evidence that both a normal clone of erythroid precursors and the abnormal anomalous clone respond to strong erythropoietic stimulation. In vivo the abnormal autonomous erythropoiesis proceeds despite the elevated hemoglobin level and decreased erythropoietin production of the polycythemic state.

SELECTED REFERENCES

Adamson, J. W. The polycythemias: Diagnosis and treatment. *Hosp. Practice* 18(1983): 49.

Berlin, N. I., et al. Polycythemia. *Semin. Hematol.* 12(1975): 335; 13(1976): 1.

Castle, W. B., and Jandl, J. H. Blood viscosity and blood volume: Opposing influences upon oxygen transport in polycythemia. *Semin. Hematol.* 3(1966): 193.

Cobb, L. A., et al. Circulatory effects of chronic hypervolemia in polycythemia vera. *J. Clin. Invest.* 39(1960): 1722.

Erslev, A. J. Erythrocyte disorders—Erythrocytosis (Section 170). In Williams, W. J., et al., eds., *Hematology,* 3d ed., New York: McGraw-Hill, 1983, pp. 673–690.

Erslev, A. J., et al. Plasma erythropoietin in polycythemia. *Am. J. Med.* 66(1979): 243.

Finch, C. A. Oxygen transport in man. *New Eng. J. Med.* 286(1972): 407.

Morpurgo, G., et al. Sherpas living permanently at high altitude: A new pattern of adaptation. *Proc. Nat. Acad. Sci. U.S.A.* 73(1976): 747.

Noble, J. A. Hepatic vein thrombosis complicating polycythemia vera. *Arch. Intern. Med.* 120(1967): 105.

Prchal, J. F., et al. Polycythemia vera: The in vitro response of normal and abnormal stem cell lines to erythropoietin. *J. Clin. Invest.* 61(1978): 1044.

Russell, R. P., and Conley, C. L. Benign polycythemia: Gaisböck's syndrome. *Arch. Intern. Med.* 114(1964): 734.

Weatherall, D. J. Polycythemia resulting from abnormal hemoglobins. *New Eng. J. Med.* 280(1969): 604.

LECTURE 21 The Leukemias

David C. Harmon

I. INTRODUCTION

A. Definition

The leukemias are neoplasms of the hematopoietic system that are variously related to the myeloproliferative disorders and lymphomas. In leukemia ("white blood") uncontrolled proliferation of a malignant clone of one cell line eventually replaces marrow, at the expense of other cell lines, with resulting cytopenias. Immature lymphocytes and myeloid cells predominate in *acute lymphocytic* and *acute myelocytic leukemias,* respectively. In the *chronic leukemias* more mature lymphoid or myeloid cells accumulate. Tissue invasion by abnormal cells eventually causes organ dysfunction and death.

B. Incidence

1. Frequency

Leukemia accounts for 4% of all cancers in the United States with 10 new cases, 5 acute and 5 chronic, arising per 100,000 people each year. Among children acute leukemia comprises nearly half of all malignancies.

2. Age of onset

Despite the relative rarity of pediatric cancer, half of the acute leukemias arise during childhood. *Acute lymphocytic leukemia* (ALL) is most commonly a disease of children, accounting for 80% of all childhood leukemias. The incidence of *acute myelocytic leukemia* (AML), which accounts for 20% of childhood leukemia, increases with age and is the commonest adult leukemia. *Chronic lymphocytic leukemia* (CLL) is almost never seen in children and uncommonly before age 40 but then steadily increases in incidence with age. *Chronic myelocytic leukemia* (CML) has a peak incidence in middle age but may occur at any age.

II. ETIOLOGY

When studied with sensitive techniques, virtually all leukemias display chromosomal abnormalities (gains, losses, and translocations) in all cells of the malignant clone. Their patterns are nonrandom.

A. Chromosomal alterations

Specific cytogenetic abnormalities are gradually being associated with specific types of leukemia—for example, the *Philadelphia chromosome,* abbreviated Ph^1 and symbolized (t9;22) (q34; q11), is associated with CML. Such alterations underlie current theories of malignant transformation and uncontrolled proliferation. Although detailed mechanisms require elucidation, it is believed that various agents operate at a number of "hot spots" within the genetic material to derepress genes responsible for proliferation or to cause failure of feedback regulation.

B. Oncogenes

Activation of cellular oncogenes and overproduction of their products is a key step in some types of neoplastic transformation. Chromosome abnormalities may accomplish this step by bringing on oncogenes with transforming ability under the transcriptional control of genes active in that specific cell type. For example, in CLL and some B cell lymphomas, the genes for κ light chain (2p12), λ light chain (22q11), or μ heavy chain (14q32) are often at break points where they may be brought into association with oncogenes such as *myc* (on chromosome 8) in Burkitt's lymphoma. The surface immunoglobulin of the malignant lymphocyte expresses the light chain type of the affected gene in such cases. It remains to be seen what role oncogenes play in leukemogenesis.

C. Host factors

Host factors may include increased susceptibility of the chromosomes themselves to alterations or of the organism to agents that cause genetic damage. Such host factors include the following.

1. Heredity

The identical twin of a patient with acute leukemia has a 25% chance of developing acute leukemia, while a fraternal twin has little excess risk.

2. Congenital chromosome abnormalities

Leukemia occurs relatively frequently in association with aneuploid chromosomes (Down's syndrome, Klinefelter's syndrome, Turner's syndrome, etc.) and with defective repair of chromosome breaks (Fanconi's anemia, Bloom's syndrome) or chromosomal fragments.

3. Immune deficiency

Immune deficiency, whether cell mediated (ataxia telangiectasia) or humorally mediated (X-linked agammaglobulinemia), may predispose to leukemia.

4. Chronic marrow dysfunction

Preleukemia refers to a clonal hematopoietic stem cell disorder with abnormal maturation and ineffective hematopoietic stem cell disorder with abnormal maturation and ineffective hematopoiesis that subsequently terminates in acute leukemia. Abnormal cell morphology and nonrandom cytogenetic abnormalities characterize many cases (e.g., trisomy 8, monosomy 7). In practice it is difficult to differentiate preleukemia from other chronic marrow disorders that are associated with cytopenias but do not invariably terminate in leukemia (e.g., aplastic anemia, Kostmann's syndrome, refractory sideroblastic anemias, and megaloblastic anemias). Paroxysmal nocturnal hemoglobinuria is a clonal disorder with some tendency to develop into acute leukemia, while the myeloproliferative disorders typically undergo a process of clonal evolution with increasingly aberrant chromosomes and abnormal maturation that ends in leukemia.

D. Environmental factors

1. Radiation and chemicals

Ionizing radiation from radiotherapy and atomic bombs can cause chromosome damage and is followed by marked increases in the incidence of acute and chronic myelocytic leukemia. Radiomimetic antitumor agents (especially Alkeran®) also have strong links to leukemia. Statistical associations implicate benzene and some environmental chemical pollutants as well. Carcinogens may act preferentially on specific DNA sites as suggested by the frequency of abnormalities of chromosomes 6 and 7 among chemotherapy-induced leukemia. Chronic immunosuppressive therapy may also increase susceptibility to leukemia (see below).

2. Viruses

Since retroviruses cause some animal leukemias, research has focused on *C-type RNA tumor viruses* in humans. Virally coded reverse transcriptase has been found in human lymphoblasts. Significantly antibody to human T cell leukemia virus has been found in most patients with a rare form of leukemia that occurs in geographic clusters. DNA sequences of this virus have been detected in the cells of the leukemic T cell clone but not in the normal B cells of affected patients. The Epstein-Barr virus also has a close association with lymphoproliferative diseases but is not yet a proved cause of leukemia.

III. PATHOPHYSIOLOGY

A. Abnormal growth in vitro

In vitro cultures of leukemic bone marrows demonstrate abnormal growth patterns. Typical findings are a low cloning efficiency, a tendency to abortive colonies, and an increased percentage of light density CFU-GMs. Most colonies still respond to CSF, though a variety of abnormalities are described. Some preleukemic marrows follow similar patterns. To date no single pattern has emerged that typifies leukemia.

B. Failure of maturation

The crucial problem is the failure to undergo maturation and to produce functional end cells. Hence in addition to showing morphologic immaturity, leukemic cells (especially in acute cases) may lack enzymes, have altered surface antigens, produce fetal hemoglobin, or perform poorly in functional assays.

C. Growth advantage of leukemic clone

Since they are immature, leukemic cells are likely to stay in the marrow and remain capable of dividing, producing more and more nonfunctional cells that eventually "pack" the marrow. Their presence may inhibit growth of normal cells, perhaps by chalones or by physical and nutritional competition. As a population the neoplastic clone has a growth advantage over normal cells even though the individual stem cells may actually divide more slowly.

D. Cytokinetics

The leukemic cell cycle generation time is ordinarily longer than normal due to an S-phase that is prolonged to 2 to 3 times normal. The cell death rate is high. Nonetheless the growth fraction is such that in acute leukemia, the tumor doubling time may be as short as 4 days. Since the diagnosis of leukemia can be made only when the total body burden exceeds 10^9 leukemic cells (approximately 1 g), a *minimum* of about 120 days (or 3–4 months) must pass between the time of the first malignant transformation and the time of diagnosis. When the number of leukemic cells exceeds 10^{12}, the acute leukemias eliminate normal-functioning bone marrow and prove rapidly fatal. Because only 10 doublings are necessary for 10^9 cells to become 10^{12}, only a brief time (i.e., 10×4 days) is needed for maximally severe symptoms to evolve. This is not true of the chronic leukemias in which slower cell division is occurring, greater numbers can be tolerated, and symptoms may be of several years' duration. Complete clinical remission occurs whenever the number of leukemic cells can be reduced to fewer than 10^9. Although the body might still contain up to 10^9 cells, ordinarily none would be detectable in blood or bone marrow. Cure can be said to occur only when all leukemic cells are gone.

E. Metabolic complications

Because of ineffective hematopoiesis and resulting high nucleic acid turnover, *uric acid production* increases. Nephrotoxic levels may accumulate, especially following the tumor cell lysis caused by chemotherapy. Massive cell lysis can also cause *hyperkalemia,* while poorly understood renal tubule toxins (possibly lysozyme) occasionally cause *hypokalemia.*

F. Causes of death

Marrow replacement by leukemic cells causes *anemia, thrombocytopenia,* and *granulocytopenia.* Bleeding presents a major threat, but infection is the major killer. Opportunistic organisms often infect leukemic patients because of diminished immunity.

IV. CLASSIFICATION

On the basis of clinical history and light microscopy alone, most leukemias can be easily divided into lymphocytic or myelocytic and acute or chronic and their respective prognoses and therapies established. The French-American-British (FAB) system assigns a letter and a number to each of the morphologic subtypes (in brackets below); however, the use of newer approaches is refining basic understanding and clinical approach.

A. Acute

1. *Acute lymphocytic leukemia* (ALL)
   a. Childhood: null cell, B cell, T cell [usually homogenous-L_1]
   b. Adult: null cell, B cell, or T cell [usually heterogenous-L_2]
   c. Burkitt's [L_3]
2. *Acute nonlymphocytic leukemia* (ANLL)
   a. Acute myelocytic leukemia (AML) [M_1 without or M_2 with maturation]
   b. Acute promyelocytic leukemia (APL) [M_3]
   c. Acute myelomonocytic leukemia (AMML) [M_4]
   d. Acute monocytic leukemia (AMoL) [M_5]
   e. Erythroleukemia [M_6]

B. Chronic

1. *Chronic lymphocytic leukemia* (CLL): B cell, T cell, hairy cell
2. *Chronic myelocytic leukemia* (CML)

C. Methods used in classification

Laboratory techniques may help in distinguishing the major types and subtypes of leukemia.

1. Light microscopy

Criteria for distinguishing the blast cells of ALL and ANLL are presented in table 21.1. Morphologic subtypes of ANLL are described in the FAB system. The more mature cells of CLL and CML are usually easily recognized.

2. Electron microscopy

Electron microscopy occasionally can reveal granules missed by light microscopy.

3. Histochemistry

Histochemical staining (table 21.2) brings out patterns useful in differentiating the acute leukemias.

Table 21.1
Morphologic Distinction of Acute Leukemia Blast Cells

Characteristic	ALL	ANLL
Size	Small	Larger
Shape	Round	Irregular
Cytoplasm	Dark blue rim	Pale blue, (granular)
Nucleus	Central, round	Eccentric, irregular
Nucleoli	Faint	"Punched out"
Auer rods	Absent	Present in 50%

Table 21.2
Histochemistry of Acute Leukemias

FAB class of leukemia	M_1	$M_{2,3}$	M_4	M_5	$L_{1,2,3}$
Peroxidase or Sudan Black	+	+ + +	+ +	+/−	−
Esterase	+	+ +	+ + +	+ + +	−/+
Lysozyme (muramidase)	−	+	+ +	+ + +	−
Periodic acid-Schiff (PAS)	−/+	+/−	+/−	+/−	+ + +/−

Table 21.3
Cell Surface Markers

	Null ALL	Pre B-ALL	B-ALL	CLL	T-cell ALL	ANLL
Surface Ig	−	−	+	+	−	−
Cytoplasmic Ig	−	+	−	−	−	−
I^A	+	+	+	+	−	+
CALLA	+/−	+/−	+/−	−	−	−
T-series	−	−	−	rare +	+	−
My Series	−	−	−	−	−	+

Note: See lecture 23.

4. Enzymes

In addition to histochemical stains, enzyme assays on blood and urine can detect lysozyme (muramidase) with the same pattern of expression as in table 21.2 and with levels correlating with the white blood cell count. *Terminal deoxynucleotidyl transferase* (TdT), a unique DNA polymerase, randomly adds deoxynucleotide units to the 3′-OH terminus of DNA without needing a template. Blasts from 95% of patients with ALL are TdT positive, while fewer than 5% of patients with ANLL have blasts positive for TdT. Some patients with CML evolving into acute leukemia have TdT positive blasts, and these often look and behave like lymphoblasts.

5. Cell surface markers

As discussed in lecture 23, immunologic methods reveal different surface antigens that depend on cell lineages (table 21.3). Surface immunoglobulin (SIg) characterizes all B cells, and in a malignant clone, only one light chain type is expressed. The finding of only one light chain type does not prove monoclonality or malignancy, but in a clinical setting it is often interpreted in that way. The nature of the *common acute lymphocytic leukemia antigen* (CALLA) remains unknown. Empirically it helps distinguish leukemias from other disorders even though it lacks complete specificity. T-series antigens are becoming better understood as monoclonal antibodies are being applied (e.g., the interleukin receptor). Myeloid (My) antigens are just now being explored.

6. Chromosomes

Presumably the several leukemias ultimately derive from the multitude of chromosomal alterations that cause neoplastic transformation. Only a handful of these are established (table 21.4).

V. ACUTE LEUKEMIAS

A. Acute lymphocytic leukemia

1. Clinical features

ALL usually presents abruptly with signs and symptoms of only a few weeks' duration.

Table 21.4
Chromosomal Alterations in Leukemia

Abnormality	Diagnosis
Philadelphia chromosome:	CML
t (9,22) (q34, q11)	90%
Variants: (22q, ___)	5%
t (15–17) (q22, q21)	APL [M_3] 50% of cases
16 inversion	APL with abnormal eosinophils
t (8,21) (q24, q22)	AML [M_2]
t (8,14/2/22)	Burkitt's lymphoma/leukemia

a. Signs of marrow depression

Bruising, bleeding, fever, pallor, and fatigue with shortness of breath relate to aspects of marrow dysfunction: thrombocytopenia, neutropenia, and anemia. A packed, expanding bone marrow can cause bone pain.

b. Signs of organ infiltration

Splenomegaly and hepatomegaly are commonly found. Lymphadenopathy occurs less often.

c. CNS involvement

A special form of tissue infiltration, central nervous system (CNS) involvement presents in three ways: (1) meningeal leukemia (arachnoidal infiltration can produce headache, nausea, vomiting, lethargy, paresis of legs, enuresis, visual disturbances, papilledema, cranial nerve palsies, seizures, and coma; (2) leukostatic thrombi (more common in AML) occurs when circulating blasts exceed 100,000/cu mm and can lead to intracerebral hemorrhage; (3) subarachnoid hemorrhage due to thrombocytopenia.

2. Laboratory features

a. Blood

Anemia is present in more than 90% of patients. The initial white cell count is variable. In nearly half the cases the white count is normal or low; it is above 20,000 in 33% and above 100,000 in 20%. Thrombocytopenia is typically present. Since blasts may or may not be seen in the blood smear, bone marrow aspiration and biopsy are essential for diagnosis.

b. Bone marrow

The bone marrow is largely replaced by lymphoblasts, which account for 50–100% of all marrow cells even when the circulating white cell numbers and the percentage of abnormal forms in the blood are low. The typical lymphoblast contains a round nucleus with diffuse chromatin and 1 or 2 nucleoli and scant basophilic cytoplasm without granules. In many cases it is impossible to distinguish lymphoblasts from myeloblasts.

c. Other tests

Since blood cell morphology alone sometimes fails to distinguish lymphoblasts from myeloblasts, the following tests are performed on the first marrow sample:

1. Terminal deoxynucleotidyl transferase (TdT) is positive in virtually all patients with ALL and negative in ANLL.
2. Periodic acid-Schiff (PAS) stain, which detects intracellular glycogen, is more often positive in ALL than ANLL.
3. Myeloperoxidase stain is negative in ALL and usually positive in ANLL.
4. Nonspecific esterase stain is negative in ALL and often positive in ANLL.
5. Electron microscopy can change the diagnosis to ANLL by detecting microgranules. Surface marker studies help distinguish lineage and prognosis (see table 21.3).
6. Chromosomes: sometimes ALL evolves from CML. A Ph^1 chromosome can suggest such lineage. It also implies a poorer prognosis.

3. Therapy

Treatment can be viewed in terms of tactics and strategy. Tactics are the means of attaining given strategic ends and vary in different institutions using different drugs, dosages, and scheduling. Strategy, however, has become constant over the last decade and falls under four headings: (1) remission induction; (2) CNS prophylaxis; (3) maintenance chemotherapy; and (4) cessation of treatment.

a. Remission induction

Induction aims at bringing the total leukemic cell number below the level of detectability (approximately 10^9) with the use of *prednisone* (a corticosteroid) and *vincristine* (a mitotic spindle inhibitor) and sometimes *anthracycline* (a DNA intercalator). *Asparaginase*, which deprives lymphoblasts of an amino acid more essential to them than to normal cells, consolidates remission. Complete remission is achieved in 95% of children and 75% of adults.

b. CNS prophylaxis

Leukemic cells will have entered the CNS by the time of diagnosis in 70% of patients. Because of the pharmacological blood-brain barrier, the cells are free to divide in spite of effective bone marrow chemotherapy. Thus, they are said to be in a "sanctuary." The resulting *meningeal leukemia,* or "leukemic meningitis," becomes apparent several months later and strikingly reduces the chance of cure. Effective prevention can be provided by administration of *methotrexate* (a folic acid antagonist) directly into the spinal fluid. Because intrathecal administration introduces the drug into the brain ventricles only in small quantities, prophylactic cranial radiation or a high dose of intravenous methotrexate sufficient to cross the blood-brain barrier may also be useful. Such therapy is undertaken as soon as the bone marrow is in remission.

c. Maintenance chemotherapy

Extended treatment aimed at reducing the number of leukemic cells from 10^9 to 0 takes 2 to 3 years in most patients. Effective drugs include *methotrexate* and *6-mercaptopurine* (a purine analogue) with pulses of vincristine, prednisone, and other agents. During this phase chronic bone marrow suppression of a modest degree is necessary to ensure effective drug activity.

d. Cessation of treatment

Current data suggest that there is no advantage to continuing chemotherapy beyond 2½–3 years. Even when bone marrow and spinal fluid remain visibly disease free, testicular biopsy occasionally may reveal another sanctuary of disease requiring radiotherapy. Otherwise treatment is terminated, and the patient is followed closely. The major complication of treatment is immunosuppression with increased susceptibility to bacterial, fungal, viral, or parasitic infections. Improved supportive care therefore adds to the cure rate.

4. Prognosis

By following these simple strategic goals, the results shown in figure 21.1 have been obtained, with over half of children apparently cured. Factors affecting the prognosis adversely are: (1) age (<2 or >9 years); (2) male sex; (3) WBC greater than 20,000/cu mm; (4) presence of mediastinal mass; (5) CNS disease; (6) T, B, or pre-B cell disease; and (7) Ph^1 chromosome. The largest group (65–75% of patients) has null-cell CALLA-positive disease, which has a good prognosis. A small group with T-cell disease combines most of the other adverse prognostic factors and has a dramatically poorer outlook. Adults do not fare as well as children, but results of more aggressive therapy protocols are promising. Almost all relapses occur within 5 years. Treatable relapsed ALL is rarely cured. Bone marrow transplantation may improve the outlook. In vitro monoclonal treatment offers a way to "clean up" marrow for autotransplantation.

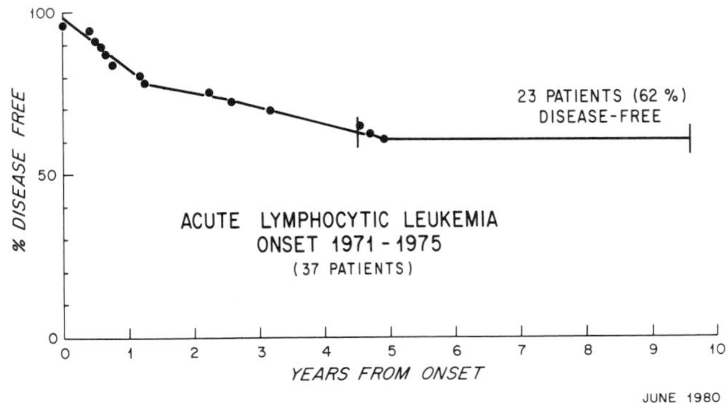

Fig. 21.1
Survival in childhood ALL. The figure summarizes experience with 37 patients seen at the Massachusetts General Hospital from 1971 to 1975. Each closed circle represents bone marrow relapse during chemotherapy. As of January 1980, 23 patients remain disease-free, although 2 patients developed recurrent leukemia following cessation of chemotherapy and required an additional 3 yr of treatment.

B. Acute nonlymphocytic leukemia

As noted above, this family is subdivided into various categories on the basis of blood cell morphology and biochemical studies; however, their distinctness from ALL places them together.

1. Clinical features

Onset is usually abrupt as in ALL with similar symptoms and clinical findings. Occasionally in an elderly patient, a smoldering leukemia makes a slow appearance over several months or years. Splenomegaly, lymphadenopathy and CNS disease are less common than in ALL. An unusual form of tissue infiltration, gum involvement, occurs in the monocytic variety.

2. Laboratory features

a. AML

Diagnosis rests on a finding of excess nonlymphoid blasts in the bone marrow aspirate and on laboratory studies described above. A typical myeloblast has an irregular nucleus with loose or finely dispersed chromatin, 2 or more nucleoli with a punched-out appearance, and a moderate amount of light-blue cytoplasm. Usually blasts are accompanied by promyelocytes but by few cells intermediate in differentiation. This is a *leukemic hiatus*. *Auer rods*, or *bodies* (needle-like red cytoplasmic inclusions consisting of lysosomal material), are pathognomonic for ANLL but are seen in fewer than 50% of patients. In general the more granules that are visible on Wright's stain, the more strongly positive will be the peroxidase and esterase stains.

b. Myelomonocytic and monocytic leukemias

The leukemic cells in myelomonocytic leukemia combine features of myelocytes and monocytes. They are faintly positive or negative for peroxidase, but histochemical, serum, and urine lysozyme are usually greatly elevated. In a few cases the blast nuclei are clearly monocytoid.

c. Promyelocytic leukemia

Characteristic cells are uniformly and densely filled with granules that stain intensely for peroxidase and often with Auer rods in large numbers. Procoagulant material released from these granules, especially after treatment accelerates cell lysis, initiate disseminated intravascular coagulation (DIC) (see lecture 28) and a severe hemorrhagic diathesis, distinctive of promyelocytic leukemia. Coagulation factors are consumed, and fibrin split products accumulate in the serum. Aggressive replacement of clotting factors and platelets is often necessary, and heparin therapy may be required. A specific chromosome translocation (15,17) can be found in 50% of cases.

d. Erythroleukemia

In its early stage this disorder (also known as Di Guglielmo's disease) is characterized by erythroid dysplasia and ineffective erythropoiesis (see lecture 5). As it progresses, the red cell precursors become bizarre and multinucleated. It finally reaches an erythromyelocytic phase marked by increasing numbers of dysplastic promyelocytes and myeloblasts, along with a population of primitive blast cells difficult to classify. Eventually most cases evolve into AML.

e. Other leukemia

Eosinophilic, basophilic, and megakaryocytic leukemias are rarely encounted leukemias in which immature eosinophils, basophils, or megakaryocytes predominate. Eosinophilic leukemia is difficult to distinguish from the hypereosinophilic syndromes (see lecture 19).

3. Therapy

As with ALL, therapy follows certain widely accepted strategic considerations.

a. Remission

Current regimens use *cytosine arabinoside* (a cycle-specific antimetabolite) and *daunorubicin* (an anthracycline antibiotic) given aggressively to induce complete marrow aplasia. In 75% of patients normal marrow regenerates within 3–6 weeks. The supportive care of patients in a prolonged phase of marrow aplasia requires meticulous attention to antibiotics and blood product replacement and can be undertaken only in major medical centers. Remission must be confirmed by the demonstration of normal bone marrow recovery.

b. Maintenance chemotherapy

With aggressive maintenance chemotherapy, 5-year disease-free survivals are achieved in approximately 25% of patients. It has not yet been determined at what point therapy can safely be terminated, nor has it been shown that specific CNS treatment is essential. Bone marrow transplantation using HLA-identical siblings produces prolonged disease-free survivals in about 50% of recipients when done during first remission in patients under 30. Since there is only 1 chance in 4 that a sibling will share HLA identity with a patient, however, marrow transplantation now can be offered to only a small portion of leukemic patients. The procedure consists of withdrawing 10^{10} marrow cells by aspiration from the donor and administering them intravenously to a recipient who has been immunosuppressed by total body irradiation and massive chemotherapy.

VI. THE CHRONIC LEUKEMIAS

A. Chronic myelocytic leukemia

1. Clinical features

CML is the least common of the major leukemias. Some would group it with the myeloproliferative disorders (see lecture 19). Often it is discovered on routine physical or blood examination during a preclinical phase that lasts 1–3 years. Fullness in the upper abdomen, due to an enlarged spleen, may be the presenting complaint. As disease advances, an enlarged spleen is found in 80–

90% of patients. Symptoms due to hypermetabolism include easy fatigue, low-grade fever, night sweats, and weight loss. Bones are often tender. Sometimes accumulation of leukemic cells form masses in the skin and elsewhere called chloromas. Eventually, as in other leukemias, bleeding, anemia, and infection cause disability and death.

2. Laboratory features

a. Blood

Leukocytosis is characteristically present with a white count in the range of 50,000–500,000/cu mm. High white counts may be recognized early from the size of the buffy coat in the hematocrit tube. Every 1% of leukocyte hematocrit is roughly equivalent to 15,000 white cells/cu mm. On blood smears neutrophils, metamyelocytes, and myelocytes predominate while some blasts appear. A greater frequency of eosinophilic and basophilic granulocytes helps distinguish CML from benign leukocytosis or leukemoid reaction. Early in the course of CML, moderate anemia is common. Red cells may display anisocytosis but seldom significant pokilocytosis as in myeloid metaplasia (where ''teardrop''-shaped cells are common). Occasional normoblasts, polychromatophilic cells, and basophilic stippling of red cells may be seen. Platelet levels are usually normal or increased, sometimes to levels above 1,000,000/cu mm, although their function is often abnormal.

b. Bone marrow

The marrow shows marked granulocytic hyperplasia with a predominance of metamyelocytes, myelocytes, and frequently increased numbers of megakaryocytes. Bone marrow cells usually resemble those in the blood so that marrow aspiration is not essential. There is no leukemic hiatus between immature and mature forms as in the acute leukemias. The M/E ratio is strikingly elevated, reaching 25 : 1 or higher.

c. Ph^1 chromosome

The great majority (95%) of patients have a Ph^1 chromosome. The clone of granulocytes having this abnormality develops a selective advantage and over a period of several years replaces normal myeloid precursors. Ultimately all granulocyte, megakaryocyte, erythroid elements, and perhaps B lymphocytes contain the abnormal chromosome. Fibroblasts do not. Thus the Ph^1 chromosome reflects the presence of a somatic cell mutation. Prognosis of the disease is generally poorer in Ph^1-negative or variant patients, in-whom death usually occurs within a year.

d. Leukocyte alkaline phosphatase

A low leukocyte alkaline phosphatase is found in 90% of patients. This distinguishes CML from leukemoid reactions and myeloid metaplasia (see lecture 19).

e. Other features

As in other conditions with high granulocyte counts, serum vitamin B_{12} and vitamin B_{12}-binding proteins (especially TC III) are markedly increased in CML. Uric acid levels are commonly elevated.

3. Course

A rapidly evolving acute phase, or blastic crisis, occurs within 3–6 years of diagnosis. Over a few weeks or months the granulocytes in the blood become increasingly immature, ultimately terminating in a blastic picture indistinguishable from acute leukemia. Further karyotypic abnormalities often accompany the change. In a third of such patients, the blasts have characteristics (positive TdT and negative peroxidase) and electron microscopic appearance of lymphoblasts. In these cases there is often a dramatic though short-lived response to ALL-type induction treatment with vincristine and prednisone, but as in the more common nonlymphoid form, the patient dies of uncontrolled blastic replacement of the marrow within a few months. Most patients live normal and productive lives for a number of years from the time of diagnosis before going into blast crisis or an accelerated phase with attendant infection and bleeding but without excessive blasts.

4. Therapy

The alkylating agent *busulfan* reduces the leukemia cell burden but rarely eradicates all cells with the Ph^1 chromosome to effect a complete remission. *Hydroxyurea* (an agent that blocks DNA synthesis) and *6-mercaptopurine* also control the disease temporarily, and radiation therapy can shrink refractory splenomegaly. Hyperuricemia can be controlled with *allopurinol*. Thus far cure has been achieved only in a few patients with marrow transplantation.

B. Chronic lymphocytic leukemia

CLL is a disease of the elderly that in many ways resembles diffuse, well-differentiated lymphocytic lymphoma (see lectures 22 and 23). It has a peculiar population distribution: rare in Orientals yet one of the most common forms of leukemia among Western peoples.

1. Clinical features

There is usually generalized lymphadenopathy and moderate splenomegaly, often of many years' duration. The disease characteristically follows an indolent, asymptomatic course, but a certain percentage of cases may become more aggressive. Frequently the patients are asymptomatic. Common complaints include fatigue, weight loss, fever, and night sweats.

2. Laboratory features

Typically the white count ranges between 20,000 and 150,000/cu mm and occasionally over 1 million. The cells are primarily mature lymphocytes with clonal B surface markers (i.e., they have surface immunoglobulin with a single light chain type). A $14q^+$ abnormality is common. In spite of the vast number of cells there is less crowding of normal bone marrow until years into the course. Thus significant thrombocytopenia, neutropenia, and anemia signify advancing disease. Common complications of CLL are immunological. Reduction of immunoglobulins and decreased numbers of granulocytes predispose to infection. Antibody response to antigenic challenge is impaired, yet autoantibodies sometimes develop. Immunohemolytic anemia may be overt, with icterus, indirect hyperbilirubinemia, brisk reticulocytosis, spherocytosis, and a positive Coombs test (see lecture 12). Less often ITP aggravates the thrombocytopenia already produced by diminished platelet production and hypersplenism (see lecture 27). Dermatologic manifestations include leukemia cutis, herpes zoster, generalized erythroderma, exfoliative dermatitis, and severe reaction to smallpox vaccination and insect bites. Patients with CLL have a high incidence of nonleukemic malignancies, such as cancer of the skin, lung, and bowel, which may be evidence favoring the view that malignant disease is prevented or controlled in normal subjects by a process of immunologic surveillance.

3. Therapy

The treatment of CLL is undertaken with prudence. In elderly patients the disease follows a slow and remarkably benign course, with mortality figures for the untreated CLL patients not differing significantly from population controls. In younger patients (ages 40–60) more aggressive disease often necessitates more aggressive treatment. It is usually wise to treat the patient's symptoms rather than the white count. Alkylating agents such as *chlorambucil* or *cyclophosphamide* are the initial choices. *Prednisone* may be added judiciously. Radiation therapy can shrink obstructing lymph nodes or a bothersome spleen. Exciting research centers on immunologic approaches to therapy using interferon or monoclonal antibodies against idiotypic determinants of the surface immunoglobulin.

4. Hairy cell leukemia

Leukemic reticuloendotheliosis (hairy cell leukemia) is a rare but malignant variant of CLL characterized by splenomegaly and pancytopenia. Characteristic cells with hairy projections can be seen on phase microscopy or identified histochemically with tartrate-resistant acid phosphatase. The most effective treatment is splenectomy. Alpha interferon has been reported to benefit some patients.

5. T-cell CLL

Adult T cell leukemia is a rare variety of CLL closely linked to the human T cell leukemia virus (HTLV) (see lecture 23). First described in Japan and the Caribbean, it presents with lymphadenopathy, skin lesions, and hypercalcemia. Mature-appearing lymphocytes with "knobby" nuclear outlines have surface markers of helper cells but functionally help to suppress nitogen-driven antibody production. Much more aggressive than an immunologically distinct chronic T cell leukemia that presents with neutropenia, HTLV-associated leukemia responds poorly to therapy and follows a more subacute course.

SELECTED REFERENCES

Blayney, D. W., et al. The human T-cell leukemia/lymphoma virus, lymphoma, lytic bone lesions, and hypercalcemia. *Ann. Intern. Med.* 98(1983): 144.

Bouroncle, B. A. Leukemic reticuloendotheliosis (hairy cell leukemia). *Blood* 53(1979): 412.

Fefer, A., et al. Treatment of chronic granulocytic leukemia with chemoradiotherapy and transplantation from identical twins. *New Engl. J. Med.* 306(1982): 63.

Foon, K. A., et al. Surface markers on leukemia and lymphoma cells: Recent advances. *Blood* 60(1982): 1.

Haghbin, M., et al. A long term follow-up of children with acute lymphoblastic leukemia treated with intensive chemotherapy regimens. *Cancer* 46(1980): 241.

Koeffller, H. P., and Golde, D. W. Human preleukemia. *Ann. Int. Med.* 93(1980): 347.

Koeffler, H. P., and Golde, D. W. Chronic myelogenous leukemia—new concepts. *New Eng. J. Med.* 301(1979): 597.

Thomas, E. D., et al. Marrow transplantation for acute nonlymphoblastic leukemia in first remission. *New Eng. J. Med.* 201(1979): 597.

Weinstein, H. J., et al. Treatment of acute myelogenous leukemia in children and adults. *New Eng. J. Med.* 303(1980): 473.

LECTURE 22 The Malignant Lymphomas I. Clinical Aspects

David S. Rosenthal

I. INTRODUCTION

A. Definitions

This lecture deals with a group of disorders known as the *malignant lymphomas*. They involve the cells of the *lymphatic system* (which are discussed in lecture 2) and thus are termed *lymphoproliferative disorders*, a category that also includes the lymphocytic leukemias, ALL and CLL, which were discussed in lecture 21, and Waldenström's macroglobulinemia, which is discussed in lecture 24. Although there are similarities among the various lymphomas, they include a wide spectrum of clinical and histological patterns.

B. Enlarged lymph nodes

One of the major clinical presentations of lymphoma is enlarged lymph nodes. Although lymphadenopathy is always ominous because it may signify malignant disease, it should be emphasized that enlarged lymph nodes are more commonly related to infectious, inflammatory, and other benign disorders. Lymph node enlargement is most commonly a secondary phenomenon—a reaction to a nearby inflammatory process or to a systemic process. Table 22.1 lists the major causes of lymphadenopathy. A careful history and physical examination is most important in evaluating a patient with enlarged lymph nodes. Infectious nodes are usually soft, tender, less than 2 cm in diameter, and located in areas that drain common infections. For example, the anterior and posterior cervical chain of the neck drains the ears and throat. Potentially malignant nodes are generally firm, hard, or rubbery, fixed to underlying tissue, multiple, nontender, greater than 2 cm in diameter, and located in unusual sites—for example, the infraclavicular area. When the diagnosis is uncertain, histologic examination of an enlarged lymph node is essential.

Because of its characteristic pathology, *Hodgkin's disease* has been separated from the other lymphomas. This fact (and limitations of our knowledge) has led to an unfortunate terminology in which the other lymphoid malignancies are grouped under the term *non-Hodgkin's lymphoma*. Research is active in this area, and new concepts of Hodgkin's disease and non-Hodgkin's lymphoma are continuously appearing in the literature. The student is urged to consider this changing field critically.

Table 22.1
Causes of Lymph Node Enlargement

Infections
Acute (infectious mononucleosis, toxoplasmosis, cytomegalovirus, generalized dermatitis, common communicable diseases)
Chronic (syphilis, tuberculosis, sarcoidosis)
Hypersensitivity reactions and connective tissue disease
Serum sickness
Rheumatoid arthritis
Systemic lupus erythematosus
Drug pseudolymphoma (diphenylhydantoin)
Primary lymphoproliferative disease
Hodgkin's disease
Non-Hodgkin's lymphoma
Leukemia (CLL, ALL, blast crisis of CML)
Waldenström's macroglobulinemia
Endocrine disorder
Hyperthyroidism
Hypoadrenalism
Hypopituitarism
Lipidoses
Metastatic cancer
Breast
Lung
Gastrointestinal

II. HODGKIN'S DISEASE

A. Introduction

In 1666 a fatal disease was described in which the lymphoid tissues and spleen appeared as a "cluster of grapes." In 1832 Thomas Hodgkin and later Samuel Wilkes described a disease characterized by gradual progressive enlargement of the lymph nodes "beginning usually in the cervical region and spreading throughout the lymphoid tissue of the body, forming nodular growths in the internal organs, resulting in anemia, and usually, fatal cachexia." The major features of these cases were (1) slow and relentless growth, the disease sometimes lasting many years and (2) characteristic histopathologic pattern (as later elucidated by Reed and Sternberg) that included the distinctive giant cell known as the *Reed-Sternberg cell* (see figure 23.3). Although it was later found that Reed-Sternberg cells occur in other disorders, pathologists now require that this cell be present before concluding that the diagnosis is Hodgkin's disease. Researchers have wondered which is the malignant cell in this disease—histiocytes, lymphocytes, or Reed-Sternberg cells. Many believe that the Reed-Sternberg cell is neoplastic and that it is admixed with presumably reactive populations of lymphocytes, eosinophils, and others. Current evidence indirectly suggests that Hodgkin's disease is a proliferative disorder of T cells (e.g., defects in cell-mediated immunity; preferential involvement of thymus-dependent portions of lymphoreticular system; increase in T cells in involved nodes). In vitro cultivation of Hodgkin's disease tissue has not yet been possible. The disorder has never been described in animals and is one of the most unusual diseases of humans. Until recently, it was considered a catastrophic, nearly always fatal illness. The advent of modern radiation therapy and chemotherapy has dramatically altered its course and prognosis. Some have now questioned whether clinically this is a malignant disease because of the excellent prognosis in early stages.

B. Epidemiology

Hodgkin's disease occurs at a rate of 2 per 100,000 population per year in the United States. However, the incidence varies widely according to age, sex, and geography. In the United States and Northern Europe, Hodgkin's disease has a peculiar bimodal age incidence with a high peak occurring between 15 and 35 and a lower peak after the age of 50. There is a slight male predominance.

Recent epidemiologic studies suggest a higher incidence of Hodgkin's disease among high school students in some areas of the United States and in relatives of patients with Hodgkin's disease. However, the statistical validity of these findings has been questioned, and more prospective data will be needed before the existence of clusters or predisposed families can be established.

Several reports suggest that there is an increased incidence or risk of the disease among siblings, especially of the same sex, that may be related to identity of HLA antigens.

C. Clinical features

Hodgkin's disease usually presents with a nonpainful swelling of a lymph node in the neck. Less commonly, the onset may be marked by fever, night sweats, and weight loss. Rarely, patients initially experience severe itching of the skin (pruritis).

Unlike the pattern in other lymphomas, Hodgkin's disease usually spreads contiguously from one lymph node region to another. For example, in a patient with early Hodgkin's disease, there may be involvement of only neck and mediastinal nodes. In patients presenting with more advanced disease, diffuse adenopathy, along with involvement of liver, marrow, lung, or other organs, may be present.

As will be noted in detail below, it is customary to speak of the several *stages* of Hodgkin's disease—and of the process of determining the stage in a given patient's course of disease as *staging*. In the early or favorable stages, it is the characteristic contiguous nature of the pattern of spread that makes staging such an important guide to treatment.

There is a close relation between the occurrence of significant symptoms and the course of Hodgkin's disease. Typical symptoms consist of a loss of more than 10% of the body weight (unrelated to dieting), persistent fever that is not due to infection, and night sweats. Generalized itching (pruritis) may be a related symptom.

D. Histologic classification

The histologic classification currently employed is known as the Rye Conference (1965) classification. This classification, which is discussed in lecture 23, includes four major types: *lymphocyte predominance, nodular sclerosis, mixed cellularity*, and *lymphocyte depletion*. The course of the disease is related to the histologic type. Patients who present with nodular sclerosis and lymphocyte-predominant types of Hodgkin's disease generally have a much better prognosis than those with mixed cellularity and lymphocyte-depleted types of Hodgkin's disease. The histologic features of the four types are discussed in lecture 23.

E. Clinical staging

In addition to the histologic type, it is important in determining prognosis and therapy to quantify the amount and distribution of disease present at the onset. Currently accepted criteria and definitions for the four clinical stages of Hodgkin's disease and non-Hodgkin's lymphoma are summarized in table 22.2.

Table 22.2
Modified Definitions of Clinical Stages (Ann Arbor Symposium 1971)

Stage	Clinical features (and terminology)
I	Involvement of a single lymph node region or involvement of a single extralymphatic organ or site
II	Involvement of two or more lymph node regions on the same side of the diaphragm alone or with involvement of limited, contiguous extralymphatic organ or tissue
III	Involvement of lymph node regions on both sides of the diaphragm (which may include the spleen and/or limited contiguous extralymphatic organ or site)
III_1	Involvement limited to spleen, splenic hilar nodes, and high abdominal nodes
III_2	Involvement of para-aortic, pelvic and iliac nodes in addition to III_1 involvement
IV	Multiple or disseminated foci of involvement of one or more extralymphatic organs or tissues, with or without lymphatic involvement

Note: All cases are further subclassified to indicate the absence (A) or presence (B) of the systemic symptoms: significant fever, night sweats, and/or unexplained weight loss of greater than 10% of normal body weight. Thus, a patient is said to be in stage IIIA or IIIB. The term *clinical stage* (CS) refers to the patient's stage as determined by diagnostic examinations and a single diagnostic biopsy. If a second biopsy or laparotomy is performed, the term *pathologic stage* (PS) is used.

Experience has shown that systematic clinical staging must include the following examinations: (1) physical examination with careful attention to all lymph node areas; (2) various routine laboratory studies; (3) computerized tomography scans of the abdomen, the latter supplying information regarding the liver and abdominal nodes; (4) a bipedal lymphangiogram, a procedure in which radio-opaque dye is injected into lymphatic channels of the feet with resulting visualization of iliac and para-aortic nodes. In some clinics laparoscopy is performed following lymphangiography. The liver and spleen are inspected, and the liver is biopsied under direct visualization. In most clinics, if the CT scans of the abdomen are negative a so-called staging laparotomy is carried out in which the abdomen is explored and suspicious nodes seen on the lymphangiogram are removed. Splenectomy is performed, and biopsies are performed of both lobes of the liver and the bone marrow. With a careful and detailed pathologic examination of the spleen, minute areas of Hodgkin's disease are often identifiable. Splenic Hodgkin's disease without evidence of disease elsewhere in the abdomen suggests that involvement of various organs (such as the spleen) may occur not only by contiguous extension but by hematogenous spread. Experience has shown that staging laparotomy alters the clinician's opinion of the patient's stage in a third of the cases and, more important, may change the plan of therapy. A final judgment whether surgical staging should be restricted to certain types of cases or whether it should be done at all will not be possible until more patients have been observed for longer periods of time. Most investigators now suggest that if the operative findings may change the therapeutic plan, then laparotomy is necessary. Clinical emergencies may arise when massive lymph node enlargement compresses vital organs. For example, a malignant node may compress the trachea or the venous return to the heart (superior vena caval syndrome) or obstruct urinary flow by extrinsic compression of the ureters. These life-threatening occurrences require immediate therapy.

F. Laboratory studies

There are no pathognomonic hematologic findings in Hodgkin's disease. Leukocytosis with lymphocytopenia is not uncommon. An elevated erythrocyte sedimentation rate (ESR) will correlate with disease activity, and serial ESR studies may be a useful way to follow the disease process. Eosinophilia and rarely monocytosis are noted. Other hematologic abnormalities such as leukopenia and thrombocytopenia usually appear with advanced disease and are either secondary to bone marrow involvement or previous therapy.

Patients frequently demonstrate defects in delayed hypersensitivity reaction and have negative tuberculin reactions even in the presence of active tuberculosis. This defect in cellular immunity is probably associated with an increased incidence of infections with unusual organisms, such as *Pneumocystis carinii*, various fungi, and herpes zoster. The impairment of cellular immunity appears to be related in part to active suppression of T lymphocyte function.

G. Course and prognosis

The factors that appear to correlate with the course of the disease are the following: (1) presence or absence of "B" symptoms; (2) age of the patient; older patients tend to do more poorly than younger patients; (3) type of histology: patients with lymphocyte predominance, nodular sclerosis, and mixed cellularity have a more favorable prognosis than those with lymphocyte depletion; and (4) clinical stage: patients in stages I and II have a more favorable prognosis than those in stages III and IV (and those in stage III have a better prognosis than those in Stage IV).

H. Therapy

Major therapeutic developments that began in the early 1960s have dramatically improved the incidence and duration of remissions. With increasing experience, methods of therapy undergo continuing modification. Future research on the etiology and pathogenesis of Hodgkin's disease may lead to new and more physiologic forms of therapy.

1. Radiation therapy

The concept of intensive, "curative" irradiation therapy for Hodgkin's disease was developed by Gilbert and Peters and later by Kaplan and Johnson. Details of therapy and expected results vary with the stage. Table 22.3 summarizes approximate 5-yr disease-free survival rates currently associated with various therapeutic programs. Radiation therapy is usually delivered into three major fields—known as the mantle, para-aortic, and pelvic or inverted Y fields (figure 22.1). In total nodal radiation therapy, treatment is given to all three fields, which encompass most of the body's lymph node regions.

Table 22.3
Five-Year Disease-free Survival Rates in Hodgkin's Disease

Stage	Therapy	Five-year disease-free survival (%)
I and IIA	Intensive radiation therapy	85–90
IB, IIB (rare)	Intensive radiation therapy	80–85
IIIA	Intensive radiation therapy or chemotherapy	60–90
$IIIA_1$	Intensive radiation therapy or chemotherapy	60–80
$IIIA_2$	Chemotherapy ± radiation therapy	60–80
IIIB	Chemotherapy ± radiation therapy	60–80
IVA and IVB	Chemotherapy alone	30–50

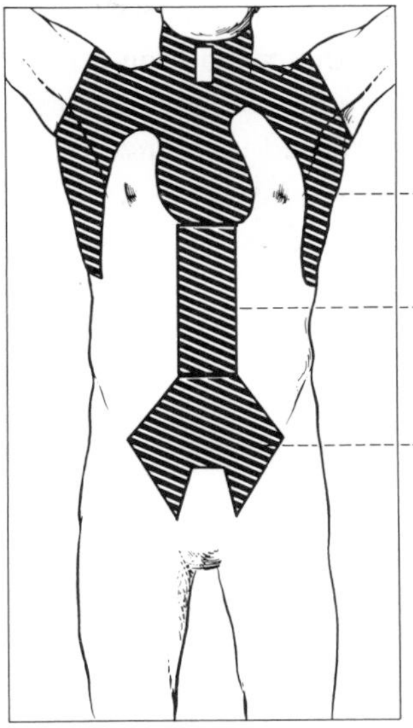

Fig. 22.1
Radiation fields in therapy of Hodgkin's disease. Shaded areas represent the three treatment fields. The *mantle field* is the uppermost field. Lungs and vocal cords are protected by lead blocks; heart and thyroid are within the field. The *para-aortic field*, or middle field, extends from the diaphragm to just above the bifurcation of the aorta. When the spleen has not been removed, this field is extended to include the entire spleen and splenic hilum. The *pelvic* or *inverted Y field* is the lowest field. It encompasses the pelvic and inguinal nodes and includes a large area of bone marrow.

2. Chemotherapy

Aggressive chemotherapy has also produced long disease-free remissions in advanced Hodgkin's disease. A program developed by DeVita and coworkers, known as MOPP (for the drug combination Mustargen® (nitrogen mustard) Oncovin® (vincristine), procarbazine, and prednisone) has resulted in complete remissions in 60–70%. However, 5-yr disease-free survival was obtained in only 50% of these cases. Recently, other combined chemotherapy programs employing Adriamycin®, bleomycin, vinblastine, and imidazole carboxamide have yielded similar results.

3. Therapeutic approach

Currently therapy is dictated by the stage of disease. The monocentric origin and the orderly spread have led to the approach of treating the known disease and the potential next site of occurrence. For example, with disease limited to the mediastinal nodes (stage I), radiation therapy to the mantle area plus an upper abdominal field would be recommended. If the disease were widespread in all nodal areas above and below the diaphragm, including the spleen, the next potential site of spread would be a parenchymal organ, and therefore one would consider chemotherapy as the primary mode of therapy.

4. Complications

The combined use of intensive radiation therapy and chemotherapy has created immediate and long-term complications. The former can be ameliorated by skillful dosage adjustment and overall management. An increased incidence of second malignancies, especially leukemia, as a consequence of combined therapy now seems well established. Careful consideration in recommending therapy must be given to these late complications and others (table 22.4).

III. NON-HODGKIN'S LYMPHOMA

A. Introduction

This is a heterogenous collection of lymphoid malignancies with some common features and many differences. Unlike Hodgkin's disease they appear to be multicentric in origin with a tendency to spread widely early in the disease. A peripheral blood leukemic phase is not uncommon (figure 22.2A), and there is some evidence that nearly all patients with non-Hodgkin's lymphoma have malignant cells in their blood regardless of the stage of disease.

B. Incidence

Non-Hodgkin's lymphoma, unlike Hodgkin's disease, is primarily a disease of older adults, with a peak incidence in the late 50s. Although it is infrequent in children and young adults, untreated it is usually an aggressive and potentially rapidly fatal disease in this age group.

C. Clinical features

Presenting signs and symptoms are extremely variable and relate to site and extent of disease. Many patients seek investigation of an enlarged node or abdominal mass. Other cases begin with com-

Table 22.4
Complications of Therapy of Hodgkin's Disease

Radiation therapy (RT)
Hypothyroidism
Pericarditis
Pneumonitis
Chemotherapy (CT)
Nausea, vomiting
Alopecia (especially with Adriamycin®)
Sterility in males (especially with alkylating agents)
Myelosuppression
Neuropathy (vincristine)
Cardiomyopathy
RT plus CT (combined modality therapy)
Second malignancies, especially acute leukemia and non-Hodgkin's lymphoma

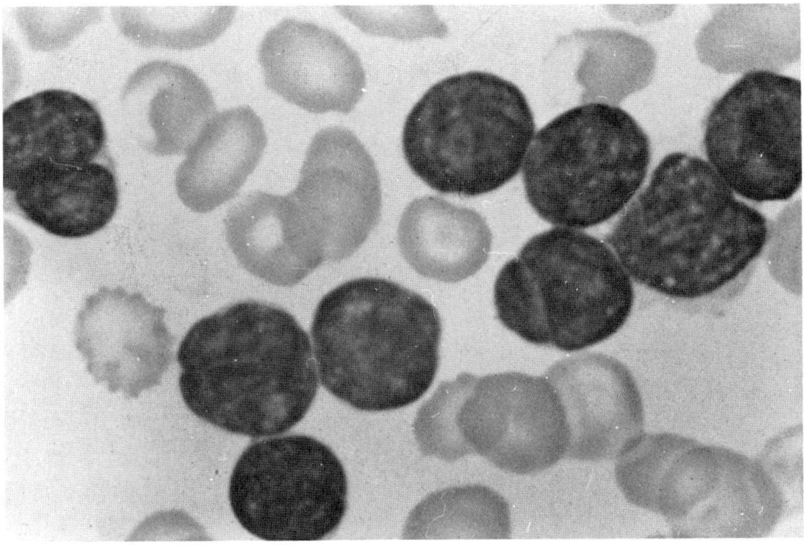

A

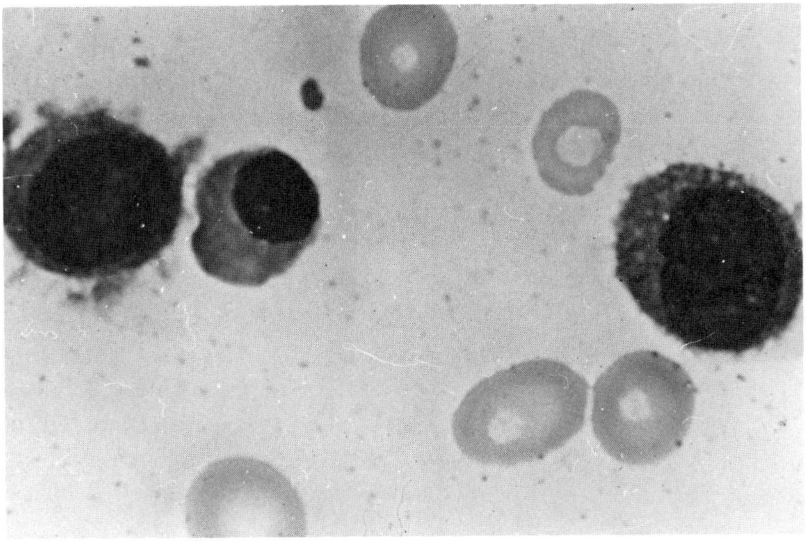

B

Fig. 22.2
Abnormal peripheral blood in lymphoproliferative disorders. A leukemic blood picture may occur during the course of non-Hodgkin's lymphoma. *A*, cells in this field (×500) have cleaved or fissured nuclei, which indicate immaturity. *B*, hairy cells with hairy cytoplasmic projections and cleaved nuclei (×500).

plaints referable to the alimentary tract, for example, a pharyngeal mass, abdominal pain, vomiting, or gastrointestinal bleeding. Systemic manifestations are usually bland: fever, sweats, and itching are uncommon; weight loss is common.

Most non-Hodgkin's lymphomas are B-cell malignancies and may be accompanied by hypogammaglobulinemia and autoimmune phenomenon such as immunohemolytic anemia or immunothrombocytopenia.

D. Classification

The classification (see lecture 23) of the non-Hodgkin's lymphomas is a complicated subject that can be approached in three ways:

1. Nodal architecture (according to Rappaport): nodular appearance *versus* diffuse histology.
2. Degree of cellular differentiation, i.e., well-differentiated lymphocytic *versus* poorly differentiated *versus* undifferentiated cell types.
3. Immunologic classification (according to Lukes): based on whether a malignant lymphoid cell is a B cell, T cell, or undefined. The majority (80%) are of B cell origin.

A recent review demonstrated that non-Hodgkin's lymphomas could be subgrouped into those major categories that had clinical significance: low-grade, intermediate-grade, or high-grade malignancies (see table 22.5). This formulation attempts to combine the three previously used classifications.

E. Clinical staging

The extent of disease at initial presentation is determined on the basis of history, physical examination, blood studies, bone marrow biopsy, and CT scan. Such studies demonstrated that less than 15% of the patients with non-Hodgkin's lymphoma are in stage I or II when first seen (compared to 30–60% in Hodgkin's disease). Thus most patients have diffuse disease from the onset, and staging laparotomy usually is of no benefit.

F. Incidence of leukemia

Unlike Hodgkin's disease, in which leukemia occurs only rarely (and then it may be as a complication of combined intensive radiation therapy and chemotherapy), leukemia is common in the non-Hodgkin's lymphomas. This fact makes the prognosis even worse. The leukemic cell type is usually similar to that seen in the involved lymph node.

G. Therapy

Chemotherapy combinations (table 22.6) in most instances give more and better remissions than single agents. Therapy with single agents may be justified, however, in favorable histologic groups (nodular).

Table 22.5
New Formulation of Non-Hodgkin's Lymphoma (Rappaport)

Categories	New symbols
Low grade	
Small lymphocytes	WDL
Similar to CLL	
Plasmacytoid features	
Follicular small cleaved lymphocyte	NPDL
Follicular small cleaved and large cell-mixed	NM
Intermediate	
Follicular predominantly large cell	NH
Diffuse small cleaved	DPDL
Diffuse mixed small and large cell	DM
Diffuse large cell	DH
Cleaved	
Noncleaved	
High grade	
Diffuse large cell immunoblastic	DH
Plasmacytoid (B cell)	
Clear (T cell)	
Polymorphous	
Epithelial cell component	
Lymphoblastic	LB
Convoluted	
Nonconvoluted	
Small noncleaved	DU
Burkitt's	
Non-Burkitt's	

Table 22.6
Chemotherapy Programs Used in Non-Hodgkin's Lymphomas

Single agents	Combination programs
Vinca alkaloids: Vincristine (Oncovin®); Vinblastine (Velban®)	CVP or COP: cyclophosphamide, vincristine (Oncovin®), prednisone
Corticosteroids: Prednisone	C-MOPP: Cyclophosphamide plus MOPP
Alkylating agents: Cyclophosphamide (Cytoxan®); Chlorambucil (Leukeran®)	B-COP: Bleomycin plus COP
Anthracycline: Adriamycin®	BACOP: Adriamycin® plus B-COP
Other drugs: Procarbazine; Methotrexate; Bleomycin	M-BACOP: high dose methotrexate plus BACOP

1. Low-grade non-Hodgkin's lymphoma

Low grade types, e.g., nodular poorly differentiated lymphocytic (NPDL), are frequently slow growing, quick to respond to relatively little chemotherapy or radiation, and frequently require little or no therapy for months to years. Unfortunately, although extremely sensitive to therapy, there is a high recurrence rate, and very few patients are free of disease for the long term. Statistics for various therapies demonstrate 55–65% 10-year survivors but only 5–15% 10-year disease-free survivors. Currently it is recommended that patients be treated conservatively for symptoms of enlarging or obstructing adenopathy. Eventually this "favorable" subgroup may convert to a "high-grade," "unfavorable," or resistant non-Hodgkin's lymphoma, with death resulting eventually.

2. High-grade non-Hodgkin's lymphoma

High-grade types, e.g., diffuse histiocytic (DH), are aggressive forms whose cells are very immature, have a high growth rate, a short natural history of disease (several months), and resist mild forms of therapy. In patients who achieve a complete remission, however, a significant proportion (40–60%) continue in remission long after stopping chemotherapy and appear to be cured. It is suspected that because these lymphomas are so rapidly growing, they can be cured by aggressive chemotherapies.

H. Unusual clinical problems

1. Burkitt's lymphoma

This extranodal lymphoma (usually affecting the jaw) was first described in Uganda by Burkitt. The histology is specific. The disorder is probably caused by an infectious DNA virus, specifically the Epstein-Barr virus, which is the same agent that causes infectious mononucleosis (see lecture 19). Specific cytogenetic abnormalities have been described involving translocation of 2, 14, 22 with 12. The disease is notably sensitive to chemotherapy.

2. Primary gastrointestinal lymphoma

This disorder, common in Mediterranean areas, is associated with an IgA gammopathy.

I. Related disorders

1. Mycosis fungoides

Mycosis fungoides is a slowly progressive neoplastic proliferation of T-lymphocytes. The disease presents with skin involvement and may remain confined there for years but in time spreads to other organs. Skin lesions are destructive. Biopsy reveals an indurated plaque with a mixed infiltrate in the upper dermis near the epidermal basement membrane. Histology is classified in lecture 23.

As the disease progresses, nodules and fungating tumors develop in the skin, and histiocytic proliferation spreads to lymph nodes, lung, spleen, liver, bone marrow, and myocardium.

2. Sézary's syndrome

Sézary's syndrome is a rare chronic disorder that is associated with diffuse erythroderma that is progressive and pruritic, exfoliative lesions, and lymphadenopathy. Characteristics of Sézary cells are described in lecture 23. Unlike the abnormal lymphocyte of CLL, which is a B cell, this is a T cell. Skin biopsy reveals an upper dermal infiltrate somewhat like that of mycosis fungoides. The T cell in both mycosis fungoides and Sézary's syndrome is usually of the helper subset (T4).

3. Waldenström's macroglobulinemia

This IgM gammopathy is a form of non-Hodgkin's lymphoma. It is discussed in lecture 24.

4. Hairy cell leukemia

This disorder, also known as leukemic reticuloendotheliosis, is characterized by pancytopenia, massive splenomegaly, and diffuse nodal involvement. It is often temporarily controlled by splenectomy alone. The "hairy cells" are immunologically similar to CLL cells, i.e., they are B cells in more than 90% of cases (see figure 22.2B).

5. Histiocytic medullary reticulosis

Histiocytic medullary reticulosis is a disorder that appears to represent a neoplastic transformation of the sinusoidal histiocytes of the lymphoreticular system. The cells retain the functional capacity of histiocytes and have a pronounced phagocytic capacity that leads to erythrophagocytosis (i.e., ingestion of red cells). Clinical features commonly include (1) acute onset and short course; (2) skin rash caused by proliferating histiocytes in skin; (3) rapidly developing anemia due to myelophthisis and to hemolysis caused by erythrophagocytosis by histiocytes proliferating in the sinusoids of the liver and spleen. Occasionally, atypical histiocytes appear in the blood smear. Lymph node biopsy reveals histiocyte proliferation throughout the stroma, but not the syncytial pattern found in the histiocytic lymphomas. Some histiocytes may resemble Reed-Sternberg cells.

SELECTED REFERENCES

Berard, C. W., et al. A multidisciplinary approach to non-Hodgkin's lymphoma. *Ann. Int. Med.* 94(1981): 218.

Berard, C. W., et al. Current concepts of leukemia and lymphoma: Etiology, pathogenesis, and therapy. *Ann. Int. Med.* 85(1976): 351.

Carbone, P. P., et al. Symposium (Ann Arbor): Staging In Hodgkin's disease. *Cancer Res.*31(1971): 1707, 1870.

Chabner, B. A., et al. Sequential staging of non Hodgkin's lymphoma. *Cancer Treat. Rep.* 61(1977): 993.

Desforges, J. F., et al. Hodgkin's disease. *New Eng. J. Med.* 301(1979): 1212.

DeVita, V. T., and Hellman, S. Hodgkin's disease and the non-Hodgkin's lymphomas. In DeVita, V. T., Hellman, S., and Rosenberg, S. A., eds., *Cancer Principles and Practice of Oncology*, Philadelphia: J. B. Lippincott, 1982, pp. 1331–1392.

DeVita, V. T., et al. Combination chemotherapy in the treatment of advanced Hodgkin's disease. *Ann. Int. Med.* 73(1970): 881.

Kaplan, H. S. *Hodgkin's Disease*, 2d ed., Cambridge, MA: Harvard University Press, 1980.

Kaplan, H. S., et al. Staging laparotomy and splenectomy in Hodgkin's disease. *Natl. Cancer Inst. Monogr.* 36(1973): 291.

Lukes, R. J., and Collins, R. D. Immunologic characterization of human malignant lymphoma. *Cancer* 34(1974): 1488.

Rappaport, H. *Tumors of the Hematopoietic System. Atlas of Tumor Pathology*, American Registry of Pathology. Armed Forces Institute of Pathology, Washington, D.C., 1966.

Rosenberg, S. A. Non-Hodgkin's lymphoma: Selection of treatment on the basis of histologic type. *New Eng. J. Med.* 301(1979): 924.

Rosenberg, S. A., and Kaplan, H. S. Evidence for an orderly progression in the spread of Hodgkin's disease. *Cancer Res.* 26(1966): 1225.

LECTURE 23 Malignant Lymphomas II. Pathology

Nancy L. Harris

I. INTRODUCTION

Malignant lymphomas are neoplasms of the cells that constitute the immune system. Although they usually arise in lymph nodes, they may occur in extranodal sites as well. Whereas normal immunologic responses involve many types of cells (i.e., they are histologically *polymorphous*), neoplasms ordinarily involve proliferation of a single cell type (i.e., they are *monomorphous*). In normal immunologic responses cellular proliferation occurs in an orderly fashion in certain compartments of the lymphoid tissues. Lymphomas, in contrast, do not respect these compartments. Thus the diagnosis of lymphoma is based on two major observations: (1) *cellular composition* and (2) *architectural pattern*. These two features distinguish reactive from neoplastic lymphoid proliferations and permit classification of lymphomas.

Understanding lymphomas is enhanced by understanding the normal immune system. The development of immunologic markers for different subtypes of lymphoid cells has facilitated diagnosis, classification, and correlation of neoplastic lymphoid cells with their normal counterparts. Since lymphomas appear to represent clones of lymphocytes arrested at particular stages of differentiation, studies of lymphoma cells have helped in elucidating the normal pathways of lymphocyte differentiation.

II. REVIEW OF IMMUNE SYSTEM

A. Architecture of normal lymph node

As noted in lecture 2 (see figure 2.3), the normal lymph node has three compartments (figure 23.1). The *cortex* is the subcapsular zone that contains primary follicles and germinal centers; this is a B cell area. The *paracortex* is the space between and deep to the follicles; this is primarily a T cell area. The *medulla* is between the paracortex and the hilus of the node; it contains the medullary cords (T and B cells, plasma cells) and medullary sinuses (histiocytes).

B. B lymphocytes

1. Origin

Removal of the cloacal bursa (bursa of Fabricius) in avian species results in absent immunoglobulin production and depletion of the outer cortex of lymph nodes of lymphocytes, with failure to develop germinal centers. The lymphocytes occupying this area are

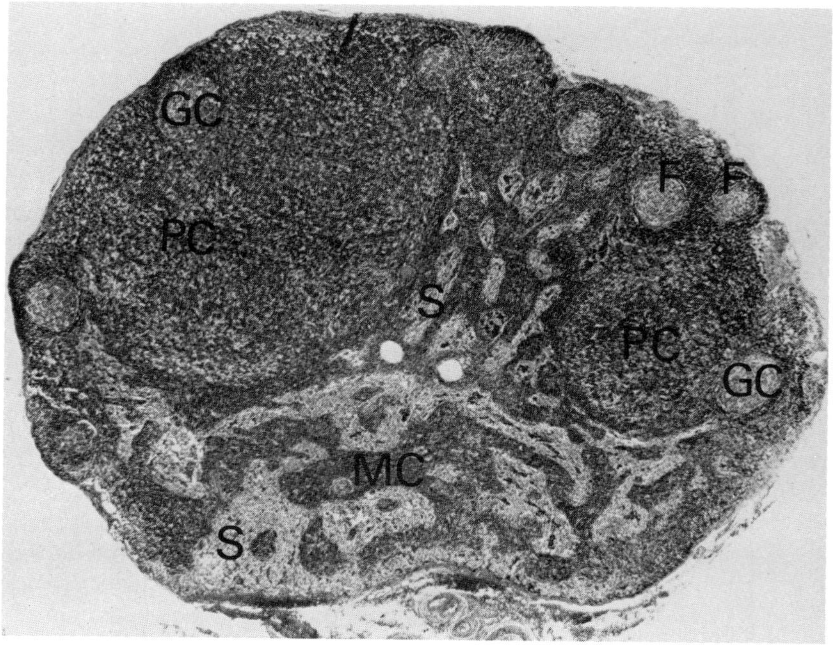

Fig. 23.1
Normal lymph node architecture. The cortex contains follicles (F) with germinal centers (GC). These are B cell regions. The paracortex (PC) contains predominantly T cells. The medullary cords (MC) contain a mixture of T and B cells and plasma cells, and the medullary sinuses (S) contain phagocytic histiocytes as well as some lymphocytes. (Compare with figures 2.3 and 2.4.)

called B cells, for bursa dependent. The mammalian equivalent of the avian bursa is not known, although the bone marrow seems to be the most likely candidate.

2. Localization

Normal B cells home to the follicular cortex of lymph nodes (see figure 2.4) and tonsils, the malphighian corpuscles of the spleen, and the submucosal gastrointestinal lymphoid follicles.

3. Function

B lymphocytes proliferate in germinal centers in response to antigenic stimuli and eventually mature into antibody-secreting plasma cells.

4. Markers

Major hematopoietic cell markers are summarized in table 23.1.

a. Surface immunoglobulin (SIg)

At most stages of differentiation B lymphocytes carry immunoglobulin molecules on their surfaces. Each normal B cell produces immunoglobulin of a single light chain type (κ or λ). During differentiation several different heavy chain classes (δ, μ, γ, or α) may be produced by a single B cell, but they all have the same type of light chain. Populations of normal human B cells carry κ *and* λ light chains in a 2:1 ratio. A neoplastic population arising from a single progenitor cell—a clone—should produce only a single light

Table 23.1
Hematopoietic Cell Markers

Marker	Abbreviations	Cell type
Surface immunoglobulin	SIg	B cells
Cytoplasmic immunoglobulin	CIg	B cells
B cell monoclonal antibodies		B cells
Sheep erythrocyte rosettes	E	T cells
Terminal deoxynucleotidyl transferase	TdT	Lymphoblasts (T or pre-B)
T cell monoclonal antibodies	T4 T8	Helper cell Suppressor/cytotoxic cells

chain: κ or λ. Thus immunoglobulin can be used to identify cells as B lymphocytes, and the presence of light chain restriction—monotypic or "monoclonal" Ig—is presumptive evidence of neoplasia. Use of fluorescence-labeled antibodies to immunoglobulin molecules permits identification of viable B lymphocytes in cell suspension. SIg can also be detected by immunofluorescence or immunoperoxidase techniques on frozen sections of lymphoid tissues.

b. Cytoplasmic immunoglobulin (CIg)

As B lymphocytes differentiate toward plasma cells, they produce larger amounts of immunoglobulin, which accumulates in the cytoplasm. This may be detected with antibodies against immunoglobulin, using the immunoperoxidase technique, in either frozen or paraffin sections or on fixed smears.

c. Monoclonal antibodies

Several monoclonal antibodies to B cell-associated antigens have been developed. Some appear to be B cell specific.

5. Morphology

a. Small lymphocytes

In the blood 5–10% of circulating small lymphocytes are B cells, as shown by SIg. On morphologic grounds these are indistinguishable from circulating T lymphocytes. *Neoplastic counterparts:* chronic lymphocytic leukemia (CLL) and small lymphocytic lymphoma.

b. Plasmacytoid lymphocytes, plasma cells

Since the plasma cell is the end stage of B cell differentiation, all cells with recognizable plasmacytoid differentiation are B lymphocytes. *Neoplastic counterparts:* plasmacytoid lymphocytes of Waldenström's macroglobulinemia, plasmacytoma, and myeloma.

c. Immunoblast

When stimulated by mitogens in vitro, small lymphocytes undergo transformation to large proliferating mononuclear cells with prominent central nucleoli and abundant, basophilic cytoplasm. These are called *immunoblasts*. B immunoblasts eventually mature into *plasma cells*. They are seen in antigenically stimulated lymph nodes, occasionally in germinal centers, and occasionally in the sinuses but more commonly in the paracortex and medulla. When stained with the immunoperoxidase technique, many contain cytoplasmic immunoglobulin. *Neoplastic counterpart:* a subset of diffuse large cell lymphoma (B immunoblastic lymphoma).

d. Follicular center cells

Germinal centers are a major site of B cell proliferation in response to antigen in vivo. The earliest event in germinal center formation is the accumulation of large, mitotically active blast cells in the centers of primary follicles. These collections enlarge, become sharply demarcated from the surrounding mantle of small lymphocytes, and develop a "starry-sky" pattern due to phagocytosis of nuclear debris by macrophages ("tingle body" macrophages).

Two types of cells can be recognized in Giemsa-stained sections at this time. *Centroblasts,* or *large, noncleaved follicle center cells,* are large cells with round, clear nuclei, 1 to 3 peripherally located nuclei, and a narrow rim of basophilic cytoplasm. *Neoplastic equivalent:* a subset of diffuse large cell lymphoma (large noncleaved or centroblastic type).

Small, noncleaved follicle center cells are smaller, primitive-appearing cells with darker nuclei, multiple small central nucleoli, and basophilic cytoplasm that may occasionally be found in germinal centers during the "starry-sky" phase. *Neoplastic equivalent:* Burkitt's tumor or undifferentiated lymphoma, non-Burkitt type.

In time large numbers of cells with irregular or cleaved nuclei appear in the germinal center. These are *centrocytes,* or *cleaved follicle center cells.* Centrocytes have a spectrum of sizes, from cells almost as large as centroblasts to cells only slightly larger than normal lymphocytes. Centroblasts appear to be precursors of centrocytes. *Neoplastic equivalents:* large-cleaved (a subset of diffuse large cell lymphoma), small-cleaved (diffuse small cleaved cell or centrocytic) lymphoma; all follicular lymphomas are composed of a variable mixture of cleaved and noncleaved cells (centrocytes and centroblasts).

C. T lymphocytes

1. Origin

Neonatal thymectomy results in defective cellular immunity and deficiency of lymphocytes in the paracortical lymph node areas. These lymphocytes are called T cells, for thymus dependent.

2. Localization

Thymus; paracortex of lymph nodes (see figure 2.4) and tonsils; periarteriolar lymphoid sheath of spleen; 80% of circulating lymphocytes.

3. Function

T lymphocytes act to help or suppress T and B cell function (antibody production) and are the effector (cytotoxic) cells of cell-mediated immunity (delayed hypersensitivity, graft rejection).

4. Markers

a. E-rosettes

Human T lymphocytes have a poorly understood ability to bind unsensitized sheep erythrocytes when incubated in the cold.

(Monoclonal antibodies to the E-rosette receptor are now available.) The E-rosette reaction can be performed only with suspensions of viable cells, but the E-rosette receptor can be stained in frozen sections with monoclonal antibody using fluorescence or immunoperoxidase techniques.

b. Terminal deoxynucleotidyl transferase (TdT)

TdT is a distinctive DNA polymerase enzyme found in thymus. Its physiological function is not known, but it serves as a marker for thymic T lymphocytes and their precursors. It is also present in early B cells, prior to the development of surface immunoglobulin. It can be detected by biochemical or immunofluorescence techniques in normal thymic T cells, the lymphocytes of thymomas—*not* in lymph node or circulating (peripheral) T cells—and in the lymphoblasts of acute lymphoblastic leukemia and lymphoblastic lymphoma.

c. Monoclonal antibodies

These detect a variety of antigens on T cell surfaces and are used to identify and subclassify T cells. They have largely replaced E-rosette determinations.

5. Morphology

a. Small lymphocyte

Blood T lymphocytes are indistinguishable on morphologic grounds from circulating B cells. *Neoplastic counterpart:* T cell CLL.

b. Cerebriform lymphocytes

In certain reactive conditions, particularly dermatologic disorders, small T cells with highly convoluted nuclei are found in the dermis, circulating blood, and paracortex of lymph nodes (dermatopathic lymphadenitis). These are thought to be activated T lymphocytes. *Neoplastic counterpart:* Sézary's syndrome, mycosis fungoides.

c. Immunoblast

On mitogenic stimulation in vitro, small T cells transform into large, mitotically active cells with prominent nucleoli and basophilic cytoplasm. These may be indistinguishable from B immunoblasts but do not show plasmacytoid differentiation. Presumptive T immunoblasts may be observed in the paracortex of virally stimulated lymph nodes, where they impart a starry-sky appearance to the node. They do not contain immunoglobulin. *Neoplastic counterpart:* a subset of diffused mixed or large cell lymphomas (T immunoblastic lymphoma); adult T cell lymphoma/leukemia.

D. Lymphocyte differentiation

As shown in figure 1.2, a common stem cell (CFU-LM) is believed to give rise to both lymphoid and myeloid cells (figure 23.2). A common lymphoid stem cell is postulated to give rise to the T and B cell lines. There are two distinct phases of development within both T and B cell lines: antigen independent and antigen dependent.

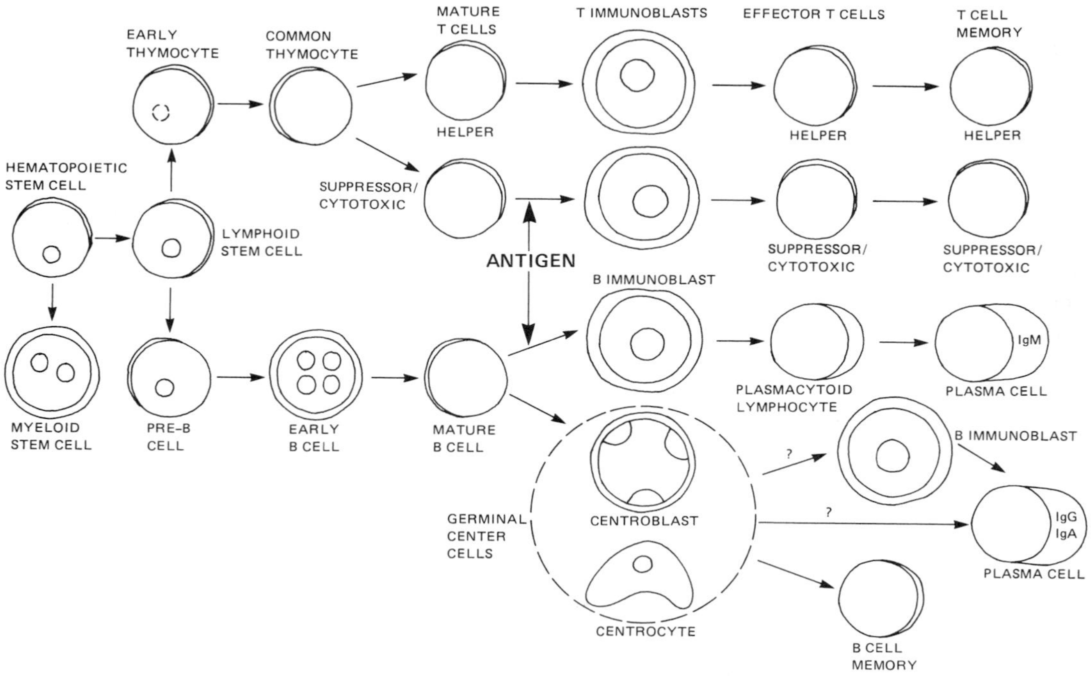

Fig. 23.2
Hypothetical scheme of lymphocyte differentiation.

Antigen-independent differentiation occurs in the primary lymphoid organs, bone marrow (or bursa equivalent) and thymus, and does not require exposure to antigen. It takes the cell from the stem cell through the pre-B cell or pre-T cell (thymocyte) stages to the so-called virgin or unstimulated mature T and B cells, which morphologically resemble small lymphocytes.

Antigen-dependent differentiation occurs in peripheral lymphoid tissues. On encountering antigen, virgin T or B cells undergo blast transformation, proliferate, and differentiate into antigen-specific T or B effector cells, which carry out immune functions. Antigen-dependent B cell differentiation may take two forms. In the primary immune response, B cells transform directly to immunoblasts and mature into IgM secreting plasma cells. Later, in the germinal center reaction, lymphocytes transform into centroblasts and centrocytes and eventually give rise to the IgG (or IgA) secreting plasma cell of the late primary or secondary immune response.

III. FEATURES OF LYMPHOMAS

As noted in lecture 22, lymphomas are divided into Hodgkin's disease and the non-Hodgkin's lymphomas. With the use of a combination of morphologic features, clinical information, and immunologic studies, we can now recognize at least 13 types of lymphomas, as well as Hodgkin's disease. Non-Hodgkin's lymphomas differ from one another as much as they do from Hodgkin's disease and thus are distinct entities. The different classification schemes lump and split these entities in a variety of ways, and the current state of the art has not produced an ultimately satisfactory lymphoma classification. Hence we will simply list the lymphomas that can be recognized at present (table 23.2). The following sections summarize morphologic and clinical features of each disease and attempt, to the extent possible, to place each in a scheme of lymphoctye differentiation, as shown in figure 23.2. The lymphomas are listed in order of their putative positions along the B and T cell differentiation pathways. Lymphomas and lymphoid leukemias are discussed together; the distinction between them is artificial, since many lymphomas can have a leukemic phase, and diseases usually classified as leukemia may not have circulating malignant cells in all cases.

A. Hodgkin's disease

1. Immunology and cell of origin

The malignant cell of Hodgkin's disease is believed to be the *Reed-Sternberg cell* and its mononuclear variants. Its lineage remains obscure. Some believe it arises from either the lymphocyte or the histiocyte/macrophage line, but definitive evidence is lacking.

The major problem in defining the malignant cell is its relative scarcity in tumor tissue, which results in difficulty in obtaining a pure cell population for study. Cell lines established from malignant effusions in terminally ill patients have shown no definitive markers of T or B lymphocytes or macrophages. Antibodies raised to some cell lines have been shown to react with Reed-Sternberg cells in tissue sections. Immunohistologic studies of tissue involved by Hodgkin's disease show that numerous benign T and B cells are present, with an increase in apparently activated T cells. Reed-Sternberg cells lack markers of T or B cells and monocytes.

2. Morphology

The morphology of Hodgkin's disease differs strikingly from that of non-Hodgkin's lymphomas, which usually consist of a relatively uniform population of neoplastic lymphoid cells. In Hodgkin's disease the neoplastic cells comprise a minority of the cells in the infiltrate, the bulk of which is usually made up of reactive lymphocytes, histiocytes, fibroblasts, eosinophils, and plasma cells. The diagnosis of Hodgkin's disease rests on finding Reed-Sternberg cells in the appropriate cellular background. Diagnostic Reed-Sternberg cells are large cells (25–50 μm in diameter) with bilobed or double nuclei, with at least two prominent inclusion-like nucleoli (figure 23.3). The symmetrical double nuclei, each with its nucleolus, give the cell a characteristic "owl's eye" ap-

Table 23.2
Major Categories of Lymphoproliferative Disease now Recognizable by Morphology and Immunologic Markers

Name (synonyms, subtypes)	Characteristic features	Markers
Hodgkin's disease	Reed-Sternberg cells Reactive lymphocytes, histiocytes, eosinophils, plasma cells	Mixed T and B cells, polyclonal
B cell neoplasms	Relatively uniform population of neoplastic lymphoid cells resembling normal B cell stages	Monotypic immunoglobulin
Acute lymphocytic leukemia ("null," common, and pre-B cell types)	Lymphoblasts: medium-sized cells, dispersed chromatin, inconspicuous nucleoli, scant cytoplasm; high mitotic rate	TdT+(Ig gene rearrangement)
Burkitt's tumor (small, non-cleaved cell)	Medium-sized cells, multiple nucleoli, basophilic cytoplasm, "starry-sky," very high mitotic rate	SIg+ (EBV+)
Small lymphocytic lymphoma (chronic lymphocytic leukemia)	Small lymphocytes, clumped chromatin; low mitotic rate	SIg+
Lymphoplasmacytoid lymphoma	Plasmacytoid lymphocytes, plasma cells, immunoblasts, low mitotic rate	SIg+CIg+(M-component)
Centrocytic lymphoma (diffuse, small-cleaved cell)	Small cleaved follicular center cells, variable mitotic rate	SIg+
Germinal center lymphomas (follicular lymphomas)	Mixture of follicular center cells; usually follicular pattern; low mitotic rate	SIg+
Large cell lymphoma (centroblastic, immunoblastic)	Monomorphous large cells with prominent nucleoli and basophilic cytoplasm; high mitotic rate	SIg+(±CIg)
Hairy cell leukemia	Small lymphocytes, "hairy" cytoplasm, low mitotic rate	SIg+
Plasmacytoma, myeloma	Plasma cells, plasmablasts; low mitotic rate	CIg+ (M-component)
T cell neoplasms	Relatively pleomorphic neoplastic lymphoid cells; not clearly resembling any normal cells	E-rosettes, T cell specific monoclonal antibodies
Acute lymphocytic leukemia, T cell type; lymphoblastic lymphoma (convoluted lymphocytic lymphoma)	Lymphoblasts: medium-sized cells, occasional nuclear convolution, inconspicuous cytoplasm; high mitotic rate	TdT+, E+, T cell antigens+
Adult T cell lymphoma/leukemia	Variable proportions of atypical lymphocytes and immunoblasts	E+, Helper cell antigens+ HTLV+ (human T cell leukemia virus)
Sézary's syndrome; mycosis fungoides (cutaneous T cell lymphomas)	Small and large lymphoid cells with "cerebriform" nuclei	E+, Helper cell antigens+
Other T cell neoplasms	Heterogenous	E+; other markers variable

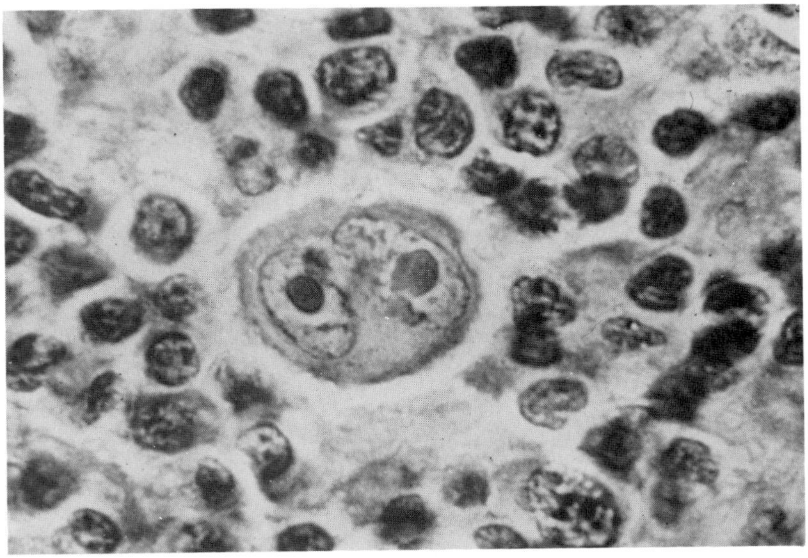

Fig. 23.3
Reed-Sternberg cell. The bilobed nucleus and double nucleoli give the cell an "owl-eye" appearance.

Table 23.3
Histologic Classification of Hodgkin's Disease

Type	Histologic characteristics	Prognosis	Approximate median survival (year)
Lymphocytic predominance	Lymphocytes, histiocytes	Most favorable	8
Nodular sclerosis	Fibrous bands, lacunar cells	Favorable	4
Mixed cellularity	Eosinophils, plasma cells	Intermediate	2.5
Lymphocytic depletion	Predominance of Reed-Sternberg cells, diffuse fibrosis	Least favorable	1.5

pearance. Mononuclear cells with similar nucleoli are also found. These are also believed to be malignant; however, since they are not reliably distinguishable from benign immunoblasts, they are not in themselves diagnostic of Hodgkin's disease.

3. Classification

As shown in table 23.3, four histologic types of Hodgkin's disease are recognized by the relative proportions of Reed-Sternberg cells, lymphocytes, other inflammatory cells, and fibrosis. In *lymphocytic predominance* lymphocytes are numerous, and Reed-Sternberg cells are hard to find. In *mixed cellularity* Reed-Sternberg cells are easily found, and the infiltrate contains numerous eosinophils and plasma cells, in addition to lymphocytes. In *lymphocytic depletion* Reed-Sternberg cells and atypical mononuclear cells constitute the predominant cells, and there is diffuse fibrosis. *Nodular sclerosis* is a special type of Hodgkin's disease,

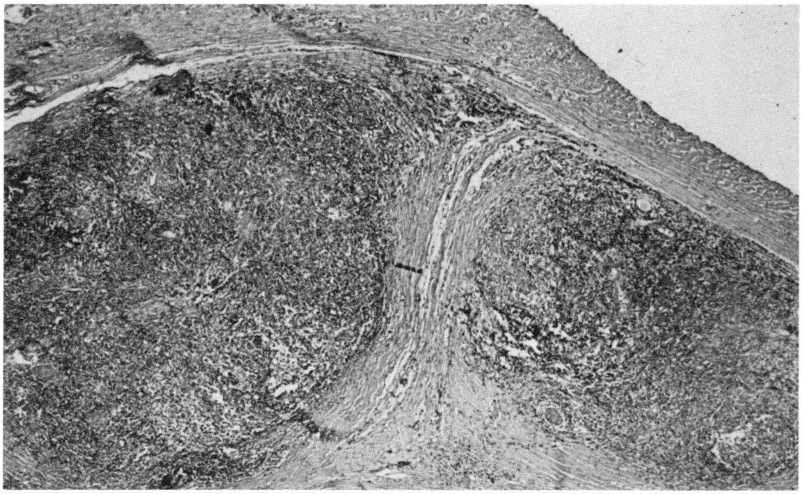

Fig. 23.4
Hodgkin's disease, nodular sclerosis type. Fibrous bands divide the tumor into nodules.

most common in young adults, in which dense, fibrous bands divide the tumor into nodules (figure 23.4). It is also characterized by a particular multinucleated variant of the Reed-Sternberg cell, called the *lacunar cell*.

4. Clinical correlations

Prior to advances in therapy, the prognosis of Hodgkin's disease was related to the histologic type, with lymphocytic predominance the most indolent and mixed cellularity and lymphocytic depletion more aggressive. Improvements in the therapy have obscured these differences. In current practice the major determinant of treatment and survival is the stage of the disease at diagnosis. For this reason there is little current controversy about subclassification.

With increased survival due to improved therapy, two recent complications have been seen: acute nonlymphocytic leukemias (ANLL) and non-Hodgkin's lymphomas. The ANLL appear related to the use of combined modality therapy (radiation therapy plus chemotherapy with alkylating agents). The non-Hodgkin's lymphomas—usually Burkett-like or immunoblastic —may result from the immuno-suppressed state associated with either Hodgkin's disease or cytotoxic therapy.

B. B cell neoplasms

1. Lymphoblastic lymphoma/leukemia (null and pre-B cell types)

In childhood ALL 80% of cases lack either surface immunoglobulin or the E-rosette receptor. About 30% of these so-called null lymphoblastic leukemias have cytoplasmic μ chains ($C\mu$) and are therefore pre-B cells. More recently the majority of both $C\mu+$ and $C\mu-$ ALL have been shown to react with monoclonal antibodies to B cells and to display immunoglobulin gene arrangement. Therefore the cells of most "null" ALL are primitive B cell precursors, which are TdT positive. Neoplasms of null and pre-B cell types usually present with diffuse bone marrow involvement and an elevated leukocyte count (common in children, infrequent in adults). Occasionally neoplasms of these cells present as a solitary tumor of bone or other sites. These are termed *null lymphoblastic lymphomas*.

2. Burkitt's tumor and Burkitt-like lymphomas

a. Immunology and cell of origin

The position of these tumors in the B cell differentiation pathway is controversial. Cells resembling Burkitt's tumor cells are not readily identified in normal lymphoid tissues. Occasional germinal center cells, particularly in children, may resemble Burkitt's tumor cells. African Burkitt's tumor and non-African cases of similar histology invariably have surface immunoglobulin, usually IgM with κ light chain but occasionally λ. In contrast to pre-B cell neoplasms, Burkitt's tumor is TdT negative. A characteristic chromosome translocation (8:14) is found in the majority of the cases. This involves translocation of a cellular oncogene (*c-myc*) from chromosome 8 to the Ig heavy chain switch region, located on chromosome 14. Epstein-Barr virus (EBV) genomes can be demonstrated in the tumor cells in most African cases and occasionally in non-African cases.

b. Morphology

Burkitt's tumor cells are similar in size to those of ALL—larger than normal circulating lymphocytes but smaller than immunoblasts and large follicular center cells. In typical Burkitt's tumor the cells are uniform in size and shape; in Burkitt-like lymphomas there is more variation in cell size and shape. The nuclei are round, with coarsely clumped, dark chromatin, multiple (2–5) nucleoli that tend to be central, and abundant cytoplasm that is basophilic on Giemsa stain. The cells are cohesive, and the abundant cytoplasm imparts a mosaic or pavement-like appearance to the infiltrate. Sharply defined cell borders are frequently seen. The mitotic rate is high and may exceed 20 per 40× field. A starry-sky pattern is usually present, imparted by numerous benign macrophages that have ingested nuclear debris.

c. Clinical features

Classic Burkitt's tumor is primarily a disease of childhood. In African (endemic) cases there is a predilection for involvement of the jaw and other facial bones. In American (nonendemic) cases, jaw tumors are uncommon. Over half of the cases present with abdominal tumors, most commonly involving the distal ileum and/or mesentery, ovaries, or kidneys. Burkitt's and Burkitt-like lymphomas account for approximately one-third of childhood non-Hodgkin's lymphomas in the United States. The M:F ratio is 2–3:1. A second peak of frequency is seen in older adults. These tumors are usually Burkitt-like. Approximately 10% of nonendemic cases have bone marrow involvement. A few present as acute leukemia with Burkitt's tumor cells (B-ALL). Untreated tumors are rapidly fatal, but the tumor is very sensitive to chemotherapy. Life-threatening tumor lysis syndrome may occur during treatment of patients with bulky disease. In children, if the tumor can be completely resected, the 2-year survival with chemotherapy may be as high as 80%. With bulky disease the survival drops to 40% at 2 years. There is no apparent different in survival between children with Burkitt and Burkitt-like lymphomas. Mortality in adults is higher. Tumors with this morphology are common in patients with the acquired immune deficiency syndrome (AIDS).

3. Small lymphocytic lymphoma (CLL)

a. Immunology and cell of origin

Over 90% of cases of typical CLL are of B cell type, with faint SIg of IgM ± IgD type. The presence of both IgM and IgD in the majority of cases favors the idea that these are "virgin" B cells, since antigen-stimulated and memory B cells are thought not to have SIgD.

b. Morphology

Tissue involvement by small lymphocytic lymphoma is indistinguishable from CLL. A diagnosis of CLL requires peripheral lymphocytosis. Typical CLL produces a diffuse infiltrate in lymph nodes. The predominant cell may be slightly larger than a normal lymphocyte, with clumped chromatin and a round nucleus (figure 23.5A). Many mitotically active large lymphoid cells may be seen in lymph nodes involved in CLL. The number of large cells does not adversely affect prognosis, but a mitotic rate greater than 30 per high power field is associated with a short survival. Bone marrow involvement is common and may be focal or diffuse.

c. Clinical features

As discussed in lecture 21, CLL is predominantly a disease of older adults. It follows a protracted course, with gradual enlargement of lymph nodes and spleen and progressive marrow and organ infiltration. Blast transformation, common in CML, is a rare but well-documented phenomenon termed *Richter's syndrome.*

B cell lymphomas of small lymphocytes without CLL may also occur. These may involve lymph nodes or extranodal sites, such as the orbit, lung, stomach, and skin, where they may be impossible to distinguish from benign lymphoid infiltrates without special studies to demonstrate monotype SIg. Some may develop CLL; others may not.

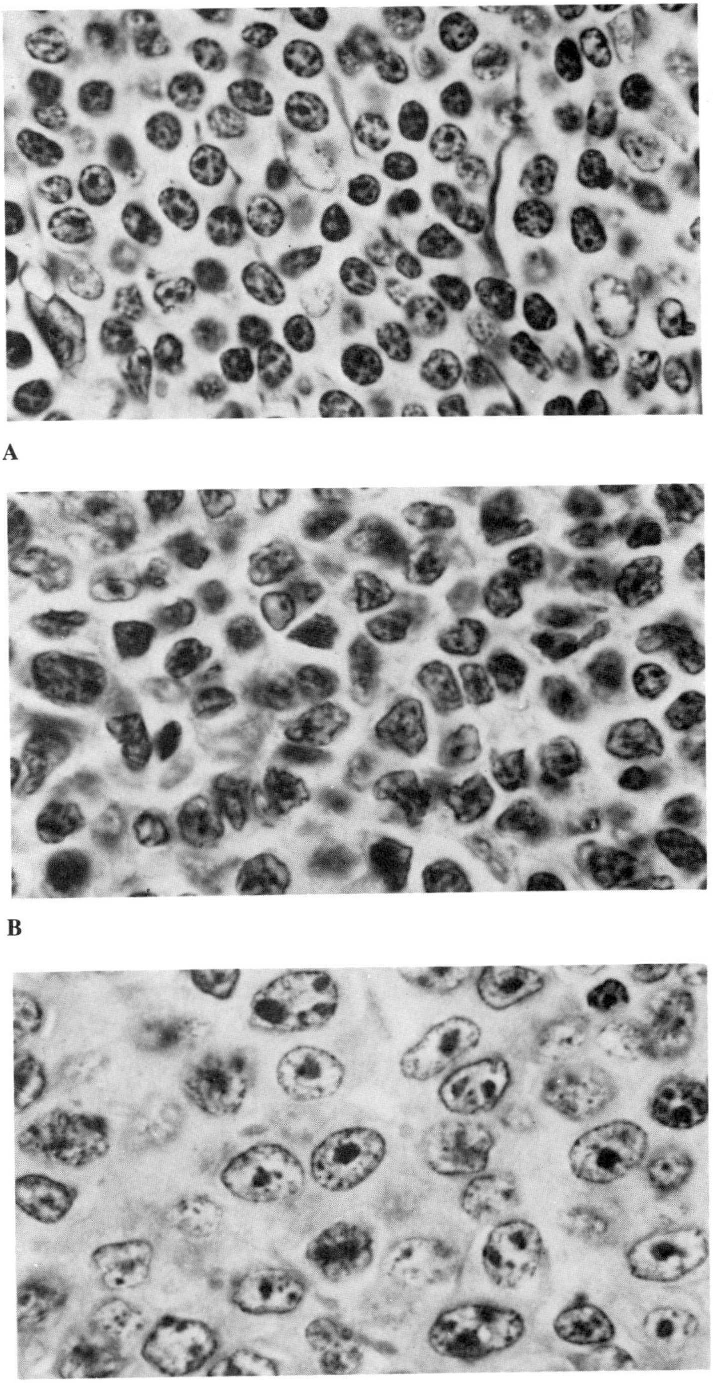

A

B

C

Fig. 23.5
Cytologic features of non-Hodgkin's lymphoma. *A*, small lymphocytic lymphoma; *B*, small cleaved cell lymphoma; *C*, large cell lymphoma, immunoblastic. Lymphomas are subclassified based on the size and shape of the nucleus, nucleoli, and cytoplasm.

4. Lymphoplasmacytoid lymphoma

a. Immunology and cell of origin

Lymphoplasmacytoid (or plasmacytoid lymphocytic) lymphomas are tumors of lymphocytes that are capable of secreting Ig, usually IgM. Thus they are analogous to the effector cells of the primary immune response. In suspension the tumor cells have abundant SIgM, in contrast to the faint SIgM of CLL; IgD is lacking; in imprints or sections some cells also have cytoplasmic Ig.

b. Morphology

The predominant cell is the small lymphocyte. A varying number of cells have abundant basophilic cytoplasm but lymphocyte-like nuclei. Some cases have typical plasma cells in addition to these plasmacytoid lymphocytes.

c. Clinical features

They occur in the same general age group as CLL. Bone marrow is frequently involved, as are lymph nodes and spleen. Leukemia may occur but is less common than in nonplasmacytoid lymphomas, and average total lymphocyte count is lower. A monoclonal serum protein, usually IgM, occurs in approximately half the cases (Waldenström's macroglobulinemia). Lymphomas that arise in patients with autoimmune disease—most notably Sjogren's syndrome—are characteristically of lymphoplasmacytoid type. Type I or type II cryoglobulinemia and/or Coombs-positive hemolytic anemia may be associated with the paraprotein. Like CLL the disease may terminate in a large cell lymphoma.

5. Centrocytic lymphomas (diffuse, small cleaved cell)

a. Immunology and cell of origin

This is a B cell tumor that is usually SIgM+, with or without IgD, but may be IgG+. The cell of origin is thought to be the small cleaved cell of the germinal center.

b. Morphology

The tumor is composed exclusively of small cleaved cells (figure 23.5B). In some cases the cells are very small, and some cells resemble small lymphocytes. Large noncleaved cells are rare or absent. The pattern is usually diffuse but may be vaguely nodular. Well-defined follicles as in folicular lymphomas are not seen. Marrow involvement and leukemia are frequent. The tumor in the marrow may be either focal and paratrabecular or diffuse. Marrow and blood involvement by centrocytic lymphoma may be indistinguishable from that by follicular lymphoma.

c. Clinical features

In contrast to follicular lymphomas, centrocytic lymphoma has a high male predominance, an increased frequency of extranodal involvement, and a relatively poor prognosis, with median survival in the range of 2–4 years instead of 7–9. Like follicular lymphomas, patients usually have widespread disease at presentation and a high incidence of peripheral blood involvement. The presence of leukemia does not adversely affect prognosis. The incidence of this tumor is higher in Europe, particularly in Italy, than in the United States.

6. Follicular lymphomas (nodular lymphomas)

a. Immunology and cell of origin

Follicular lymphomas are germinal center B cell tumors (figure 23.6A). They are SIg+ having either IgM, IgC, or IgA.

b. Morphology

Like germinal centers follicular lymphomas are composed of a mixture of centrocytes and centroblasts. The predominant cell is usually a centrocyte, which may range in size from small to large. Centroblasts are in the minority but are always present. In most classification schemes, follicular lymphomas are classified according to the predominant cell type. However, 85% or more of the cases are of "small" or "mixed small and large" type; these have a very similar prognosis in most series.

Marrow involvement is frequent; tumor cell aggregates are characteristically paratrabecular. The follicular pattern may not be

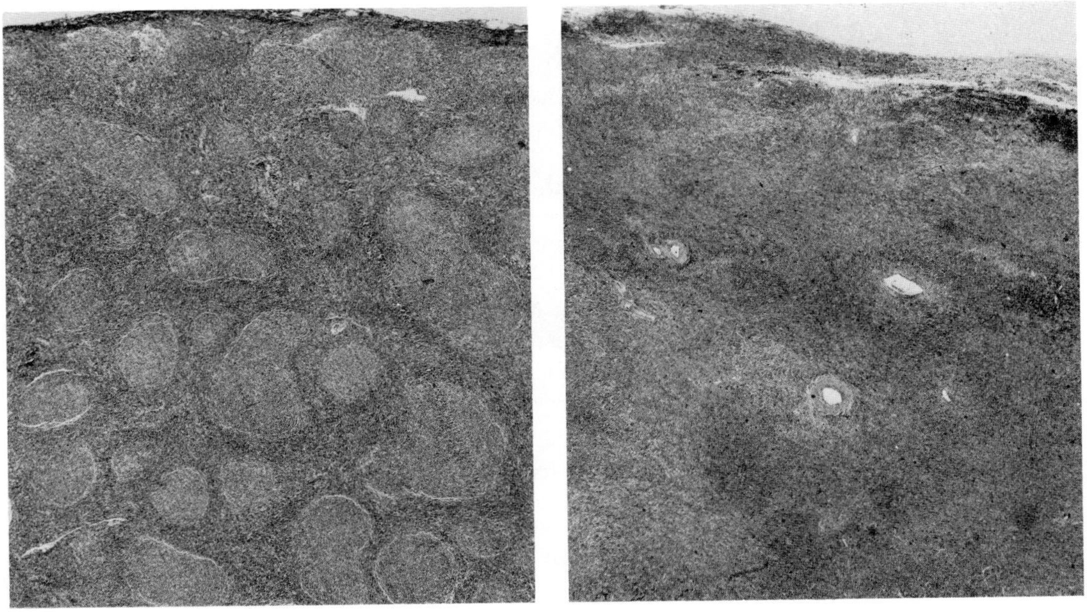

A B

Fig. 23.6
Architectural features of non-Hodgkin's lymphoma. *A*, follicular lymphoma; *B*, diffuse large cell lymphoma. Note that the neoplastic infiltrates obliterate the normal nodal architecture. (Compare with figure 23.1.)

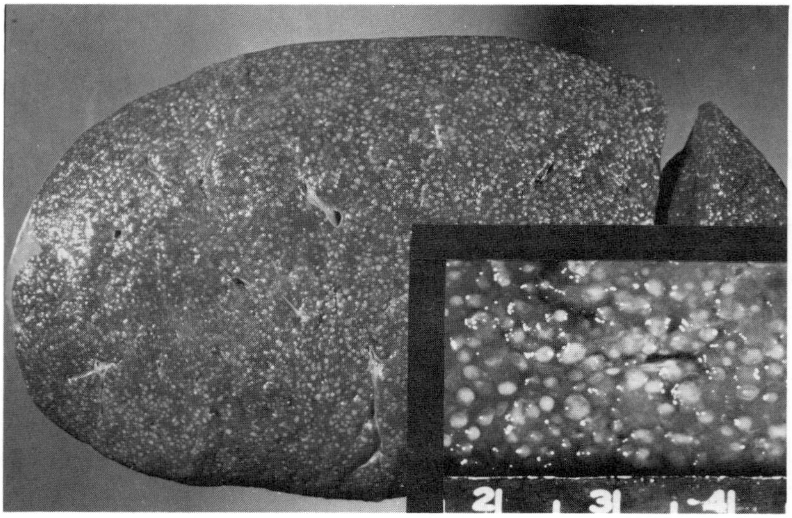

A

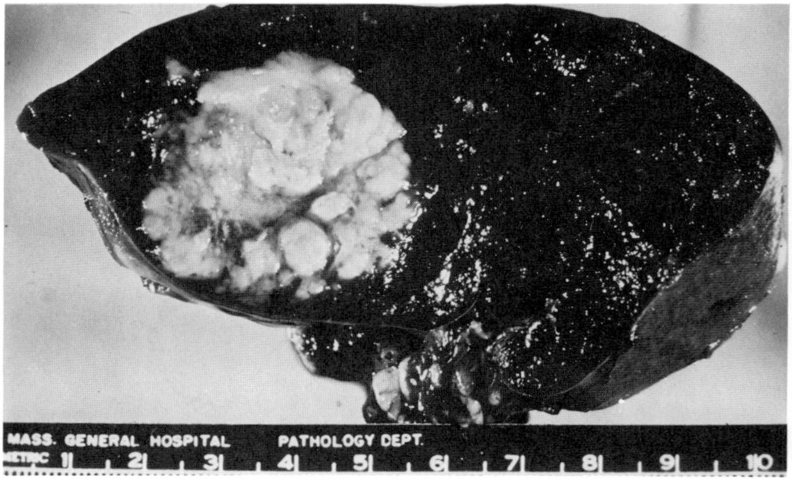

B

Fig. 23.7
Gross features of non-Hodgkin's lymphomas in the spleen. *A,* follicular lymphoma; *B,* diffuse large cell lymphoma. The neoplastic cells of the follicular lymphoma "home" to the normal B cell regions of the white pulp, while the large cell lymphoma forms a destructive, invasive tumor mass.

apparent on marrow biopsy, and the cells may appear smaller than in the node. Thus classification of lymphoma should not be attempted on marrow biopsy alone. The gross appearance of the enlarged spleen is shown in figure 23.7A.

Follicular lymphomas tend to progress to a larger cell type and/or a diffuse pattern. It is not uncommon to see variation in cytologic composition from one nodule to another in the same biopsy or from one biopsy to another in a given patient. If we think of the centroblast as the proliferating cell, which normally matures into centrocytes, then this natural history can be explained as follows. In the usual follicular lymphoma, the tumor cells retain their ability to mature all the way to centrocytes, and these cells tend to form follicles. Thus, only a few centroblasts remain. These are actively dividing. With time the tumor cells either gradually lose their ability to mature or begin to proliferate more rapidly, so that fewer centrocytes accumulate and the relative number of centroblasts increases. Concomitantly the tumor shows less tendency toward nodularity. Clinically the tumor becomes more aggressive, and histologically an increase in large noncleaved cells is seen. The overall picture is interpreted as progression from a follicular small cell or mixed lymphoma to diffuse large cell lymphoma, but in reality it simply represents a transition to a more aggressive phase of the original tumor. The fact that the same immunoglobulin chains can be demonstrated in such cases on the original follicular lymphoma and on the subsequent diffuse large cell lymphoma supports this interpretation.

c. Clinical features

Follicular lymphomas are a distinct clinical entity. They constitute 40–50% of adult non-Hodgkin's lymphomas in the United States. The incidence is much lower in Europe. They are rare under age 20. The sex incidence is approximately equal. Patients present with painless adenopathy, which is frequently generalized yet asymptomatic. Involvement of the bone marrow is common at diagnosis, occurring in up to 75% of patients. Follicular lymphoma is a predominantly nodal disease, with less than 20% presenting in extranodal sites. The long natural history (7–8 yr median survival) appears largely unaffected by treatment.

7. Large cell lymphoma

a. Immunology and cell of origin

Up to 80% of tumors designated histiocytic lymphoma in the Rappaport classification are of B cell origin, as demonstrated by the presence of surface or cytoplasmic immunoglobulin. In addition many Ig-negative large cell lymphomas react with anti-B cell monoclonal antibodies.

b. Morphology

Large cell lymphomas are subclassified according to the predominant cell, which may resemble either a large cleaved or noncleaved follicular center cell or an immunoblast (figure 23.5C). B immunoblastic lymphomas may or may not have plasmacytoid features. The majority of large cell lymphomas are of noncleaved or immunoblastic type, and both types of cells may be present in some cases. The gross appearance of the spleen is shown in figure 23.7B.

c. Clinical features

Diffuse large cell lymphomas (figure 23.6B) are clinically distinct from follicular lymphomas. These tumors constitute 30–40% of adult non-Hodgkin's lymphomas and are thus comparable numerically to follicular lymphomas of small cleaved and mixed cell type. The M/F ratio is greater than 1. The age range is broad, and large cell lymphoma is more common in young adults than is follicular lymphoma. Large cell lymphoma constitutes 25–30% of childhood lymphomas. Patients typically present with a rapidly enlarging, often symptomatic mass at a single nodal or extranodal site. The disease is much more likely to be localized than is follicular lymphoma, and extranodal presentation is more common. Untreated, large cell lymphomas are rapidly progressive and fatal, but if a complete response can be obtained with therapy, long-term disease-free survival (? cure) may be possible (see lecture 22). This is in contrast to follicular lymphomas, which show a continuous slow mortality rate with time regardless of therapy.

8. Hairy cell leukemia

a. Immunology and cell of origin

Most cases of hairy cell leukemia are SIg+ B cell lymphomas. The presence of tartrate-resistant acid phosphatase in hairy cells is characteristic, but it is neither necessary nor sufficient for the diagnosis. There is no recognized normal counterpart to the hairy cell.

b. Morphology

The hairy cell has an oval or bean-shaped nucleus with chromatin slightly less clumped than that of a normal lymphocyte. The abundant, pale cytoplasm has a syncytial appearance in tissue sections; hence nuclei appear widely separated in contrast to the closely packed nuclei of small lymphocytic lymphomas. The bone marrow is almost always involved and because of increased reticulin is not readily aspirated. The spleen is usually involved and may be massive. Tumor involves the red pulp; the white pulp is usually atrophic.

c. Clinical features

Hairy cell leukemia is a disease of adults. As noted in lecture 21, patients present with pancytopenia and may or may not have circulating neoplastic cells. The diagnosis is best made on marrow biopsy. A marked defect in cell-mediated immunity is seen despite normal T cell subsets. Atypical mycobacterial infections as well as other infections are common. The course may be protracted.

Long, spontaneous remissions occur. It does not respond to conventional lymphoma chemotherapy. Splenectomy is often followed by prolonged clinical improvement.

9. Plasmacytoma/ multiple myeloma

a. Immunology and cell of origin

The plasma cell of multiple myeloma represents the terminally differentiated B cell of the late primary or secondary immune response, which secretes IgG or IgA rather than IgM. Neoplastic plasma cells in myeloma lack SIg and have only cytoplasmic immunoglobulin.

b. Morphology

Typical cells resemble mature or immature plasma cells, with no admixture of lymphoid cells. An "anaplastic" stage resembling large cell lymphoma may be a preterminal event.

c. Clinical features

Clinical features are described in lecture 24.

C. T cell neoplasms

1. T lymphoblastic lymphoma (LBL) and T cell ALL

a. Immunology and cell of origin

Most cases of lymphoblastic lymphoma are of T cell origin. About 20% of cases of ALL have T cell markers. Both neoplasms represent primitive thymic T cells. Analysis with monoclonal antibodies indicates that the cells of T-ALL are at a more primitive stage of development than those of T-LBL. The cells of both tumors are TdT^+, usually form E-rosettes, and react with many monoclonal anti-T cell antibodies.

b. Morphology

Involved lymph nodes or thymus contain a diffuse proliferation of small to medium-sized lymphoid cells with finely dispersed chromatin and inconspicuous nucleoli. Some cells have fine nuclear grooves or convolutions. In contrast to Burkitt's tumor, the cytoplasm is scant and only moderately basophilic; the cells appear noncohesive. In imprints the cells are indistinguishable from the lymphoblasts of childhood ALL. No normal adult tissue counterpart of this cell has been described.

c. Clinical features

Lymphoblastic lymphoma is a disease of adolescents and young adults. It constitutes less than 5% of all non-Hodgkin's lymphomas but up to 40% of childhood lymphomas. Patients present with rapidly enlarging, symptomatic mediastinal (thymic) masses and/or supradiaphragmatic lymphadenopathy. Untreated, it is rapidly fatal, usually terminating in acute leukemia. CNS involvement is common. Combination chemotherapy may be beneficial, but the prognosis is not as good as that for common ALL.

2. Adult T cell lymphoma/leukemia

a. Immunology and cell of origin

In the late 1970s Japanese workers noted that the majority of non-Hodgkin's lymphomas and CLL seen in certain areas of Japan were of T cell type. Since the clinical spectrum includes both nodal disease and blood involvement, this disease is now known as adult T cell lymphoma/leukemia, to distinguish it from childhood T cell ALL. A unique human retrovirus has been identified in cultured cells from both the Japanese patients and also from black patients with a similar disorder from the Caribbean and southeastern United States. Antibody to this human T cell lymphoma/leukemia virus (HTLV) is found in the blood of patients with the disease in all 3 areas but is not found in the blood of most normal individuals. Close relatives of patients and individuals residing in southern Japan have an increased incidence of antibodies to HTLV. The virus isolated from human tumor cells causes cord blood T cells to transform into continuously growing cell lines, mimicking the effect of Epstein-Barr virus on B cells. Current evidence supports the conclusion that ATL/L is a true virus-induced neoplasm. The surface marker phenotype is that of mature helper T cells.

b. Morphology

The histologic picture of HTLV-associated lymphomas and leukemia is variable. The neoplastic cells range from small lymphocytes to pleomorphic giant cells resembling Reed-Sternberg cells. There are no distinctive histologic features that permit a definite diagnosis of ATL to be made on paraffin-embedded sections alone. The diagnosis rests on the combination of morphology, immunologic studies, and documentation of HTLV infection, in the form of serum antibodies and/or virus identification in tumor cells.

c. Clinical features

Most cases have been reported in southern Japan, the Caribbean, and the southeastern United States. Patients are adults of all ages. The majority are leukemic and have widespread disease involving lymph nodes, liver, and spleen at the time of diagnosis. Skin infiltration and hypercalcemia (due to osteoclast activation) are common. Patients usually respond poorly to therapy and die in 1–2 years.

3. Mycosis fungoides/Sézary's syndrome (MF/SS)

a. Immunology and cell of origin

The neoplastic cell of MF/SS is a T lymphocyte of the helper subset. A few patients with clinical features indistinguishable from MF have antibodies to HTLV, but most do not.

b. Morphology

The characteristic cell of MF is a large lymphocyte with a highly convoluted (cerebriform) nucleus. This cell infiltrates the epidermis, producing microabscesses. In SS the circulating cell is a small cerebriform lymphocyte. As a terminal event a large cell lymphoma may develop; this probably represents a failure of maturation of the large MF cells rather than development of a second neoplasm.

c. Clinical features

Chronically progressive cutaneous disease leads to eventual visceral lymphoma and death. Symptoms are alleviated by various therapies, but the disease is not curable. Recently monoclonal anti-T cell antibodies have been used therapeutically.

4. Other T cell lymphomas

Many reports of single cases and series of cases of lymphomas with T cell markers have appeared. These have been given a bewildering variety of names. Since there is no marker for malignancy in T cells that is analogous to the light chain restriction in B cell neoplasms, these reports are difficult to evaluate. As noted, morphologic features alone are not reliable for defining the T cell origin of a lymphoma. To make a definite diagnosis of T cell neoplasia, a *homogeneous population of morphologically malignant cells* must be shown to have a specific T cell marker. Since both the well-characterized T cell tumors (ATL/L and MF) and many other cases reported as T cell tumors are characterized by a heterogeneous nodal infiltrate, this requirement is difficult to satisfy. T cell lineage is most readily proved in tumors with a leukemic phase, and it is for this reason that lymphoblastic lymphoma, ATL/L, and MF/SS can be accepted as T cell neoplasms. In addition to these entities there are many well-documented cases of "T CLL"—the relationship of these tumors to ATL/L-HTLV remains to be elucidated. The study of T cell disorders is an interesting and difficult area that requires much further study.

SELECTED REFERENCES

Foon, K., et al. Surface markers on leukemia and lymphoma cells: Recent advances. *Blood* 60(1982): 1.

Jaffe, E. S., et al. The pathologic spectrum of adult T-cell leukemia/lymphoma in the United States. *Am. J. Surg. Pathol.* 8 (1984): 263.

Kaplan, H. S. *Hodgkin's Disease,* 2d ed., Cambridge, MA: Harvard University Press, 1980.

Lennert, K. *Histopathology of Non-Hodgkin's Lymphomas: Based on the Kiel Classification,* New York: Springer-Verlag, 1981.

Lukes, R. J., and Butler, J. J. The pathology and nomenclature of Hodgkin's disease. *Cancer Res.* 26(1966): 1063.

Multiple authors — The non-Hodgkin's lymphoma pathologic classification project. National Cancer Institute–sponsored study of classification of non-Hodgkin's lymphomas: Summary and description of a working formulation for clinical usage. *Cancer* 49(1982): 2112.

Murphy, S. B. — Childhood non-Hodgkin's lymphoma. *New Eng. J. Med.* 299(1978): 1446.

Rosenberg, S. A. — Non-Hodgkin's lymphoma: Selection of treatment on the basis of histologic type. *New Eng. J. Med.* 301(1979): 924.

Weissman, I. L., et al. — The lymphoid system. *Human Pathol.* 9(1978): 25.

LECTURE 24 Plasma Cell Disorders and the Dysproteinemias

W. Hallowell Churchill, Jr.

I. NORMAL IMMUNOGLOBULINS

The immunoglobulins of normal blood serum are a heterogeneous group of proteins with antibody activity. The concentrations of immunoglobulins that comprise the normal range reflect the antigen exposure that all of us experience. This normal range differs among different populations and rises with age, most markedly in the first few years of life.

A. Classes

On the basis of certain structural features that are detected by reactivities with antisera prepared against proteins of homogeneous structure, the immunoglobulins have been shown to consist of five major classes of molecules: *IgG, IgA, IgM, IgD,* and *IgE.* Subclasses based on immunologic reactivities have also been found. Thus, a given IgG molecule, for example, may be either IgG1, IgG2, IgG3, or IgG4. There are two such IgA and IgM subclasses. Even within a subclass, molecules are structurally and electrophoretically heterogeneous.

B. Structure

1. Arrangements of H and L polypeptide chains

IgG molecules consist of two kinds of polypeptides, *H chains* (for heavy) and *L chains* (for light), that are arranged symmetrically with respect to the long axis of the molecules. Thus, each half-molecule has one H and one L chain (figure 24.1). In any given molecule, the two H chains are structurally identical, as are the two L chains. Papain cleaves IgG molecules near the hinge (interchain disulfide bridge) point. Two kinds of fragments result: (1) Fab (for antigen-binding) fragments, consisting of the L chains and about half the H chains; and (2) Fc (for crystallizable) fragments, which contain the remaining portions of the H chains. The structure of non-IgG immunoglobulins generally resembles that of IgG. IgM molecules occur chiefly as pentamers. A portion of IgA is dimeric. The monomer resembles IgG except for the class specificity of the H chain.

2. Classes, subclasses, and types

Class specificity resides in the H chain. Each of the major immunoglobulin classes has a distinctive kind of H chain. These are termed γ, α, μ, δ, and ϵ, the Greek letters corresponding to the Roman letters designating the groups. Four varieties of γ chains occur: γ_1, γ_2, γ_3, and γ_4. These are the basis for the subclasses of IgG. Finally, all L chains are κ or λ; corresponding immunoglobulins are classified as type K and type L. It should be noted

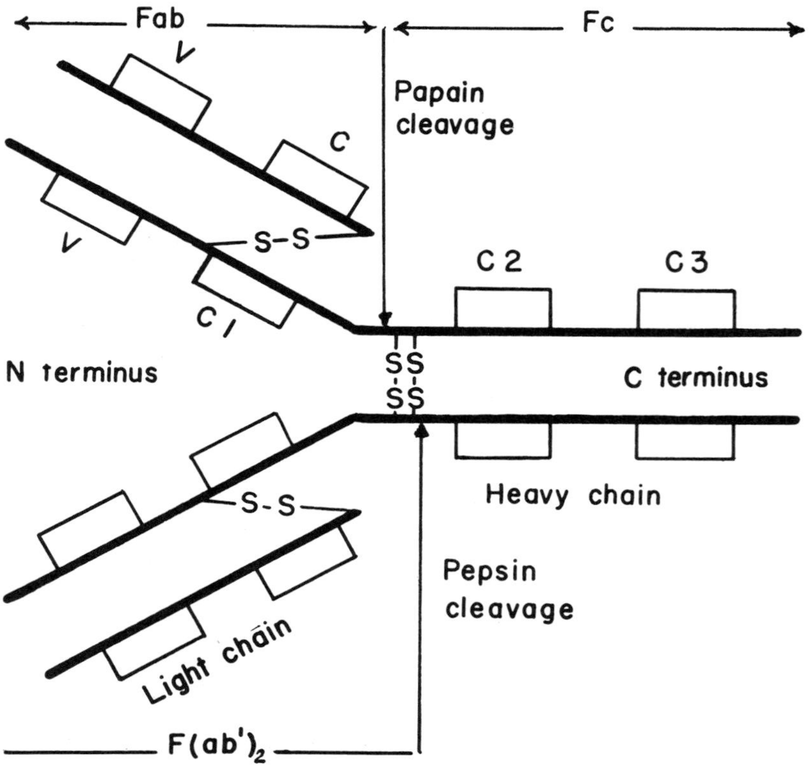

Figure 24.1
Schematic diagram of structure of IgG molecule.

that an individual immunoglobulin molecule contains only one class of H chain and one type of L chain.

IgM in its usual pentameric form and the dimeric form of IgA have one *J chain* (mol. wt. 22,000) per polymer. Moreover, in bodily secretions, IgA exists in a special form (*secretory IgA*) that, in addition to a J chain, has a protein moiety (mol. wt. 55,000) called the *secretory component*.

3. Constant and variable portions

When given IgG molecules were compared, it was found that the C-terminal halves of the L chains and the corresponding parts of the H chains have similar amino acid sequences within a given class or subclass. However, the remaining N-terminal portions (V_H and V_L) are *variable* in structure (figure 24.1). The variability is believed to be related to antibody specificity. Each light chain has two interchain disulfide bridges, one in V_L, the other in the *constant* region C_L. Similarly, there is an intrachain disulfide bridge in V_H and one in each of the three constant domains, C_H1, C_H2, and C_H3. The various biological properties of IgG molecules reside in one or another of these domains.

Table 24.1
Properties of Imunoglobulins

	IgG	IgA	IgM	IgD	IgE
Molecular weight	15,000	180,000 or 390,000[a]	900,000	150,000	200,000
Sedimentation coefficient	7S	7S or 11S[b]	19S	7S	8S
Concentration in plasma (mg/100 ml)	600–1,500	60–290	50–200	3	0.05
Biologic half-life (days)	20[b]	6	5	3	2
Complement fixation	+	0	+	0	0
Passive cutaneous anaphylaxis	+	0	0	?	?
Reagenic antibody	0	0	0	0	+
Placental transfer	+	0	0	0	0

a. Secretory IgA.
b. Half-life of IgG1.

C. Concentrations in serum

The bulk (80–85%) of total serum immunoglobulin is IgG. The normal concentrations per 100 ml in adults are IgG, 600–1,500 mg; IgA, 60–290 mg; IgM, 50–200 mg; IgD, approximately 3 mg; and IgE, only 0.05 mg. The ratios of IgG1 : IgG2 : IgG3 : IgG4 are approximately 70 : 24 : 3.5 : 2.5. The ratio of K to l type molecules in the serum immunoglobulins is 2 : 1. Other properties are summarized in table 24.1.

II. HYPOGAMMA-GLOBULINEMIA

A decreased serum concentration of the immunoglobulins may result from decreased synthesis (congenital agammaglobulinemia) or increased catabolism and/or loss (nephrotic syndrome or exudative enteropathy).

III. HYPER-GAMMA-GLOBULINEMIA

An increased serum concentration of one or more immunoglobulins may result from hyperplasia or neoplasia of B lymphocytes or their derivatives, plasma cells.

A. Types

Hypergammaglobulinemia is divisible into two types with different clinical and biochemical features: *monoclonal* and *polyclonal gammopathies*.

1. Monoclonal gammopathy

In the monoclonal type, proliferating plasma cells produce one (or at most a few) structurally homogeneous immunoglobulin molecule. Monoclonal gammopathies involve greatly increased concentrations of one or a few immunoglobulins, which are referred to as *M-components*. A complete M-component belongs to a single immunoglobulin class, subclass, and type and is similar in structure to normal immunoglobulin molecules. Since molecular weights of complete M-components are usually 160,000 or higher, they are largely restricted to circulating plasma and extracellular fluid. They appear in the urine in significant amounts only in the presence of glomerular damage. However, fragments of immunoglobulin molecules (e.g., free L chains) are produced in some patients, and a given patient may have a complete M-component, an incomplete M-component (L chain), or both. Unlike complete M-components, free L chains are found primarily in the urine. They occur in plasma in significant concentrations only in the presence of renal failure or when production is massive. If both complete and incomplete M-components are found in the same patient, the free L chains are usually identical to those in the complete molecule. Of the many M-components of different patients that have so far been studied, no two have been structurally identical. Significantly antibody or antibody-like activity has been found in some M-components. This demonstration provides further evidence that the structural information derived from study of these monoclonal proteins can be extrapolated to normal antibodies. However, the most direct evidence for this hypothesis comes from the demonstration that antibody response to certain pneumococcal polysaccharides is monoclonal.

2. Polyclonal gammopathy

Polyclonal hypergammaglobulinemia results from the proliferation of plasma cells that are producing many different immunoglobulins. Usually it occurs in response to antigenic stimulation.

B. Laboratory features

Laboratory abnormalities may be divided into (1) those due to hyperglobulinemia per se (rouleaux of red cells, elevated erythrocyte sedimentation rate, and positive Sia water test) and (2) those that distinguish between monoclonal and polyclonal gammopathies (i.e., electrophoretic procedures).

1. Elevated serum globulin

Normal serum contains 3.5–4.5 g albumin/100 ml and 3.0–4.0 g globulin/100 ml. Increased production of immunoglobulins usually elevates the total serum globulin level.

2. Erythrocyte sedimentation rate

An increased sedimentation rate of red cells in plasma reflects the presence of plasma substances that aggregate red cells. The most common cause is an increase in the concentration of fibrinogen; however, hypergammaglobulinemia of moderate to severe degree can also be a cause.

3. Sia water test

The Sia water test is a simple procedure for demonstrating the presence of euglobulins (proteins insoluble at low ionic strength). A positive result indicates hypergammaglobulinemia, which may be polyclonal or monoclonal.

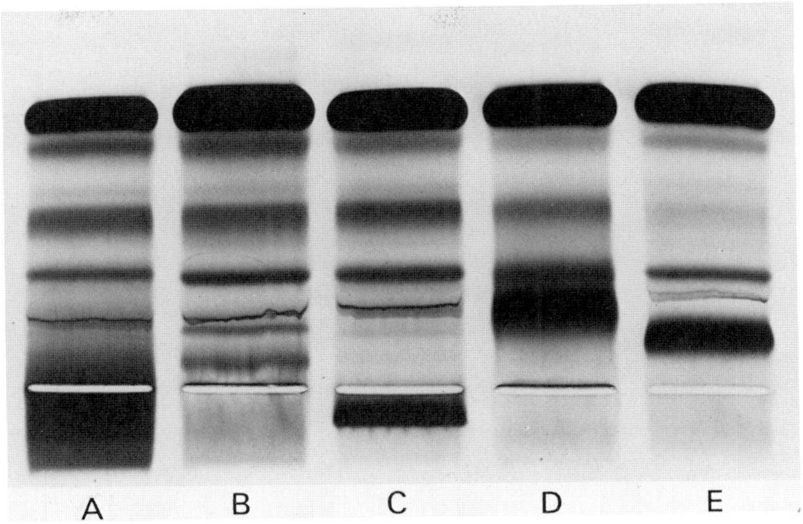

Fig. 24.2
Agarose gel electrophoresis of serum protein: *A*, diffuse hypergammaglobulinemia; *B*, normal plasma, showing fibrinogen just anodal to origin; *C*, IgG M-component; *D*, IgA M-component; *E*, IgM M-component.

4. Electrophoretic demonstration of M-components

Serum electrophoresis is the best screening test for diseases of immunoglobulin-producing cells (figure 24.2). M-components appear on zone electrophoresis (paper, agarose, agar, cellulose acetate) as narrow bands with sharp leading and trailing edges (figure 24.2C–E). In contrast the hypergammaglobulinemia of polyclonal grammopathies gives a diffuse pattern (figure 24.2A). On immunoelectrophoresis M-components produce a localized distortion or blister of the normal arc of the immunoglobulin class or type to which they belong (figure 24.3). The immunoelectrophoretic patterns of patients with polyclonal gammopathies show an increase in density and length of the normal IgG, IgA, and IgM arcs without local distortions. Zone electrophoresis of serum and of urine (concentrated about 30-fold) is the simplest means of detecting M-components (figure 24.2). For positive identification and typing, immunoelectrophoresis using antisera to κ and λ chains and other appropriate monospecific antisera is required. Such procedures also distinguish between free L chains and intact M-components. Protein electrophoresis and immunoelectrophoresis of serum and urine together should be able to identify virtually all monoclonal proteins encountered. If the screening protein electrophoresis is normal, it is most unusual to find a significant abnormality on the immunoelectrophoresis.

5. Bence Jones protein

Over 120 years ago Henry Bence Jones reported on the presence of "animal matter" in the urine of a patient with "fragilitas et mollities ossium," later called multiple myeloma. The material

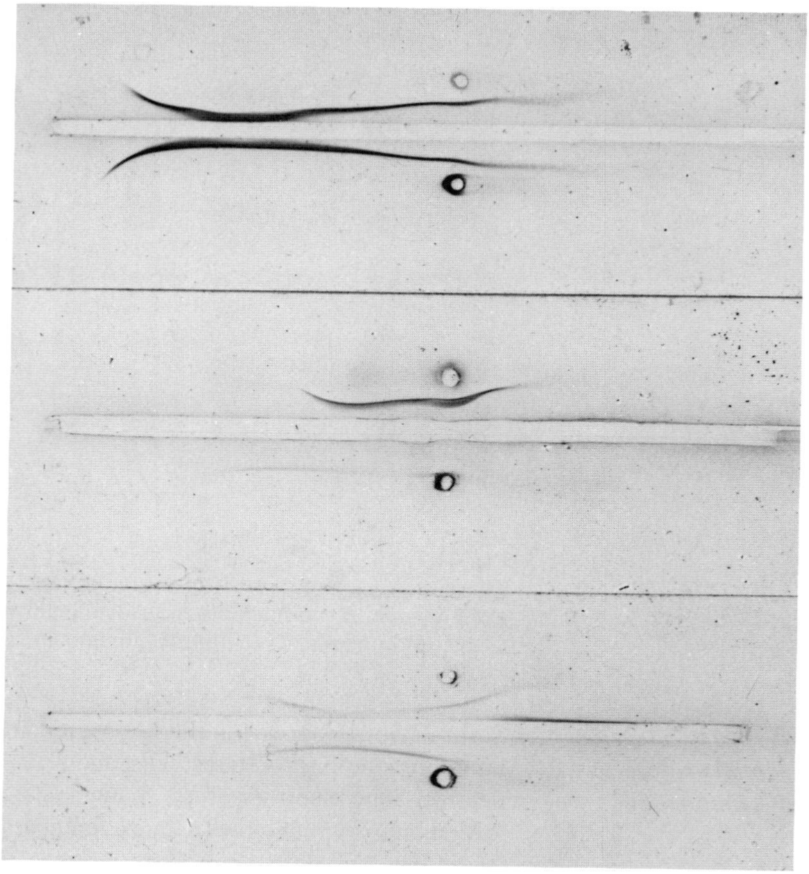

Fig. 24.3
Immunoelectrophoretic appearance of M-components. The anode was at the right. The antisera used to develop patterns were (from top to bottom) anti-IgG, anti-IgM, anti-IgA. All lower wells contained normal serum. Upper wells contained (top to bottom) IgG myeloma serum, serum from a patient with Waldenström's macroglobulinemia, and IgA myeloma serum. Note that M-components produce distortion and thickening of normal arcs.

precipitated on heating of the urine to 50–60°C and redissolved as the temperature was raised to the boiling point. Later work identified Bence Jones protein as free L chains. The characteristic behavior of free L chains on heating has been used as a screening test for multiple myeloma for over a century; however, the heat test is relatively insensitive and may be falsely negative. Also, excretion of L chains occurs not only in multiple myeloma but in other of the M-component disorders to be discussed below. "Stick tests" for proteinuria (such as Albustix®) are positive only in the presence of albumin and may be negative if only L chains are present.

C. Clinical consequences

1. Hyperviscosity

Hypergammaglobulinemia of any type when sufficiently severe may cause plasma hyperviscosity with sludging of blood in the capillaries. This effect is aggravated by the formation of red cell rouleaux. Sludging may lead to: hypergammaglobulinemic purpura; visual disturbances with dilation and segmentation of retinal veins, hemorrhages, and sometimes papilledema; CNS symptoms (e.g., vertigo, convulsions); and right-sided congestive heart failure. Increased excretion of light chain may cause proximal renal tubular acidosis, or acute renal failure.

2. Cryoglobulinemia

An immunoglobulin that reversibly precipitates (or gels) in the cold (4°C) is called a *cryoglobulin*. Cryoglobulins are usually M-components, but the phenomenon of cold precipitability can occur in polyclonal hypergammaglobulinemia. The proteins may be of any immunoglobulin class, including L chains alone, or may consist of a complex between immunoglobulins of different classes or between immunoglobulins and other serum proteins. Circulating antigen-antibody complexes may behave like cryoglobulins. Cryoglobulin formation may be looked upon as an extreme example of cold-facilitated molecular aggregation. When cryoglobulin precipitates in vivo, Raynaud's phenomenon, frank thrombosis, and gangrene may occur in exposed areas.

3. Interference with coagulation

M-components may interfere with normal blood coagulation by (1) complex formation with specific clotting factor (e.g., factor VIII); (2) interference with polymerization of fibrin monomer; or (3) coating platelets, thereby inducing a defect in platelet aggregate formation so that a poor primary hemostatic plug is formed despite a normal platelet count (see lectures 26–28). The latter is most common with IgM paraproteins.

4. Anemia, leukopenia, and thrombocytopenia

Coating of blood cells by M-components may accelerate their destruction. In myeloma and related diseases, anemia also results from bleeding, marrow replacement, uremia, and folate and/or vitamin B_{12} deficiency. In polyclonal hypergammaglobulinemia, chronic inflammation contributes to anemia by suppressing iron utilization.

D. Classification

A. Polyclonal gammopathies
B. Monoclonal gammopathies (malignant)
   1. Myeloma
   2. Waldenström's macroglobulinemia
   3. Heavy chain diseases
      a. Gamma (γ) chain disease
      b. Alpha (α) chain disease
      c. Mu (μ) chain disease
   4. Light chain disease
C. Monoclonal gammopathies of unknown significance
   1. Benign monoclonal gammopathy of unknown significance
   2. M-components associated with other disorders

IV. SPECIFIC DISORDERS

A. Polyclonal gammopathies

An otherwise normal individual develops diffuse hypergammaglobulinemia about 10–14 days following a sufficient antigenic stimulus. An increase in many or all immunoglobulins may occur reactively in many disorders, among them bacterial pneumonia; abscess; granulomatous disease; certain chronic infectious diseases (e.g., lymphogranuloma venereum, in which the agent is a chlamydia; kala-azar, in which hypergammaglobulinemia may be marked); and connective tissue disorders (e.g., systemic lupus erythematosus) and chronic hepatocellular disease (in both of which the causes of diffuse hypergammaglobulinemia are obscure). It may represent an immune response to foreign intracellular antigens released from damaged tissues.

B. Monoclonal gammopathies (malignant)

1. Multiple myeloma

The most common disease associated with monoclonal protein is multiple myeloma, a neoplastic proliferation of plasma cells in various stages of maturity. This disease rarely presents with multiple localized plasmacytomas but is usually widely disseminated at the time of presentation. An isolated plasmacytoma is more likely to meet the clinical criteria for monoclonal gammopathy of unknown significance than is multiple myeloma. The clinical picture reflects the effects of (1) infiltration of organs by plasma cells and (2) the associated monoclonal gammopathy.

Table 24.2
Clinical Features of Multiple Myeloma

	IgG myeloma	IgA myeloma	IgD myeloma	Light chain disease
Mean age at diagnosis	56	62	64	52
M:F ratio	1:1	1:1	3:1	1:1
κ:λ ratio	2:1	2:1	1:9	1:35
Incidence of Bence Jones protein (%)	60	70	92	100
Amyloid disease			↑	↑
Extraosseous involvement			↑	

a. Clinical features

Clinical features are summarized in table 24.2. The peak incidence is between ages 55 and 65, except for light chain disease, which may occur earlier. Except for IgD myeloma in which men exceed women by a 3:1 ratio, the distribution between the sexes is equal. The incidence of different heavy chain types roughly parallels their relative concentration among normal globulins. Light chain distribution is similar to that of normal light chains with 2 κ to every λ light chains. Untreated the median survival is 18 months. Survival is directly related to the state at onset and other prognostic factors, but with adequate treatment it is generally 3–5 years.

(1) Effects on blood

Almost all patients have a normochromic-normocytic anemia. As noted, this anemia has multiple causes. Moderate leukopenia and thrombocytopenia are common. The blood smear typically shows rouleaux formation. When marrow is heavily infiltrated, the blood smear may display a leukoerythroblastic reaction (see lecture 19). Rarely, plasma cells appear in the blood. This usually signifies a late stage of disease.

(2) Bone marrow

Aspirated bone marrow containing more than 15% plasma cells is suggestive of myeloma. The morphology or ultrastructure of individual cells is usually not diagnostically helpful. Increase in plasma cell number is not diagnostic because some benign illnesses (e.g., chronic liver disease) can display marked plasmacytosis. The most suggestive finding is sheets of plasma cells.

(3) Effect on bone

Bone abnormalities associated with multiple myeloma range from diffuse osteoporosis, present in about half the patients, to osteolytic lesions in the skull and long bones of the axial skeleton. Presence of osteolytic lesions usually signifies advanced disease. Osteolytic lesions heal following treatment in less than a third of patients. Pathogenesis of bone disease is thought to involve production of an *osteoclast-activating factor* by plasma cells. Hypercalcemia, found in about 10% of patients, is usually associated with severe bone disease.

(4) Renal impairment There is some evidence that some, but not all, light chains have toxic effects on proximal tubules, causing a proximal tubular leak. The finding of large amounts of proteinuria and/or of the nephrotic syndrome may be a manifestation of amyloid of the kidney. Good medical management with prevention of dehydration is a crucial element in preventing the occurrence of renal failure in patients with myeloma.

(5) Associated immunoglobulin abnormalities All but 1–2% of patients have a monoclonal protein that can be identified in the sera and/or in the urine. The levels of normal immunoglobulins are usually reduced in multiple myeloma. Why should there be a relative deficiency of normal immunoglobulins in patients with myeloma? It is known that mononuclear cells from patients with myeloma inhibit the pokeweed-driven synthesis of immunoglobulin by normal B cells. This suppressive activity is a property of the adherent mononuclear cell fraction. At least for IgG, increased amounts of IgG monoclonal protein enhance the catabolism of normal IgG. These changes presumably contribute to the known tendency of patients with myeloma to have difficulty with infections. There is no evidence that gamma globulin replacement therapy in these patients is of clinical value.

(6) Chemical changes in body fluids Other significant changes include hypercalcemia, which is invariably associated with extensive bony disease, hyperuricemia, and a rise in serum creatinine.

b. Cell kinetics and prognostic features Because myeloma cells produce a discrete protein, it is possible to estimate quite precisely cell mass at different stages of myeloma. The per cell production rate of IgG can be established in vitro. Turnover studies establish the whole body catabolic and synthetic rates. Division of the whole body rate by the per cell rate yields the total number of cells. Data of these kinds have been extrapolated to suggest that the amount of monoclonal protein produced by 35 gm of tissue is the limit of what can be detected by immunoelectrophoresis.

Most symptomatic patients have about 10^{12} tumor cells. Death may occur when the cell number reaches the range of 3.5 to 5×10^{12} cells. In a 70 kg patient, that corresponds to 5–7% of the body weight. Multivariate analysis permits a correlation of clinical data with direct measurement of tumor cell mass. These studies have shown that low-risk, low-tumor-burden patients lack bone disease and have hemoglobins over 8.5 g/100 ml and normal serum calciums. Poor risk, high-tumor-burden patients, on the other hand, have bone disease, high serum calciums, and anemia with hemoglobins below 8.5 g/100 ml. At intermediate risk are patients that have some, but not all, of the characteristics of high-risk patients. Recently additional prognostic features such as labeling index, β_2-microglobulin, and rate of progression of disease have been used as discriminating characteristics. Characterizing subgroups of myeloma patients is becoming increasingly important in selection of chemotherapy.

c. Treatment

Drugs effective in myeloma include L-phenylalanine mustard (Alkeran®), cyclophosphamide (Cytoxan®), prednisone, vincristine, BCNU, and Adriamycin®. The standard therapy against which other therapy is compared is still Alkeran® and prednisone. Recent studies have suggested that combination chemotherapy may enhance survival in selected clinical groups, as, for example, high-risk, high-tumor-burden patients. Indolent or slowly progressive myeloma should not be treated. Treatment can safely be withheld in these patients without changing the overall prognosis. This is important because there is clearly an increased incidence of secondary leukemias following prolonged therapy with either Alkeran® or Cytoxan®.

2. Macroglobulinemia of Waldenström

This disorder, also known as primary macroglobulinemia, is a neoplastic proliferation of lymphocytoid plasma cells that may be considered a variant of lymphocytic lymphoma (see lecture 22) in which the abnormal cell is an activated B lymphocyte. Marrow and other organs are infiltrated with immunoglobulin-producing cells, and tissue mast cells are increased.

a. Clinical features

The peak age incidence occurs at 60–70. There is a slight predilection for males. Survival averages 2–5 years but occasionally is much longer. The clinical picture is determined by the tumor cell infiltration and the effects of IgM. Infiltration usually causes hepatosplenomegaly and lymphadenopathy (which is unusual in multiple myeloma). Bone involvement (in contrast to multiple myeloma) is rare. Neurologic symptoms, such as peripheral neuropathy, are common. Manifestations of the abnormal protein are (1) presence of an IgM M-component; (2) hyperviscosity of the blood; (3) retinal hemorrhage and mucosal bleeding; (4) Bence Jones proteinuria in at least 10% of cases (which is less common than in multiple myeloma); and (5) the renal disease, usually glomerular rather than tubular.

b. Therapy

As in multiple myeloma, therapy consists mainly of cytolytic agents such as chlorambucil (Leukeran®), cyclophosphamide (Cytoxan®), and L-phenylalanine mustard (Alkeran®). In the face of incipient blindness from retinal hemorrhage, intractable congestive failure, or other severe manifestations of the hyperviscosity syndrome, intensive plasmapheresis may be useful. Unlike the abnormal proteins of multiple myeloma, the IgM of macroglobulinemia is largely within the blood and thus can be substantially diminished by plasmapheresis.

3. Heavy chain diseases

These rare disorders are characterized by neoplastic proliferation of plasma and reticulum cells with hepatosplenomegaly and soft tissue tumors in some instances. The course is rapidly downhill with fever, unveal edema, hyperuricemia, and debilitation. Several variants have been reported.

a. Gamma (γ) chain disease

In this disorder, also known as Franklin's disease, an identical M-component is found in serum and urine. Study shows it to be γ chains or more commonly some fragment of γ chains. Sometimes a group of amino acids has been deleted from the normal sequence. Normal immunoglobulins are low in concentration, and these patients are susceptible to infection. Lytic bone lesions are not found.

b. Alpha (α) chain disease

Alpha chain disease is the most common of the heavy chain diseases. Typical cases have abdominal lymphoma with a serum and urine M-component related to the H chain (α type) of IgA (see lecture 22). Patients have been mainly of North African or Eastern Mediterranean origin. Outside the Mediterranean area, α chain disease occurs in a rarer pulmonic form. Peak incidence is in the second and third decades of life, with 50% more males affected than females. In some early stages the course of this disease is modified by antibiotics.

c. Mu (μ) chain disease

A few cases of chronic lymphocytic leukemia have had serum M-components consisting only of μ chains. Unlike the situation with other heavy chain diseases, the abnormal protein is not found in the urine. Large vaculated plasma cells may be found in the bone marrow.

C. Monoclonal gammopathies of unknown significance

1. Benign monoclonal gammopathy of unknown significance

M-components may occur in some individuals without any symptoms or signs of disease. This situation is termed *benign monoclonal gammopathy* or *benign M-type hypergammaglobulinemia*. These M-components are usually low in concentration (< 2 gm/100 ml) and show no gradual increase with time (as occurs in multiple myeloma and macroglobulinemia). The incidence of this "disorder" approaches 1% in healthy populations and 6% among octogenarians. Many of these patients will evolve into multiple myeloma.

2. M-components associated with other disorders

Low concentrations of M-components have been reported in the serum of patients with chronic lymphocytic leukemia and lymphomas, cold agglutinin disease, and certain bacterial infections. Whether these will evolve in the direction of lymphoma is not clear.

V. SERUM PROTEIN ELECTROPHORESIS

It is the purpose of this brief section to provide a guide to the interpretation of serum electrophoretic patterns and the assessment of the value and limitations of this simple and widely used technique in the interpretation of clinical problems. Discussion of abnormalities in M-component diseases will not be repeated.

A. Proteins in serum

Over 100 serum proteins are known, and the list continues to grow. Many occurring in trace amounts are of great biologic importance. The proteins visible on clinical serum electrophoresis are a small fraction of the number present and represent only those occurring in sufficiently high concentration to form distinct stainable bands (table 24.3). A popular electrophoretic medium is agarose gel; cellulose acetate is also used. Agarose has the advantage of transparency. It also allows distinct separation of transferrin and β-lipoprotein (figure 24.4). If Ca^{++} is included in the buffer, a slow C3 band can be visualized. If one desires to quantify proteins, chemical or immunochemical techniques must be used. Such methods are now available for 40 to 50 serum proteins.

Table 24.3
Proteins Visible on Agarose Gel Electrophoresis

Protein	Function	Concentration in normal serum (mg/100 ml)	Mol. wt.
Prealbumin	Thyroxine-binding	10–40	70,000
Albumin	Colloid osmotic pressure; transport	3,500–5,000	69,000
α_1-Antitrypsin	Protease inhibitor	200–400	45,000
α_2-Macroglobulin	Protease inhibitor	150–400	720,000
Haptoglobin	Hemoglobin binding	50–200	85,000
Transferrin	Fe transport	200–400	90,000
β-Lipoprotein	Lipid transport	300–900	>2,000,000
C3	Complement component	100–200	220,000
IgG	Antibody	600–1,500	160,000

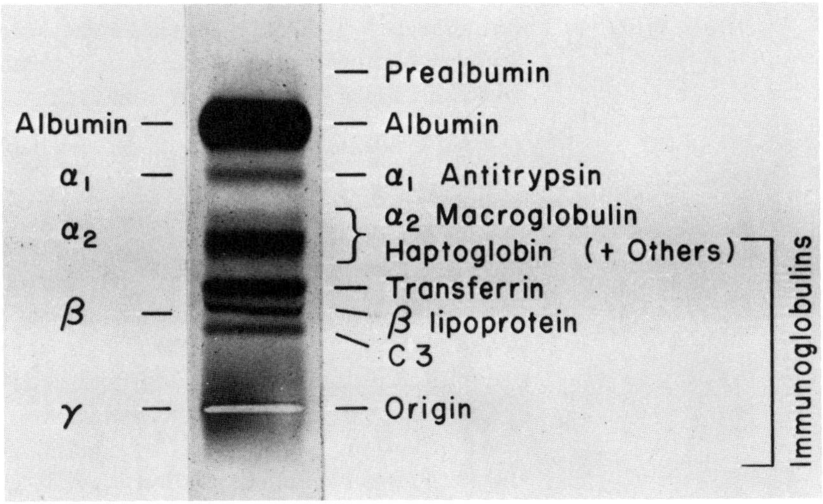

Fig. 24.4
Agarose gel electrophoresis pattern of normal human serum. The anode is at the top and the electrophoresis buffer is pH 8.6, 0.05 M barbital.

Table 24.4
Changes in Serum Proteins in Disease

Disease state	Pre-alb	Alb	α_1-at	α_2-glob[a]	Tf	Lip	C3	IgG
Acute inflammation	↓	↓	↑	↑	↓	± ↑	± ↑	0
Chronic inflammation	↓	↓	± ↑	± ↑	↓	± ↑	± ↑	↑
Obstructive jaundice	0	0	0	0	0	↑	↑	0
Chronic liver disease	↓	↓	± ↓	↓	↓	± ↓	± ↓	↑
Nephrotic syndrome	↓	↓ ↓	± ↓	↑ ↑	↓	↑ ↑	0	± ↓
Hemolytic anemia	0	0	0	↓	0	0	0	0
Iron deficiency	0	0	0	0	↑	0	0	0
Acute glomerulonephritis	0	0	0	0	0	0	↓	± ↑
Systemic lupus erythematosus	↓	↓	↑	± ↓	↓	0	± ↓	↑

Note: 0 = no change; ↓ = decrease; ↑ = increase; ± ↑ = variable increase, etc.
a. Changes in α_2-globulin are due mainly to alterations in haptoglobin concentration, except in the nephrotic syndrome, where the increase is due largely to α_2-macroglobulins.

B. Patterns in disease

Table 24.4 summarizes the changes observed on agarose gel electrophoresis of fresh serum from patients with various disease states. Abbreviations in table 24.4 refer to zones and bands described in figure 24.4 and table 24.3. These patterns may overlap in a given patient. For example, the patterns of chronic liver disease and obstructive jaundice often coexist. If a patient with hemolytic anemia also has an inflammatory process, α_1-antitrypsin may be elevated, but haptoglobin does not rise correspondingly. Thus, the α_2-globulin area appears relatively less dense. Changes in lupus erythematosus are variable because the disease is variable in its expression and severity. A low C3 usually indicates severe disease with renal or other parenchymatous involvement. Whether haptoglobin is relatively or absolutely decreased depends on the presence or absence of hemolytic anemia.

1. Acute inflammation

The pattern of acute inflammation is probably the most common in any hospital population. In general, it is nonspecific and occurs in a wide variety of acute inflammatory or necrotic processes, for example, postsurgery, after an acute myocardial infarction, in malignant tumors with necrosis, after pneumonia, or after endotoxin administration. The noted changes occur within a day or two of the insult and persist for 5–7 days, except that C3 does not rise until after the first week and the increase is only moderate.

The pattern of chronic inflammation or necrosis is variable because of varying contributions by continuing acute inflammation and varying antigenic stimulation (the latter resulting in a rise in immunoglobins).

2. Obstructive biliary disease

In obstructive biliary disease (or any jaundice with increased conjugated bilirubin), the bilirubin complex binds to albumin and causes a shift in electrophoretic mobility of the albumin toward the anode. Drugs (such as aspirin) can cause the same phenomenon because the altered albumin is more acidic than unaltered albumin.

3. Chronic liver disease

In chronic liver disease, α_2-globulin is often decreased because of decreased haptoglobin owing to concomitant hemolytic anemia. The increase in immunoglobulins is particularly marked in the slow β area (because of the marked increase in IgA usually present in this disorder).

4. Nephrosis

The nephrotic pattern is one of the most striking of those listed. The increase in α_2-globulin chiefly represents α_2-macroglobulin. In this disorder, there is a general increase in the synthesis of nonimmunoglobulin protein and an increase in the catabolism of all proteins in rough proportion to their molecular weights. The usual cutoff is at about 200,000–300,000. Thus, β-lipoprotein (mol. wt. >200,000) and α_2-macroglobulin (mol. wt. 720,000) are markedly increased in concentration and most other proteins are reduced. IgG is usually reduced, but if normal, one should suspect preexisting hypergammaglobulinemia.

5. Iron deficiency

The only change in iron deficiency is the increase in transferrin, which is reflected in the rise in total iron-binding capacity (lecture 6). An artifactual increase in this band may result from extensive hemolysis in vitro since hemoglobin A has the same mobility. Small amounts of hemoglobin arising from hemolysis in vitro cause a backward slurring of the α_2-area owing to formation in vitro of hemoglobin-haptoglobin complex.

6. Acute glomerulonephritis

In uncomplicated acute glomerulonephritis, the decrease or absence of the C3 band is striking. This persists for up to 4–6 weeks. One must be certain that (1) Ca^{++} is present in the electrophoresis buffer and (2) the serum sample is fresh. On storage of serum, particularly at elevated temperatures, C3 converts to a large fragment, C3c, that travels just ahead of transferrin. The increase in immunoglobulin often seen in this condition results from the previous streptococcal infection.

7. Lupus erythematosus

The pattern in systemic lupus erythematosus usually shows a pronounced increase in slowly migrating IgG. Signs of acute inflammation are also usually present; decreases in α_2-globulin and C3 were discussed above.

8. Others

Other situations need only brief mention. Hemoconcentration and hemodilution may be detected by changes in total protein concentration. A decrease in total protein and a general decrease in individual proteins is associated with protein-losing enteropathy. All bands and zones show either an increase or decrease. Specific deficiency states show an absence of single bands or zones (e.g., of albumin, α_1-antitrypsin, transferrin, β-lipoprotein, C3, and the immunoglobulins).

SELECTED REFERENCES

Alper, C. A. Plasma protein measurements as a diagnostic aid. *New Eng. J. Med.* 29(1974): 287.

Axelson, U., and Hallen, J. Review of 54 subjects with monoclonal gammopathy. *Brit. J. Haematol.* 15(1968): 417.

Durie, B. G. M., et al. Pretreatment tumor mass, cell kinetics, and prognosis in multiple myeloma. *Blood* 55(1980): 364.

Durie, B. G. M., et al. Human myeloma *in vitro* colony growth: Interrelationships between drug sensitivity, cell kinetics, and patient survival duration. *Blood* 61(1983): 929.

Greipp, P. R., and Kyle, R. A. Clinical, morphological, and cell kinetic differences among multiple myeloma, monoclonal gammopathy of undetermined significance, and smoldering multiple myeloma. *Blood* 62(1983): 166.

Kyle, R. A. Long term survival in multiple myeloma. *New Eng. J. Med.* 308(1983): 314.

Kyle, R. A. Monoclonal gammopathy of undetermined significance: Natural history in 241 cases. *Amer. J. Med.* 64(1978): 814.

Kyle, R. A., and Greipp, P. R. Idiopathic Bence Jones proteinuria. *New Eng. J. Med.* 306(1982): 564.

McIntyre, O. R. Multiple myeloma. *New Eng. J. Med.* 301(1979): 193.

Solomon, A. Bence Jones proteins and light chains of immunoglobulins. *New Eng. J. Med.* 306(1982): 605.

LECTURE 25 Histiocytoses and Lipidoses

Allen C. Crocker

I. INTRODUCTON

This lecture is concerned with two entirely dissimilar types of disorders, both of which display notable pathology within the reticuloendothelial system (RES). The syndromes under discussion provide a useful basis for consideration of the range of functions and special reactivity of the RES system, especially its histiocytic elements. The two principal areas of concern are (1) the *histiocytoses*, which are reflections of a disturbed histiocytic reaction, and (2) the *lipidoses* and *mucopolysaccharidoses,* in which the histiocyte may be a locus of expression of an inborn error of metabolism.

II. HISTIOCYTOSES

The histiocytoses or histiocytosis syndromes (which include the *Schüller-Christian* and *Letterer-Siwe syndromes*) are relatively uncommon disorders that are usually seen in childhood, although occasionally in adult life, with a sporadic incidence not evidently correlating with environmental factors. The clinical picture suggests an overresponse to some as yet unidentified stimulus. Clinical involvement may be mild, or a predicament may develop that resembles a diffuse reticuloendothelial cell malignancy with fatal outcome. The latter situation displays many biologic analogies with the lymphomas.

A. Characteristics of lesions

1. Histology

The process, wherever it occurs, is fundamentally a disseminated granuloma, of which the primary cell type is the histiocyte. Other reactive elements are also present, including eosinophils, lymphocytes, neutrophils, fibroblasts, plasma cells, and giant cells.

2. Sites of predilection

As might have been predicted, typical lesions occur most notably in tissues rich in reticuloendothelial elements. The medullary cavity of bone is the most common site. Relatively prominent and dynamic involvement also occurs in lymph nodes, lungs, liver, and spleen. Significant lesions also occur frequently in skin and meninges. The thymus is commonly involved by histiocytic infiltration, either focal or general.

3. Etiology

Extensive studies have failed to yield consistent evidence for the presence of bacteria, fungi, or viruses in the lesions. The process is not contagious for humans or transmittable to animals. There has never been multiple incidence in one family. This is not the case in the distantly related familial syndromes—"lymphohistiocytosis," "familial reticuloendotheliosis with eosinophilia," and so forth. There is accumulating evidence that the basic disorder may be a complex disturbance in immune regulation.

4. Natural history

It is notable that the lesions of these syndromes are potentially reversible under favorable circumstances, with a subsidence of the active proliferative phase, sometimes spontaneously, though with residual fibrosis and sometimes disruption of local organ architecture. A specific correlation between age and degree of dissemination of the granulomatous process is observed in children. Infants (especially in the 6–18 month range) have the most severe involvement, older children often showing only one or more lesions localized in bone.

5. Response to therapy

The granulomas are sensitive to radiotherapy in low dosage, but such treatment is usually restricted to large or painful lesions in bone or for the circumstance of diabetes insipidus. Suppressive effects can be seen with antitumor chemotherapy, but caution is appropriate regarding the use of potentially teratogenic and/or oncogenic agents in the treatment of nonmalignant disease. The most effective agent appears to be vinblastine. Regrettably this medication will not reverse the aggressive disease sometimes seen in infants. For many children the most appropriate management is good general support, with attention to transfusion, improved nutrition, and antibiotics where needed. At this time there is no single specific treatment for the histiocytosis syndromes.

6. Tendency toward lipidization

The histiocytes may form masses of "foam cells" with vacuolated cytoplasm. Tissue cholesterol levels may rise to 10% of the wet weight. This is especially common in thymus, meninges, bone, and skin.

B. Typical clinical pictures

The most frequent type of lesion is an expanding granuloma in the medullary cavity of bone. This produces destruction of normal bone, often with local pain and swelling, and may lead to pathologic fracture. The spread of involvement beyond these single or multiple bone lesions may be very broad, with a variety of cutaneous eruptions (small vesicles, papules, nodules, and confluent lesions), enlargement of the lymph nodes and abdominal viscera, diabetes insipidus due to involvement in the meninges, or deeper and pulmonary infiltration (figure 25.1).

Nomenclature for the several clinical forms of disease expression is imprecise, drawing loosely on early publications. For the five characteristic disease pictures listed below, it is customary to employ the term *eosinophilic granuloma* for the first, *Schüller-Christian syndrome* for the second and third, and *Letterer-Siwe syndrome* for the fourth and fifth.

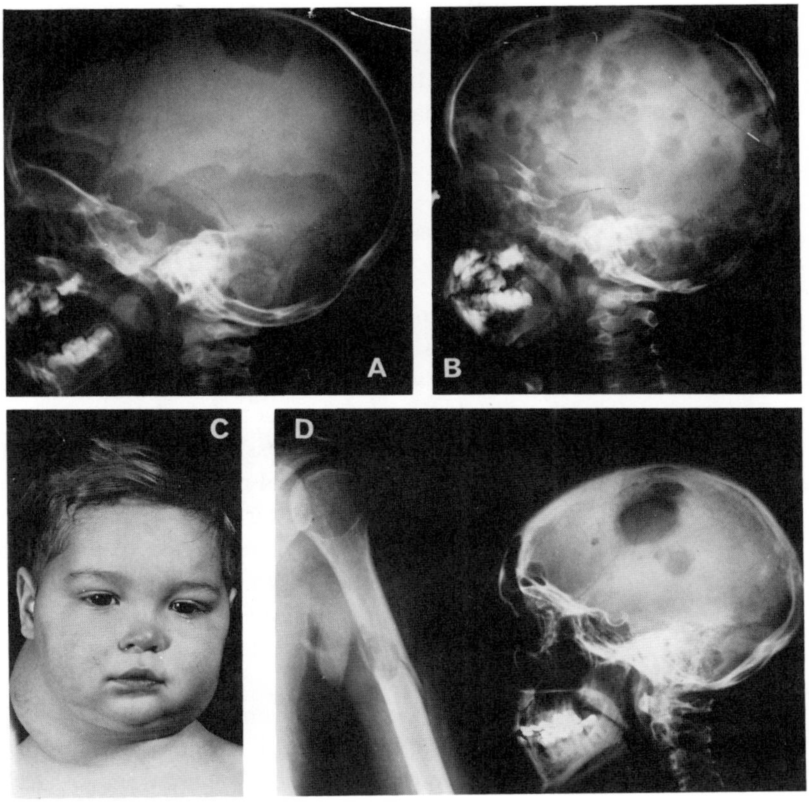

Fig. 25.1
Granulomatous lesions in the histiocytoses: *A*, extensive lytic lesions in the calvarium of a 2-year-old girl with Schüller-Christian syndrome; *B*, the same child, now 4 years old, with repair of some of the earlier lesions, but many new areas of involvement; *C*, severe lateral cervical adenopathy in a 2-year-old boy with Letterer-Siwe syndrome; *D*, osteolytic lesions in the humerus (with pathologic fracture) and skull of a 36-year-old woman with Schüller-Christian syndrome.

1. Bone lesions only

About half of the patients show only bone lesions. The most frequent locations are the axial skeleton (skull, spine, pelvis, ribs, shoulder girdle) and proximal long bones (femurs, humeruses).

2. Bone lesions plus minor additional involvement

Examples of such limited extension would be localized eruption in the skin or mucous membranes, diabetes insipidus, and secondary anemia.

3. Bone lesions plus moderate visceral involvement

This form is characterized by diffuse scaly papular skin lesions, seborrhea-like eruptions on the scalp and in the ear canals, gingival inflammation, pulmonary infiltration, mild hepatomegaly, and granulomas around the orbits, middle ears, and pituitary.

4. Major visceral involvement

This form displays greater hepatomegaly, splenomegaly, adenopathy, serious pulmonary infiltration, confluent or petechial skin eruption, bone marrow suppression, and, often, fever.

5. Special local progression

When expression of disease is particularly advanced and disabling in one system, the picture can include cystic disease of the lung, severe hepatic involvement, or massive lateral cervical adenopathy.

III. LIPIDOSES AND MUCOPOLY-SACCHARIDOSES

A. Pathophysiology

The clinical and pathologic pictures in these diseases, the so-called storage or foam cell diseases, are consequences of a heritable enzymopathy—usually a single gene-determined disorder producing deficient activity of a specific enzyme system. Most commonly the expression of disease reflects a homozygous abnormality with autosomal recessive transmission. Rarely, it is X-linked or dominant. The characteristic anatomic manifestation of the metabolic disorder is alteration of histiocytes by accumulation in their cytoplasm of metabolites in membrane-limited organelles, probably secondary lysosomes (figure 25.2). Amassed materials are assumed to be at least in part of local biosynthetic origin.

B. Clinical pictures

Several dozen syndromes have been described within the categories of lipidoses and mucopolysaccharidoses, and new ones are still being identified. In addition, separate subgroups or phenotypes with special or distinct features occur among many of the principal disease types. Hence, the following discussion will be

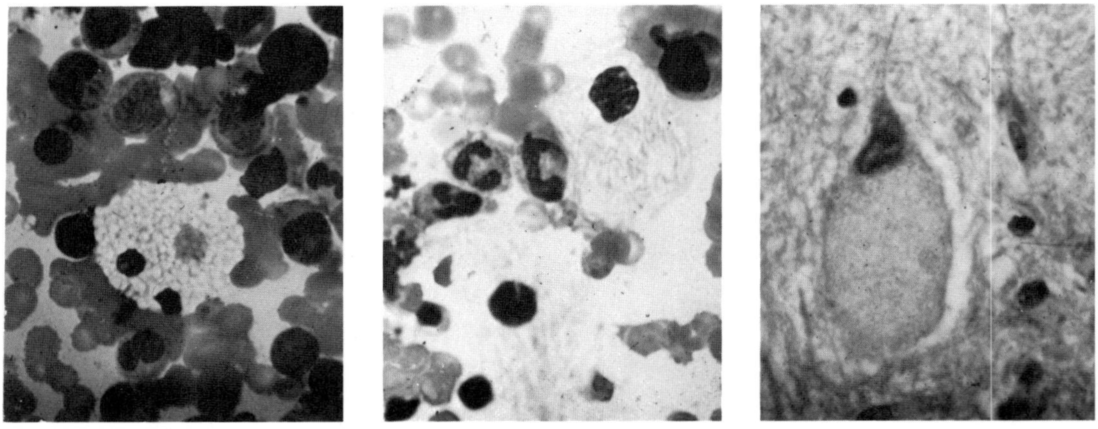

A B C

Fig. 25.2
Cellular changes in the lipidoses: *A*, vacuolated foam cell in the marrow of Niemann-Pick disease; *B*, Gaucher cells in the bone marrow, showing the fibrillated appearance of the cytoplasm; *C*, a distended neuron in the gray matter of a child with Tay-Sachs disease.

limited to a consideration of principles. It is possible to anticipate the most significant pathology for a particular syndrome by (1) considering the normal physiologic role of the substance whose metabolism is compromised and (2) remembering that for most of these diseases, expression of the handicap occurs primarily in four systems: solid viscera; skeleton; central nervous system; and circulating white cells.

1. Changes in solid viscera

The presence of foam cells in the tissues of liver, spleen, lymph nodes, lungs, or kidneys causes them to be abnormally firm and pale in appearance, with increased weight and volume. Resulting functional handicaps are variable. The most common are hypersplenism, impaired renal function, and chronic nutritional failure.

2. Changes in skeleton

Many effects follow from the presence of foam cells in the medullary cavity. Volume of the marrow mass increases, and there ensue defects in bone modeling with growth, thinning of cortices, pathologic fractures, and aseptic necrosis. There may also be (in the mucopolysaccharidoses) basic alterations in cartilage and bone, with resultant abnormal face and body form and an atypical pattern of growth.

3. Changes in central nervous system.

The most conspicuous feature is distention of neurones with the formation of membranous bodies in the cytoplasm that are presumably analogous to those in visceral foam cells (figure 25.2). In time, cell death occurs with neuronal loss, gliosis, and thickening of meninges. Characteristically there is also reduction in white matter (myelin) from either primary or secondary mechanisms. There are numerous examples of differences in the types of chemical alteration affecting the brain and viscera of the same patient. Such variations presumably reflect critical differences in substrate availability. It is puzzling that some phenotypes of diseases in which brain involvement ordinarily occurs display no CNS abnormalities whatever (e.g., as seen in Niemann-Pick, Gaucher, and Farber diseases).

4. Changes in white cells

In many of the syndromes, lymphocytes and monocytes show cytoplasmic vacuoles that appear to be congested lysosomes (figure 25.3). Metachromatic granules (Alder bodies) may also appear in these cells, sometimes presenting in dried smears as granules without vacuoles (Mittwoch bodies). Rarely, in the mucopolysaccharidoses, an increase in granule prominence in neutrophils (Reilly bodies) causes them superficially to resemble basophils.

C. Features of the lipidoses

The presumed primary enzymatic defects in all of the major lipidoses have been identified since 1966, and assay systems have been developed that permit accurate diagnosis and investigations concerning possible replacement therapy. Some of the results appear in table 25.1. These enzymes commonly diffuse from cells or

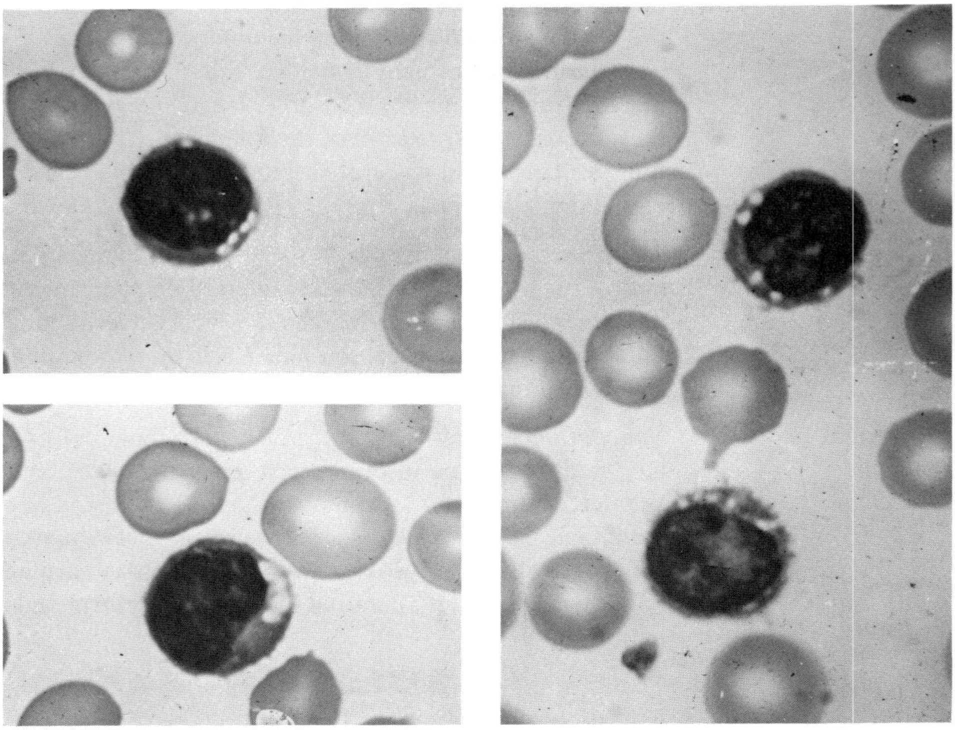

Fig. 25.3
Lymphocytes with vacuolated cytoplasm in Niemann-Pick disease.

Table 25.1
Chemical Findings in the Major Lipidoses

Syndrome	Substance accumulated	Enzyme deficiency
Gaucher	Glucocerebroside	Glucocerebroside β-glucosidase
Niemann-Pick	Sphingomyelin	Sphingomyelinase
Krabbe	Galactocerebroside	Galactocerebroside β-galactosidase
Metachromatic leukodystrophy	Sulfatide	Sulfatidase
Fabry	Ceramide trihexoside	α-galactosidase A
Tay-Sachs	G_{M2}-ganglioside	Hexosaminidase A
Generalized gangliosidosis	G_{M1}-ganglioside	β-galactosidase
Wolman	Cholesterol ester, triglyceride	Esterase
Refsum	Phytanic acid	Phytanic acid hydroxylase
Farber	Ceramide	Acid ceramidase

Table 25.2
Pattern of Enzyme Deficiency in a Typical Lipidosis

Level of enzyme	Homozygous individual	Heterozygous individual
Liver	Decreased	
CNS, gray matter	Decreased	
Circulating white cells	Decreased	Moderately decreased
Serum	Decreased	Moderately decreased
Urine	Decreased (?)	
Skin fibroblast culture	Decreased	Moderately decreased
Amniotic fluid (soluble fraction)	Decreased (?)	
Amniotic fluid cells (assayed in culture)	Decreased	Moderately decreased (?)

Note: Question mark indicates that data may be inconclusive.

are released by cell turnover. Following the characterization of the enzyme defect, it has been found that a reduced level of enzyme is present in body fluids (serum and urine) as well as in solid viscera and white blood cells. Table 25.2 lists the sequence (reading from the top) in which enzyme data usually become available during the investigation of a new disease. As shown in the table, heterozygously involved individuals may have partially reduced enzyme levels in various tissues or fluids without functional handicap. Such data can provide information that is useful in genetic counseling. In spite of the relative abundance of new information on these enzymopathies, many obscure points remain regarding the pathogenesis of the lipidoses.

D. Features of the mucopolysaccharidoses

The mucopolysaccharidoses parallel the lipidoses in a number of ways. Both manifest various analogous visceral and central nervous system phenomena. There is stockpiling of mucopolysaccharides in histiocytes in Hurler disease and related conditions (the Hunter, Sanfilippo, Scheie, and Maroteaux-Lamy phenotypes). Beyond this, there are special features attributable to (1) *extracellular molecular effects*—such as changes in connective tissue ground substance, heart valves, joint capsule, and cornea, and (2) *parenchymal cell pathology*—particularly of myocardium and renal tubules. Effects of these involvements include recurrent inguinal and umbilical hernias, chronic congestive heart failure, restriction of joint movement, and corneal clouding. One also finds a peculiar chronic nasal discharge, hearing handicap, and the formation of juxtasellar arachnoid cysts. A feature of special interest is the formation of granular intracellular inclusions in cultured fibroblasts (figure 25.4), which can be cleared by addition of cell-free corrective factors from various biologic sources (including media fluid from cell cultures of different phenotypes). The renal tubular involvement is presumed to be the origin of mucopolysac-

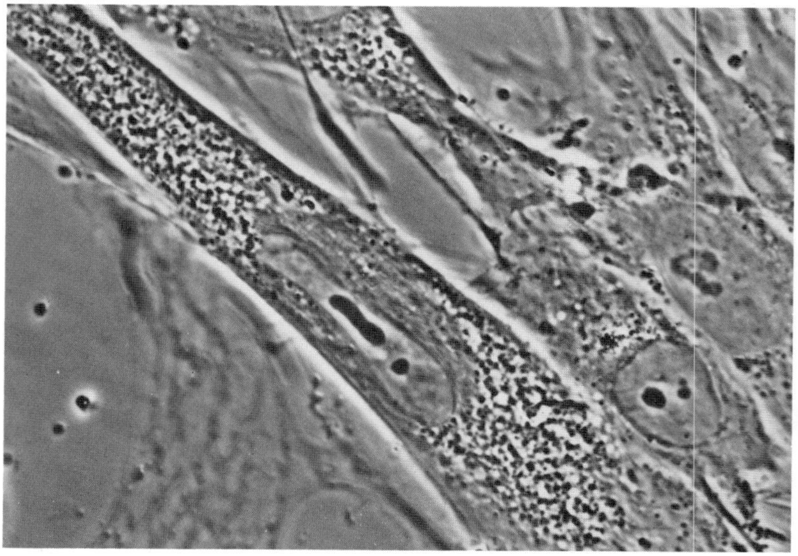

Fig. 25.4
Granule-packed fibroblasts growing in the culture of a skin biopsy from a child with the Hunter phenotype of the mucopolysaccharidoses. Phase contrast microphotograph.

Table 25.3
Chemical Findings in the Major Mucopolysaccharidoses

Syndrome	Substance accumulated	Enzyme deficiency
Hurler	Dermatan and heparan sulfates	α-L-iduronidase
Hunter	Dermatan and heparan sulfates	Iduronate sulfatase
Sanfilippo A	Heparan sulfate	Heparan N-sulfatase
Sanfilippo B	Heparan sulfate	N-acetyl-α-D-glucosaminidase
Morquio	Keratan sulfate and chondroitin 4- and 6-sulfates	Hexosamine 6-sulfatase
Maroteaux-Lamy	Dermatan sulfate	Arylsulfatase B

charide leakage into the urine, which constitutes an important biochemical marker of the mucopolysaccharidoses. The most prominent phenotypes are summarized in table 25.3.

E. Differential diagnosis of presenting signs

1. Vacuolated lymphocytes

Vacuolated lymphocytes in blood are seen in (1) Niemann-Pick disease (all phenotypes); (2) Wolman disease; (3) Swedish form of Batten disease, (4) generalized gangliosidosis; (5) G_{MI}-gangliosidosis, type 2; (6) I-cell disease; and (7) fucosidosis.

2. Elevated urinary acid mucopolysaccharides

Elevated urinary levels of acid mucopolysaccharides occur in (1) mucopolysaccharidoses (regularly in Hurler, Hunter, Sanfilippo, Scheie, and Maroteaux-Lamy phenotypes; irregularly in Morquio disease); (2) multiple sulfatase deficiency metachromatic leukodystrophy; (3) rarely in other constitutional disorders with skeletal handicaps (e.g., familial exostoses).

3. Cherry-red maculae

A cherry-red spot is seen in the macula of the ocular fundus in (1) Tay-Sachs disease; (2) Niemann-Pick disease, Group A; (3) generalized gangliosidosis; and (4) rarely in metachromatic leukodystrophy and Farber disease.

4. Elevated serum acid phosphatase

An increase of the serum phosphatase level in childhood patients is found in (1) Gaucher disease; (2) osteopetrosis; (3) the late form of osteogenesis imperfecta; and (4) rarely in Niemann-Pick disease.

SELECTED REFERENCES

Crocker, A. C. — The histiocytosis syndromes. In Fitzpatrick, T. B., et al, eds., *Dermatology in General Medicine*, 3d ed., New York: McGraw-Hill Book Co., 1984, in press.

Greenberger, J. S., et al. — Results of treatment of 127 patients with systematic histiocytosis. *Medicine* 60(1981): 311.

McKusick, V. A. — *Heritable Disorders of Connective Tissue*, 4th ed., St. Louis: Mosby, 1972.

Milunsky, A., ed. — *The Prevention of Genetic Disease and Mental Retardation*, Philadelphia: W. B. Saunders, 1975.

Multiple authors — Disorders of lysosomal enzymes (Part 5). In *The Metabolic Basis of Inherited Disease*, 5th ed., Stanbury, J. B., et al., eds., New York: McGraw-Hill Book Co., 1983, pp. 751–969.

LECTURE 26 Hemorrhagic Disorders I. Protein Interactions in the Clotting Mechanism

Robert D. Rosenberg

I. INTRODUCTION

The normal process of *hemostasis* begins when vascular endothelium is damaged. Exposed subendothelial structures attract platelets and induce their loose *aggregation*. These components in turn initiate the *generation of thrombin*, which aggregates platelets irreversibly and causes the laying down of *clot*, a platelet-fibrin network that is an effective barrier against further escape of blood and a scaffold for repair of vessel damage. Simultaneously, *limiting processes* are activated that confine hemostasis to the site of injury. Finally, *lysis* of the platelet fibrin network occurs when vascular endothelium is regenerated.

Typical transformations of the hemostatic system are depicted in figure 26.1. An enzyme precursor, or *zymogen*, is normally present in the blood, but possesses essentially no biological activity. The protein is transformed to a trypsin-like protease (i.e., it is activated) either by a conformational change or by scission of peptide bonds via action of a converting enzyme. The rate of this reaction may be accelerated by a nonenzymatic protein cofactor, which may act either by altering zymogen conformation (figure 26.1, type 1) or by binding converting enzyme and zymogen close together on a phospholipid surface (figure 26.1, type 2).

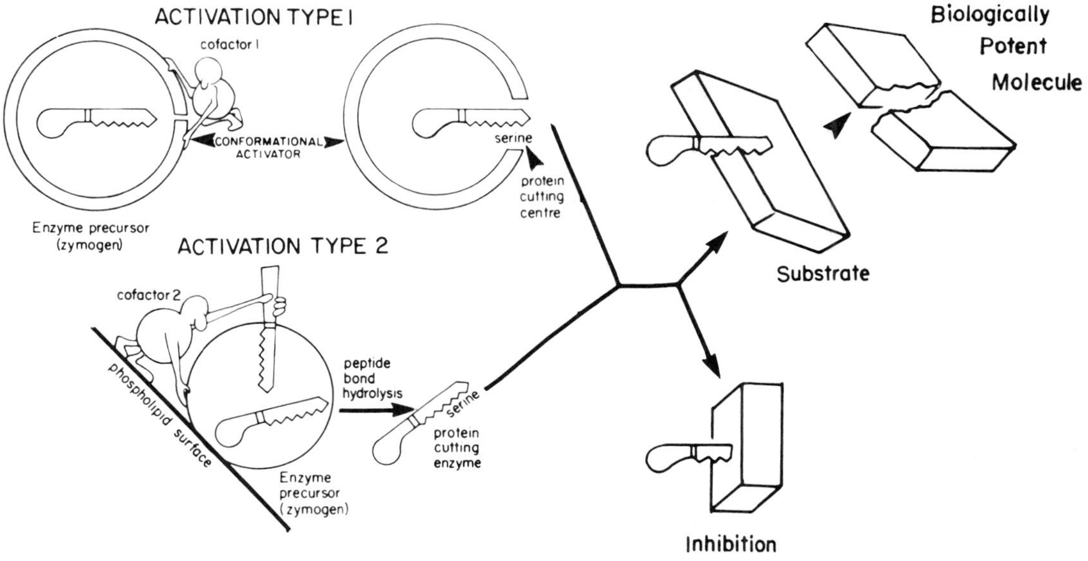

Fig. 26.1
Activation mechanisms for zymogens of the hemostatic reaction.

During evolution, homologous sets of cofactors and zymogens arose through gene duplication and mutation. This resulted in the development of a linked series of reactions in which a zymogen is converted to a *serine protease* (i.e., a protease that contains an essential serine residue at its active site) that then catalyzes a subsequent precursor-protease transition. In fact, activation of zymogens in the initial stages of the hemostatic system is accomplished by conformational alteration induced by components (cofactors) that are exposed when vascular endothelium is damaged. But in later stages, activation occurs by proteolytic cleavage of the next zymogen in the sequence. Early reactions tend to occur on surfaces exposed by vascular injury; later reactions are thought to take place on phospholipid surfaces of aggregated platelets. This linked, multistage system permits both amplification and modulation of the initial stimulus that sets the hemostatic mechanism into action. (The soluble clotting factors are by international convention designated by Roman numerals, though various synonyms were used earlier. The factors and their several synonyms are summarized in table 26.1.)

The hemostatic system consists essentially of two discrete series of proteolytic reactions. The first is the *clotting*, or *coagulation mechanism*, the end product of which is *thrombin*. The second is the *fibrinolytic mechanism*, the end product of which is *plasmin*. The major role of thrombin is to initiate formation of the fibrin clot by cleaving specific peptide bonds in the plasma protein *fibrinogen*. Plasmin breaks down the clot by hydrolyzing different peptide bonds in the fibrin molecule. These two serine proteases may also interact with plasma components that neutralize their enzymatic activities. These inhibitory species contain peptide sequences similar to those in fibrinogen and other natural substrates of the two enzymes. However, when thrombin or plasmin interacts with these inhibitors, bond hydrolysis is hindered and a stable complex is formed. Thus, similar biochemical mechanisms are responsible for the initiation and suppression of hemostatic system activity.

In this lecture, we shall summarize the biochemistry of these processes, especially the pathways for generation of thrombin, formation of the fibrin clot, mechanisms of fibrinolysis, and the several limiting reactions. The platelet and its role in hemostasis will be discussed separately in lecture 27.

II. GENERATION OF THROMBIN

The generation of thrombin can be subdivided into two major sets of reactions: (1) the *activation of factor X* and (2) the subsequent *conversion of prothrombin to thrombin*. These processes are precisely regulated by a series of complex interactions that include the *protein C-thrombomodulin mechanism*.

Table 26.1
Glossary of Coagulation Factor Nomenclature

Coagulation factors (international nomenclature)	Synonyms
I	Fibrinogen
II	Prothrombin
III	Tissue factor, tissue thromboplastin
IV	Calcium (Ca^{++})
V	Proaccelerin Labile factor Ac-globulin
VII	SPCA Convertin Stable factor
VIII	Antihemophilic globulin (AHG) Antihemophilic factor (AHF) Antihemophilic factor A
IX	Plasma thromboplastin component (PTC) Antihemophilic factor B
X	Stuart factor (Stuart-Prower)
XI	Plasma thromboplastin antecedent (PTA) Antihemophilic factor C
XII	Hageman factor Antihemophilic factor D
XIII	Fibrin stabilizing factor (FSF) Laki-Lorand factor
Prekallikrein	Fletcher factor
High-molecular-weight kininogen	Fitzgerald factor
Antithrombin	Antithrombin III
Antiplasmin	
α_2-Macroglobulin Protein C Protein S	

Note: Not all coagulation factors have been given roman numerals. Roman numerals were assigned in order of discovery and do not imply place in sequence of reactions. There is no factor VI. This book follows the common practice of referring to factor I as fibrinogen, factor II as prothrombin, factor III as tissue factor, and factor IV as Ca^{++}.

A. Activation of factor X

Two distinct pathways exist for the conversion of the factor X zymogen to its corresponding serine protease, factor Xa (note that by convention the suffix "a" indicates that a factor is in "activated" form). These are the *intrinsic coagulation cascade* and the *extrinsic coagulation cascade*. Activation of each cascade is initiated when damaged vascular endothelium and blood come in contact with components that are normally hidden. Both pathways seem essential for the generation of adequate amounts of factor Xa in vivo.

1. Intrinsic coagulation cascade

a. Activation of factor XII

The activation of the intrinsic coagulation cascade is sparked when blood is exposed to collagen, basement membrane, or microfibrillar substance. Factor XII, a single polypeptide chain zymogen of mol. wt. 80,000, is normally present in plasma. It binds to these subendothelial structures and undergoes a conformational transition to factor XIIa, which contains an active serine center. Alternatively, factor XII can be converted to factor XIIa by proteolytic cleavages that produce a diverse spectrum of products of mol. wt. 25,000–75,000. Once formed, factor XIIa is able to hydrolyze prekallikrein and factor XI as well as plasminogen and thus activate the kinin-generating coagulation and fibrinolytic mechanisms (figure 26.2).

Prekallikrein is a single polypeptide chain zymogen of mol. wt. 85,000. It circulates in the blood as a 1:1 stoichiometric complex with a cofactor termed *high-molecular-weight kininogen* (mol. wt. 120,000). Factor XIIa can cleave the prekallikrein zymogen and convert it into the serine protease *kallikrein*, which has a heavy and a light polypeptide chain of mol. wt. 52,000 and 33,000, respectively. The presence of high-molecular-weight kininogen

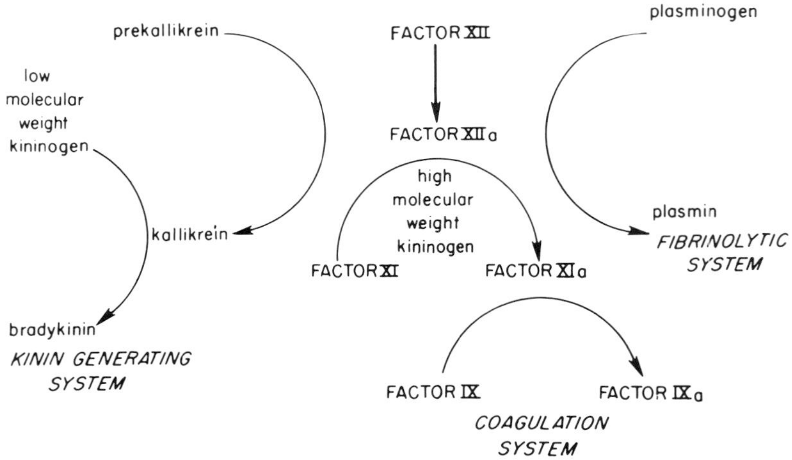

Fig. 26.2
Consequences of factor XII activation.

cofactor is essential for the rapid generation of kallikrein from prekallikrein. Once formed, kallikrein is able to cleave the single polypeptide chain of high-molecular-weight kininogen and release from the center of the molecule the decapeptide *bradykinin*, a potent substance that lowers blood pressure, increases capillary permeability, and acts as a vasodilator. Kallikrein itself exhibits chemotactic activity for neutrophils and monocytes, recruiting them into sites of tissue injury.

b. Activation of factor XI

Factor XI is a zymogen formed by two identical polypeptide chains of mol. wt. 80,000 that are connected by disulfide (S–S) bonds. It circulates in plasma as a 1:1 stoichiometric complex with high-molecular-weight kininogen. Factor XIIa can convert the factor XI zymogen into the serine protease factor XIa by the scissioning of specific bonds within each of the polypeptide chains of the zymogen. This gives rise to two sets of fragments of mol. wt. 50,000 and 30,000 that are held together by disulfide bonds. Thus, factor XIa structurally is a two-headed dimeric enzyme. High-molecular-weight kininogen must be present if factor XIa is to be rapidly generated in significant quantities. Once formed, factor XIa initiates activation of the remainder of the intrinsic coagulation cascade with the eventual formation of factor Xa (figure 26.3).

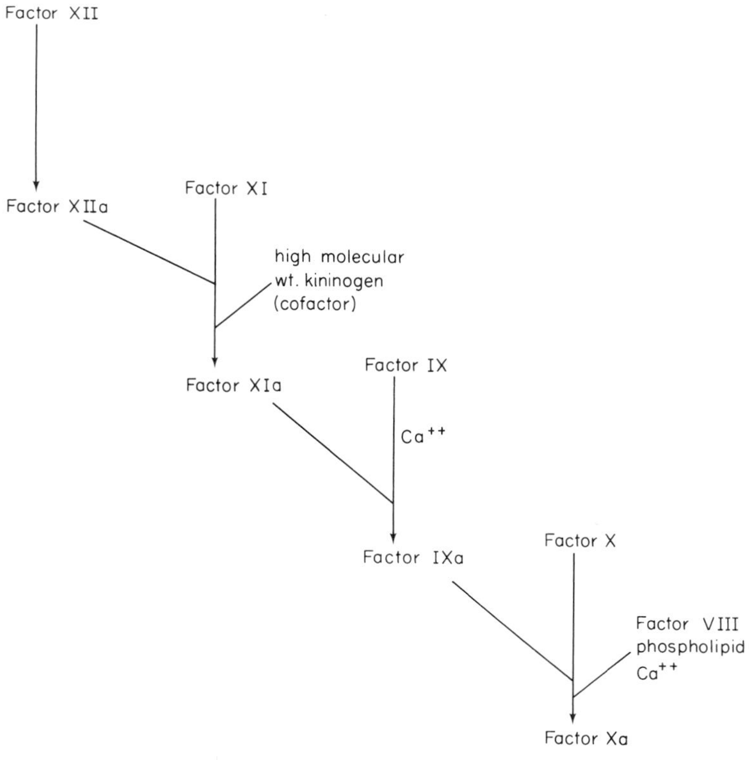

Fig. 26.3
The intrinsic coagulation cascade.

Factor XIIa also activates *plasminogen*, a zymogen normally present in the blood, to form the serine protease *plasmin*, which can lyse the fibrin clot (see below). Since factor XIIa can convert plasminogen to plasmin, it can initiate systemic fibrinolysis. It is still unclear whether factor XIIa can directly activate plasminogen or whether this is accomplished indirectly via generation of kallikrein as well as factor XIa, both of which subsequently cleave the zymogen. It is of interest that kallikrein, plasmin, and factor XIa (all generated by factor XIIa) can produce in turn additional factor XIIa by proteolytic cleavage of the factor XII zymogen. *High-molecular-weight kininogen* is a critical cofactor in this process. These multiple pathways autocatalytically magnify the initial stimulus activating factor XII and thereby produce greater amounts of enzyme. However, the species generated is a low-molecular-weight form of factor XIIa, which cannot bind to surfaces and is relatively impotent in activating the coagulation mechanism. This type of factor XIIa is a powerful mobilizer of the fibrinolytic as well as the kinin-generating system. Thus, the amplication process described previously orients the hemostatic mechanism toward clot resolution and kinin formation as opposed to fibrin deposition.

c. Activation of factor IX

Once generated, factor XIa can interact with a zymogen termed factor IX (a single polypeptide chain of mol. wt. 55,000) and convert it to the serine protease factor IXa (figure 26.4). The initial step in activation is scission of a specific bond within the zymogen to form an inactive two-chain disulfide-linked intermediate that has heavy and light chains of mol. wt. 38,000 and 16,000, respectively. In a later step, a polypeptide of mol. wt. 9,000 is split from the newly formed N-terminal of the heavy chain. The product is the serine protease factor IXa.

Preservation of the original N-terminal region of the zymogen within the structure of factor IXa is a critical feature of the activation mechanism. This area contains a number of *γ-carboxyglutamic acid* residues (abbreviated Gla residues) whose presence is due to a vitamin K-dependent postribosomal modification in which preexisting specific glutamyl residues are γ-carboxylated. These unique amino acid moieties are responsible for the binding of factor IXa to phospholipid or platelet surfaces in association with Ca^{++} ions. Therefore, these residues are essential for the subsequent surface-dependent activation of factor X. The maintenance of these γ-carboxyglutamic acid moieties within factor IXa parallels the situation occurring when prothrombin is transformed to thrombin. In the latter case, these residues are absent from the enzymatic end product. The γ-carboxyglutamic acid residues in factor IXa may localize this enzyme to the area of hemostatic injury and allow it to interact with factor X bound to the same sur-

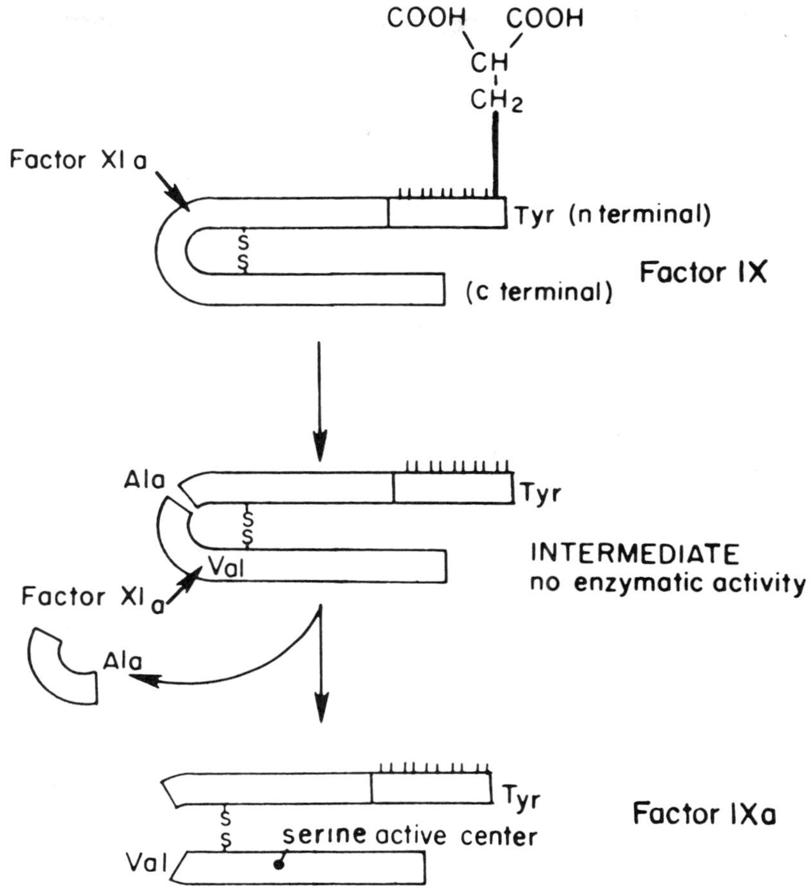

Fig. 26.4
The activation of factor IX.

face. The absence of the same residues in thrombin facilitates diffusion of the enzyme from this locale and permits it to act upon platelets as well as fibrinogen at some distance from the site of hemostatic system activation.

d. Activation of factor X

When factor IXa is formed, it converts the factor X zymogen to the serine protease factor Xa. Factor X (mol. wt. 55,000) circulates in plasma as a two-chain species whose primary structure is homologous to that of the factor IX intermediate. The site at which the newly synthesized single-chain factor X is scissioned to form this two-chain zymogen is unknown. The mechanism of activation of this latter component is virtually identical to the second step of factor IX conversion depicted in figure 26.4 Additional scissions at the C-terminal of the heavy chain of factor Xa can occur when high levels of reactants are utilized, but this represents a biologically unimportant set of side reactions.

e. Factor VIII and von Willebrand's factor

In vivo, the activation of factor X by factor IXa must occur at a rapid rate and yet be localized to the site of hemostatic injury. This is accomplished by the action of a cofactor termed factor VIII in association with Ca^{++} ions and a phospholipid or platelet surface (see figure 26.3). The interactions responsible for the formation of a *factor IXa–factor VIII–factor X–Ca^{++}–phospholipid complex* are poorly understood, but must be similar to those required for stabilization of the analogous factor Xa–factor V–prothrombin–Ca^{++}–phospholipid complex. Acceleration of factor X activation is probably achieved by close approximation of enzyme and substrate on the surface as well as by a conformational change in factor X that renders it more susceptible to enzymatic attack. Localization of factor Xa generation is attained by formation of the multimolecular complex only at sites of injury and by the presence of γ-carboxyglutamic acid residues on the enzyme. These structures bind factor Xa to the phospholipid surface via Ca^{++} ions and prevent it from diffusing away from the locale.

Factor VIII, the cofactor required for rapid conversion of factor X, is difficult to separate from a related but immunologically distinct protein, *von Willebrand's factor*. This latter substance has a multimeric (polymeric) structure with the molecular weights that range up to 5×10^6. The stable protomeric unit of this multimeric structure is a dimer that consists of disulfide-bonded polypeptide chains of mol. wt. 240,000. This species is able to assemble into larger aggregates via labile disulfide bridges. The protomeric units also bear oligosaccharide chains similar in structure to blood group substance (e.g., galactose and sialic acid groups are the penultimate and ultimate residues).

Von Willebrand's factor binds to a specific platelet receptor, glycoprotein I, and mediates the adhesion of platelets to subendothelial structures such as collagen. A similar interaction between this plasma protein and the platelet receptor is required for the ristocetin-induced aggregation of these cellular elements. The larger multimeric forms of von Willebrand's factor are essential for its biologic action upon platelets. This appears to be due to the high affinity of this form of the protein for the platelet receptor as well as its subsequent ability to bridge the distance between these cellular elements and induce platelet association. The lower-molecular-weight forms of von Willebrand's factor exhibit this ability to only a minimal extent. The oligosaccharide chains attached to the protomeric unit are also critical with respect to platelet interactions. Removal of the terminal sialic acid and galactose residues dramatically reduces the activity of von Willebrand's factor. Furthermore, the desialyated form of the protein has a short survival time within the circulation owing to its removal by hepatocytes. It is of interest that individuals with a congenital decrease in the function of von Willebrand's factor may exhibit reductions in the levels of this protein or abnormalities in its biological activity. In the latter case the multimeric forms of von Willebrand's factor may be decreased, and the monomeric subunits may possess incomplete oligosaccharide chains. These phenomena may explain some of the clinical abnormalities of platelet function that are an integral part of von Willebrand's disease.

Factor VIII has a mol. wt. of about 270,000 and circulates in the blood bound to von Willebrand's factor. Given the relative concentrations of these two components, it is apparent that only about 3% of the von Willebrand's factor molecules can be complexed to factor VIII. Current data suggest that factor VIII is predominantly bound to high molecular weight multimers of von Willebrand's factor and that these complexes can be dissociated with reducing agents, high ionic strength, or Ca^{++} ions.

f. Comparison of von Willebrand's disease and factor VIII deficiency

It is revealing to contrast the abnormalities noted in von Willebrand's disease with those in factor VIII deficiency. Patients with the former disorder suffer abnormalities in platelet function as well as reductions in factor VIII activity. Patients with the latter abnormality have normal platelet function but exhibit defects in the intrinsic coagulation cascade. These findings support the view that von Willebrand's factor is a carrier of factor VIII. This view is strengthened by the observation that transfusion of plasma from individuals with severe factor VIII deficiency into patients with von Willebrand's disease promptly restores the latter's factor VIII activity to normal. This is accomplished by providing a source of endogenous von Willebrand's factor that can associate with the endogenous factor VIII.

2. Extrinsic coagulation cascade

Factor X can also be activated by the addition to plasma of *tissue extracts* (figure 26.5). Two discrete components interact in this mechanism.

a. Tissue factor

The first is *tissue factor*, a membrane-bound glycoprotein on the surfaces of various somatic cells, especially subendothelial struc-

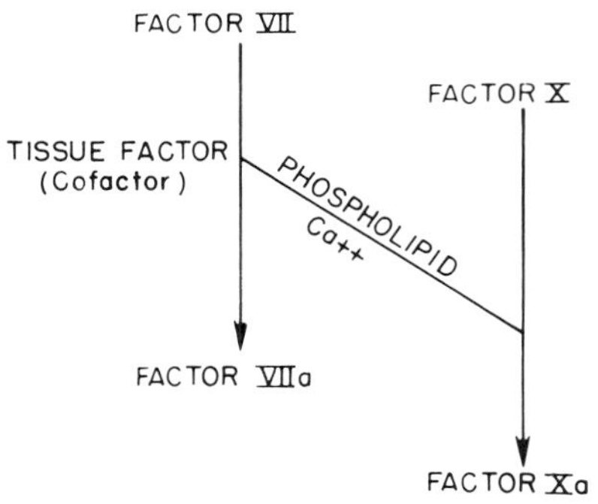

Fig. 26.5
The extrinsic coagulation cascade.

tures such as smooth muscle cells and fibroblasts. Surfaces of cells that are normally in contact with plasma (endothelial cells, leukocytes, etc.) also possess tissue factor. However, the tissue factor present on these surfaces is usually inaccessible unless proteolytic enzymes or membrane damage exposes it.

b. Factor VII

The second required component is factor VII (mol. wt. 60,000). It is comprised of a single polypeptide chain and is structurally homologous to factor II (prothrombin), factor IX, and factor X. Damage to the vascular surface exposes tissue factor, which interacts with factor VII. The phospholipid component of tissue factor appears critical for complex formation. When the complex has formed, factor VII is converted into an active serine protease, probably by conformational changes rather than peptide bond scission. Both factor VII and factor X are bound to the tissue factor complex via phospholipid–Ca^{++}–γ-carboxyglutamic acid residues interactions similar to those described above. Factor X is then rapidly converted to factor Xa. The transformation process occurs via proteolytic cleavage identical to those occurring in the intrinsic activation of factor X.

c. Control mechanisms

The extrinsic pathway exhibits both positive and negative control mechanisms. For example, generation of factor Xa results initially in the specific cleavage of factor VII to form a disulfide-linked two-chain molecule. This new molecular species binds more tightly to tissue factor and has ~80-fold greater potency with respect to factor X activation. As greater quantities of factor Xa are produced, additional peptide cleavage of the two-chain form of factor VII renders this species inactive.

B. Activation of prothrombin (the common pathway)

Prothrombin is a single chain zymogen (mol. wt. 65,000) with two triple-loop structures termed *kringles* (after a Danish pastry of similar configuration) within its N-terminal region (figure 26.5). The kringles divide this area of the prothrombin molecule into two semi-independent domains termed F_1 and F_2 regions. The F_1 region also contains 10 unique γ-carboxyglutamic acid residues, of which 6 are present as 3 pairs. These moieties are also formed by a vitamin K-dependent postribosomal process. *Coumarin drugs* act as anticoagulants by opposing the action of vitamin K and preventing this process of γ-carboxylation from taking place. A similar result occurs with factors VII, IX, and X.

Once the intrinsic and extrinsic coagulation cascades have generated factor Xa in sufficient amounts, it can convert prothrombin to the disulfide-linked two-chain serine protease thrombin. This is accomplished by scissioning Arg_{273}-Thr_{274} and/or Arg_{155}-Ser_{156} and releasing the N-terminal polypeptides F_{1+2} or F_1 and F_2. In a subsequent step of the activation mechanism, factor Xa cleaves Arg_{322}-Ile_{323} in the remaining C-terminal region of pro-

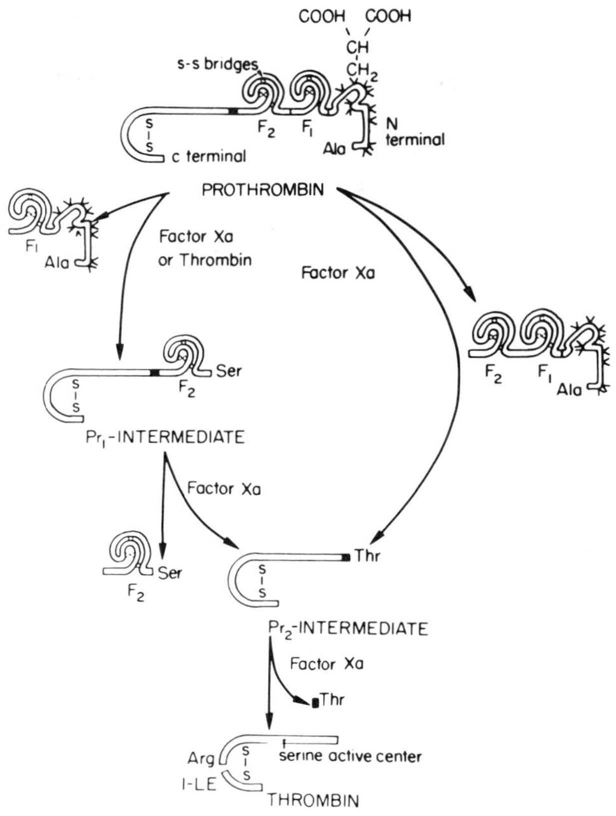

Fig. 26.6
The common pathway of thrombin generation.

thrombin and generates a two-chain component with enzymatic activity. Release of a 12-amino acid polypeptide from the N-terminal of the latter species may also occur.

In vitro thrombin generation via this sequence of events proceeds slowly, requiring many hours. In vivo, the process is dramatically accelerated by the action of the cofactor V (a glycoprotein of mol. wt. 270,000) in conjunction with Ca^{++} and a phospholipid or platelet surface.

Prothrombin has two specialized features within the N-terminal region that play an essential role in its conversion to thrombin (figure 26.6). First, the γ-carboxyglutamic acid residues of the F_1 region have great avidity for Ca^{++} ions and are critical sites in the interaction of the zymogen with the phospholipid or platelet surface. During coumadin ingestion, prothrombin is synthesized without a full complement of these unique residues. Hence, the zymogen cannot bind tightly to appropriate surfaces and cannot be rapidly activated to thrombin. Similar functional defects are noted with factors VII, IX, and X synthesized during the same time period. Second, the F_2 region contains a factor V-binding site. Thus, the cofactor can interact with the zymogen. A specific receptor on the platelet surface binds factor V tightly and thereby links factor Xa to this cellular element. The factor Xa–factor V–platelet complex specifically interacts with the prothrombin molecule, bringing prothrombin and factor Xa into close approximation and increasing their chances for interaction. Furthermore, the binding of prothrombin to the factor V–platelet complex probably induces a conformational alteration in the zymogen that renders it more susceptible to proteolysis by factor Xa. The result of these multiple interactions is a 10,000–15,000-fold acceleration in the rate of conversion of prothrombin to thrombin so that this process can take place in a matter of seconds (figure 26.6).

Two regulatory mechanisms may aid in the in vivo control of thrombin generation. On the one hand, thrombin proteolyzes factor V and thereby renders it 50–100 times more potent. This favors an augmentation in thrombin production. On the other hand, thrombin generated within the multimolecular complex diffuses out into the blood and is eventually able to release the F_1 fragment from circulating prothrombin. This altered zymogen binds to the factor V–Ca^{++}–phospholipid complex or to the factor V–factor Xa–platelet complex with lower affinity and can only be slowly converted to thrombin.

C. Relations among cascades and common pathway of thrombin generation

We have considered various control mechanisms that may operate *within* each of the three discrete elements of the hemostatic system. However, certain specific interactions *among* the intrinsic cascade, the extrinsic cascade, and the common pathway are also important in regulating coagulation.

1. Effect of thrombin on factor VIII

The first intersystem control mechanism is based on the ability of thrombin to increase dramatically the potency of factor VIII. Indeed, without prior thrombin activation, this protein is virtually unable to act as a cofactor in the factor IXa-dependent conversion of factor X to factor Xa. Little is known of the molecular details of this interaction. It is known that thrombin must hydrolyze a specific arginine-*x* bond in factor VIII in order to activate this component.

2. Interactions between factors Xa and IX

The second intersystem control mechanism depends on the capacity of the factor VII–tissue factor complex to convert factor IX to factor IXa and subsequently factor X to factor Xa. This is accomplished at about half the rate of direct transformation of factor X to factor Xa under the conditions normally present in blood.

The third intersystem control mechanism involves the interaction between factor Xa and factor IX. Factor Xa can proteolyze factor IX and convert it into a serine protease. The capacity of the extrinsic cascade to bypass the earliest phases of the intrinsic cascade may explain the minimal hemorrhagic complications noted in factor XI deficiency.

These three intersystem control mechanisms allow the extrinsic cascade to activate the more complex and slower-acting intrinsic cascade. This would permit the intrinsic cascade to produce additional thrombin.

3. Interactions between factors XIIa and VII

A fourth intersystem control mechanism depends on the proteolysis of factor VII by factor XIIa. This results in the production of a disulfide-linked two-chain form of factor VII with increased affinity for tissue factor and an enhanced potency as an activator of factor X. Thus, activation of the intrinsic cascade can augment the thrombin-generating ability of the extrinsic cascade.

The existence of these multiple intersystem control mechanisms suggests that the intrinsic and extrinsic cascades are linked in a complex kinetic fashion. Indeed interactions between the two pathways are probably essential for the generation of adequate amounts of thrombin in vivo. This surmise is supported by the clinical observation that patients with an isolated congenital defect in either cascade exhibit profound bleeding diatheses.

D. Protein C–thrombomodulin mechanism

Protein C is one of several vitamin K–dependent glycoproteins (other than the four classical ones). It consists of a heavy chain of mol. wt. 41,000 and a light chain of mol. wt. 21,000, which are joined by a single disulfide bridge. To perform its biological function, protein C is converted to the serine protease *protein Ca* by thrombin. This process involves the scissioning of a single Arg_{12}-Leu_{13} bond at the N-terminal end of the heavy chain with release of an activation peptide of mol. wt. ~1,400. Both protein C and protein Ca possess γ-carboxyglutamic acid residues on their light chains that are required for the binding of either protein to Ca^{++} ions and cell membranes.

Thrombin is the only physiological serine protease that can convert protein C to protein Ca. The rate of this reaction is quite slow when blood is allowed to clot under in vitro conditions. This observation raised questions about the biologic role of protein C within the body; however, perfusion of protein C and thrombin through the vascular tree of animals resulted in a 20,000-fold increase in the rate of conversion of zymogen to serine protease. Since this process can be saturated with either excess protein C or thrombin, it seems likely that a receptor is present on the endothelium that can dramatically accelerate the reaction.

This hypothesis was substantiated by isolating the putative receptor—a protein of mol. wt. 74,000—from rabbit lung. Addition of thrombin to this receptor, termed *thrombomodulin*, leads to the avid formation of a 1:1 stoichiometric complex of enzyme and cofactor that rapidly activates protein C in the presence of Ca^{++} ions. It should be noted that thrombin attached to thrombomodulin can be neutralized by antithrombin at a rate equivalent

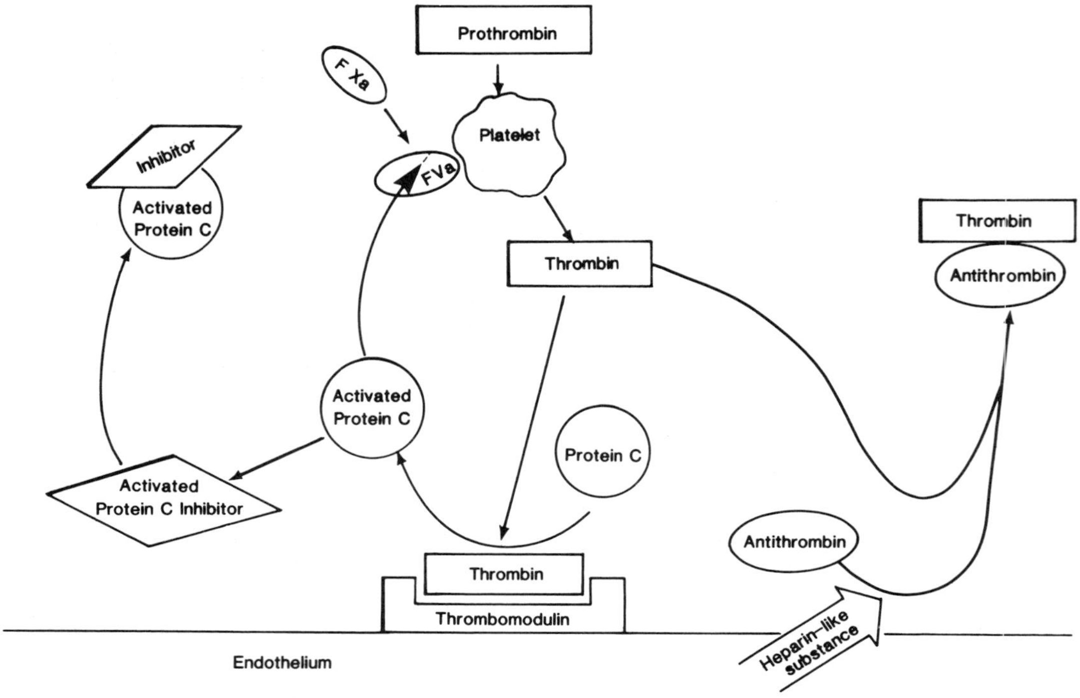

Fig. 26.7
Natural anticoagulant functions of the protein C–thrombomodulin and heparin-antithrombin systems.

to that of free enzyme (see below). However, the thrombin-thrombomodulin complex exhibits a greatly diminished ability to clot fibrinogen, activate factor V, or trigger platelet activation.

Once evolved, protein Ca functions as a potent inhibitor of the cofactors factor V–Va and factor VIII–VIIIa (figure 26.7). Its first site of action is located at the surface of the platelet where factor V–Va bound to specific sites acts as a receptor for factor Xa. This multimolecular prothrombinase complex rapidly converts prothrombin to thrombin. Protein Ca functions as a naturally occurring anticoagulant by specifically scissioning factor V or factor Va. Factor Va seems particularly sensitive to destruction by protein Ca especially under in vivo conditions where the levels of this enzyme are exceedingly low. Thus protein Ca possesses the necessary specificity to prevent assembly of the prothrombinase complex and thereby suppress production of thrombin.

This inhibitory effect of protein Ca is modulated by a variety of additional interactions. On the one hand a slow rate of cleavage of factor V–Va allows factor Xa to bind to the unaffected cofactor. thereby protecting this protein against any subsequent action of protein Ca. On the other hand various plasma proteins appear to be involved in the protein Ca-dependent destruction of factor V–Va on the platelet surface. For example, another vitamin K–dependent protein, *protein S*, enhances the binding of protein Ca to phospholipid-containing membranes and accelerates the cleavage of factor Va by this serine protease. The complement component, *C4b binding protein*, complexes with protein S and may be involved in regulating its function.

Thus several interactions are probably responsible for determining the rate of translocation of protein Ca from its site of production on the endothelium to the surface of the platelet. One might expect that small amounts of protein Ca remain bound to the endothelial cell surface by γ-carboxyglutamic acid residues on this serine protease. In this manner protein Ca could also regulate the factor Va-dependent thrombin generation, which is known to occur on the endothelial cell surface in a fashion analogous to that described for the platelet membrane.

The second site of action of protein Ca occurs at a locale where fator VIIIa regulates the interaction between factor IXa and factor X. At present little is known concerning the biochemical details of the protein Ca-dependent cleavage of this cofactor or of the biologic surface where these events take place; however, this inhibitory process would limit the generation of factor Xa and thereby prevent production of thrombin.

Clinical observations indicate that the protein C-thrombomodulin mechanism functions under in vivo conditions to suppress hemostatic system activity. Several families have been described who have congenital reductions of about 50% in the antigenic levels of protein C and who exhibit repeated thrombotic episodes. In other kindreds individuals heterozygous for protein C deficiency have minimal symptoms, whereas those who are homozygous for this trait die in infancy with massive venous thrombosis and purpura fulminans. These data suggest that other factors such as the density of thrombomodulin on the endothelium, the levels of protein S within the blood, the amounts of Factor V–Va present of the platelet surface, etc., are likely to modulate the effects of protein C deficiency.

III. FORMATION OF FIBRIN CLOT

A. Structure of fibrinogen

Fibrinogen is a plasma protein (mol. wt. 340,000) composed of 3 pairs of polypeptide chains designated Aα, Bβ, and γ. The 6 chains are held together by numerous disulfide bridges. As shown in figure 26.8, the N-terminal regions of all chains are maintained by several disulfide bridges in a rigid, symmetrical configuration at one end of the molecule. This region of the fibrinogen molecule is referred to as the N-terminal disulfide knot or *N-DSK region*. It is part of a larger nodular structure, termed the *E domain*, that is made up of intertwined polypeptide chains. The 6 chains emerge

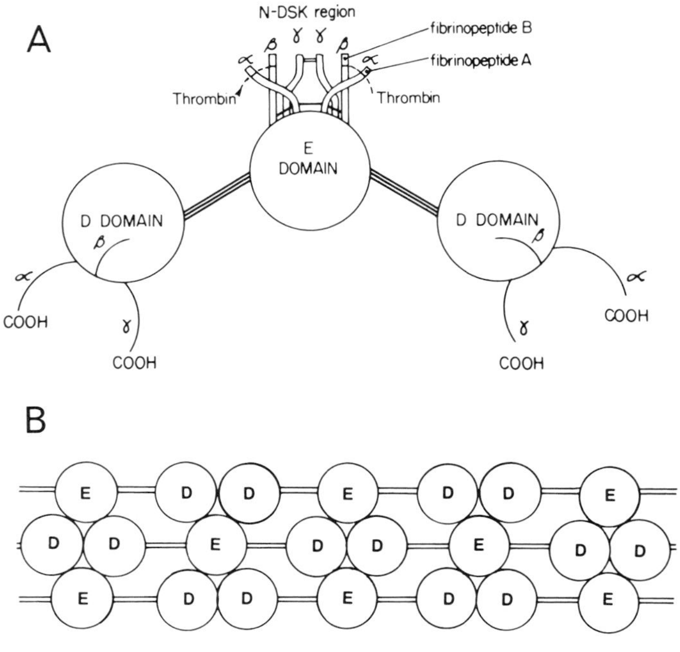

Fig. 26.8
Structures of fibrinogen (*A*) and fibrin clot (*B*).

from this area of the molecule to form 2 lateral bundles of 3 each, each bundle containing single Aα, Bβ, and γ polypeptide chains. The C-terminal region of each of these bundles intertwines to form 2 separate nodular structures termed the *D domains*. The C-terminal regions of the Aα and γ chains are in a particularly exposed position within the D domain. The last 12 residues of the C-terminal segment of the γ chain constitute the major domain by which fibrinogen binds to the platelet membrane. The final phases of platelet aggregation require the interaction of divalent fibrinogen with exposed glycoprotein IIb/IIIa receptors of separate platelets in order to bridge the distance between these cellular elements (lecture 27).

B. Conversion of fibrinogen to fibrin

Once thrombin is evolved, it cleaves the 2 sets of Aα and Bβ chains within the N-DSK region and thereby converts fibrinogen to fibrin (figure 26.8). Initially this enzyme clips a pair of *arginine-glycine* bonds into the Aα chains (Arg_{16}-Gly_{17}), with release of the highly acidic *fibrinopeptide A* (mol. wt. 1,800) and conversion of fibrinogen to *fibrin I monomer*. Subsequently thrombin cleaves another set of arginine-glycine bonds within Bβ chains (Arg_{14}-Gly_{15}), liberating the highly acidic *fibrinopeptide B* (mol. wt. 1,500) with concomitant generation of *fibrin II monomer*, which rapidly polymerizes to form a thrombus. Release of fibrinopeptide A from fibrinogen initiates fibrin polymerization. Indeed, snake venoms such as *reptilase* can liberate only fibrinopeptide A, but are still capable of generating a fibrin clot. Such venoms can be employed to assay for fibrinogen in the presence of heparin (see lecture 28) and to anticoagulate patients by lowering fibrinogen levels. Fibrinopeptide B release also promotes fibrin polymerization, but its function is unclear. Sensitive radioimmunoassays for both types of fibrinopeptides appear to be useful indicators of ongoing thrombosis and can be expected gradually to come into clinical use.

C. Polymerization of fibrin

Release of fibrinopeptides appears to unmask specific sites on α and γ chains within the D domains that are responsible for fibrin polymerization. This process may result from simple reduction in negative charge or from more complex molecular transformations induced by liberation of the fibrinopeptides. Once formed, fibrin may undergo two different fates.

1. Interaction of fibrin and fibrinogen: paracoagulation

On one hand, single molecules of fibrin (or low-molecular-weight fibrin polymers) may interact with fibrinogen to form *soluble fibrin-fibrinogen complexes* or *SFC*. (These complexes also form when fibrin associates with certain plasmin-induced degradation products or fibrinogen.) This phenomenon is termed *paracoagulation*. Patients with hyperactive coagulation systems exhibit elevated levels of SFC as assayed by a variety of techniques. Assay methods are of two types: (1) methods based on immunologic identification of soluble fibrinogen-like material at molecular weights that are multiples of 340,000 and (2) methods in which fibrin is discharged from SFC by disruption of hydrophobic and electrostatic bonds. This may be accomplished by addition of *protamine sulfate* or *ethanol* to plasma, or by *cryoprecipitation*. The discharged fibrin subsequently polymerizes into fine strands. Unfortunately, procedures for demonstrating paracoagulation are variable and thus not wholly satisfactory for detection of ongoing thrombosis or disseminated intravascular coagulation.

2. Insolubilization of fibrin polymers

On the other hand, fibrin polymers may gradually grow in size and become insoluble. The resulting fibrin clot is held together by hydrophobic as well as electrostatic interactions. Therefore, its gel structure can be disrupted by addition of denaturing agents such as *urea* and *monochloroacetic acid*. In the next step of the coagulation mechanism (discussed below), covalent cross-links are introduced between polymerized fibrin molecules. Disruption of the clot by denaturants is then no longer possible.

D. Activation of factor XIII: cross-linking of fibrin

The covalent cross-linking of fibrin is accomplished by a *transamidination* reaction catalyzed by *factor XIIIa*. Factor XIII, the precursor of this enzyme, is found in plasma, on platelet surfaces, and in other tissues. *Plasma* factor XIII is a *tetramer* composed

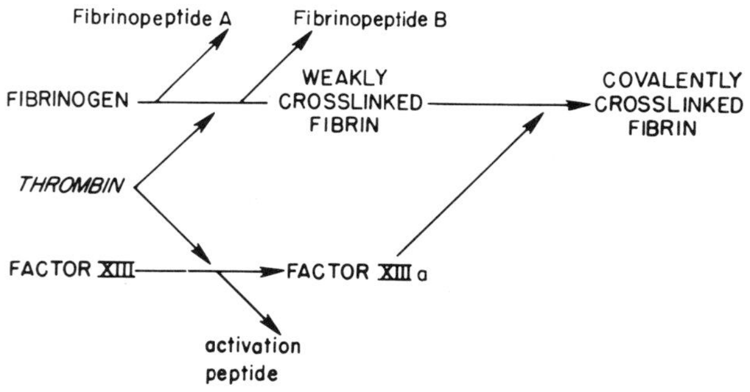

Fig. 26.9
Formation of the cross-linked fibrin clot.

of two pairs of identical subunits termed *a* and *b* (mol. wt. 80,000). *Platelet* factor XIII is a *dimer* comprised of 2 *a* subunits.

Once it is generated, thrombin hydrolyzes a specific arginine-glycine bond in the N-terminal segment of the *a* chain of both plasma and platelet factor XIII, with release of a peptide of mol. wt. 4,500. In platelet factor XIII, this process generates enzymatic activity. In plasma factor XIII, a subsequent dissociation of *a* and *b* subunits that requires Ca^{++} is required for exposure of an -SH group that is the active enzyme center. Either form of factor XIIIa can stitch neighboring fibrin polymers together by covalently joining the side chains of specific lysine residues with the side chains of certain glutamine acceptors. The critical areas cross-linked are within the C-terminal regions of the α and γ chains in the D domains of fibrin. As discussed above, these areas are brought into close proximity during fibrin polymerization. It is of interest that these regions are relatively inaccessible to factor XIIIa unless fibrinogen is transformed to fibrin. Thus thrombin must, in parallel, convert fibrinogen to fibrin as well as activate factor XIII if a stable clot is to be formed (see figure 26.9).

The cross-linked clot is mechanically stronger and better able to withstand the brunt of collisional events within the vascular system. It is also less likely to be rapidly dissolved by the fibrinolytic mechanism. The physiologic importance of fibrin cross-linking is emphasized by the occurrence of bleeding diatheses in patients with defects in this mechanism.

IV. FIBRINOLYTIC SYSTEM

The *fibrinolytic system* is in part responsible for dissolution of the fibrin clot. In this section we shall discuss the manner in which this is accomplished and describe abnormalities in this mechanism that can lead to thrombosis.

A. Transformation of plasminogen to plasmin

A pivotal component of this mechanism is the zymogen *plasminogen* (mol. wt. 81,000). A scheme of its structure is shown in figure 26.10. A major section of the N-terminal region of this protein is

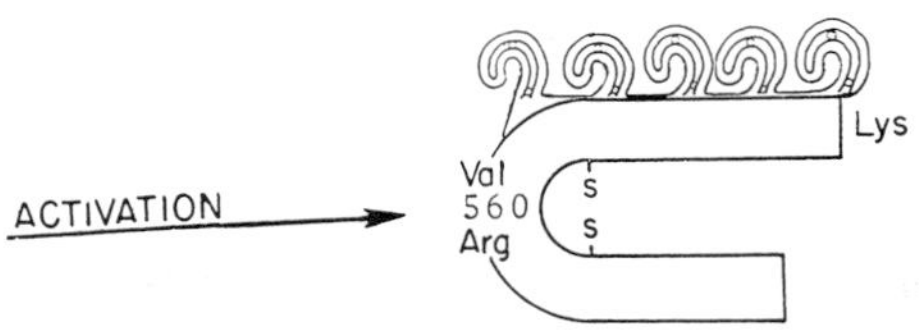

Fig. 26.10
Structure of plasminogen and its mechanism of activation.

composed of a series of five triple loop structures (kringles) resembling those found on the nonthrombin portion of prothrombin (see above). These unique features appear to represent specific binding sites on plasminogen that permit this zymogen to interact with and become concentrated within the fibrin meshwork. Furthermore, antifibrinolytic amino acids such as ϵ-aminocaproic acid bind to these areas of plasminogen. This interaction causes a marked conformational alteration in plasminogen that significantly limits the ability of this zymogen to be converted to active enzyme.

The central event in the fibrinolytic system is the transformation of the single-chain plasminogen to the enzymatically potent two-chain serine protease *plasmin*. This conversion is accomplished by scission of the zymogen at the Arg_{560}–Val_{561} bond as depicted in figure 26.10. The initial generation of plasmin frequently permits this enzyme to act upon plasminogen and induce several additional proteolytic cleavages within the zymogen at Lys_{77}–Lys_{78}, Arg_{68}–Met_{69}, and so forth prior to its activation. These auxiliary scissions result in the release of a fragment of mol. wt. 10,000 that has been termed the *preactivation peptide*. However, this series of additional bond cleavages takes place to a minimal extent when plasminogen is converted to plasmin in the presence of protease inhibitors such as antiplasmin or antithrombin. Thus, the physiologically relevant pathway of plasminogen-to-plasmin conversion probably required only a scission of the Arg_{560}–Val_{561} bond. The serine protease generated by this process still possesses the 5 kringle structures. These binding sites are critical for the interaction of plasmin with its natural substrate fibrin as well as for the rapid neutralization of this enzyme by antiplasmin (discussed below).

B. Plasminogen activators

Four types of naturally occurring substances can convert plasminogen to plasmin.

1. Endothelial cell activators: major activation pathway

The activation of plasminogen is initiated by the proteolytic action of *urokinase* or *tissue-type plasminogen activator*. Urokinase (mol. wt. 54,000) transforms plasminogen to plasmin in the absence of a cofactor and may be responsible for the continuous fluid phase generation of the latter enzyme. Tissue-type plasminogen activator (mol. wt. 70,000) has a high affinity for fibrin, which it employs as a cofactor during the conversion of plasminogen to plasmin and appears to be involved in the generation of the latter enzyme on fibrin polymers, as well as within the interstices of the clot. Both types of macromolecules are immunologically distinct and appear to be synthesized by a wide variety of cellular elements, including microvascular and macrovascular endothelial cells. Thrombin binds to endothelial cells, inhibits the synthesis of urokinase, and stimulates the production of tissue-type plasminogen activator. The last effect may be mediated in part by the generation of protein Ca. Both plasminogen activators are readily released into the blood by *physiologic* stimuli such as exercise, *pharmacologic* stimuli such as nicotinic acid or hypoglycemic agents, and *pathologic* stimuli such as hypotensive shock. These macromolecules are partially responsible for keeping the microcirculation open and free of fibrin deposits.

2. Factor XIIa: minor activation pathway

Activation of factor XII not only triggers the coagulation cascade and kinin-generating mechanism, it also converts plasminogen to plasmin. Thus the event that triggers clot formation by activation of factor XII also sets in motion a mechanism for its ultimate resolution.

3. Poorly characterized activators

A number of poorly characterized activators are found in the lysosomes of heart, kidney, and other organs. These substances are insoluble and have little physiologic significance; however, at times of extensive organ damage, these activators can be released into the blood. This phenomenon may be responsible for the frequent occurrence of systemic fibrinolysis in patients with widespread trauma.

4. Streptokinase: use of fibrinolytic agents

Streptokinase, a bacterial protein, has been administered to patients in an effort to dissolve established thrombi in coronary and pulmonary vessels. *Urokinase* has been employed for the same purpose. If used early enough, the infusion of streptokinase into the coronary artery may lyse existing thrombi and prevent myocardial infarction. The use of *tissue-type plasminogen activator* has recently been advocated in place of streptokinase since it can be infused into a vein, would be expected to dissolve fibrin clots, but should not induce a systemic fibrinolytic state with potential hemorrhagic consequences (see below). The cloning of the tissue-type plasminogen activator gene is likely to make this form of therapy widely available in the next few years.

C. Function of the fibrinolytic system

Under normal conditions, fibrinolysis is a precisely regulated process (figure 26.11). It is initiated by the incorporation of plasminogen within the fibrin clot as these polymers are deposited onto the vascular endothelium. This is due to the specific interaction of the

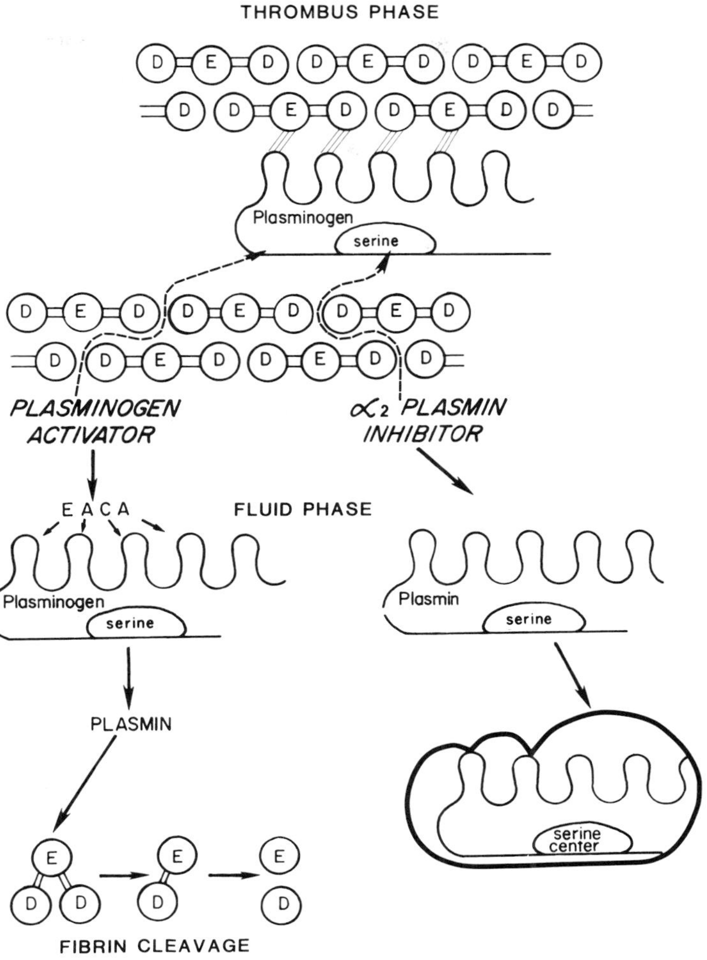

Fig. 26.11
Regulation of the fibrinolytic mechanism. The pharmacologic agent ε-aminocaproic acid is designated EACA.

kringle structures of the zymogen with the fibrin meshwork. In this locus, plasminogen is sequestered away from protease inhibitors normally present in the blood and in direct proximity to the fibrin substrate. Diffusion of plasminogen activators from the blood or endothelium into the clot transforms the zymogen into plasmin. The resultant enzyme remains bound to its substrate by interaction of the kringle structures with the fibrin strands and therefore can only be slowly neutralized by antiplasmin. In this manner, a gradual but effective lysis of the clot occurs. Leukocytes incorporated into the clot also elaborate proteases that may directly hydrolyze the fibrin meshwork. Outside the area of the clot, activators of the fibrinolytic system are relatively impotent. This is due, in large measure, to the presence of antiplasmin, which can rapidly neutralize plasmin as it is formed. Thus, fibrinolytic activity is restricted to the region of the resolving clot. However, in disease states, excessive release of activators occurs, and large amounts of plasmin are generated. This gradually overwhelms the capacity of antiplasmin to limit the fibrinolytic process, and free enzyme, as well as plasmin–α_2-macroglobulin complexes, is found within the circulation. These two entities induce systemic fibrinolysis with proteolysis as well as inactivation of proteins such as factor V, factor VIII, and fibrinogen.

D. Degradation of fibrinogen by plasmin

The effect of plasmin on the fibrinogen molecule has been extensively investigated. It is of interest because it is the basis for a variety of tests for detecting systemic fibrinolysis. Figure 26.12 shows the sequential proteolysis of the fibrinogen molecule. The lysis of fibrin within the clot structure is thought to proceed similarly.

Exposed N-terminal regions of the Bβ chains of fibrinogen in the E domains as well as C-terminal regions of the Aα chains of fibrinogen in the D domains are cleaved initially. The remaining portion of the molecule is termed the *X fragment.* This limited degree of proteolysis appears to occur continuously in normal individuals since about 25% of circulating fibrinogen molcules are in this form. Next, plasmin cleaves one of the two bundles that connect the D and E domains with liberation of the D domain fragment and a binodular structure termed the *Y fragment.* Later, plasmin is able to clip the second of the two bundles connecting the D and E domains within the Y fragment and liberate these nodules as individual species called *D* and *E fragments.*

The X, Y, D, and E fragments, called *fibrinogen split products*, have characteristic biological properties. The X fragment partially retains its ability to be activated by thrombin to form fibrin. However, this happens more slowly than with normal fibrinogen. The Y, D, and E fragments cannot be clotted by thrombin and the thrombin-dependent conversion of fibrinogen to fibrin is slowed by these fragments. This effect may be due to direct inhibition of thrombin or to interference with normal fibrin polymerization. These fibrinogen split products also inhibit platelet aggregation. Thus, the X, Y, D, and E fragments are capable of suppressing the hemostatic mechanism at several loci.

Various other biologic actions are ascribed to the fragments X, Y, D, and E, including potentiation of the hypotensive effect of bradykinin, chemotactic properties with respect to monocytes as well as neutrophils, and an ability to impair the immunologic mechanism.

The clinical assays of fibrinogen split products include the *thrombin time*, which detects abnormalities in fibrin polymerization (and is most sensitive to X, Y, and D) as well as *immuno-*

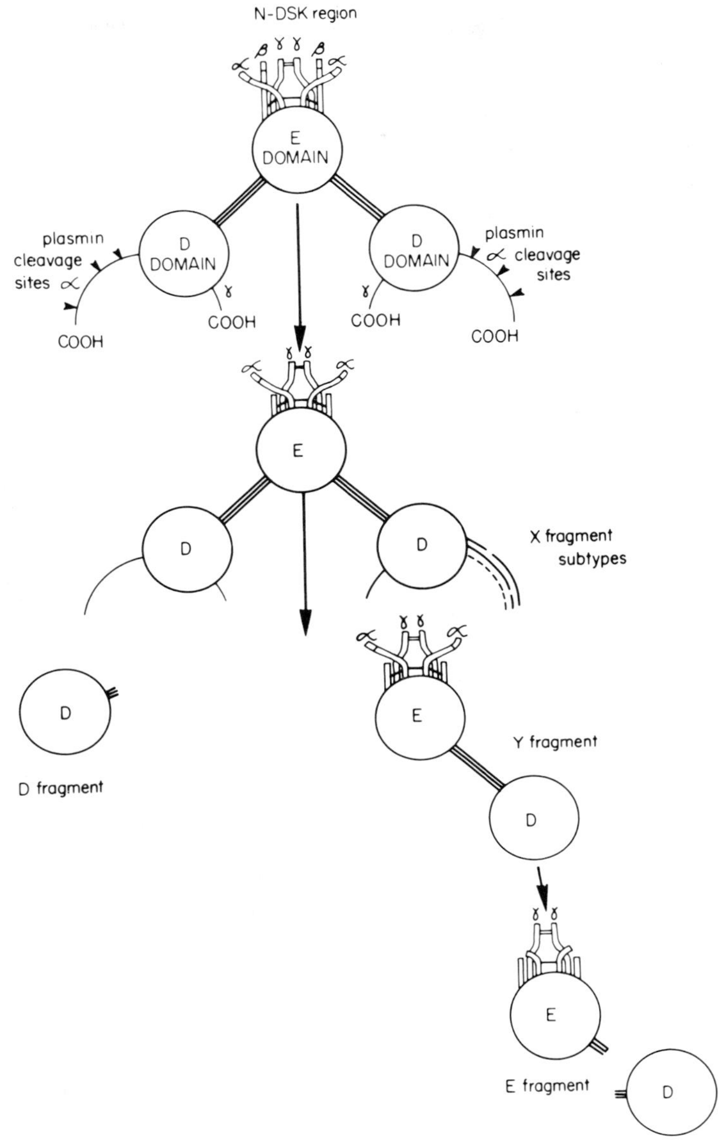

Fig. 26.12
Degradation of fibrinogen by plasmin.

logic tests, which measure nonclottable fibrinogen-like material (mainly Y, D, and E).

E. Relations between coagulation and fibrinolytic systems

Three major links connect the coagulation and fibrinolytic systems: (1) activation of factor XII initiates transformation of plasminogen proactivator to plasminogen activator, which, in turn, converts plasminogen to plasmin; (2) plasmin can cleave factor XII and thus generate the activated form of the zymogen; and (3) generation of activated protein C stimulates fibrinolysis by unknown mechanisms.

F. Defects in fibrinolytic system resulting in thrombosis

Multiple episodes of venous thromboembolic disease have occurred in several families with *congenital abnormalities* of the fibrinolytic system (i.e., functional defects in the plasminogen molecule, reductions in the release of plasminogen activator, and alterations in the structure of fibrinogen). Presumably thrombotic phenomena in these patients are due to a reduced ability to lyse small fibrin clots and prevent extension. It has been suggested that plasmin may serve as a natural anticoagulant.

Plasmin cleaves a set of Arg_{42}-Ala_{43} bonds within the Bβ chains of fibrin I monomer, releasing *Bβ 1-42* and thereby converting fibrin I monomer to fragment X, which is further degraded to form the soluble cleavage products mentioned previously.

Radioimmunoassays for fibrinopeptide A, fibrinopeptide B, and Bβ 1-42 have been used in studies of intravascular coagulation and venous thrombosis. These have shown in patients receiving hypertonic saline to terminate pregnancy that immediately after intrauterine infusion fibrin I monomer is generated by thrombin-mediated proteolysis of fibrinogen. Thereafter fibrin I monomer is either cleaved by thrombin to liberate fibrinopeptide B or proteolyzed by plasmin to release Bβ 1-42. Hence the relative rates at which thrombin and plasmin cleave the Bβ chain of fibrin I monomer could determine the occurrence of thrombosis. These techniques indicate that compared to normal controls, individuals who develop venous thrombosis have levels of fibrinopeptide A that are considerably higher than the concentrations of Bβ 1-42 during the 4 days preceding the onset of thrombosis. These observations lend credence to the hypothesis that a sustained imbalance between the procoagulant effects of thrombin and the anticoagulant actions of plasmin upon fibrin I monomer may lead to thrombotic disorders in humans. The precise molecular defects responsible for these phenomena are still unknown but probably include abnormalities in the regulatory mechanisms governing the release of plasminogen activators or their inhibitors from cellular sites.

V. LIMITING REACTIONS

As we have seen, the hemostatic mechanism consists of a series of linked proteolytic reactions that sequentially generates various serine proteases. The kallikrein and complement mechanisms operate similarly. When these three mechanisms are activated at sites of injury, it is necessary to localize their actions in order to avoid propagation of their effects throughout the vascular system. If this were not the case, limited vascular damage would lead to widespread thrombosis, systemic fibrinolysis, and profound changes in vascular permeability. Nature has designed the following diverse mechanisms to localize activity and prevent such an explosive outcome.

A. Blood flow

Rapid movement of blood within vascular channels serves to dilute high concentrations of procoagulants or profibrinolytic components generated locally at sites of injury. Indeed, infusion of serine proteases of the coagulation system into experimental animals does not induce venous thrombosis unless blood flow is stopped within a vein segment during periods of induced hypercoagulability. Stasis alone does not produce a venous thrombosis. Thus, normal blood remains fluid in the face of some degree of hypercoagulability if it continues to flow freely.

B. Hepatic clearance of activated components

If coagulation system serine proteases or plasminogen activators are experimentally injected into the portal vein, the liver removes them before they reach the systemic venous circulation. This probably occurs via interactions of protein inhibitors on hepatic cell surfaces. The liver and RES also remove soluble fibrin complexes from the circulation. Liver disease (cirrhosis, viral hepatitis, etc.) can impair this clearance mechanism and may cause systemic fibrinolysis as well as widespread thrombosis.

C. Localization of enzyme generation

To activate hemostatic system zymogens at adequate rates, *multimolecular complexes* must be sequentially formed between zymogens, cofactors, enzymes, Ca^{++}, and an altered surface (that furnishes phospholipid). In the absence of these complexes, generation of serine proteases is minimal. In addition to dramatically accelerating enzyme production, these complexes also localize events to sites of vascular damage.

D. Specific destruction of cofactors or activated cofactors

The protein C-thrombomodulin mechanism suppresses the generation of thrombin by reducing the production of this enzyme by specific proteolysis of cofactors or activated cofactors (see discussion above).

E. Modulation of fibrin polymerization

The conversion of fibrin I to fibrin II by the action of thrombin results in thrombus formation. This transformation is avoided when fibrin I is converted to fragment X by the action of plasmin (see discussion above).

F. Plasma protease inhibitors

Several plasma proteins can dampen the activity of proteolytic enzymes generated in the coagulation, fibrinolytic, and kinin-generating systems. Molecular species that exert these effects and are reasonably well characterized include *antithrombin* (*antithrombin III*), *antiplasmin,* α_2*-macroglobulin,* α_1*-antitrypsin,* and *C1 inactivator*. (The first three are the most important and will be discussed in some detail below.)

1. Deficiency states

Inherited deficiencies of four of these proteins are known to result in human disease: (1) antithrombin deficiency is found in patients with severe thrombotic disease; (2) antiplasmin deficiency has been observed in a family with a bleeding diathesis, presumably secondary to unrestricted local fibrinolysis; (3) C1 inactivator deficiency is associated with hereditary angioneurotic edema; and (4) α_1-antitrypsin deficiency is present in patients with severe emphysema and liver disease. To date, there have been reports of an inherited deficiency of α_2-macroglobulin but without overt clinical symptoms.

Based upon the pathophysiologic consequences of inherited deficiencies as well as biochemical data, it appears that antithrombin, antiplasmin, and α_2-macroglobulin constitute critical modulators of the hemostatic mechanism. The structure and function of these three components are discussed in the following sections. The remaining plasma proteins—α_1-antitrypsin and C1 inactivator—are of greater importance in the inhibition of competent, kinin-generating, and leukocyte-derived serine proteases. However, these two species are capable of neutralizing proteolytic enzymes of the hemostatic system to some degree and may represent a second line of defense against activation of this physiologic mechanism. These latter protease inhibitors are not discussed further.

2. Antithrombin: mechanism of action of heparin

The major inhibitor of the coagulation cascade is antithrombin (mol. wt. 56,000). It is also the essential cofactor for the action of *heparin* (figure 26.13), a naturally occurring sulfated mucopolysaccharide of mol. wt. 5,000–50,000 that is employed clinically as an anticoagulant. This polymer is composed of alternating residues of hexosamine and hexuronic acid. The hexosamine residues are glucosamines that may be N-sulfated, N-acetylated, or ester-sulfated. Alternatively, they may have no substituents at one or more of these positions. The hexuronic acid residues can be glucuronic acid, iduronic acid, or ester-sulfated iduronic acid. Thus, a great variety of possible hexosamine-uronic acid sequences may exist within a heparin molecule. It is thought that the monosaccharide sequence iduronic acid–N-sulfated or N-acetyl glucosamine 6-0-sulfate–glucuronic acid–N-sulfated glucosamine 3,6-0-sulfate–iduronic acid 2-0-sulfate–N-sulfated glucosamine 6-0-sulfate represents the major antithrombin binding

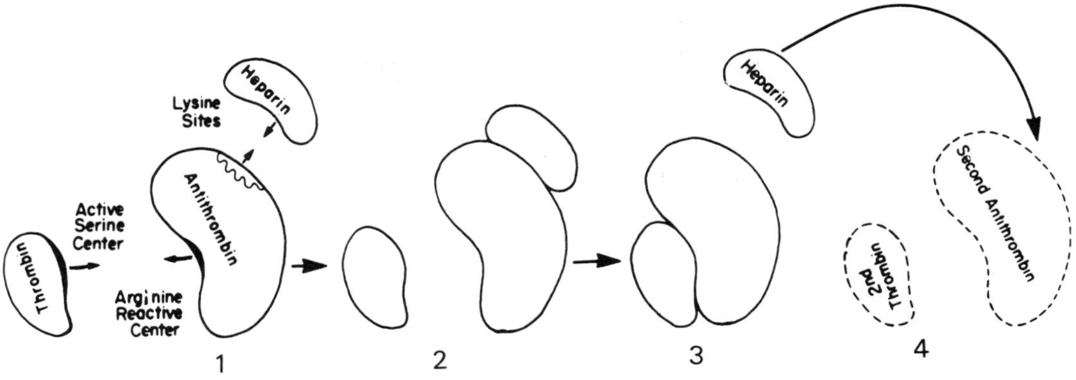

Fig. 26.13
Mechanism of heparin action.

site on heparin. Heparin has been isolated from a variety of organs and is also found in mast cells and basophils. *Heparan sulfate*, a chemical relative with some anticoagulant properties, has recently been located on the surface of the platelet as well as the vascular endothelium.

In the absence of heparin, antithrombin neutralizes the activity of thrombin by slowly forming a 1:1 complex of enzyme and inhibitor. In the presence of the sulfated mucopolysaccharide, the rate of complex formation is increased 2,000–10,000 fold, and neutralization of thrombin is virtually instantaneous. Formation of an enzyme inhibitor complex in the presence and absence of heparin is dependent on the active serine center of thrombin. If this residue is blocked, interaction between thrombin and antithrombin is inhibited. The reactive site of the inhibitor, which binds the active serine center of thrombin, contains an arginine residue. Modification of this group on antithrombin virtually eliminates the ability of the protein to inhibit thrombin in the presence or absence of heparin.

In view of the highly acidic nature of heparin, one would expect that positive groups on antithrombin (e.g., ε-aminolysyl residues) form the binding site for this negatively charged anticoagulant. Chemical alteration of these residues prevents binding of heparin to this protein and suppresses the acceleration of inhibitor action by the anticoagulant. However, the slow, progressive neutralization of thrombin by antithrombin is not appreciably affected. Furthermore, heparin functions as a catalyst in this reaction. Relatively small amounts dramatically accelerate the interaction of considerably larger amounts of thrombin and antithrombin. This occurs because of the displacement of heparin from antithrombin during formation of the thrombin-antithrombin complex. Thus, the mucopolysaccharide is available to bind to free inhibitor and cyclically promote subsequent rounds of interactions.

In summary, antithrombin neutralizes the activity of thrombin by complex formation via a reactive site (arginine)–active center (serine) interaction. If small amounts of heparin are added to the system, it preferentially binds to the lysyl residues on antithrombin. The resulting heparin-antithrombin complex rapidly inactivates thrombin. This most probably is due to a heparin-dependent conformational alteration of the inhibitor, which renders the reactive site arginine more accessible to the active serine center of thrombin. Once thrombin-antithrombin complex formation has occurred, heparin is released and is again available for binding to free inhibitor. Thus, the mucopolysaccharide is capable of catalyzing numerous subsequent rounds of thrombin-antithrombin complex formation.

This mechanism of inhibitor action implies that antithrombin neutralizes all the serine proteases of the coagulation cascade and that heparin accelerates each of these interactions. This hypothesis has been shown to be valid with respect to factor IXa, factor Xa, factor XIa, and factor XIIa. The behavior of the remaining enzymes of the hemostatic system, that is, factor VIIa and protein C, are anomalous in this regard. The activities of these serine proteases are not affected by antithrombin in the presence or absence of heparin. Similarly designated enzymes generated in physiologic systems that are separate from but linked to the hemostatic mechanism (e.g., complement system, kallikrein system) are only minimally affected by this inhibitory process.

The availability of heparin-like substances on endothelium permits antithrombin to be selectively activated at blood-surface interfaces where enzymes of the hemostatic mechanism are generated. Thus the plasma protease inhibitor is critically placed to neutralize these enzymes and thereby protect natural surfaces against thrombus formation. Moreover the catalytic nature of heparin would ensure the continual regeneration of the nonthrombogenic properties of these natural surfaces. Once the antithrombin bound to vessel wall mucopolysaccharide complexes with enzyme, the enzyme-inhibitor complex would be liberated into circulation. The heparin-like material would again be available to recruit free antithrombin and thereby continually renew the ability of the surface to resist the attack of serine proteases of the hemostatic cascade.

It is noteworthy that the factor VII–tissue factor and protein C-thrombomodulin interactions operate virtually independently of the endogenous heparin-antithrombin mechanism. On the one hand this may permit the extrinsic pathway of thrombin generation to function as a "spark" to mobilize the intrinsic pathway of thrombin generation. On the other hand it may allow the protein C-thrombomodulin mechanism to utilize thrombin that escapes neutralization by the endogenous heparin-antithrombin mechanism to suppress thrombin production by specific destruction of cofactors or activated cofactors.

3. Antiplasmin

The principal inhibitor of the fibrinolytic mechanism is a plasma protein termed *antiplasmin* (mol. wt. 67,000). Two forms have been isolated with slightly different physiochemical properties, but the biologic significance of this microheterogeneity remains unclear. Plasmin is rapidly neutralized by antiplasmin by formation of 1:1 stoichiometric complex of enzyme and inhibitor. The mechanism appears to be similar to that discussed for the thrombin-antithrombin reaction and involves an interaction between the serine active center of plasmin and a reactive site on antiplasmin. However, accessory areas on the plasmin molecule such as the kringles are also critical for the rapid formation of enzyme-inhibitor complexes. The addition of low-molecular-weight ligands such as ϵ-aminocaproic acid (EACA) that bind to these regions of plasmin can reduce the rapid rate of this interaction 10–50-fold (figure 26.11). Antiplasmin has also been observed to inactivate factors IXa and XIIa, albeit at a relatively slow rate. Thus, it may be partially involved in suppressing plasminogen-to-plasmin conversion as well as opposing the action of the enzyme when formed.

Sufficient levels of antiplasmin are normally present to inactivate half the plasmin that can theoretically be generated within the blood. Provided that this level of zymogen conversion is not exceeded in the fluid phase, plasmin neutralization is rapid, as well as complete, and systemic fibrinolysis is prevented. As noted, plasmin formed within the fibrin clot structure is sequestered from the action of protease inhibitors. This appears to be due to the interaction of the enzyme with the fibrin strands via its kringle structures. Under these conditions, plasmin can only be slowly neutralized by antiplasmin and is capable of gradually lysing the fibrin meshwork (figure 26.11).

In pathologic states such as disseminated intravascular coagulation or during infusion of urokinase for therapeutic purposes, considerably more than half the circulating plasminogen may be converted to plasmin. Once the capacity of antiplasmin has been exceeded, excess proteolytic enzyme is bound to α_2-macroglobulin. Since a small percentage of the plasmin bound within this complex remains active, systemic fibrinolysis is able to take place. Thus antiplasmin appears to be the major barrier against the action of the fibrinolytic system.

4. α_2-Macroglobulin

The proteolytic inhibitor *α_2-macroglobulin* is capable of neutralizing a wide variety of proteolytic enzymes such as plasmin, trypsin, thrombin, kallikrein, elastase, collegenase, and cathepsins. However, the rates of inactivation are relatively modest compared with those of the other protease inhibitors.

This plasma protein is composed of two equivalent half-molecules of mol. wt. 360,000 that are held together by noncovalent interaction. Each half-molecule consists of two peptide chains of mol. wt. 180,000 that are linked by disulfide bridges. The various endopeptidases are inactivated by formation of either 1:1 or 2:1 stoichiometric complexes of enzyme and inhibitor. The initial phase of this process most probably requires an interaction between the active center of the protease and a reactive site on α_2-macroglobulin. Thereafter, a complex alteration in the spacing of the four subunits that make up the protease inhibitor is apparent. The latter event may be triggered by interactions between unique internal pyroglutamic acid moieties that are part of the structure of α_2-macroglobulin.

This latter transition has two major consequences. First, enzyme molecules trapped within α_2-macroglobulin are able to function in a limited fashion as proteases. Second, the endopeptidases bound to the α_2-macroglobulin are protected against the action of other circulating protease inhibitors that would completely inactivate these enzymes. The enzyme–α_2-macroglobulin complexes are cleared by the RES in 15–30 min.

The primary in vivo function of this inhibitor may be to preserve a portion of the biologic activity of bound enzyme within the circulatory system and allow this bound enzyme to express its activity for a specified period of time in the presence of other plasma inhibitors. For example, plasmin bound to α_2-macroglobulin may play a critical role in the normal process of fibrinolysis, whereas thrombin bound to this inhibitor may be important in activating small amounts of cofactors such as factor V or factor VIII. Thus, these sequestered enzymes may be capable of maintaining coagulation-fibrinolytic system activity at some basal level and thereby keeping the hemostatic system poised and ready for action.

5. Other inhibitors of the hemostatic system

Two new protease inhibitors of the hemostatic system have recently been described. The first (mol. wt. 57,000) slowly inactivates protein Ca generated within the blood. It is unclear whether alterations in the levels of this component can alter the function of the protein C-thrombomodulin mechanism. The second (mol. wt. 40,000) is produced by endothelial cells and platelets and rapidly neutralizes the action of urokinase or tissue-type plasminogen activator. Congenital elevations in the latter protease inhibitor may lead to thrombosis.

VI. SOURCES OF CLOTTING PROTEINS

A. Liver

The liver is the site for production of prothrombin, factor VII, factor IX, factor X, factor XI, factor XII, plasminogen and protease inhibitors such as antithrombin-heparin cofactor, and α_2-macroglobulin. Factor V may also be synthesized in the liver.

1. Role of vitamin K

The biosynthesis of the 5 *homologous proteins* prothrombin, factor VII, factor IX, factor X, and protein C has a unique common feature. After these polypeptide chains are released from the ribosome, as suggested earlier, specific glutamic acid residues in the N-terminal region of these 5 proteins are γ-carboxylated. This process requires *vitamin K* as well as a poorly characterized microsomal enzyme carboxylating system. If these proteins are not so modified, they are functionally inactive.

2. Coumadin

Coumadin is a widely used anticoagulant that functions by interfering with the vitamin K–dependent γ-carboxylation process and thus prevents formation of functionally active prothrombin, factor VII, factor IX, factor X, and protein C.

B. Endothelial cells

Endothelial cells are the sites of production of von Willebrand's factor, tissue factor, plasminogen activator, and possibly factor V.

C. Kidney

The kidney may be an auxiliary site for the synthesis of plasminogen.

SELECTED REFERENCES

Aoki, N., et al. Fibrinolysis. *Semin. Thromb. Hemostasis* 10(1984): 1.

Davie, E. W., et al. The role of serine proteases in the blood coagulation cascade. *Adv. Enzymol.* 48(1979): 277.

Esmon, C. T. Protein C. *Semin. Thromb. Hemostasis* 10(1984): 109.

Jackson, C., and Nemerson, Y. Blood coagulation. *Ann. Rev. Biochem.* 49(1980): 769.

Ratnoff, O. D., and Saito, H. Surface-mediated reactions. In Piomello, S., and Yachnin, S., eds., *Current Topics in Hematology*, New York: Alan R. Liss, 1979, 2:1–57.

Rosenberg, R. D., and Rosenberg, J. S. Natural anticoagulant mechanisms. *J. Clin. Invest.* 74 (1984): 1.

LECTURE 27 Hemorrhagic Disorders II. Platelets and Purpura

Robert I. Handin

I. INTRODUCTION

A. Definition

Platelets, or *thrombocytes,* are cell fragments that adhere to injured blood vessel walls, form cellular aggregates or *hemostatic plugs,* and secrete a variety of potent biologic mediators. These properties allow them to perform several important functions: (1) they form hemostatic plugs that help to stanch the flow of blood from damaged blood vessels; (2) they provide a surface that promotes activation of coagulation system plasma proteins (see lecture 26); (3) they help maintain the integrity of the vascular endothelium; and (4) they give rise to mediators that initiate repair of the vessel wall and may regulate vascular tonicity and inflammatory reactions. Bleeding disorders arise when there are too few platelets to perform these functions or when platelets are present but defective.

B. Evolutionary aspects

Humans and other higher vertebrates possess a complicated hemostatic mechanism that requires both platelets and soluble coagulation proteins. Hemostasis is less complex in some primitive animals. For example, the ancient arthropod *Limulus polyphaemus,* the horseshoe crab, possesses a single blood cell, the *amebocyte,* which is a combination phagocyte and platelet and a source of coagulation proteins. When a particle of foreign material enters the circulation, the wandering amebocytes are attracted to the area and adhere to the particle, forming cellular aggregates. The amebocyte also secretes a clottable protein, roughly equivalent to mammalian fibrinogen, which then immoblizes the invader and repairs tissue damage.

C. Functions

1. Relations between platelets and plasma proteins

The two functions—*formation of intercellular aggregates* and *production of coagulable proteins*—later became increasingly complex and were segregated by evolution into separate systems consisting of cellular elements and soluble plasma proteins.

When we later consider disorders of the platelet, the close relation of platelet function and coagulation protein function should be remembered. There are many examples of this relation. Various coagulation reactions require addition of phospholipid. Synthetic phospholipids can be used in vitro; the platelet is a major source in vivo. In addition, certain coagulation proteins are absorbed onto the platelet surface and secreted from platelet granules. There is evidence that some of the coagulation reactions may actually occur on the platelet rather than in the plasma. Conversely, platelets need plasma proteins such as fibrinogen and von Willebrand's factor in order to function normally.

2. Relations between platelets and endothelium

Platelets help in some manner to *maintain integrity of vascular endothelium* and may *stimulate proliferation* of *arterial smooth muscle*. When the platelet count is low, capillary permeability increases and blood cells spontaneously pass between endothelial cells and to the outside of the vascular lumen. Clinically, this gives rise to *petechiae,* tiny, pinpoint hemorrhagic lesions that do not disappear when pressure is applied. Isolated organs also survive better when perfused with fluids containing a few platelets.

The endothelial cell may itself be the source of certain *coagulation proteins* (e.g., factor VIII, von Willebrand's factor, and plasminogen activators) or of biologically active materials like prostacyclin (prostaglandin I_2), a potent vasodilator and inhibitor of platelet function. Thus, hemostasis must be viewed as a complex web of events involving plasma proteins, platelets, and components of the vessel wall that are not totally separable. In addition to the obvious importance of the system in limiting blood loss after vascular injury, its components may be importantly related to such diverse phenomena as graft survival, vessel repair, thromboembolism, and the pathogenesis of atherosclerosis.

D. Production and destruction

1. Source of platelets

The platelet is a small fragment of a giant bone marrow precursor cell, the *megakaryocyte*.

a. Megakaryocyte formation

The earliest recognizable megakaryocyte progenitor is the *megakaryoblast,* which arises from the same pluripotent stem cell as the erythrocytic and granulocytic series (figure 27.1). As the megakaryoblast matures into a *promegakaryocyte,* it increases the amount of nuclear chromatin without concomitant cytoplasmic division, a process known as *endomitosis*. Although the average megakaryocyte has 8 nuclear lobes (or nuclear units), normal bone marrow contains megakaryocytes in various stages of development and may include cells with from 2 to 32 nuclear units. When platelet production is increased, there is an increase in the total number of megakaryocytes, the volume of each megakaryocyte, and the number of nuclear lobes per megakaryocyte. In stressed marrow, the modal value of nuclear units may rise to 16–32.

b. Platelet formation

The promegakaryocyte begins to develop cytoplasmic granular material when it has 16–32 nuclei. *Demarcation membranes* then develop as invaginations from the megakaryocyte's plasma membrane. They define the outer limit of each mature platelet, which arises as a fragment of cytoplasm. In fixed stained marrow it is

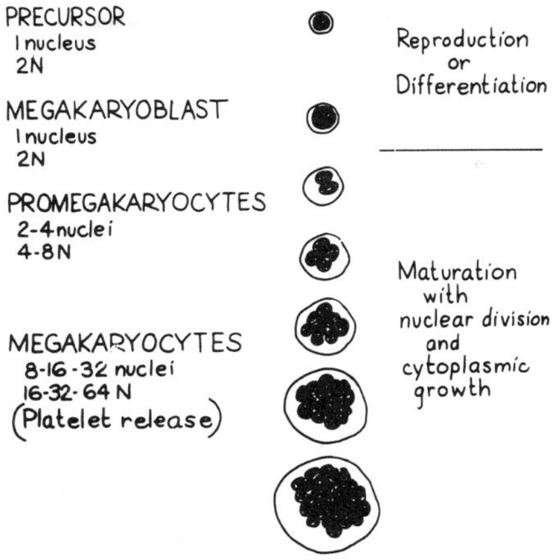

Fig. 27.1
Schematic diagram of the differentiation and maturation of megakaryocytes.

common to see "budding" of platelet fragments from megakaryocytes. This is probably an artifact because phase contrast microscopy of unfixed marrow shows simultaneous fragmentation of the entire megakaryocyte into about 50 platelets per nuclear unit per day. Since platelets arise from a common stem cell (lecture 1), it is not surprising that there are abnormalities of megakaryocyte morphology in the myeloproliferative disorders (lecture 19) and leukemias (lecture 21). Dysplastic megakaryocytes (with small rounded nuclei) have also been noted in the refractory anemias (lectures 5 and 6).

As noted below, platelets contain various organelles and granules. Their final organization probably occurs in the marrow. Circulating platelets vary in size and in granule and organelle content and density. The origin and significance of this heterogeneity are controversial. There is evidence that increased megakaryocyte number and ploidy causes the generation, on a random basis, of platelet heterogeneity with increased numbers of large, dense platelets. There is also evidence that platelets undergo "remodeling" while in the circulation with variable loss in membrane and granule contents giving rise to smaller and less dense platelets. Platelet granule contents, important for normal hemostatis, are not replenished during the platelet life span. Disorders of granule morphology and granule packaging and platelet membrane proteins can cause defective hemostasis.

2. Regulation of production

There are normally 150,000–350,000 platelets/mm^3 of blood. The platelet count is precisely controlled, presumably by a humoral mechanism similar to those thought to regulate the concentration of erythrocytes (lecture 1) and granulocytes (lecture 17).

a. Evidence for thrombopoietin

The evidence that such a hormone (thrombopoietin) controls platelet production was long based on the study of a single patient whose chronic thrombocytopenia was believed due to lack of thrombopoietin. Following an infusion of normal plasma, there is an increase both in the number and in the degree of maturation of the marrow megakaryocytes, and the platelet count returns to normal for several days. However, there is recent evidence that this patient had accelerated platelet destruction that was temporarily arrested by plasma infusion, rather than a marrow production defect. In addition, plasma collected from patients with marrow suppression and thrombocytopenia due to alcohol ingestion can produce thrombocytosis (higher than normal platelet count) when infused back into the patients after their recovery. Finally, when thrombocytopenia is produced experimentally by antibody infusion or exchange transfusion, platelet production is stimulated in the marrow. An experimental model that correlates incorporation of ^{75}Se-methionine into platelet proteins with platelet production confirms some of the clinical observations just mentioned. Following infusion of serum from a thrombocytopenic animal (that is rich in thromobopoietin) rabbits with suppressed thrombopoiesis incorporate more ^{75}Se-methionine into their platelets.

b. Role of thrombopoietin

The mechanism by which thrombopoietin stimulates platelet production is not clearly defined. Theoretically, thrombopoietin could work in several ways: it could *stimulate stem cells* committed to thrombopoiesis; it could *accelerate endomitosis* or *maturation;* or it could *produce large megakaryocytes* that yield an increased number of platelets. All three events are observed in marrow of patients with an increased rate of platelet production. Current evidence suggests that the thrombopoietin level of plasma is determined not only by the platelet count of blood but by the total platelet mass.

3. Regulation of destruction: role of spleen

After platelets leave the marrow, they are taken up by the spleen. They then equilibrate slowly with the circulating platelet pool. When the spleen enlarges from any cause (see table 2.1), the trapping of a higher proportion of platelets in the spleen may cause thrombocytopenia. The marrow may respond to thrombocytopenia resulting from splenic sequestration by increasing platelet production.

The presence of a *splenic platelet pool* complicates the interpretation of platelet survival studies. For example, after infusion of platelets labeled with ^{51}Cr, about one-third of the labeled platelets enter the splenic pool. A small percentage of the circulating platelets are consumed in hemostasis and rapidly removed from the circulation, but most of the platelets circulate for 8–10 days and die of "old age." This leads to an almost linear decline in the level of circulating radioactivity. With splenic enlargement, the life span of the circulating platelets remains normal and the loss of radioactivity remains linear, but the initial recovery of radioactivity decreases. This is in contrast with the fate of the red cells in patients with splenomegaly, in whom there is usually a decrease in erythrocyte life span (see figure 11.1). When platelets are randomly consumed in large numbers as a result of disordered coagulation or antibody attack, there is an exponential loss of circulating radioactivity with a decrease in life span. Thus, the *initial yield* of radioactivity, the *pattern of removal,* and the *total life span* must all considered when interpreting platelet survival data.

E. Morphology

1. Light microscopy

The mature platelet is a highly developed, motile, secretory cell with a complex internal architecture that cannot be fully appreciated by light microscopic examination of blood films. On a dried, Wright's-stained smear, the platelet appears as an irregularly shaped, small, refractile bit of pale blue cytoplasm with a few azurophilic granules. In fact, until the late nineteenth century, this bit of stained material was considered debris derived from degeneration of other blood cells or an unusual microorganism. Thus, there was doubt or ignorance of the existence of platelets.

2. Electron microscopy

Transmission electron micrographs (figure 27.2) demonstrate complex internal structure. The *outer (plasma) membrane* evidently invaginates into the platelet interior to form an extensive canalicular system. Just beneath the membrane is a *microtubule cytoskeleton* that may help maintain the platelet in a normal disk configuration. The platelet also contains visible actin, microfilaments, myosin, glycogen deposits, and a few mitochondria. The most prominent ultrastructural feature is an array of granules of varying sizes and electron densities. Those called *dense bodies* contain ADP, ATP, serotonin, and calcium. The less dense α *granules* include two populations of granules, one of which, the *platelet lysosomes,* contains various hydrolytic enzymes. The other contains platelet pools of fibrinogen and fibronectin, factor V, von Willebrand's factor, a lectin-like protein called thrombospondin, and three platelet-specific proteins—β-*thromboglobulin, platelet factor 4*, and *platelet-derived growth factor* (PDGF), a potent mitogen. With appropriate stimulation, the contents of all of these granules are selectively discharged to the exterior by the canalicular system, an event called the *release reaction.*

F. Role in clotting

1. Primary and secondary

The platelet maintains its normal discoid shape in the circulation unless it encounters damaged endothelium or exposed subendothelium. This triggering event rapidly leads to a series of am-

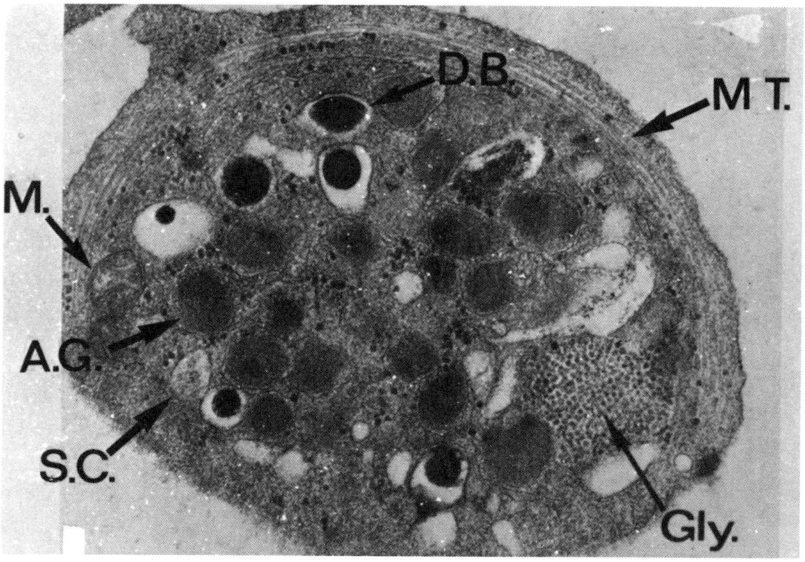

Fig. 27.2
Internal architecture of a normal platelet as demonstrated by transmission electron micrograph ($\times 15{,}000$): MT, circumferential band of microtubules; BD, dense body (which contains ADP and serotonin); AG, α granule (which contains fibrinogen and a heparin-neutralizing protein); M, mitochondrion; Gly, glycogen; SC, surface-connected; OCS, open canalicular system. (Reprinted with permission from J. A. White, in T. H. Spaet, ed., *Progress in Hemostasis and Thrombosis,* Vol. 2, New York: Grune & Stratton, 1974, p. 53)

plifying reactions that begins with *adhesion* of platelets to exposed subdothelial *collagen* and is followed by a *change in shape* and *degranulation.* ADP released from adherent platelets or damaged tissues and red cells causes adjacent platelets to adhere to the initial platelet layer and each other, forming a *primary hemostatic plug.* In addition small amounts of thrombin are generated by the plasma coagulation system, which is also activated by contact of blood with the damaged vessel wall. Thrombin and collagen, as well as ADP in high concentration, all cause platelets in the primary plug to degranulate with release of additional ADP, vasoactive amines, and lysosomal enzymes and generation of the potent aggregating agent and vasoconstrictor thromboxane A_2 (TXA_2). Thus, there is a positive feedback loop with thrombin causing further release of ADP and generation of TXA_2 by platelets. The platelet plug is now fused into a tightly packed syncytial mass referred to as a *definitive* or *secondary hemostatic plug.* Plasma fibrinogen facilitates aggregation and acts as an adhesive protein. It binds to receptor sites on activated platelets and links them together to form the intial hemostatic plug or platelet aggregate. Later, as higher concentrations of thrombin are generated, fibrinogen in plasma is converted to fibrin strands, which help solidify the platelet plug.

A number of *limiting reactions* exist that normally prevent massive platelet deposition in the wake of a trivial injury. These include (1) continued flow of blood past the growing platelet plug, which removes loosely adherent platelets and dilutes the concentration of ADP and other mediators; (2) actions of plasma enzymes that degrade ADP to adenosine, which is a competitive inhibitor of platelet aggregation; and (3) production by endothelial cells of the platelet inhibitory prostaglandin PGI_2.

2. Associated biochemistry

The initial hemostatic event appears to be the *binding of mediators,* such as ADP and thrombin, to receptors on the platelet membrane. The adhesion of platelets to collagen requires that collagen be in a native fibrillar quaternary structure. There may be multiple sites of interaction between collagen and platelets. In other cases binding may be a simple biomolecular interaction of a specific aggregating agent (agonist) and a discrete receptor protein. Well-defined receptors for the platelet agonists thrombin, ADP, epinephrine, and TXA_2 and the antagonists prostaglandin I_2 and D_2 have been described. Next there is *transformation of shape*—from discoidal to spheroidal—and *extension of pseudopods,* reactions mediated by the platelet contractile proteins actin and myosin.

Agents that promote platelet aggregation (e.g., thrombin, epinephrine) also inhibit platelet *adenylate cyclase,* the enzyme that maintains high levels of cyclic 3′,5′-adenosine monophosphate (cyclic AMP). Both of these labile intermediates enhance aggregation and release. TXA_2 is also a potent vasoconstrictor (figure 27.3). Finally platelets have *protein kinases,* partly controlled by the level of cyclic AMP, which catalyze the phosphorylation of specific platelet proteins. For example, there is a cyclic AMP-dependent protein kinase that phosphorylates the light chain on myosin and facilitates the actin-myosin interaction that controls shape change and degranulation. Another protein kinase (protein kinase C), which is regulated by diglycerides released from the hydrolysis of platelet membrane phosphatidyl inositol, phosphorylates a 40,000-dalton platelet protein. This phosphorylation reaction accompanies platelet activation and secretion. Agents that induce aggregation increase intracellular Ca^{++}, which controls several of these biochemical events. Pharmacologic manipulation of any of these reactions may result in inhibition or stimulation of platelet function.

3. Role of endothelial cells

Although we have focused on the platelet, there is substantial evidence for a role for *endothelial cells* in regulating hemostasis. For example, they convert endogenous arachidonate or platelet-derived endoperoxide into the potent platelet inhibitor PGI_2 (pros-

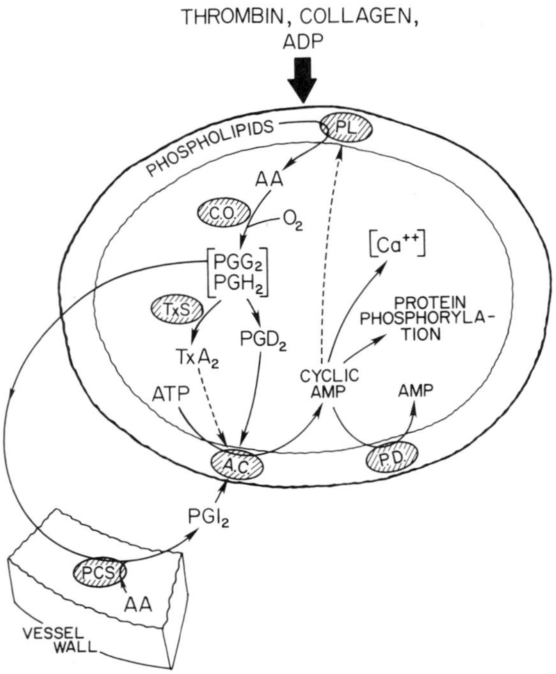

Fig. 27.3
Outline of biochemical mechanisms underlying platelet aggregation and release reaction. PL: phospholipases; CO: cyclooxygenase; TXS: thromboxane synthetase; AC: adenylate cyclase; PD: phosphodiesterase; PCS: prostacyclin synthetase.

tacyclin), which may limit the size of hemostatic plugs. This balance between platelet and endothelial products may be critical for normal hemostasis.

4. Platelet coagulant activity

The long-recognized fact that platelets can accelerate certain coagulation reactions (like prothrombin conversion) has been referred to as *platelet factor 3* activity. This property is due to the binding of factor V from platelets or plasma to the platelet membrane. When activated, factor Va serves as a receptor for factor Xa, which converts prothrombin to thrombin on the platelet surface (figure 27.4). The severity of bleeding in factor V deficiency has been related to *intraplatelet* factor V content, and patients have been described with a bleeding disorder who lack the platelet binding site for factor Va. Platelets may play an important regulatory role in initiating coagulation reactions since platelets can release and bind Va without the production of thrombin (see lecture 26). In addition Xa bound to the platelet may be protected from the inhibitory effect of antithrombin and on this site can accelerate prothrombin conversion 10,000-fold.

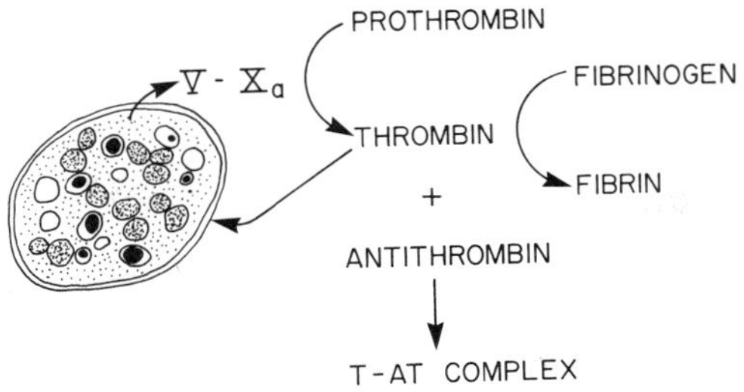

Fig. 27.4
Platelet binding of factors V and Xa and prothrombin conversion.

II. PLATELET DISORDERS

A. Quantitative disorders

Bleeding is commonly secondary to a reduction in the platelet count (*thrombocytopenia*), and a *thrombic tendency* may be associated with elevation in the count (*thrombocytosis*). We shall survey causes of these conditions in the following discussion. *Diagnosis* of these conditions depends on an accurate platelet count. The count can be estimated in a good Wright's-stained blood smear, each platelet in an oil immersion field representing approximately 10,000 platelets/mm^3 of blood. Platelets are counted more precisely in a hemocytometer with a phase microscope. However, this procedure is accurate to only 10–20% even when expertly performed. Thus, minor changes in the platelet count are as likely to reflect technical factors as a true variation. Accurate automated techniques now becoming available can count platelets in whole blood and permit greater accuracy. The evaluation of quantitative platelet disorders also depends on accurate information on spleen size and bone marrow morphology.

1. Thrombocytopenia

With such information, most cases of thrombocytopenia can be classified (as outlined in table 27.1) according to probable mechanism into (1) production defects (i.e., marrow failure); (2) distribution defects; (3) dilutional loss; and (4) abnormal destruction (nonimmune or immune). Figure 27.5 is a flowsheet for the evaluation of thrombocytopenia. It should be remembered that complex situations may occur in which multiple factors contribute to the low platelet count.

a. Production defects

Reduction in platelet production can be best correlated with an absolute reduction in total *megakaryocyte mass*. However, mass is tedious to measure, requiring careful examination of serial microscopic sections of marrow, and hence is not widely employed. Clinicians usually estimate megakaryocyte mass by inspection of a needle biopsy section or a bone marrow aspirate smear. A low-power ($\times$ 10) field of a needle biopsy section contains an average of 5 megakaryocytes.

Table 27.1
Classification of the Thrombocytopenias

Decreased production	
A. Hypoproliferation (see lecture 3)	Toxic agents (see table 3.1) Radiation, infection Constitutional factors (Fanconi's anemia, etc.) Idiopathic aplastic anemia Paroxysmal nocturnal hemoglobinuria Myelophthisis (tumor, fibrosis, etc.)
B. Ineffective thrombopoiesis	Megaloblastic anemia (see lectures 4–5) Di Guglielmo's syndrome Familial thrombocytopenia
Abnormal distribution	Congestive splenomegaly Myeloid metaplasia, lymphoma Gaucher's disease
Dilutional loss	Massive blood transfusion
Abnormal destruction	
A. Consumption	Disseminated intravascular coagulation, vasculitis Thrombotic thrombocytopenia (TTP)
B. Immune mechanism	Idiopathic thrombocytopenic purpura (ITP) Drug-induced thrombocytopenia Chronic lymphocytic leukemia, lymphoma, LE Neonatal thrombocytopenia Posttransfusion purpura

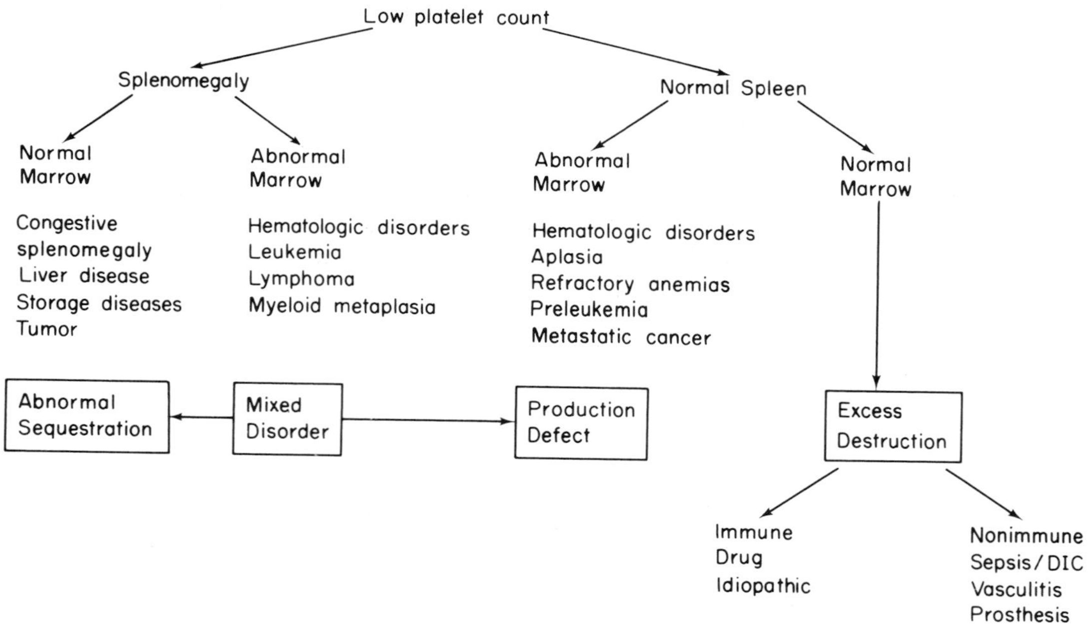

Fig. 27.5
A schematic approach to the clinical evaluation of patients with thrombocytopenia.

Normally, in addition to a reduction in the number of megakaryocytes, decreased platelet production is often associated with other bone marrow abnormalities: for example, thrombocytopenia due to aplastic anemia is associated with marrow hypocellularity that may involve all cell lines (lecture 3), and thrombocytopenia due to myelophthisis is associated with tumor cells, fibrosis, or leukemic cells (lecture 3).

In contrast with these hypoproliferative states, the mild thrombocytopenia associated with megaloblastic anemia is due to *ineffective thrombopoiesis* (lecture 4). The marrow contains an increased number of megakaryocytes often with megaloblastic morphology and megaloblastosis of other cell lines. Congenital or familial thrombocytopenia is also associated with plentiful but ineffective megakaryocytes.

b. Distribution defects

As noted in lecture 2, splenomegaly enlarges the splenic platelet pool and may thereby cause thrombocytopenia (figure 27.6). If marrow function is normal, this redistribution does not cause severe thrombocytopenia or bleeding—even in massive splenomegaly when recovery of ^{51}Cr-labeled platelets is as low as 10–15%. In some myeloproliferative disorders (e.g., CML), platelet production in marrow can be great enough to produce thrombocytosis despite massive splenic enlargement. Interestingly, patients with myeloid metaplasia have a complex combination of abnormal platelet production from dysplastic megakaryocytes, splenic sequestration, and production of platelets from extramedullary sites such as liver and spleen.

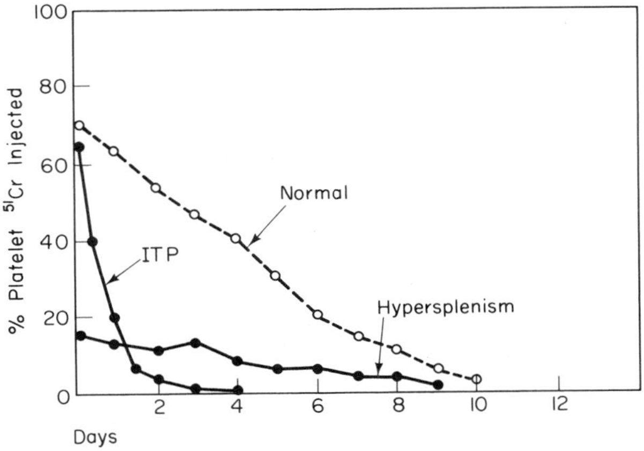

Fig. 27.6
Recovery and subsequent life span of isotopically labeled platelets infused into a normal individual and a patient ITP. Note that platelet recovery is reduced in patients with splenomegaly (and hypersplenism), but platelet life span is normal. Patients with ITP have normal recovery and shortened life span. (Reprinted with permission from R. Aster, in W. J. Williams et al., eds., *Hematology,* New York: McGraw-Hill, 1972, chapter 140, pp. 1159–1161.

c. Dilutional loss

Patients who receive many blood transfusions within a short time period may develop *dilutional thrombocytopenia* because infused blood does not contain viable platelets. As noted in lecture 16, platelets are no longer viable after blood is stored for more than a few hours at 4°C. Thrombocytopenia may persist for several days until the marrow synthesizes a sufficient number of new platelets. These patients are treated by infusion with fresh platelets.

d. Abnormal destruction

(1) Classification

As mentioned above, few platelets are consumed in the normal maintenance of hemostasis. However, platelets can be destroyed so rapidly that the marrow cannot compensate and thrombocytopenia develops. The major causes are (1) platelet consumption, due to disseminated intravascular coagulation (see lecture 28); (2) damage to platelets by abnormal vessel walls (vasculitis) or foreign surfaces; and (3) removal of platelets that have been coated by an antiplatelet antibody. Immune thrombocytopenia may occur with no obvious associated illness.

Accelerated platelet destruction is associated with an increase in megakaryocytes in an otherwise normal marrow aspirate and a normal-sized spleen. There is also decreased ^{51}Cr-platelet life span and failure to respond to platelet transfusions. There is an increased percentage in the blood smear of large platelets, which are termed *megathrombocytes*. There is debate over whether they are truly large, young platelets or whether they arise from a spreading artifact. While it would be useful to have a clinical index of young platelets that would illuminate platelet kinetics as the reticulocyte illuminates red cell kinetics, evaluation of the number of megathrombocytes in a blood smear is highly subjective. The most striking megathrombocytes are seen in myeloproliferative disorders; megaloblastic anemia; severe thrombocytopenia ($<50{,}000/mm^3$); and in rare inherited platelet disorders such as the Bernard-Soulier syndrome (see below).

(2) Immune thrombocytopenia

Nonimmune causes of platelet destruction are clinically obvious, but evaluating the patient with immune thrombocytopenia can still be a difficult task. Often the diagnosis is made by exclusion. In some types of immune thrombocytopenia, antigenic determinants and the stimulus for antibody production are well known. In others, neither antigen nor stimulus has been identified, and the diagnosis must rest on clinical findings.

Platelets do have several surface antigenic systems capable of interacting with antibody (figure 27.7). They share histocompatibility antigens (HLA) with lymphocytes and other tissues and have some of the ABO antigens (see lecture 15). In addition, the platelet has a unique PLA antigenic series. Platelets also contain

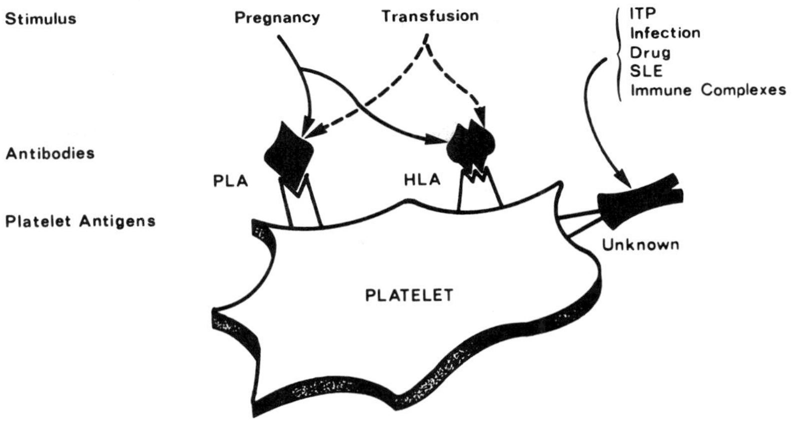

Fig. 27.7
Platelet surface antigens and the circumstances in which they elicit anti-platelet antibody.

receptors for the F_c portion of immunoglobulin that can bind altered IgG or immune complexes. Final confirmation of the diagnosis of immune thrombocytopenia requires detection of antibody directed against platelet antigens or deposition of an antigen-antibody complex on the platelet.

The most important pathophysiologic effect of a platelet antibody is to sensitize the platelet so that its subsequent clearance from the circulation and phagocytosis by splenic or liver macrophages is accelerated. IgG alone on the platelet surface can lead to sequestration and phagocytosis, as does IgG on the red cell surface in immunohemolytic anemia (see lecture 12). However, certain platelet antibodies (e.g., HLA antibodies) elicited by chronic transfusion or multiple pregnancies fix complement. In addition, deposition of drug-antibody complexes onto the platelet can cause complement fixation and direct platelet lysis. The relative importance of sensitization with IgG antibody alone, platelet opsonization with C3, or activation of the entire complement sequence varies with the type of antibody stimulus. It also changes with time in a single patient.

e. Special forms of immune thrombocytopenia

(1) Drug-induced thrombocytopenia

A large number of drugs can induce thrombocytopenia. A few are frequent offenders—for example, quinine, quinidine, sulfonamides, Sedormid®, and antibiotics like Keflin®. Patients usually show a rapid fall in platelet count while they are taking the sensitizing medication. There is then a prompt rise in platelet count within 7–10 days of drug withdrawal, though this time may be prolonged with drugs such as gold thiomalate or diphenylhydantoin (Dilantin®) that are metabolized and eliminated slowly.

Heparin has been implicated in an increasing number of cases of thrombocytopenia. The incidence varies from 3 to 25% of patients receiving heparin and may vary with the source of heparin or production lot. Some cases arise by an immune mechanism and others by a direct effect of certain heparin fractions on the platelet. Heparin thrombocytopenia is unique in that patients may develop paradoxical thrombosis that *improves* after heparin withdrawal.

The offending drug usually acts as a hapten, and the ensuing drug-antibody complex binds to the platelet, fixes complement, and causes intravascular lysis or damage (with subsequent removal by the RES). Quinidine-induced thrombocytopenia has been studied most extensively. In this disorder, passive transfer of immune serum to a normal individual, followed by drug challenge, produces transient thrombocytopenia. This drug-dependent antibody can be detected by quantitative complement fixation techniques. Unlike the situation in drug-induced hemolysis (lecture 13), drug-induced platelet antibodies are not usually directed against specific platelet antigens, nor do drugs coat platelets and then elicit and interact with circulating antibody.

A unique and significant case was reported several years ago in which a patient was sensitized to a *metabolite* of a common analgesic acetaminophen (Tylenol®) rather than to the drug itself. This case illustrates the difficulties of excluding a diagnosis of drug-induced thrombocytopenia in a given patient or of trying to make a laboratory diagnosis without strong suspicions of which drug or metabolite to test. The sudden onset of thrombocytopenia that remits shortly after discounting a particular drug remains the best clinical proof of drug-induced thrombocytopenia.

(2) Neonatal thrombocytopenia

Newborn infants often have abnormalities in the vitamin K–dependent synthesis of coagulation factors, but they usually have a normal platelet count. Most cases of thrombocytopenia arise in sick, premature infants with sepsis or DIC; but some infants are otherwise normal. In some of these cases, the mother's platelets lack the PLA-1 antigen, which is carried by 98–99% of the population. This produces a syndrome analogous to erythroblastosis fetalis (lecture 16). The PLA-1-negative mother carrying a PLA-1-positive fetus develops antibody against this antigen that is transmitted through the placenta to the fetus, so that the child is born with temporary thrombocytopenia. The platelet count returns to normal in 13–28 days as the level of antiplatelet antibody (7S IgG) declines. The infant is susceptible to intracranial hemorrhage and requires temporary platelet infusions. The mother is the ideal platelet donor; her PLA-1-negative platelets, washed free of antibody-containing plasma, can be safely transfused to the child for several days.

(3) Posttransfusion purpura

Since only 1–2% of the population lacks the PLA-1 antigen, PLA-negative donors commonly become sensitized during pregnancy or after blood transfusions. This is analogous to sensitization with uncommon red cell antigens (e.g., Kell and Duffy). This has little effect on the recipient of an incompatible transfusion except for rapid destruction of the "mismatched" platelets.

Rarely, PLA-1-negative individuals, usually multiparous females who have received blood containing PLA-1-positive platelets, develop profound thrombocytopenia 7–10 days after the transfusion. The mechanism of this *posttransfusion purpura* is not clear. Probably PLA-1 antigen in transfused blood is absorbed onto PLA-1-negative platelets, which are then destroyed by antibody. In 10–14 days, the platelet count returns to normal as the patient clears the foreign antigen. The patient then continues to produce PLA-1-negative platelets that coexist with anti-PLA-1 antibody. Although rare, it has been fatal, and is difficult to treat since all platelets are incompatible.

(4) Idiopathic thrombocytopenic purpura

In the group of disorders termed *idiopathic thrombocytopenic purpura* (ITP), the cause of accelerated platelet destruction is more elusive than in the syndromes discussed above. In most cases an antibody is directed against platelets, although the actual stimulus for antibody production is usually not known. It was shown decades ago that some women with ITP deliver children with transient neonatal thrombocytopenia, which differs from neonatal isoimmune thrombocytopenia in that the mother does not lack PLA-1 antigen. This suggestion of transplacental passage of a causative humoral agent was bolstered by Harrington's demonstration that infusion of plasma from patients with ITP into normal individuals lowers the platelet count and that the active principle is a 7S IgG.

Tests for platelet antibody analogous to the red cell Coombs or direct antiglobulin test have been developed to measure platelet surface IgG and C3. They reveal the presence of IgG or C3 in most, but not all, patients with ITP. The majority of antibodies in patients with ITP are directed against determinants on glycoprotein (Gp) IIIa. The epitopes are distinct from the PLA-1 antigen, which is also on Gp IIIa. Despite the fact that fibrinogen binds to sites on Gp IIIa, most antibodies do not impair platelet aggregation or inhibit fibrin formation. Despite these laboratory aids, the diagnosis must rest as well on clinical observation and occasionally on platelet kinetic studies. ITP may present as an acute, transient disorder or as a chronic, lifelong condition.

Acute ITP is a self-limited condition that occurs mainly in children following a viral infection (e.g., rubella, cytomegalovirus, viral hepatitis, infectious mononucleosis, various unidentified viruses). Thrombocytopenia, often severe, may lead to mucosal bleeding and petechiae. However, mortality is low, and recovery usually occurs in 2–6 weeks. A viral antigen-antibody complex may be absorbed onto platelet surfaces. Complete recovery follows clearance of these complexes. The few who do not recover in 6 months enter a chronic phase and resemble the patients described below.

Chronic ITP, a disorder of young and middle-aged women, is associated with an autoantibody against unknown platelet antigens. The patients may present with a long history of easy bruising and skin hemorrhage, or with a more acute picture. Some patients have other diseases, such as systemic lupus erythematosus, lymphoproliferative disorders (CLL or lymphoma), or immunohemolytic anemia (the combination being termed *Evans's syndrome*). The risk of intracranial hemorrhage and other serious complications is much higher in adults with chronic ITP than in children with acute ITP. Treatment consists of corticosteroids, splenectomy, or immunosuppressive drugs. Most patients who respond to corticosteroids will respond well to splenectomy, entering a long or permanent remission during which platelet counts are normal despite persistent antibody activity and accelerated platelet destruction. Nonresponders may develop refractory thrombocytopenia and require immunosuppressive drugs.

2. Thrombocytosis

Elevation of the platelet count to levels over 1,000,000/mm^3 may not cause signs or symptoms per se. However, counts above 1,000,000 can cause hemorrhage *and* thrombosis. Elevation of the platelet count may be reactive or it may occur autonomously. In the former case it is termed *thrombocytosis*; in the latter, *thrombocythemia*.

a. Reactive

High platelet counts occur commonly in association with malignancy, inflammation, hemolysis, the postsplenectomy state, and bleeding. It may also be associated with iron deficiency even when active bleeding is not occurring. The highest platelet counts, sometimes reaching several million per cubic millimeter, occur immediately after splenectomy. Reactive thrombocytosis is benign and does not lead to bleeding or thrombosis.

b. Autonomous

As noted, platelet counts may also be elevated as a manifestation of a myeloproliferative disorder (lecture 19). This is termed *essential*, or *autonomous, thrombocythemia*. Total megakaryocyte mass is usually markedly increased in this situation. Platelets in some of these disorders may have qualitative defects. Defects in membrane glycoprotein content and loss of specific receptors and enzymes such as lipoxygenase have been described. Autonomous thrombocytosis can lead to massive thrombosis and requires intensive treatment aimed at lowering the platelet count and inhibiting excess platelet reactivity.

B. Qualitative disorders

Patients with a normal platelet count and a clinical picture suggesting a platelet abnormality are said to have a *qualitative*, or

Table 27.2
Test Results in Qualitative Platelet Disorders

	Aggregation								
	ADP		Epinephrine						
Disorder[a]	1°	2°	1°	2°	Collagen	Ristocetin	5-HT uptake	Release of ADP, ATP, 5-HT	VIII_{AGN}
Adhesion									
von Willebrand's disease	N	N	N	N	N	↓	N	N	↓
Bernard-Soulier syndrome	N	N	N	N	N	↓	N	N	N
Primary aggregation									
Thrombasthenia	↓	↓	↓	↓	↓	N	N	N	N
Secondary aggregation and release									
Aspirin(-like) defect	N	↓	N	↓	↓	N	N	↓	N
Storage pool disease	N	↓	N	↓	↓	N	↓	N/↓	N

Note: Abbreviations: 1°, first phase; 2°, second phase; N, normal; ↓, decreased; 5-HT, 5-hydroxytryptamine (serotonin); VIII_{AGN}, factor VIII antigen (i.e., factor VIII as determined by immunoassay).
[a]The bleeding time is prolonged in all of the listed disorders.

functional, platelet disorder (see table 27.2). As noted above, platelet functions may be subdivided into three major reactions—adhesion, aggregation, and release. Specific defects have been described in each reaction. Collectively, they comprise a major cause of easy bruising and minor bleeding tendency.

1. Evaluation of platelet function

Diagnosis of qualitative disorders depends on suitable platelet function tests that seek to reproduce in vitro the hemostatic events occurring in vivo.

a. Bleeding time

The overall reaction sequence mediated by platelets is simulated by the *bleeding time* (BT), a most useful test of platelet function. A small incision is made on the skin of the forearm and the time recorded that is required for cessation of blood flow. Mechanical aids such as a plastic template help standardize the incision and improve precision. Normal BT is 4.5 ± 3.0 min. It should be remembered that the BT can be prolonged by quantitative *and* qualitative platelet disorders. A patient with normal platelet count and normal BT is unlikely to have a significant platelet abnormality. Since the BT does not become prolonged until the platelet count falls below 100,000/mm^3, the presence of moderate thrombocytopenia and severely prolonged BT should suggest the possibility that a qualitative platelet disorder coexists with thrombocytopenia.

b. Aggregation

Platelet plug formation is also studied in turbidimetric assays of the time course and extent of *platelet aggregation* following addition to platelet-rich plasma of *ADP, collagen*, or *epinephrine*, in-

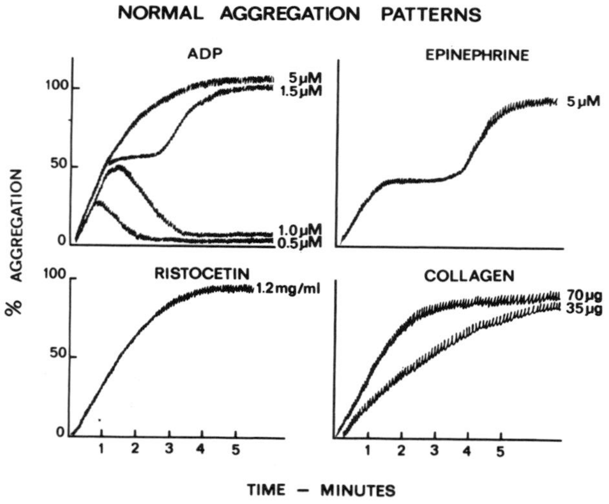

Fig. 27.8
Aggregation patterns of normal platelets after challenge with various aggregating agents. Note that a biphasic pattern can be obtained with certain concentrations of ADP and with epinephrine. The secondary wave, which corresponds to the platelet release action, is abolished by drugs such as aspirin.

creased light transmittance through the cuvette indicating platelet aggregation. As shown in Figure 27.8, when ADP (1 μM) is added, a few aggregates form, which may then disaggregate. As [ADP] is increased, a point is reached (at ~1.5 μM) at which a second wave of aggregation occurs. This is due to release of ADP from the platelets. The second wave of aggregation coincides with the platelet release reaction as shown by other data. A similar biphasic curve occurs on addition of epinephrine. However, incubation with collagen produces monophasic aggregation because endogenous platelet ADP is released following adhesion of platelets to collagen fibrils. Collagen itself does not cause aggregation directly. Some stimuli continue to induce aggregation after platelet function has been partially inhibited. For example, high doses of collagen induce aggregation after aspirin therapy blocks thromboxane production, and thrombin causes aggregation even after thromboxane generation and ADP secretion have been blocked.

c. Release reaction

Released *adenine nucleotides* and *serotonin* (5-hydroxytryptamine) are convenient assay parameters for the platelet release reaction. In addition, it is possible by incubating platelets with ^{14}C-adenine to estimate the pool of adenine nucleotides in platelet granules. Granule-bound ADP and ATP, termed *storage pool* ADP and ATP, are to be distinguished from *metabolic pool* ADP and ATP in the cytoplasm. Since ^{14}C-adenine is readily converted to metabolic pool nucleotides and excluded from granules, relative sizes of the two pools can be estimated by measuring and comparing total and radioactive adenine nucleotides. As will be noted below, this procedure identifies patients in whom failure to achieve normal secondary aggregation is due to a reduced adenine nucleotide pool in the granules, rather than a defect in release per se. It is also possible to measure release of granule constituents using radioimmunoassays for platelet-specific protein, β-thromboglobulin, or PF-4. This is of practical importance since selective deficiencies of granule contents have been discovered.

d. Adhesion

Platelet adhesion—that is, the interaction of platelets with a foreign or nonplatelet surface—has been difficult to quantify. Platelets can be perfused through small rings made from endothelium-free blood vessels to quantify adhesion to subendothelium. This technique can dissociate adhesion to the vessel wall from aggregation of platelets to adherent platelets and can vary the concentration of plasma cofactors and shear stress, which can both affect adhesion.

e. Interaction of platelets with factor VIII/von Willebrand's factor

Measurement of the effect of von Willebrand's factor (VWF) on adhesion is based on the fact that platelets exposed to plasma deficient in VWF do not adhere normally to vascular subendothelium. The interaction of VWF with the platelet can also be

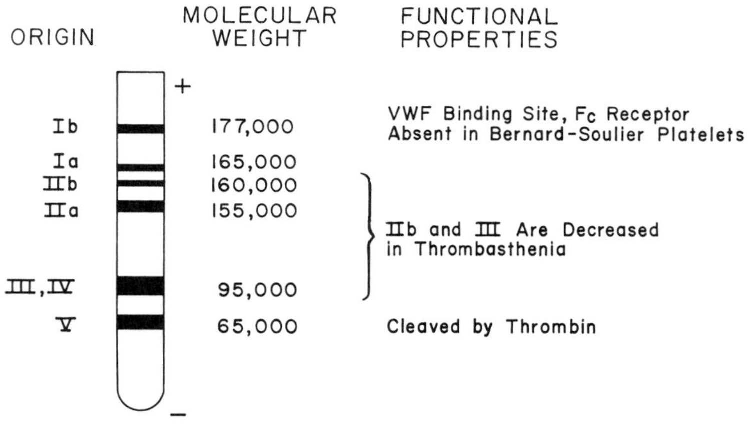

Fig. 27.9
SDS-polyacrylamide gel electrophoresis of platelet membrane glycoproteins and glycoprotein functions.

studied by measuring the effect of the antibiotic *ristocetin* on platelet aggregation. Patients whose platelets are not aggregated by ristocetin either lack *von Willebrand's factor* activity or the platelet receptor for VWF (see lectures 26 and 28).

f. Biochemical tests

Aggregation and release require normal membrane structure and intact platelet metabolism. Functional platelet abnormalities can be correlated with metabolic defects sufficiently often to merit special testing of patients with platelet dysfunction. The glycoprotein pattern of platelet membranes is depicted in figure 27.9. Two specific defects, Glanzmann's thrombasthenia and the Bernard-Soulier syndrome, are caused by membrane glycoprotein defects. Arachidonic acid metabolism can be assessed by (1) measuring the burst in oxygen consumption or production of thromboxane A_2 by radioimmunoassay or radiochemical techniques induced by aggregating agents or (2) measuring aggregation with arachidonic acid. Defects relating to adenylate cyclase activity or contractile protein function have not been described, although loss of specific receptors that couple to adenylate cyclase has been described.

2. Platelet defects

a. Adhesion defects

(1) Von Willebrand's disease

The most common cause of defective adhesion is *von Willebrand's disease*, an autosomal-dominant disorder in which a plasma deficiency in factor VIII/VWF decreases platelet adhesion to vessel walls. Platelet aggregation and release are normal. Patients have a lifelong history of mucosal bleeding, epistaxis, and bruising. They have a prolonged BT and abnormal factor VIII/VWF-dependent platelet tests, for example, decreased aggregation in response to ristocetin. They also have decreased factor VIII/VWF as measured by both immunoassay and clotting assay. Normal hemostasis can be restored by infusion of plasma (or plasma fractions) rich in factor VIII/VWF. Until recently, the molecular basis for these heterogeneous abnormalities remained unclear. As discussed in lecture 26, VWF activity resides in a series of large glycoprotein polymers with estimated mol. wts. as high as 20 million. Normal plasma contains a heterogeneous collection of these VWF polymers of varying size and biologic activity. The high-molecular-weight polymers promote platelet adhesion most effectively, although polymers of all sizes have antigenic determinants and are detected in the immunoassays. VWF has binding sites for the antihemophilic factor (factor VIII), which promotes blood coagulation. The two molecules are products of separate genes, but they associate and circulate together as a high-molecular-weight complex.

In classic or *type I* von Willebrand's disease, the most common form, all three of the measurable factor VIII/VWF parameters (VIIIc activity, VIIIc: AGN, and VWF protein and ristocetin cofactor) are decreased in parallel due to an inability to release VWF oligomers from endothelial cells. Variants have been described in which the amount of protein and the binding of factor VIII are normal, although the ability to promote adhesion is defective. In *type II* von Willebrand's disease the large VWF multimers are missing from plasma. Type II subtypes are defined by differing plasma and platelet multimeric patterns, unique functional characteristics of VWF, or structural abnormalities of VWF. In *type IIA* large VWF multimers are present in both plasma and platelets owing to a failure of subunits to polymerize fully. In *type IIB* unregulated binding of large VWF polymers to the platelet surface causes their depletion from plasma. In *type IIC* VWF is structurally defective. *Type III* is the most severe form of von Willebrand's disease and the most uncommon. Ristocetin cofactor and VWF antigen are undetectable in plasma. Other von Willebrand's variants have been described, including patients with a recessively inherited disorder and patients with a platelet defect that promotes VWF binding and mimics IIB von Willebrand's disease. So-called acquired von Willebrand's disease may be due to an antibody that reacts with factor VIII/VWF or to the absorption of VIII/VWF to abnormal circulating or splenic lymphocytes in patients with lymphoproliferative disorders. Von Willebrand's disease and related syndromes have turned out to be common causes of minor and sometimes major bleeding. Therapy consists of infusions of factor VIII/VWF as needed.

(2) Bernard-Soulier syndrome

Bernard-Soulier syndrome is a rare, inherited disorder in which platelet adhesion is decreased and platelets do not respond to ristocetin despite normal plasma levels of factor VIII/VWF. The defect appears to be lack of a specific receptor protein on the platelet membrane that binds factor VIII/VWF. Loss of this receptor function is accompanied by a selective deficiency in glycoprotein Ib (figure 27.9). These patients are distinctive because they often have mild thrombocytopenia and large megathrombocytes in the blood smear. Therapy requires infusion of normal platelets, *not* plasma.

b. Aggregation defects

(1) Primary

Failure of the platelet to respond to an aggregating agent such as ADP occurs in a rare but serious autosomal recessive disorder called *(Glanzmann's) thrombasthenia* (weak platelets). The platelets do show a disk-sphere transformation in response to aggregating stimuli and can undergo a release reaction; however, they do not aggregate and hence do not form normal hemostatic plugs. The platelets do not support clot retraction, although they contain normally functioning contractile proteins. Membranes lack the IIb and IIIa complex, which contains binding sites for fibrinogen, fibronectin, and thrombospondin. Fibrinogen is critical for aggregate formation and forms bridges between platelets by binding to these receptor sites.

(2) Secondary

A heterogeneous group of congenital and acquired platelet defects has been described. The consistent features are a prolonged BT accompanied by absence of secondary platelet aggregation with ADP and epinephrine and a poor response to collagen. Patients typically show normal platelet aggregation with ristocetin as well as normal levels of factor VIII/VWF by coagulation assay and immunoassay. The two major groups of patients with this syndrome are those with a deficiency in platelet storage pool nucleotides and those with an abnormality in the release mechanism.

c. Release defects

(1) Aspirin effect

Most patients with qualitative platelet disorders have defects in secondary aggregation and release, their platelets responding to exogenous ADP, but failing to release granular or endogenous ADP. The most common cause of this release defect is the ingestion of medications such as *aspirin* (acetylsalicyclic acid). Aspirin specifically acetylates the platelet cyclooxygenase system and thus decreases production of the prostaglandin endoperoxide intermediates of thromboxane A_2 that stimulate aggregation and release. A few patients have an inherited deficiency in this enzyme system with similar functional platelet abnormalities. It should be emphasized that many nonsteroidal anti-inflammatory drugs inhibit cyclooxygenase. Aspirin is particularly potent as a platelet inhibitor as it irreversibly activates the enzyme and platelets cannot synthesize new enzyme. Other cells recover from aspirin inhibition in 4–8 hr by synthesizing new enzyme.

(2) Storage pool disease

Patients who have a normal release mechanism but granules that lack releasable stores of ADP and serotonin or other constituents have so-called *storage pool disease*. The defect can occur as an isolated autosomal dominant disorder or in association with a wide variety of diseases (e.g., leukemia, alcoholic intoxication). In addition to long BT and defective secondary aggregation, these patients have (1) decrease in total platelet ADP and ATP; (2) increase in specific labeling of the metabolic pool of platelet nucleotides; (3) decreased uptake followed by excess leakage of radiolabeled serotonin; and (4) decreased content of nondense granule constituents.

d. Acquired defects

Metabolic states such as *uremia* may also decrease platelet function. Platelets appear to be affected by such unexcreted metabolites as the *phenolic acids* and *guanidinosuccinic acid*. In addition, there is evidence that uremic plasma stimulates vascular walls to synthesize excess quantities of PGI_2.

The fact that many drugs interfere with platelet function has been exploited in the development of antithrombotic drugs such as *dipyridamole* (Persantine®) that act by inhibiting platelet phosphodiesterase. Correlation is still not good between antithrombotic effect and antiplatelet effect, some drugs showing distinct antithrombotic effects but no discernible effects on hemostatic tests when given in usual doses. Thus, while pharmacologic manipulation of platelet function is a desirable goal, means for testing antithrombotic effect of drugs remain limited.

III. VASCULAR DEFECTS

Despite progress in studies of the hemostatic role of plasma proteins and platelets, until recently the role of the blood vessel was ignored. One of the first responses to injury is contraction of smooth muscle in the vessel wall. In addition, endothelial cells may produce materials needed in hemostatic reactions and blood vessel repair is influenced by materials released from platelets. Abnormalities in the repair process may be important in the pathogenesis of atherosclerosis and thromboembolism.

Some patients with purpuric bleeding have normal platelet functions and no evidence of coagulation abnormality. These disorders, by elimination, are assumed to arise within the blood vessel itself. This situation can result from a defect in the connective tissue framework of blood vessels, as commonly seen in *senile purpura*. A similar disorder occurs in patients taking large doses of *corticosteroids* and in patients with *connective tissue disorders* (e.g., pseudoxanthoma elasticum, Ehlers-Danlos syndrome, and vitamin C deficiency or scurvy). Blood vessels also may become distended and burst in *hyperviscosity* states such as macroglobulinemia. *Rickettsia* can cause direct vascular injury, and *endotoxin-induced damage* follows infection with meningococci and other gram-negative organisms. Finally, patients with *vasculitis* (inflammation of the vessel wall) may have loss of endothelium, which promotes platelet consumption and in some cases results in vessel thrombosis.

SELECTED REFERENCES

Bellucci, S., et al. Inherited platelet disorders. In Brown, E. B., ed., *Progress in Hematology*, New York: Grune & Stratton, 1983, 13:223–264.

Fedorko, M. E., and Lichtman, M. A. Megakaryocyte structures, maturation, and ecology. In Colman, R. W., ed., *Hemostasis and Thrombosis: Basic Principles and Clinical Practice*, Philadelphia: J. B. Lippincott, 1982, pp. 210–224.

Harker, L., and Slichter, S. The bleeding time as a screening test for evaluation of platelet function. *New Eng. J. Med.* 287(1972): 155.

Kelton, J. G. The measurement of platelet-bound immunoglobulins: An overview of the methods and the biological relevance of platelet-associated IgG. In Brown, E. B., ed., *Progress in Hematology*, New York: Grune & Stratton, 1983, 13:163–199.

Multiple authors Platelet function and its disorders. In Colman, R. W., ed., *Hemostasis and Thrombosis: Basic Principles and Clinical Practice*, Philadelphia: J. B. Lippincott, 1982, pp. 343–524.

Zimmerman, T. S., et al. Factor VIII/von Willebrand's factor. In Brown, E. B., ed., *Progress in Hematology*, New York: Grune & Stratton, 1983, 13:279–309.

LECTURE 28 Hemorrhagic Disorders III: Disorders of Primary and Secondary Hemostasis

Robert I. Handin and Robert D. Rosenberg

I. INTRODUCTION

Hemorrhagic disorders are usually caused by specific abnormalities of primary or secondary hemostasis. In most cases the defect can be localized to one of the two major systems (platelets or coagulation proteins), but in certain instances both systems are involved. In this lecture we summarize the diagnostic approach to these disorders and their therapy. In addition we briefly discuss inherited disorders associated with thromboembolism, the so-called hypercoagulable or prethrombotic states. Since diagnosis in the coagulation field is dependent on assay procedures, we emphasize specific patterns of abnormal laboratory findings. In particular we distinguish between information derived from so-called *screening tests* that are readily available and information obtained from the more definitive *special tests,* which may be available only in major centers.

II. DISORDERS OF PRIMARY HEMOSTASIS: PRINCIPLES

A. Diagnostic features

As discussed in lecture 27, platelets participate in blood coagulation by adhering to areas of vessel injury and forming cellular aggregates or hemostatic plugs. This is the process referred to as *primary hemostasis*. In addition, platelets interact with vascular endothelium to prevent the egress of red blood cells and plasma proteins. Patients can bleed because of a decrease in the number of circulating platelets, or from a variety of congenital and acquired defects that prevent platelets from undergoing normal adhesion, aggregation, or release.

1. Type of bleeding

Patients with defective primary hemostasis have the characteristic bleeding pattern outlined in table 28.1. They demonstrate *ecchymoses* (bruises) and *petechiae* that appear on arms or thighs without antecedent trauma. They also bleed from mucous membranes and often have menorrhagia, gastrointestinal bleeding, repeated nosebleeds (epistaxes), and gingival bleeding following the brushing of teeth. This pattern, when part of the patient's history, is to be contrasted with the joint, muscle, or retroperitoneal hemorrhage of insidious onset that occurs in patients with coagulation protein defects—that is, defects of secondary hemostasis.

Table 28.1
Nature of Bleeding in Primary and Secondary Hemostatic Disorders

Parameter	Primary hemostatic disorders	Secondary hemostatic disorders
Bleeding source	Usually capillary	Usually small artery
Lesion	Cutaneous and musocal petechiae and/or ecchymoses	Often intramuscular and deep hematomas
Preceding trauma	Unusual	Frequent, but delayed onset of bleeding
Complications of venepuncture	Superficial ecchymoses around venepuncture site	No superficial ecchymoses, but hemorrhage may occur if firm external pressure not maintained long enough

2. History

A careful history is often helpful since many platelet disorders are inherited and some are associated with a systemic disorder. For example, patients with *oculocutaneous albinism* have an associated functional platelet defect; patients with *Wiskott-Aldrich syndrome* are usually thrombocytopenic. The family history may provide clues to the diagnosis since most platelet disorders are inherited as autosomal dominant traits, while the major coagulation protein disorders—deficiencies of factors VIII and IX—are sex-linked recessive abnormalities. Although inheritance is important, a negative family history does not exclude a platelet defect since many patients with platelet dysfunction have acquired abnormalities due to drug ingestion or metabolic disorders such as uremia.

3. Laboratory tests

From the history and physical examination, it is usually possible to diagnose a platelet defect and predict its severity. Confirmation of this impression requires two simple *screening tests*—the *platelet count* and the *bleeding time* (BT).

As noted in lecture 27, further laboratory evaluation of the patient with a low platelet count will focus on the mechanism of thrombocytopenia by assessing marrow production of platelets, the size of the splenic platelet pool, and the morphology of the platelet on the blood smear. The patient with a normal platelet count and a prolonged BT should be tested in order to define the nature of the primary hemostatic defect. This abnormality may be localized to one or more stages of the platelet mechanism—platelet adhesion, primary aggregation, and secondary aggregation or release.

A schematic approach to the patient with a prolonged BT—including the quantitative and qualitative platelet disorders—is outlined in figure 28.1. The laboratory tests employed to evaluate the various stages of platelet plug formation are based on the physio-

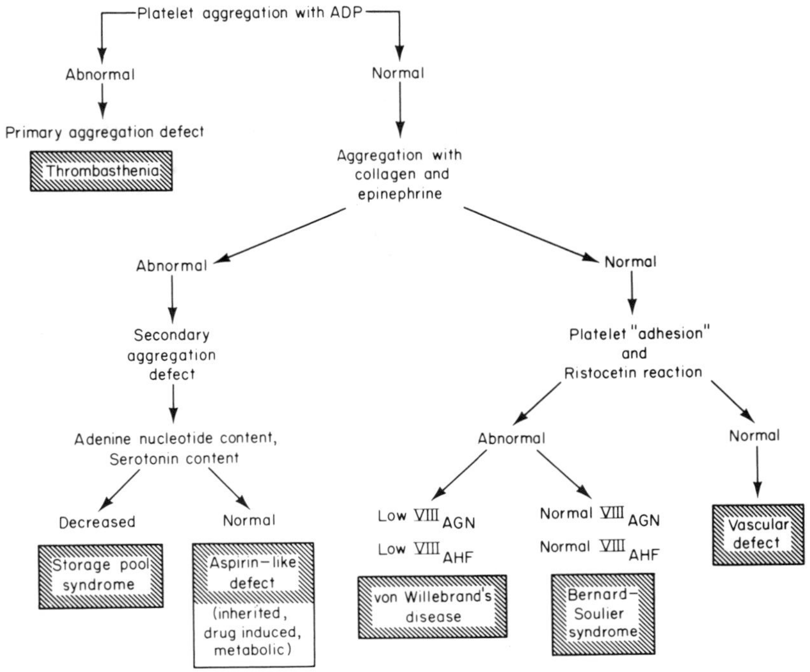

Fig. 28.1
Evaluation of a patient with a prolonged bleeding time and normal platelet count.

logic principles outlined in lecture 27. Figure 28.1 summarizes the sequence in which they should be used.

4. Classification

Disorders of primary hemostasis were summarized in lecture 27. Qualitative platelet disorders are listed in table 27.2.

III. DISORDERS OF SECONDARY HEMOSTASIS

A. Introduction

Disorders of secondary hemostasis are due to alterations in the protein component of the coagulation system. The two most important initial steps in diagnosing these abnormalities are a careful *history* and certain *screening laboratory tests*.

1. Importance of history

The history should take note of the age of onset of symptoms, their relation to trauma (e.g., responses to dental extractions or surgical procedures, including circumcision), description of hemorrhagic phenomena, their association with other illnesses, genetic factors, dietary history, and recently ingested drugs. Table 28.1 summarizes some characteristics of bleeding in secondary hemostatic disorders and contrasts them with those in primary hemostatic abnormalities. Other features of these states (e.g., genetics, sex predilection, pattern of laboratory test results) will be outlined below.

2. Screening tests and special tests

In most cases, four screening tests will identify the general locus of a hemostatic abnormality: (1) the *prothrombin time* (PT); (2) the *partial thromboplastin time* (PTT); (3) the *thrombin time* (TT); and (4) the *fibrin stability test*. These tests are available in most hospitals and are simple to perform. They should be done before more specific tests—often termed *special tests*—are chosen to pinpoint the defect responsible for a particular bleeding disorder. Special tests include assays of plasma fibrinogen, fibrin split products, various individual coagulation factors, specific inhibitors, plus other more specialized measurements that may be available only in major centers.

B. Major screening tests

1. Prothrombin time (PT)

The principle of the PT is outlined in figure 28.2. A commercial preparation of phospholipid and tissue factor is added to an aliquot of the patient's citrated plasma. The mixture is recalcified, and the stop watch is started when Ca^{++} is added. The clotting time (i.e., time required for a clot to form) is determined and compared with results obtained with plasma from a normal subject. The normal PT is 11–13 sec.

The PT is prolonged by deficiencies of the coagulant activity of

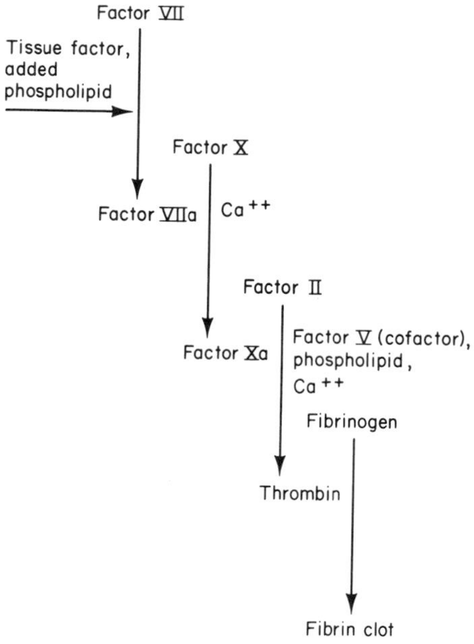

Fig. 28.2
Factors influencing the prothrombin time.

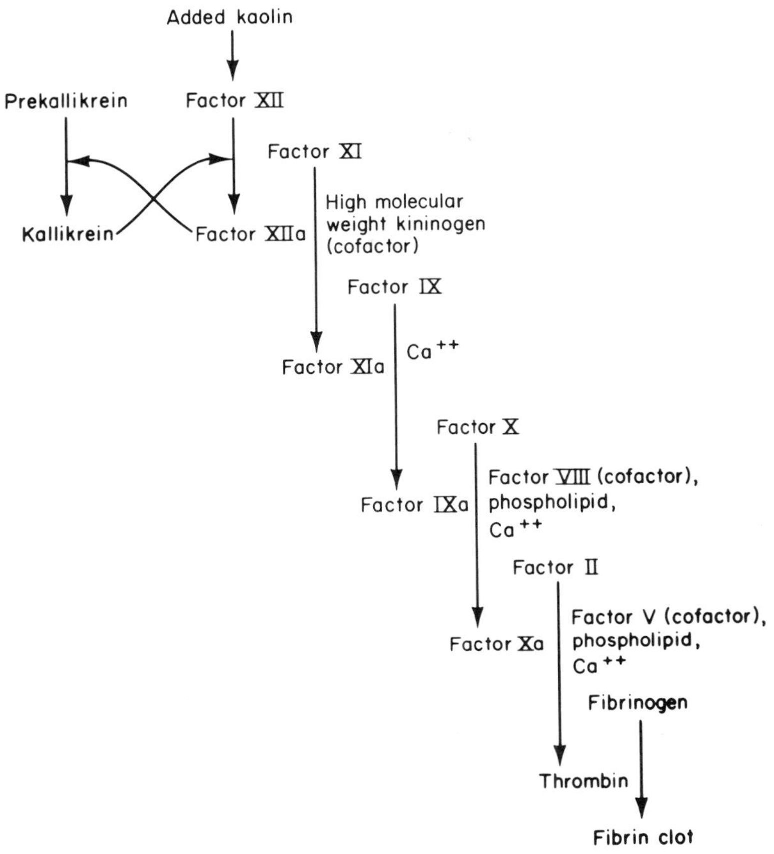

Fig. 28.3
Factors influencing the partial thromboplastin time.

factors VII, X, II, V, and *fibrinogen.* It is not affected by variations in factors VIII, IX, XI, XII, XIII, prekallikrein, high-molecular-weight kininogen, or platelets.

2. Partial thromboplastin time (PTT)

The PTT is summarized in figure 28.3. Kaolin or celite is first incubated with an aliquot of patient's citrated plasma for 3 to 5 min. Phospholipid is then added and the mixture is recalcified at time zero. Clotting time is noted and compared with results obtained with normal plasma. The normal PTT is 28–35 sec.

The PTT is prolonged by deficiencies of the coagulant activity of prekallikrein, high-molecular-weight kininogen, *factors XII, XI, IX, VIII, X, V, II,* and *fibrinogen.* It is unaffected by variations in factors VII, XIII, and platelets.

3. Thrombin time (TT)

Exogenous thrombin is added to an aliquot of citrated patient's plasma. Clotting time is measured and compared with the time obtained with normal plasma. The concentration of thrombin utilized is adjusted (with normal plasma) to give clotting time of approximately 15 sec. The TT measures the ability of thrombin to catalyze the *transformation of fibrinogen to fibrin* and the capacity of that fibrin to undergo *polymerization*. It is not affected by factors II, V, VII, VIII, IX, X, XI, XII, XIII, prekallikrein, high-molecular-weight kininogen, or platelets. *Heparin* in the patient's blood sample may cause erroneous results since it accelerates neutralization of exogeneously added thrombin. The physician may be unaware that his patient has received this drug, for example, following infusion of heparin in low concentration to maintain patency of an intra-arterial catheter. Indeed, heparin in such low doses in the presence of conditions that reduce its clearance (i.e., liver or renal disease) can completely anticoagulate the patient. Heparin in blood samples is detected by neutralizing its effect on the TT with *protamine* or measuring the time required for plasma to clot after addition of *reptilase*. This snake venom is not inhibited by heparin (see lecture 26). Thus, differences between TT and reptilase time (RT) indicate the presence of this mucopolysaccharide. RT may be useful in the assay of split products or fibrinogen levels in patients receiving heparin.

4. Fibrin stability test

Plasma from the patient is recalcified and allowed to clot. The clot is suspended in an excess of 5M urea or 1% monochloracetic acid, which disrupts hydrophobic and electrostatic interactions. The normal clot does not dissolve rapidly because covalent peptide cross-links have been introduced between the fibrin molecules. An abnormal clot that is not fully cross-linked is rapidly lysed by these agents. This test provides a measure of *factor XIII* activity as well as the availability of fibrin cross-linking sites. This screening procedure is valuable because other tests fail to detect abnormalities in this phase of the hemostatic mechanism.

C. Special tests

1. Plasma fibrinogen

Fibrinogen is measured by (1) quantifying the greatest plasma dilution at which a clot is still produced by exogenous thrombin; (2) photometrically measuring clottable protein; or (3) immunologic techniques that utilize specific antifibrinogen antisera. The normal fibrinogen level is 200–400 mg/100 ml.

2. Fibrinogen or fibrin breakdown products ("split products")

Plasmin degradation of fibrinogen produces diverse fragments. Some of these polypeptides are no longer clottable by thrombin, but retain the immunological characteristics of fibrinogen. Therefore, mixture of blood sample with large amounts of thrombin removes clottable fibrinogen but not nonclottable fragments. Such samples must be collected in the presence of a plasmin inhibitor. (i.e., ε-aminocaproic acid or Amicar®) to prevent fibrinolysis in vitro. If samples of this type are incubated with specific antisera or staphylococcal clumping agent, it is readily possible to detect and quantify nonclottable fibrinogen fragments that were generated in vivo.

3. Specific factor assays

Specific assays are available for each of the coagulation proteins—factors II, V, VII, VIII, IX, X, XI, XIII, prekallikrein and high-molecular-weight kininogen. These tests are based on the ability of patient's plasma to correct results obtained with a plasma known to be deficient in the factor to be measured. The procedures themselves are similar to the PTT and PT assays.

D. Diagnostic approach

The four screening procedures described above permit classification of disorders of secondary hemostasis into the following six *patterns* or *syndromes*.

1. Fibrin stabilization abnormal; other tests normal

In this rare syndrome, all clotting tests are normal but one: the fibrin clot is soluble in solvents such as urea or monochloracetic acid. Abnormal clot solubility is due to a reduction in the number of covalent cross-links between fibrin molecules. Underlying abnormalities may include (1) inherited factor XIII deficiency; (2) antibodies that specifically inhibit factor XIII; (3) structural alterations in the cross-linking sites within fibrinogen-fibrin; or (4) antibodies specifically directed against these regions. Choice of therapy depends on the nature of the defects in a given patient. Specialized techniques are necessary to delineate the defect.

2. TT abnormal; PT and PTT often abnormal

This constellation of test results (with other tests normal) can be caused by the following abnormalities in the conversion of fibrinogen to fibrin and its subsequent polymerization.

a. Neutralization of thrombin

Heparin in the blood sample may neutralize exogenously added thrombin and prolong the TT.

b. Quantitative alterations in fibrinogen level

Significant reductions in plasma fibrinogen usually prolong the TT. As noted above, fibrinogen levels are readily assayed by various techniques. *Hypofibrinogenemia* rarely results from an *inherited disorder* (congenital afibrinogenemia or hypofibrinogenemia). More commonly, it is due to *consumption* of fibrinogen during *disseminated intravascular coagulation,* or *DIC,* which is discussed below. If plasma fibrinogen is sufficiently depressed, hemorrhage can occur. *Hyperfibrinogenemia* is observed in *pregnancy, infection,* and other *stress* situations. It occasionally prolongs the TT because fibrinogen in high concentrations can trap fibrin within soluble complexes and thereby inhibit fibrin polymerization. This abnormality occurs in vitro and has little pathophysiologic significance. It does not cause bleeding.

c. Qualitative abnormality of fibrinogen

Qualitative abnormalities of fibrinogen (*dysfibrinogenemia*) may prolong TT and cause bleeding. Reported examples are due to genetically determined amino acid substitutions at critical sites near the fibrinopeptide region. Diagnosis requires comparison of immunologic and clotting activity assays of fibrinogen.

d. Interfering substances

The presence of substances that interfere with fibrin polymerization can prolong the TT and cause bleeding. High concentrations of *split products* generated during intense fibrinolysis or DIC are common causes of this syndrome. As noted, these fibrin(ogen) derivatives are detected by various techniques. Occasionally, high concentrations of a monoclonal immunoglobulin encountered in multiple myeloma interfere with fibrin polymerization (lecture 24).

3. PTT abnormal; PT and other tests normal

Defects responsible for this syndrome are within the intrinsic cascade of the coagulation system. They may be divided into two groups.

a. Group with no bleeding

Patients in the first group do not bleed. These relatively rare patients may have deficiencies of *factor XII, prekallikrein,* or *high-molecular-weight kininogen.* Each of these states is identifiable by appropriate factor assays utilizing plasmas from patients known to be deficient for the specific coagulation component. At present, it is unclear why these three deficiency states do not lead to hemorrhage. Perhaps low levels of these proteins are adequate for hemostasis in vivo but insufficient for artificial activation of coagulation by kaolin during the PTT assay. Alternatively, activation of the coagulation system may occur in vivo at the factor XI level; the proteins under discussion may be physiologically important only with respect to kinin generation and fibrinolysis.

b. Group with significant bleeding

Patients in the second group have significant bleeding and are more common than patients in the first group. Indeed, whenever the PTT is abnormal, it should be assumed that the patient has a tendency to bleed until it has been proved otherwise. Underlying disorders include deficiencies of *factors VIII, IX,* or *XI,* and *von Willebrand's disease.* Specific factors assays define the precise etiology. However, as noted below, diagnosis is aided by data on mode of transmission, sex, BT, and other clinical findings. We briefly summarize the four major disorders in this group.

(1) Factor VIII deficiency

Deficiency of factor VIII (*hemophilia A*) is inherited as a sex-linked recessive trait. Incidence is approximately 1/10,000 of the population. It is the most common inherited coagulation disorder. The disorder is thought to be caused either by a defective factor VIII protein or impaired conversion of a precursor to a molecule to a species with full biologic activity. Severe cases (factor VIII level, <1% of normal) often bleed in infancy at circumcision and have multiple episodes of hemarthrosis. Moderately affected individuals (factor VIII level, 1–5%) have occasional hemarthroses, but usually lack crippling deformities. Mild cases (factor VIII level, 5–25%) rarely suffer bleeding episodes and often are not diagnosed until they bleed after dental or surgical procedures. Efforts to detect the *carrier state* in clinically unaffected females by measurement of factor VIII activity have been unsuccessful owing to wide variations of factor VIII concentration in the general population. Many normal individuals have low levels of factor VIII (~50–60%) similar to those in female carriers. Our ability to detect carriers has improved significantly with the development in recent years of antisera that can quantify the VIII_{AHF} antigen. These new reagents have permitted accurate detection of carriers and the intrauterine prenatal diagnosis of hemophilia. These tests have also demonstrated that most patients with decreased VIII_{AHF} activity have a parallel decrease in VIII_{AHF} antigen.

The availability of factor VIII concentrate (cryoprecipitate) has dramatically altered the care of patients with severe factor VIII deficiency. It is now possible to control bleeding in the hospitalized patient and, when necessary, to prepare affected individuals for surgical procedures. New home care programs have also improved the lot of these patients. Training of family members to give intravenous infusions of factor VIII concentrate permits prompt therapy at the onset of a bleeding episode or immediately after trauma. This has significantly decreased the need for hospitalization and reduces the incidence of crippling deformities. Treatment of hemophilia is not without hazard since these patients may develop viral hepatitis, the acquired immunodeficiency syndrome (AIDS), and inhibitor antibodies in association with transfusions.

(2) Von Willebrand's disease

This disease is also associated with reduced levels of factor VIII/VWF activity. As noted in lecture 27, the two proteins are separate gene products that associate in plasma as a complex. Most forms of von Willebrand's disease are inherited as an autosomal trait. Type I or classical von Willebrand's disease is the only disorder known to cause a prolonged PTT–normal PT syndrome that is associated with a long BT. It is discussed more fully in lectures 26 and 27. Variant forms of von Willebrand's disease (e.g., type IIa and IIb) often have normal levels of VIIIc and a normal PTT.

(3) Factor IX deficiency

Deficiency of factor IX (*Christmas disease, hemophilia B*) is inherited as a sex-linked recessive trait. It resembles factor VIII deficiency with respect to mode of transmission and clinical manifestations. The incidence, however, is only 1–2/100,000 of the population. Affected individuals appear to have either normal levels of inactive protein or reduced levels of active zymogen. The carrier state is more often associated with reduced levels of factor IX activity than in the case with factor VIII deficiency. An immunoassay is available to aid in the classification of factor IX disease and in carrier detection. In addition the factor IX gene has been cloned and a closely linked genetic polymorphism identified that may permit intrauterine diagnosis without the need for fetoscopy. Rarely, acquired factor IX deficiency is due to selective urinary loss of this protein in the nephrotic syndrome. Concentrates containing factors II, VII, IX, and X are available for treatment of hemorrhagic episodes or preparation of patients for surgical procedures. These preparations must be used with care since they contain activated enzymes such as factor Xa or thrombin and can produce thrombotic phenomena. They can also transmit serum hepatitis.

(4) Factor XI deficiency

This deficiency is inherited as an autosomal recessive and is particularly prevalent among Jews of Eastern European descent. It is the third most common coagulation disorder following deficiencies of factors VIII and IX. Based on indirect immunoassays it appears to be associated with reduced levels of functional protein rather than the presence of an altered inactive protein. The hemorrhagic diathesis tends to be mild. Often, bleeding occurs late in life or after surgical or dental procedures. Factor XI concentrates are not available; in most instances, plasma infusion effectively controls hemorrhage.

4. PT abnormal; PTT and other tests normal

Defects responsible for this syndrome are located within the extrinsic limb of the coagulation system. Tissue factor is prevalent throughout the vascular tree and disorders due to its lack have not been described. Therefore, *factor VII deficiency* is a unique cause of this syndrome.

Inherited deficiency of factor VII is exceedingly rare (1/500,000 of the population). It is transmitted as a recessive autosomal trait. An acquired form of this syndrome can be observed early in *vitamin K deficiency,* at the onset of *coumadin therapy,* or in *mild liver disease.* This is explained by the fact that factor VII has the shortest half-life of all coagulation proteins (~3–5 hr). Cessation in production of the vitamin K-dependent proteins (factors II, VII, IX, X) is manifested initially as factor VII deficiency.

5. PTT abnormal; PT abnormal; other tests normal

Defects responsible for this syndrome are of two types. The first includes rare inherited *deficiencies of the proteins of the common pathway,* that is, *factor II, V,* and *X,* which appear to be due to the production of altered inactive forms of each protein species. Transmission is autosomal recessive, and the incidence is approximately 1/500,000–1,000,000 of the population. Definitive diagnosis requires specific factor assays.

In the second group are *multiple defects of the coagulation mechanism.* Unlike the congenital syndromes, these are relatively common. The major causes are (1) vitamin K deficiency; (2) transfusion of frozen rather than fresh plasma; and (3) liver disease.

Vitamin K deficiency may be due to ingestion of coumadin, intestinal malabsorption of fat, chronic diarrhea, or parenteral feedings without vitamin K supplementation. Lack of this vitamin results in reduced γ-carboxylation of specific glutamyl residues located on factors II, VII, IX and X (see lecture 26) with decreased biologic activity of these coagulation proteins. Parenteral administration of as little as 1 mg of vitamin K restores normal hemostatic function promptly (in 4–40 hr). Several families have been described who appear vitamin K deficient but on close examination have adequate vitamin stores with defective carboxylation. They have low levels of the four vitamin K–dependent proteins.

Transfusion with large amounts of *frozen* or *fresh plasma* often occurs during surgery when extensive blood replacement is required. Liquid plasma stored for more than several hours has reduced levels of factors V and VIII. *Liver disease* is associated with multiple defects, as discussed below.

6. Inhibitor syndrome

The hallmark of this syndrome is an abnormal PTT (or rarely an abnormal PT) that cannot be corrected in vitro by incubation for 30 min of patient plasma plus an equal volume of normal plasma. The PT and PTT are prolonged only when specific coagulation factors drop to below 40% of their normal levels. Therefore, the failure of added normal plasma to correct the abnormality rules out a deficiency state and implicates a circulating inhibitor. Inhibitors are of two types.

a. Antibody inhibitors

One type is an *antibody* directed specifically against a particular coagulation component. The effects of these immunoglobulins are time dependent. Their most common target is *factor VIII*. Inhibitors of factor VIII are found in (1) 5–10% of patients with factor VIII deficiency (these individuals may have no circulating factor VIII protein, and transfusions of factor VIII may stimulate antibody production); (2) systemic lupus erythematosus; (3) women during the postpartum period; and (4) certain elderly individuals. Precise diagnosis requires specific inhibitor assays. Treatment depends on the inhibitor level. If the titer is low, massive infusion of factor VIII concentrate can promptly correct the abnormality. In many instances, however, infusion of factor VIII stimulates subsequent antibody production and results in a higher inhibition titer. If the titer is high, infusion of factor VIII will have little effect. Various experimental procedures have been utilized to treat active bleeding, for example, immunosuppressive drugs and concentrates containing activated intermediates such as factor Xa. Inhibitors against other coagulation proteins occur rarely.

b. Nonspecific inhibitors

A second type of inhibitor may not be an immunoglobulin. These consist of molecules that appear instantaneously to neutralize many coagulation factors. Such inhibitors are present in many clinical disorders, including acute leukemia, lymphoma, and other states in which leukocyte turnover is rapid. These substances may be positively charged (cationic) lysosomal proteins from leukocytes that act in vitro by competing with coagulation proteins for negatively charged phospholipid surfaces. In one recent study, a specific antibody that bound to phospholipids was described that had the characteristics of a nonspecific inhibitor. Alterations of the plasma/phospholipid ratios utilized in the PTT or PT may dramatically influence the apparent titer of these inhibitors. A considerable excess of phospholipid is in contact with the blood in vivo. Also, when platelets are substituted for phospholipid, the abnormality disappears. Hence, it is not surprising that these inhibitors have little effect on the hemostatic system and do not cause bleeding. It is important to be able to distinguish these substances from inhibitors of the first type, which are of great clinical significance.

IV. MIXED DISORDERS

Three major types of disorders exhibit dual defects that suppress the activity of both the primary and secondary hemostatic mechanisms.

A. Von Willebrand's disease

The pathophysiology of this disease has been discussed earlier in this lecture as well as in lectures 26 and 27. As we have seen, it is due to a defect in platelet adhesion secondary to alteration in von Willebrand's factor quantity or functional competence. In some cases (Type I von Willebrand's disease) there may also be a decrease in the level of factor VIII coagulant activity (VIIIc). If the concentration of factor VIIIc activity is only modestly reduced, the patient exhibits ecchymoses, petechiae, and other evidence of mucosal bleeding. If factor VIIIc activity is profoundly depressed, the patient may present with clinical symptoms similar to those of the patient with severe classic hemophilia.

B. Disseminated intravascular coagulation

We have seen that the sequential activation of coagulation factors and platelets is a response to localized vascular injury. Several limiting reactions dampen and restrict the activity of the hemostatic mechanism. These include (1) dilution by blood flow; (2) hepatic clearance; (3) adsorption of coagulation factors to the fibrin-platelet meshwork; and (4) circulating inhibitors such as antithrombin. The presence of activated coagulation factors in the circulation leads to a *hypercoagulable state,* which, if unchecked, can produce *thrombosis*.

1. Causes

Patients with a number of serious illnesses often develop rapid and massive activation of the coagulation sequence that overwhelms the normal body defenses. As a result, they consume circulating platelets as well as coagulation proteins and develop a severe hemorrhagic disorder called *disseminated intravascular coagulation* or *DIC*. DIC is not a specific disease but a disorder triggered by a number of factors (table 28.2) that can be grouped into four categories: (1) conditions that introduce tissue factor into the circulation (e.g., tissue necrosis); (2) damage to endothelial sur-

Table 28.2
Pathogenesis of Disseminated Intravascular Coagulation

Causative factors	Examples
Liberation of tissue factor	Obstetrical catastrophes
	Hemolysis
	Tissue damage
	Neoplasms
	Fat embolism
	Snake bite
Stagnant blood flow	Kasabach-Merritt syndrome
Endothelial damage	Heat stroke
	Aortic aneurysm
	Hemolytic-uremic syndrome
	Acute glomerulonephritis
	Microangiopathic hemolytic anemia
	Rocky Mountain spotted fever
Infection	Bacterial: staphylococcus, streptococcus, pneumococcus, meningococcus, gram-negative sepsis
	Viral: arboviruses, varicella, variola, rubella
	Parasitic: malaria, kala-azar
	Mycotic: acute histoplasmosis

faces; (3) stagnation of blood flow; and (4) infection of various types. These stimuli activate both limbs of the coagulation cascade so that thrombin is generated and fibrinogen is rapidly converted to fibrin. This leads to irreversible aggregation of many circulating platelets and production of microemboli. Red cells are destroyed in the resulting fibrin meshwork with production of microangiopathic hemolytic anemia (lecture 13). The major body defense is activation of the fibrinolytic system with resulting lysis of emboli in the microcirculation. This leads to the increased level of fibrin degradation products. There may also be indiscriminate degradation of remaining fibrinogen or other coagulation proteins along with fibrin debris.

2. Diagnosis

Patients usually present with an identifiable serious illness that may be accompanied by hypotension, acidosis, and infection. There may be evidence of skin necrosis over the digits, nose, and genitals, or diffuse ecchymoses and mucous membrane bleeding. The laboratory diagnosis of DIC is uncomplicated: the blood smear shows microangiopathic red cell changes and variable degrees of thrombocytopenia; there is prolongation of PT, PTT, and TT and low levels of fibrinogen.

Fibrin degradation products—detectable by immunologic or staphylococcal clumping assays—are greatly elevated in DIC, but they are present in lesser amounts in other conditions. When fibrin monomer is generated, it can either form insoluble polymers of fibrin or bind to plasma fibrinogen to produce a relatively soluble complex. These fibrinogen-fibrin monomer complexes can be precipitated by the addition of protamine or ethanol, a phenomenon called *paracoagulation*. This has been proposed as a test to distinguish DIC from primary fibrinolysis, a much less common disorder. However, the test is nonspecific and insensitive.

3. Therapy

Treatment of DIC should be directed at correcting the triggering event. Patients with no bleeding or thrombosis require careful observation. Patients with diffuse hemorrhage may need intensive support with plasma, platelets, and red cell transfusions. There is some controversy about the efficacy of heparin in treating this syndrome. While heparin will usually suppress hemostatic system activity in DIC, regulation of the dose and prevention of heparin-induced hemorrhage is difficult. Many patients with DIC can be managed with plasma and platelets alone. Heparin can be lifesaving in the occasional patient who presents with predominantly thrombotic manifestations of DIC, which can lead to tissue ischemia and gangrene.

C. Liver disease

Since the liver is involved in the synthesis and catabolism of hemostatic system components, it is not surprising that liver dysfunction is often associated with bleeding. Although the liver is a major source of coagulation proteins, it should be kept in mind that chronic liver failure induces a number of nonhematologic abnormalities that may contribute to bleeding. Portal hypertension causes abnormal vascular channels to develop in the stomach and esophagus that are fragile and easily ruptured. There are also changes in gastric mucus composition and increased acid secretion that may cause peptic ulceration. Finally, portal hypertension causes splenomegaly and concomitant thrombocytopenia that exacerbates mechanical causes of bleeding.

1. Pathophysiology

It is established that factors II, V, VII, IX, and X are synthesized in the liver; factors XI and XII may be. Four of these proteins—factors II, VII, IX, and X—require vitamin K for normal activity. As we have noted, this vitamin is an essential cofactor for a unique carboxylation reaction in which a second carboxyl group is attached to a number of glutamic acid residues on these proteins. This postsynthetic modification permits the proteins to bind calcium and participate in coagulation reactions. Biliary tract obstruction and poor bile flow can lead to hemorrhage by *impairing vitamin K assimilation*. However, there is *impaired synthesis of coagulation factors* in most patients with liver disease despite adequate vitamin K stores because of hepatic cell failure. The decreased synthetic rate of coagulation proteins in stable liver failure is reflected by a moderately prolonged PT and PTT that is improved only slightly by vitamin K. The liver also synthesizes the major inhibitors of coagulation proteins, α_2-macroglobulin and antithrombin. A marked *reduction in inhibitor levels* might increase the rate of coagulation reactions. Moderate *thrombocytopenia* (50,000–80,000 platelets/mm^3) is often due to associated splenomegaly. Liver disease can also *impair clearance of activated coagulation factors,* although the mechanisms and cells involved in normal liver are not clearly defined. There is often *increased plasma fibrinolytic activity* because of failure to clear plasminogen activators secreted in the microcirculation. Thus, laboratory studies may show a mild increase in plasma fibrinolytic activity or a slight elevation in the concentration of fibrin degradation products. However, intense fibrinolysis or overt DIC may occur with sudden prolongation in the PT and PTT as well as further fall in platelet count, fall in fibrinogen level, and increase in fibrin degradation products. These abnormalities exacerbate bleeding due to local mechanical effects by superimposing a systemic bleeding disorder.

In sum, patients with liver disease have a complex coagulation disorder that may be in constant flux, and there is precarious and limited hemostatic reserve.

2. Therapy

Treatment of bleeding in liver disease is complicated. Transfused platelets are sequestered in the spleen, and the large protein and salt loads that accompany plasma infusion are poorly tolerated. Prothrombin complex concentrates rich in factors II, VII, IX, and X that have become available recently are of limited value because they do not provide adequate replacement of other needed coagulation factors. Furthermore, these products are contaminated with hepatitis virus and may contain traces of activated forms of the coagulation factors that can trigger thrombosis. The use of heparin or other anticoagulants to suppress the hemostatic mechanism in patients with DIC, secondary to liver disease, is dangerous because these drugs may induce bleeding. This is probably caused by the associated thrombocytopenia, secondary to splenomegaly, as well as to the erratic catabolism of these drugs due to liver dysfunction.

V. PRETHROMBOTIC OR HYPERCOAGULABLE STATES

There are no simple screening tests for identifying patients at increased risk for developing thrombosis; however, some promising clinical research procedures can detect the limited activation of the coagulation system associated with thromboembolism. These tests are immunoassays that measure released platelet membrane or granule proteins, small activation peptides released from coagulation factors or coagulation factor inhibitor complexes that are formed during thrombosis. For example, patients with deep venous thrombosis have increased circulating levels of fibrinopeptide

A, prothrombin fragment 1 + 2, and thrombin-antithrombin complex as a consequence of thrombin generation and clot formation. These abnormalities revert to normal when suitable anticoagulant therapy is administered. Similar abnormalities have been noted in other patients with active thrombosis or embolism as well as in patients with so-called prethrombotic states, i.e., patients who are currently asymptomatic but may develop thrombosis at a later date. Interestingly these changes that reflect significant activation of the coagulation mechanism are not associated with any change in the usual screening tests of hemostasis (PT, PTT, TT, bleeding time, and platelet count).

Although the etiology of thrombosis is still uncertain in the vast majority of patients, the following three well-defined genetic abnormalities qualify as prethrombotic or hypercoagulable states.

A. Antithrombin deficiency

The first is *antithrombin deficiency,* an autosomal dominant disorder that occurs once in 2,000 individuals. Affected patients have recurrent venous thrombosis and pulmonary emboli. They are usually symptomatic by the third decade of life and require prophylactic treatment at times of surgery or trauma and lifelong anticoagulation after the onset of symptoms. The diagnosis is made by demonstrating decreased immunologic or functional antithrombin in plasma. Although most patients have a mild to moderate decrease in the quantity of antithrombin, a few variants have been described in which defective heparin binding or activation by heparin has been noted.

B. Protein C deficiency

A second genetic disorder that leads to venous thrombosis and embolism is *protein C deficiency.* A reduction in plasma level of this vitamin K–dependent inhibitor of factor V and VIII activity is inherited as an autosomal dominant trait. The rare occurrence of homozygous deficiency of protein C permits massive activation of the coagulation system and fatal DIC in the neonatal period has been reported.

C. Abnormal plasminogen

Finally, several families have been described who have an *abnormal form of plasminogen* that cannot be readily activated to plasmin and a high incidence of venous thrombosis and embolism. The variant form of plasminogen has altered electrophoretic mobility and has been partially separated from the normal plasminogen molecule. There are also some less well-characterized families with venous thromboembolism and defective fibrinolysis who fail to release tissue-type plasminogen activator from blood vessels after a provocative challenge such as forearm ischemia or vigorous exercise.

SELECTED REFERENCES

Gardiner, J. E., and Griffin, J. H. Human protein C and thromboembolic disease. In Brown, E. B., ed., *Progress in Hematology,* New York: Grune & Stratton, 1983, 13:265–278.

Multiple authors Disorders of hemostasis. Chapter 140–160 in Williams, W. J., et al., eds., *Hematology,* 4th ed., New York: McGraw-Hill, 1983, pp. 1288-1488.

Multiple authors Hemorrhagic disorders (Part I). Thrombolic disorders (Part II). In Colman, R. W., et al., eds., *Hemostasis and Thrombosis: Basic Principles and Clinical Practice,* Philadelphia: J. B. Lippincott, 1982.

Index